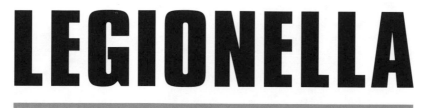

LEGIONELLA

Current Status and Emerging Perspectives

Sponsors

National Center for Infectious Diseases
Centers for Disease Control
Atlanta, Georgia

Environmental Systems Monitoring Laboratory
Environmental Protection Agency
Cincinnati, Ohio

American Society for Microbiology
Washington, D.C.

Organizing Committee
James M. Barbaree, Chairman

Robert F. Breiman
Christopher Bartlett
Alfred P. Dufour
Paul H. Edelstein
Barry I. Eisenstein

David W. Fraser
Marcus A. Horwitz
Jean R. Joly
Frederick S. Nolte

Scientific Review Committee
Robert F. Breiman, Chairman

James M. Barbaree
Robert F. Benson
Mitchell L. Cohen
Paul H. Edelstein
Barry I. Eisenstein
Barry S. Fields
Marcus A. Horwitz

Jean R. Joly
Frederick S. Nolte
William E. Pasculle
Joseph F. Plouffe
John S. Spika
Robert M. Wadowsky
Robert Yee

Consultants:
Robert C. Good
Karl Bettelheim

Technical Assistant:
Elvy Wood

Contributors
Miles, Inc., Pharmaceutical Division
Auburn University
PathCon Laboratories
Costar Corporation

LEGIONELLA

Current Status and Emerging Perspectives

EDITORS:

James M. Barbaree
Botany and Microbiology Department
Auburn University, Alabama

Robert F. Breiman
Centers for Disease Control and Prevention
Atlanta, Georgia

Alfred P. Dufour
U.S. Environmental Protection Agency
Cincinnati, Ohio

American Society for Microbiology
Washington, D.C.

Cover photograph courtesy of Barry S. Fields

Copyright © 1993   American Society for Microbiology
                     1325 Massachusetts Ave., N.W.
                     Washington, DC 20005

Library of Congress Cataloging-in-Publication Data

Legionella: current status and emerging perspectives/ editors, James
  M. Barbaree, Robert F. Breiman, Alfred P. Dufour.
       p.   cm.
     "The 4th International Symposium on Legionella was held in
  Orlando, Florida, January 26–29, 1992"—Pref.
     Includes index.
     ISBN 1-55581-055-1
     1. Legionnaires' disease—Congresses.   2. Legionella pneumophila
  —Congresses.   I. Barbaree, James M.   II. Breiman, Robert F.
  III. Dufour, Alfred P.   IV. International Symposium on Legionella
  (4th : 1992 : Orlando, Fla.)
     [DNLM: 1. Legionella—congresses.   2. Legionnaires' Disease—
  congresses.   WC 200 L5132]
  QR201.L44L43   1993
  616.2'41—dc20
  DNLM/DLC
  For Library of Congress   92-48890
                                                           CIP

CONTENTS

II. MOLECULAR AND CELL BIOLOGY OF *LEGIONELLA*

III. *LEGIONELLA*-PROTOZOA INTERRELATIONSHIPS

VI. SUMMARIES OF STRATEGY SESSIONS

VII. OVERVIEW

PREFACE

It has been almost 2 decades since the catastrophe of the 1976 Legionnaires' convention in Philadelphia. The epidemic that occurred there will never be forgotten. Perhaps one of the most remarkable events that followed was the response of the international scientific community. They put forth an organized effort in the research and surveillance on the agent and the disease, *Legionella* and Legionnaires disease. As expertise in the laboratory and clinics spread to different parts of the world and epidemics and sporadic cases were recognized, the numbers of scientists working on *Legionella* increased progressively. To address the delivery and exchange of information with a deliberate focus on *Legionella*, the First and Second International Symposia were held in Atlanta, Georgia, USA, and a third one in Israel. These meetings, and others such as the *Legionella* Colloque in Lyon, France, in 1985, were very successful in delivering information and addressing issues concerning the agent and disease.

To continue efforts to provide current information and perspectives on future research, another International Symposium on *Legionella* was held in Orlando, Florida, January 26–29, 1992. Topics at the forefront were the application of molecular methods for subtyping species and investigating virulence mechanisms, recent epidemiologic findings, and the ongoing question of the role of sampling environmental sites in the absence of disease. The symposium provided an update on all aspects of *Legionella* and a forum for discussing approaches for the control of disease due to this ubiquitous aquatic bacterium.

Key scientists around the world were consulted for their input into the planning of the meeting. Through the efforts of the Scientific Review Committee, the program was established to include sections on clinical and epidemiologic aspects of legionellosis, molecular and cell biology of *Legionella*, detection and characterization of legionellae, and prevention and control of legionellosis. In addition, there were three forums called "strategy sessions" on the topics of prevention and control, the evolution of chemotherapy and diagnostic tests, and prospects for vaccine development.

The meeting was dynamic and productive, with active participation in discussions during all presentations, including the posters and the strategy sessions. This book is a compendium of information delivered at the meeting and provides the reader with the current status and emerging perspectives concerning *Legionella*.

Thanks are extended to everybody who helped in the planning and delivery of the meeting, as well as to the participants. Included in this group are the individuals, sponsors, and contributors listed at the front of this volume. A special note of thanks is given to our wives for their patience, to Frederick Nolte for his assistance in the acquisition of funds, and to Elvira Wood for her dedication and invaluable contributions to the meeting and program.

James M. Barbaree, Ph.D.
*Botany and Microbiology
    Department
Auburn University, Alabama*

Robert F. Breiman, M.D.
*Centers for Disease Control and
    Prevention
Atlanta, Georgia*

Alfred P. Dufour, Ph.D.
*U.S. Environmental Protection
    Agency
Cincinnati, Ohio*

1976: Lessons Learned

WALTER R. DOWDLE

Centers for Disease Control and Agency for Toxic Substances and Disease Registry, Atlanta, Georgia 30333

Like every other year, 1976 began in January, and as in many other Januarys, an influenza epidemic was under way. Fort Dix, New Jersey, had a modest outbreak in a training unit. One soldier died. Marty Goldfield, Director, New Jersey State Health Laboratories, isolated multiple influenza viruses. Those he could not identify he sent to the Centers for Disease Control (CDC). Of the nine sent to CDC, five were common influenza A viruses and four, much to our surprise, were determined to be swine influenza viruses, one from a soldier who died. Sporadic cases of swine influenza had occurred in humans from time to time, but no human-to-human transmission had been documented since 1918. At that time, an influenza virus closely related to the swine virus caused over 20 million deaths. Over the next 2 weeks at CDC, the tests were repeated and paired sera from Fort Dix were examined; the results clearly showed that human-to-human transmission had occurred.

On Sunday, February 14, a beautiful sunny day in Atlanta, we met with representatives from the Food and Drug Administration, the Army, the National Institutes of Health, and the New Jersey Health Department to consider these findings and how to proceed. I remember that meeting well. It was organized, thoughtful, and conducted without fanfare. I remember it well because it was the last time that we were really in control of events. Swine influenza very quickly tended to take on a life of its own.

There were meetings of the Advisory Committee on Immunization Practices, meetings with the military, meetings with panels of experts, meetings with the public, and meetings with the media, culminating in a meeting with President Ford in March. I was not there, but Albert Sabin and Jonas Salk were there, as were other illustrious advisors of the time. They advised President Ford to request from Congress $135 million to develop and mount an immunization campaign against a virus that possibly threatened an outbreak on the scale of the 1918 pandemic.

Justification for the swine flu immunization program was based on the arguments of its supporters that (i) totally new influenza A viruses emerged approximately ever 10 years, causing pandemics and replacing the current strain; (ii) the 10-year cycle was nearly over, the last one having been in 1968 and the one before that 1957; (iii) influenza viruses recycled, and it could be time for the viruses of 1918, which resembled the swine flu virus; and (iv) whereas no one could predict with certainty whether a swine influenza pandemic would occur, it was prudent that public health agencies be prepared.

I won't go into details, since this is not a discourse on swine flu, but will simply provide some background. I can say that there is no way to recreate the atmosphere of the time. It was one of fear, uncertainty, doubt, and a commitment to do the right thing.

By summer, with no further evidence of the virus, criticism of the program began to mount. Dr. Sabin changed his mind and became vocal in his opposition. Other critics became equally vocal. The insurance companies would not insure the vaccine manufacturers because of unknown, but possible, adverse reactions to the vaccine. Manufacturers would not produce the vaccine because they were not insured. The result was a stalemate, and a vicious one at that.

To break the stalemate, President Ford introduced the Tort Claims Act to indemnify the pharmaceutical companies against claims arising from the swine flu program. But the bill would not move through Congress, and opposition continued to mount. In the last weekend of July in this very hot summer of an election year, a stymied swine influenza campaign, vocal critics of every persuasion, and a hostile press came the first reports of three deaths from Pittsburgh that had been described initially as influenza-like.

Early Monday morning, August 2, we met to consider the reports from Pittsburgh. By Monday evening, EIS officers and supervisory epidemiologists from CDC were in Pittsburgh, Harrisburg, and Philadelphia. Over the next few days, the picture became clearer: the patients presented with chest pains, high fever, lung congestion, and suspected "viral pneumonia." The numbers continued to mount as reports came in from throughout the state. All patients had attended a Legionnaires' meeting in Philadelphia during the weekend of

July 21.

Epidemiologically the illness did not appear to be influenza, and early laboratory data did not suggest influenza. But members of Congress read the newspapers, and they thought that it was influenza. If this was swine flu, they didn't want any part of it; they didn't want to be blamed in November for holding up the immunization campaign. In a matter of days, the Tort Claims bill was passed and the swine flu program was on its way.

The media turned its attention to this mysterious disease affecting Legionnaires in this year of the bicentennial celebration in Philadelphia of the signing of the Declaration of Independence. Legionnaires disease led the nightly news on all three networks for over a week, with reports of each new case identified. Hundreds of articles appeared in newspapers and weekly magazines—the press went wild. CDC was seen in a very heroic light, leading the charge. The media implied that the mystery would be solved in a matter of weeks.

By September, when CDC still had not identified the etiology, all those nice words that we had heard on the networks and read in the newspapers began to fade. David Frazier and his group of epidemiologists, who did an outstanding piece of work, had by now reported that they did not know the cause, but whatever had happened in Philadelphia had happened just outside the Bellevue Stratford hotel or in the lobby. Few people believed that; in fact, some snickered. The atmosphere was beginning to turn sour.

In the midst of all this, word began to reach us in late August and early September that a highly lethal epidemic of hemorrhagic fever was occurring in northern Zaire and southern Sudan. It took over a month to get an invitation into Zaire, but we finally did, with the second group going into Sudan under World Health Organization auspices.

The working conditions in Zaire were extremely difficult, as now, with severe economic difficulties at the time. Under Carl Johnson's leadership in Zaire and with the superb work back in the laboratory in Atlanta, the etiology was identified. The agent is now known to be Ebola virus, which is related to the Marburg virus that had earlier caused a lethal outbreak in monkeys.

Although the reservoir for Ebola virus has never been fully determined, the epidemiology at the time was rapidly worked up, the infection was shown to be associated with hospital and clinical transmission, and the outbreak was stopped, all in a matter of weeks. This was one of the most rapid and successful investigations into one of the most lethal diseases known to humans. An estimated 390 people had died in Zaire, 10 times the number in Philadelphia. The report in *Morbidity and Mortality Weekly Report* a few weeks later resulted in a paragraph in a few newspapers, but few took note of it at all.

I've always found this to be puzzling. Why so little interest? Was it because it takes more than 390 deaths in Zaire to equal 34 deaths in the United States? Was it because the investigation was successful and noncontroversial, with the closing of the hospital now over? Or was it because the media were too preoccupied with swine flu, the yet unsolved mystery of Legionnaires disease, and the election year to take much notice? Whatever the reason, by October and early November, the news media became even more strident regarding Legionnaires disease. CDC was accused of incompetence, focusing too much on epidemiology, ignoring the medical needs of the Legionnaires, chasing an infectious agent when common sense said that it was a toxin, and taking too few and the wrong kinds of specimens. Moreover, some claimed that nickel was the answer or that the outbreak was a communist plot. Finally, the Bellevue Stratford was unfairly "run out of business."

Once again there were meeting after meeting and consultant after consultant. The most memorable consultants were 11 distinguished pathologists who reviewed all of the medical histories, the slides, and the laboratory findings. After 2 full days of this process, they concluded that they could not determine the etiology; they reported that "it could be a toxin, it could be a virus, but it definitely could not be a bacteria."

That didn't help. There were increasing numbers of congressional hearings, threats, cheap shots, critics coming out of the woodwork, and numerous wild theories. Several members of Congress and not a few well-known scientists took this opportunity to further their careers.

Meanwhile, with the swine flu program back on track, vaccination began on October 1. Ten days later, three elderly people who had received the vaccine died. This immediately sparked rumors of deaths and reports of deaths from elsewhere. Once again, the nightly news and the press had a field day. When we finally convinced the media that people in their 80s and 90s die every day with or without the flu shot and the number of deaths was not unexpected, the program slowly got back on track. From that time on, nearly 50 million doses of vaccine were given in 10 weeks.

Reports of Guillain-Barré syndrome (GBS) began to surface in late November and early December, while the campaign was still in progress. Larry Schonberger at CDC, who did a brilliant job of analyzing and reanalyzing the data, made a strong case that GBS was associated with vaccination. After two quick back-to-back meetings with CDC staff and several consultants, it was concluded on the basis of 36 cases that GBS was epidemiologically related to the vaccine. On December 16, 1976, 11 months after swine flu was reported, CDC requested that the immunization program be stopped.

Christmas of 1976 was not a season of great joy around CDC. The swine flu program was no longer, there were continuing reports of GBS, and the Legionnaires disease investigation had apparently failed.

Fortunately, Joe McDade is a compulsive type. Because he wanted to put a few loose ends together before the end of the year, he reviewed his earlier guinea pig slides stained for rickettsia and on December 28, 1976, he found not rickettsia but the Legionnaires bacillus. The rest is history, with publication of the findings in *Morbidity and Mortality Weekly Report* and of the full report of the epidemiology and etiology in *New England Journal of Medicine*.

The title of this presentation is "1976: Lessons Learned." I haven't mentioned any lessons yet, but I think some are obvious. But before talking about lessons learned, I would like to provide a brief epilogue concerning the early months of 1977.

First, a new influenza virus did appear. It was not swine influenza; it was the H1N1 virus of 1950. It did not cause a pandemic, although it did circle the globe. This new 1977 virus did not displace the then current influenza A virus; in fact, these two viruses have continued to cocirculate for 15 years, which is totally unprecedented. The influenza A virus that was "threatening to change in 1976" is still here, 24 years later; it has not been replaced. So much for the natural patterns of the influenza viruses.

Second, in the midst of continued research into Ebola virus, Lassa fever, and Marburg viruses, two of our custodial staff died of a hemorrhagic disease. The etiology was not any of the above but rather the agent of Rocky Mountain spotted fever, the rickettsia that we had worked with for many years. How did the infection occur? We have never been certain.

Third, in the heady days of winter and spring, with McDade's and Shepard's findings of the Legionnaires bacillus associated with Pontiac fever, St. Elizabeth's, and other unresolved outbreaks, the learning curve outside CDC was still in effect. A bacterium as the cause of Legionnaires disease was not universally accepted by the media—and thus by the public, our scientific friends, members of Congress, and those with a conspiratorial bent. The findings still had only modest play in the press. The toxin supporters wouldn't believe it, those with axes to grind wouldn't accept it, and there were still some who held out for chlamydia.

The special session on Legionnaires disease at the American Society for Microbiology in May 1977 was filled to capacity. However, at the conclusion of the presentations, there were no shouts of "Author! Author!" but rather polite applause and a series of critical comments and questions from the floor.

Later in the fall, Senators Richard Schweiker, Edward Kennedy, and Jacob Javitz held a hearing at CDC. It was quite an event, with many news people and many cameras, lights, and microphones. Bill Foege, Dave Frazier, and I testified. Senator Kennedy started the questioning with a comment. He stated that this was a remarkable finding and that surely a Nobel Prize was in order, a sentiment echoed by the other two senators in their statements. It was at this time that the lights went out and the cameras stopped.

There was a small paragraph in the paper that evening that a hearing had been held—nothing else. On television, there was nothing on the national news, and the local station had an interview with Senator Kennedy on his plans to run for President in 1980—nothing else. And for years, when people learned I was from CDC, the predictable comment was, "You never did find out what caused Legionnaires disease, did you?"

What were the lessons learned in 1976? In regard to swine flu, I hope we learned that nature does not follow the rules of scientific dogma. We deal in biology, not physics, and in biology, we must expect the unexpected. An influenza pandemic could occur any time; then again, it may not. Second, with any vaccine, even one as innocuous as a killed influenza virus, one must expect rare adverse reactions to emerge with the inoculation of enough people. Possibly GBS is a generic problem with vaccination of adults, not necessarily with just swine influenza. Third, there are numerous lessons learned and relearned from Legionnaires disease itself, but perhaps the most important is never to confuse our limited knowledge with what there is yet to learn. At no time did any consultant suggest that the etiologic agent of Legionnaires disease was a bacterium. In fact, on the basis of the lack of staining, the pathological findings, the patients' clinical histories, and the epidemiology, we were told, as the 11 pathologists concluded, that "it could be a virus, it could be a toxin, but it definitely was not a bacteria." We now know why.

Legionnaires disease also taught us the inadequacy of our understanding of the mechanisms of host-parasite relationships and the role of the environment as a reservoir for infectious disease, much of which will be discussed at this conference. But perhaps the fundamental lesson is that infectious diseases have not been eliminated. Indeed, the prevailing thought in the early 1970s was that science had conquered infectious diseases. Funding and research emphasis began shifting, and appropriately so, to more chronic diseases. But think what has happened since 1976: the worldwide finding of legionella and associated infections; human immunodeficiency virus types

1 and 2 and AIDS; numerous opportunistic infections; hemorrhagic dengue in the New World; salmonella infections; cholera, invading the New World for the first time in over 100 years; measles and its changing epidemiology; and the increasing number of outbreaks of multidrug-resistant strains of tuberculosis. I could go on, and I'm sure you also have a list.

As the world's population grows, travel increases, and poverty expands, I predict that infectious diseases will bring many more surprises.

I'd like to leave you with one more story about 1976. Shortly after the Ebola outbreak, our investigative team there bled nearly the entire population of a small village in northern Zaire in search of subclinical Ebola infections. They didn't find any. But 10 years later another CDC team found, among those same sera, samples from several young adults in that village who already had been infected with the AIDS virus—at the very time the CDC was looking for Ebola. It all sounds a little Dickensonian, doesn't it? Without knowing it, while investigating one outbreak, the seeds of a far greater plague were already being sown. Think about it. How many more surprises are out there?

I. CLINICAL AND EPIDEMIOLOGIC ASPECTS OF LEGIONELLOSIS

A. Clinical and Laboratory Diagnosis

STATE OF THE ART LECTURE

Laboratory Diagnosis of Legionnaires Disease: an Update from 1984

PAUL H. EDELSTEIN

Department of Pathology and Laboratory Medicine and Department of Medicine, University of Pennsylvania School of Medicine, and Clinical Microbiology Laboratory, Hospital of the University of Pennsylvania, Philadelphia, Pennsylvania 19104-4283

Laboratory diagnosis of Legionnaires disease remains problematic, having changed little since 1984. The disease is still difficult to diagnose, and it is likely that we continue to miss diagnoses despite the use of optimal test techniques. In contrast to the situation in 1984, it is likely that more physicians are aware of the existence of Legionnaires disease and know how to treat it. However, little progress has been made in persuading the general laboratory community to perform cultures for *Legionella* species; we find an unfortunate persistence of the sole use of serologic diagnosis, often with invalidated and improperly performed techniques.

It has also been recognized that Legionnaires disease is difficult, if not impossible, to distinguish clinically from other common causes of pneumonia (15, 18, 41). This fact tends to lower test-positive predictive values, as more people with non-epidemic-associated pneumonia are being tested for the disease.

The relatively few advances in the diagnosis of Legionnaires disease include the availability of a commercial radioimmunoassay for urinary antigen, a DNA probe assay for primary detection of *Legionella* isolates in respiratory tract specimens, and a monoclonal antibody for bacterial detection (1, 8, 11, 17, 25, 36). The major change in the United States has been the commercialization, or privatization, of diagnostic testing and of production of diagnostic reagents and kits. While this trend has resulted in the introduction of all three major diagnostic techniques since 1984, it has also resulted in the use of poorly validated immunologic reagents for both serologic diagnosis and bacterial-antigen detection. Thus, while major advances have been made in some spheres, in others we may be somewhat worse off than when immu-

noserologic testing was being performed exclusively by specialized research and public health laboratories.

SEROLOGIC DIAGNOSIS

Serologic diagnosis of Legionnaires disease remains an important diagnostic method (10). European and North American laboratories still use different methods of antigen preparation, with the former using formolized yolk sac-grown bacteria and the latter using heat-killed, plate-grown bacteria (10, 22, 23, 26, 52). Significant advances have been made in defining the specificity of the formolized antigen, but no similar effort has been made for the heat-killed antigen (2, 32, 45). For the heated-antigen methods, there remains considerable variability in the use of yolk sac for antigen suspension and serum dilution (10). It has become apparent that serologic diagnosis of non-*Legionella pneumophila* serogroup 1 disease is likely less specific than it is for *L. pneumophila* serogroup 1 infections and that use of the polyvalent pools can lead to nonspecific results.

Serologic diagnosis of *L. pneumophila* serogroup 1 disease can be accomplished by either microagglutination or indirect immunofluorescence methods. Using immunofluorescence and either type of antigen preparation, the sensitivity of seroconversion for *L. pneumophila* serogroup 1 disease has been documented to be in the 70 to 80% range, based on culture-proven cases; a similar sensitivity has been found for microagglutination (20, 21, 23, 52). The specificity of these methods is in the range of 99 to 99.6%. However, these figures are considerably different for use of single-antibody tests and for detection of antibody to *Legionella* species or serogroups other than *L.*

pneumophila serogroup 1. The background frequencies of elevated titers in a normal population are 1 to 3% for the formolized antigen at a titer of 16 and 1 to 36% for heated antigen at a titer of 128 (2, 21–23, 26, 45, 53, 54). This difference in background seroprevalence means that single-titer results for the formolized yolk sac-grown antigen are more reliable than those for the heated antigen.

Relatively few comparisons of different antigen preparations have been carried out. Wilkinson and Brake compared the sensitivity of the boiled plate-grown *L. pneumophila* serogroup 1 antigen versus that of a formolized plate-grown antigen made from the same bacterium (51). The formolized antigen used was not yolk sac grown, and hence the conclusion of equivalent sensitivity does not apply to comparison with the yolk sac-grown bacterium. Fallon and Johnston found that heated plate-grown and formolized yolk sac-grown antigens were equivalent in sensitivity and specificity, but the study was a limited one (14).

Early studies of the specificity of the antigen preparations were performed by using serum samples from patients with mycoplasma or *Coxiella* infections but not from patients with common causes of bacterial pneumonias, such as *Streptococcus pneumoniae*, enteric gram-negative rods, *Pseudomonas aeruginosa,* or mycobacteria. Since it is now evident that Legionnaires disease cannot be readily clinically distinguished from other common causes of pneumonia, it is very important to do specificity studies with more appropriate control groups. Such studies have now been done for the formolized antigen; the results show minimal cross-reactivity except for *P. aeruginosa* infections (2, 23, 32). However, such a study has never been done with the heated plate-grown antigen. Numerous serologic cross-reactions have been reported for the heat-killed antigen, including cross-reactions with *P. aeruginosa,* several *Rickettsia* species, *Coxiella burnetii,* enteric gram-negative rods, *Bacteroides* spp., and *Haemophilus* spp. (5, 10, 45, 50, 53). In contrast, for the formolized antigen, only cross-reactions with *P. aeruginosa, Citrobacter freundii,* and *Campylobacter jejuni* have been reported (3, 19, 23). Although there is no direct proof, there is considerable evidence that the formolized antigen preparation is considerably more specific than and equal in sensitivity to the heated antigen.

Diagnosis of non-*L. pneumophila* serogroup 1 *Legionella* infections by serologic means is not as easy as was thought in 1984. Proper validation of test sensitivity has not been done because of the limited number of culture-proven cases. More problematic is test specificity, which is lower than for *L. pneumophila* serogroup 1 tests. Bornstein et al. (2) and McIntyre et al. (32), using a control population of patients with non-*Legionella* pneumonia, showed that several non-*L. pneumophila*

serogroup 1 formolized antigens were not as specific as the *L. pneumophila* serogroup 1 antigen. Such studies have not been done for heated antigens, but it is not likely that their specificity is greater than for the *L. pneumophila* serogroup 1 antigen. This consideration mandates exceptionally cautious use of non-*L. pneumophila* serogroup 1 antigens in the absence of adequate background seroprevalence rates in the population being studied. At the very least, more stringent criteria for seroconversion need to be established for these other serogroups and species. Currently, authorities in the United States and the United Kingdom advise against the routine use of non-*L. pneumophila* serogroup 1 antigens.

Use of polyvalent antigenic pools for serologic diagnosis was the result of the recognition of limited cross-reactivity between *L. pneumophila* serogroup 1 and other *Legionella* antigens (54). However, it has become apparent that seroconversions with polyvalent pools always need confirmation with the monovalent components to avoid false-positive test results (10, 13).

There are several important goals for serologic diagnosis of Legionnaires disease. It is now time for proponents of heat-killed antigens to either prove that these antigens are as specific as the formolized ones or adopt use of the latter. Also, major efforts must be made to study and improve the serologic diagnosis of non-*L. pneumophila* serogroup 1 *Legionella* infections. Laboratories that use commercially prepared serologic reagents dissimilar from the reference standards should demand evidence of equivalence of performance or choose other suppliers. Finally, use of polyvalent screening pools, without monovalent confirmation of positive tests, should be abandoned.

ANTIGEN DETECTION

Two major advances in antigen detection have been made since 1984: a monoclonal *L. pneumophila* antibody for use with direct immunofluorescence and a test for *L. pneumophila* serogroup 1 antigenuria, both of which are commercially available. The monoclonal antibody is species specific, thus precluding the use of polyvalent pools (11, 17). It remains unknown whether the monoclonal antibody is more sensitive or specific than a polyvalent *L. pneumophila* serogroup 1 to 4 pool. Unfortunately, the sensitivity of direct fluorescent antibody (DFA) testing remains highly variable (from 25 to 70%), although its specificity remains in the 99 to 99.3% range. The sensitivity and specificity of the DFA test for non-*L. pneumophila* species are still unknown, and it is wise to remain skeptical about the specificity of reagents for non-*L. pneumophila* species. The urinary antigen test has demonstrated very high specificity (>99.5%) and sensitivity (80 to 90%) for detection of *L. pneumophila* serogroup 1 Legionnaires disease (1, 25). Its major drawbacks are its radiometric format and the inability to detect infections caused by other serogroups and species. There is also disquieting preliminary evidence of low sensitivity in community-acquired, culture-negative, seropositive cases of Legionnaires disease (37). The test has been used to detect antigen in pleural fluid, although this appears to have little advantage over detection of urinary antigen (35).

Detection of *L. pneumophila* serogroup 1 antigenuria by enzyme-linked immunosorbent assay (ELISA) has been reported to be more sensitive than culture in one large prospective study (42). This finding is contrary to results presented in a previous report and needs confirmation (25).

A reverse passive agglutination assay for *L. pneumophila* antigenuria is now commercially available. However, the performance characteristics of the assay make it unreliable for clinical use (28).

A major goal for antigenuria detection is commercial development of a multivalent reagent, which has worked so well in one laboratory (44). Other goals are more prospective studies comparing culture and antigenuria detection, commercialization of nonradiometric tests, and production of genus-specific monoclonal antibodies for use in DFA or ELISA detection of antigen and enhanced sensitivity of DFA methods.

CULTURE DIAGNOSIS

Culture diagnosis remains the "gold standard" for other diagnostic methods and probably continues to be the most sensitive means of diagnosis when it is performed early in the course of disease. However, this method is not widely used, and when it is, it is done very poorly. A 1989 survey of U.S. clinical microbiology laboratories found that 32% of otherwise sophisticated laboratories were unable to grow a pure and heavy culture of *L. pneumophila* (4). Added to the already long list of extrapulmonary sites culture positive for *Legionella* species are bone marrow, prosthetic heart valves, and sternal wounds (7, 16, 29, 46). Any "culture-negative" infection should be cultured for legionellae, regardless of site or the presence of pneumonia. Blood culture for detection of *L. pneumophila* has been shown to be positive in about 30% of patients with severe Legionnaires disease (9, 40) and can be accomplished by using a variety of techniques (6, 39, 40). Buffered charcoal-yeast extract agar enriched with α-ketoglutarate (BCYEα medium) has been found to be an excellent isolation medium for *Nocardia*, *Cryptococcus*, *Blastomyces*, *Histoplasma*, *Coccidioides*, *Francisella*, *Bordetella*, and *Brucella* species (38, 48). Supplementation of BCYEα medium with albumin has been reported

to enhance the yield of *L. bozemanii* and *L. micdadei*, but not of *L. pneumophila*, from guinea pig spleens; whether this finding is of clinical benefit is unclear (33). Development of new selective media will become necessary because of increasing resistance of contaminating flora to the presently used selective agents and because of susceptibility of some *L. pneumophila* strains to cefamandole (49).

Identification of *Legionella* spp. is becoming ever more complex, as new species that can be differentiated from other species only by DNA-DNA hybridization studies are discovered. Some newer biochemical identification techniques may be useful in this regard but need further study (24, 31, 47). A commercial, nonradioisotopic DNA hybridization kit for species identification has been developed in Japan and appears to be very useful (12).

NUCLEIC ACID DETECTION

New since 1984 is a commercial genus-specific DNA probe for primary detection of *Legionella* species in clinical specimens. Its sensitivity of about 50 to 60% and specificity of about 99% place it in the same category as DFA testing (8, 36). Changes in product formulation have increased the product's specificity without affecting sensitivity, as an earlier formulation led to reports of a pseudoepidemic of Legionnaires disease (27, 36). Polymerase chain reaction assays appear to be more sensitive than the DNA probe for clinical and environmental specimens, but whether they will be as sensitive as culture, and whether inhibitors present in sputum can be dealt with, is unclear (30, 34, 43).

REFERENCES

1. **Aguero-Rosenfeld, M. E., and P. H. Edelstein.** 1988. Retrospective evaluation of the Du Pont radioimmunoassay kit for detection of *Legionella pneumophila* serogroup 1 antigenuria in humans. *J. Clin. Microbiol.* **26:**1775–1778.
2. **Bornstein, N., N. Janin, G. Bourguignon, M. Surgot, and J. Fleurette.** 1987. Prevalence of anti-legionella antibodies in a healthy population and in patients with tuberculosis or pneumonia. *Pathol. Biol.* **35:**353–356.
3. **Boswell, T. C. J., and G. Kudesia.** 1992. Seropositivity for legionella in campylobacter infection. *Lancet* **339:**191.
4. **College of American Pathologists.** 1989. Bacteriology survey, Specimen D-12, final critique. College of American Pathologists Survey Program. College of American Pathologists, Skokie, Ill.
5. **Collins, M. T., F. Espersen, N. Høiby, S. Cho, A. Friis-Møller, and J. S. Reif.** 1983. Cross-reactions between *Legionella pneumophila* (serogroup 1) and twenty-eight other bacterial species, including other members of the family *Legionellaceae*. *Infect. Immun.* **39:**1441–1456.
6. **David, C., O. Bajolet, A. Wynckel, E. LeMagrex, and O. Toupance.** 1990. Isolement chez une transplantée rénale de *Legionella pneumophila* par le système d'hémoculture Isolator. *Presse Med.* **19:**1460.
7. **deTruchis, P., E. Dournon, E. Gluckman, J. L. Touboul, C. Mayaud, and G. Akoun.** 1988. Maladie de légionnaires avec pancytopénie et isolement de légionelles

par hémocultures et cultures de moelle osseuse. *Presse Med.* **17**:34–35.

8. **Doebbling, B. N., M. J. Bale, F. P. Koontz, C. M. Helms, R. P. Wenzel, and M. A. Pfaller.** 1988. Prospective evaluation of the Gen-Probe assay for detection of legionellae in respiratory specimens. *Eur. J. Clin. Microbiol. Infect. Dis.* **7**:748–752.

9. **Dournon, E., P. Rajagopalan, and M. Assous.** 1986. Bacteremia in Legionnaires' disease. *Isr. J. Med. Sci.* **22**:759.

10. **Edelstein, P. H.** 1992. Detection of antibodies to *Legionella*, p. 459–446. *In* N. R. Rose, E. Conway de Macario, J. L. Fahey, H. Friedman, and G. M. Penn (ed.), *Manual of Clinical Laboratory Immunology,* 4th ed. American Society for Microbiology, Washington, D.C.

11. **Edelstein, P. H., K. B. Beer, J. C. Sturge, A. J. Watson, and L. C. Goldstein.** 1985. Clinical utility of a monoclonal direct fluorescent reagent specific for *Legionella pneumophila*: comparative study with other reagents. *J. Clin. Microbiol.* **22**:419–421.

12. **Ezaki, T., Y. Hashimoto, H. Yamamoto, M. L. Lucida, S. L. Liu, S. Kusunoki, K. Asano, and Y. Yabuuchi.** 1990. Evaluation of the microplate hybridization method for rapid identification of *Legionella* species. *Eur. J. Clin. Microbiol. Infect. Dis.* **9**:213–218.

13. **Fallon, R. J., and W. J. Abraham.** 1982. Polyvalent heat-killed antigen for the diagnosis of infection with *Legionella pneumophila*. *J. Clin. Pathol.* **35**:434–438.

14. **Fallon, R. J., and R. E. Johnston.** 1987. Heterogeneity of antibody response in infection with *Legionella pneumophila* serogroup 1. *J. Clin. Pathol.* **40**:569–572.

15. **Fang, G., M. Fine, J. Orloff, D. Arisumi, V. L. Yu, W. Kapoor, J. T. Grayston, S. P. Wang, R. Kohler, R. R. Muder, Y. C. Yee, J. D. Rihs, and R. M. Vickers.** 1990. New and emerging etiologies for community-acquired pneumonia with implications for therapy. A prospective multicenter study of 359 cases. *Medicine* **69**:307–316.

16. **Ferrer, A., J. Lloveras, G. Codina, and N. Martin.** 1987. Aislamiento de *Legionella pneumophila* en medula ósea. *Med. Clin.* (Barcelona) **88**:346–347.

17. **Gosting, L. H., K. Cabrian, J. C. Sturge, and L. C. Goldstein.** 1984. Identification of a species-specific antigen in *Legionella pneumophila* by a monoclonal antibody. *J. Clin. Microbiol.* **20**:1031–1035.

18. **Granados, A., D. Podzamczer, F. Guidol, and F. Manresa.** 1989. Pneumonia due to *Legionella pneumophila* and pneumococcal pneumonia: similarities and differences on presentation. *Eur. Respir. J.* **2**:130–134.

19. **Gray, J. J., K. N. Ward, R. E. Warren, and M. Farrington.** 1991. Serological cross-reactions between *Legionella pneumophila* and *Citrobacter freundii* in direct immunofluorescence and rapid microagglutination tests. *J. Clin. Microbiol.* **29**:200–201.

20. **Harrison, T. G., E. Dournon, and A. G. Taylor.** 1987. Evaluation of sensitivity of two serological tests for diagnosing pneumonia caused by *Legionella pneumophila* serogroup 1. *J. Clin. Pathol.* **40**:77–82.

21. **Harrison, T. G., and A. G. Taylor.** 1982. A rapid microagglutination test for the diagnosis of *Legionella pneumophila* (serogroup 1) infection. *J. Clin. Pathol.* **35**:1028–1031.

22. **Harrison, T. G., and A. G. Taylor.** 1982. Diagnosis of *Legionella pneumophila* infections by means of formolized yolk sac antigens. *J. Clin. Pathol.* **35**:211–214.

23. **Harrison, T. G., and A. G. Taylor.** 1988. The diagnosis of Legionnaires' disease by estimation of antibody levels, p. 113–135. *In* T. G. Harrison and A. G. Taylor (ed.), *A Laboratory Manual for Legionella.* John Wiley & Sons, New York.

24. **Horbach, I., D. Naumann, and F. J. Fehrenbach.** 1988. Simultaneous infections with different serogroups of *Legionella pneumophila* investigated by routine methods and Fourier transform infrared spectroscopy. *J. Clin. Microbiol.* **26**:1106–1110.

25. **Kohler, R. B.** 1986. Antigen detection for the rapid diagnosis of mycoplasma and legionella pneumonia. *Diagn. Microbiol. Infect. Dis.* **4**:47S–59S.

26. **Lattimer, G. L., and B. A. Cepil.** 1980. Legionnaires' disease serology. Effect of antigen preparation on specificity and sensitivity of the indirect fluorescent antibody test. *J. Clin. Pathol.* **33**:585–590.

27. **Laussucq, S., D. Schuster, W. J. Alexander, W. L. Thacker, H. W. Wilkinson, and J. S. Spika.** 1988. False-positive DNA probe test for *Legionella* species associated with a cluster of respiratory illnesses. *J. Clin. Microbiol.* **26**:1442–1444.

28. **Leland, D. S., and R. B. Kohler.** 1991. Evaluation of the L-CLONE *Legionella pneumophila* serogroup 1 urine antigen latex test. *J. Clin. Microbiol.* **29**:2220–2223.

29. **Lowry, P. W., R. J. Blankenship, W. Gridley, N. J. Troup, and L. S. Tompkins.** 1991. A cluster of legionella sternal-wound infections due to postoperative topical exposure to contaminated tap water. *N. Engl. J. Med.* **324**:109–113.

30. **Mahbubani, M. H., A. K. Bej, R. Miller, L. Haff, J. DiCesare, and R. Atlas.** 1990. Detection of *Legionella* with polymerase chain reaction and gene probe methods. *Mol. Cell. Probes* **4**:175–187.

31. **Mauchline, W. S., and C. W. Keevil.** 1991. Development of the BIOLOG substrate utilization system for identification of *Legionella* spp. *Appl. Environ. Microbiol.* **57**:3345–3349.

32. **McIntyre, M., J. B. Kurtz, and J. B. Selkon.** 1990. Prevalence of antibodies to 15 antigens of legionellaceae in patients with community-acquired pneumonia. *Epidemiol. Infect.* **104**:39–45.

33. **Morrill, W. E., J. M. Barbaree, B. S. Fields, G. N. Sanden, and W. T. Martin.** 1990. Increased recovery of *Legionella micdadei* and *Legionella bozemanii* on buffered charcoal yeast extract agar supplemented with albumin. *J. Clin. Microbiol.* **28**:616–618.

34. **Nowicki, M., N. Bornstein, B. Jaulhac, Y. Piemont, H. Monteil, and J. Fleurette.** 1992. *Program Abstr. 1992 Int. Symp. Legionella,* p. 22, abstr. II–29.

35. **Oliverio, M. J., M. A. Fisher, R. M. Vickers, V. L. Yu, and A. Menon.** 1991. Diagnosis of Legionnaires' disease by radioimmunoassay of *Legionella* antigen in pleural fluid. *J. Clin. Microbiol.* **29**:2893–2894.

36. **Pasculle, A. W., G. E. Veto, S. Krystofiak, K. McKelvey, and K. Ursalovic.** 1989. Laboratory and clinical evaluation of a commercial DNA probe for the detection of *Legionella* spp. *J. Clin. Microbiol.* **27**:2350–2358.

37. **Plouffe, J. (Ohio State University).** 1991. Personal communication.

38. **Raad, I., K. Rand, and D. Gaskins.** 1990. Buffered charcoal-yeast extract medium for the isolation of brucellae. *J. Clin. Microbiol.* **28**:1671–1672.

39. **Reinhardt, J. F., C. Nakahama, and P. H. Edelstein.** 1987. Comparison of blood culture methods for recovery of *Legionella pneumophila* from the blood of guinea pigs with experimenal infection. *J. Clin. Microbiol.* **25**:719–721.

40. **Rihs, J. D., V. L. Yu, J. J. Zuravleff, A. Goetz, and R. R. Muder.** 1985. Isolation of *Legionella pneumophila* from blood with the BACTEC system: a prospective study yielding positive results. *J. Clin. Microbiol.* **22**:422–424.

41. **Roig, J., X. Aguilar, J. Ruiz, C. Domingo, E. Mesalles, J. Manterola, and J. Morera.** 1991. Comparative study of *Legionella pneumophila* and other nosocomial-acquired pneumonias. *Chest* **99**:344–350.

42. **Ruf, B., D. Schürmann, I. Horbach, F. J. Fehrenbach, and H. D. Pohle.** 1990. Prevalence and diagnosis of *Legionella* pneumonia: a 3-year prospective study with emphasis on application of urinary antigen detection. *J. Infect. Dis.* **162**:1341–1348.

43. **Starnbach, M. N., S. Falkow, and L. Tompkins.** 1989. Species-specific detection of *Legionella pneumophila* in water by DNA amplification and hybridization. *J. Clin. Microbiol.* **27**:1257–1261.

44. **Tang, P. W., and S. Toma.** 1986. Broad-spectrum en-

zyme-linked immunosorbent assay for detection of *Legionella* soluble antigens. *J. Clin. Microbiol.* **24:**556–558.

45. **Taylor, A. G., T. G. Harrison, M. W. Dighero, and C. M. P. Bradstreet.** 1979. False positive reactions in the indirect fluorescent antibody test for Legionnaires' disease eliminated by use of formolized yolk-sac antigen. *Ann. Intern. Med.* **90:**686–689.

46. **Tompkins, L. S., B. J. Roessler, S. C. Redd, L. E. Markowitz, and M. L. Cohen.** 1988. Legionella prosthetic-valve endocarditis. N. Engl. J. Med. **318:**530–535.

47. **Vesey, G., P. J. Dennis, J. V. Lee, and A. A. West.** 1988. Further development of simple tests to differentiate the legionellas. *J. Appl. Bacteriol.* **65:**339–345.

48. **Vickers, R. M., J. D. Rihs, and V. L. Yu.** 1992. Clinical demonstration of isolation of *Nocardia asteroides* on buffered charcoal-yeast extract media. *J. Clin. Microbiol.* **30:**227–228.

49. **Vickers, R. M., J. E. Stout, L. S. Tompkins, N. J. Troup, and V. L. Yu.** 1992. Cefamandole-susceptible strains of *Legionella pneumophila*. *J. Clin. Microbiol.* **30:**537–539.

50. **Wang, E. L., B. Manson, M. Corey, K. Bernard, and C. G. Prober.** 1987. False positivity of *Legionella* serol-

ogy in patients with cystic fibrosis. *Pediatr. Infect. Dis. J.* **6:**256–259.

51. **Wilkinson, H. W., and B. J. Brake.** 1982. Formalin-killed versus heat-killed *Legionella pneumophila* serogroup 1 antigen in the indirect immunofluorescence assay for legionellosis. *J. Clin. Microbiol.* **16:**979–981.

52. **Wilkinson, H. W., D. D. Cruce, and C. V. Broome.** 1981. Validation of *Legionella pneumophila* indirect immunofluorescence assay with epidemic sera. *J. Clin. Microbiol.* **13:**139–146.

53. **Wilkinson, H. W., C. E. Farshy, B. J. Fikes, D. D. Cruce, and L. P. Yealy.** 1979. Measure of immunoglobulin G-, M-, and A-specific titers against *Legionella pneumophila* and inhibition of titers against nonspecific, gram-negative bacterial antigens in the indirect immunofluorescence test for legionellosis. *J. Clin. Microbiol.* **10:**685–689.

54. **Wilkinson, H. W., A. L. Reingold, B. J. Brake, D. L. McGiboney, G. W. Gorman, and C. V. Broome.** 1983. Reactivity of serum from patients with suspected legionellosis against 29 antigens of Legionellaceae and *Legionella*-like organisms by indirect immunofluorescence assay. *J. Infect. Dis.* **147:**23–31.

Legionella Antigenuria: Six-Year Study of Broad-Spectrum Enzyme-Linked Immunosorbent Assay as a Routine Diagnostic Test

P. TANG AND C. KRISHNAN

Central Public Health Laboratory, Ontario Ministry of Health, Toronto, Ontario M5W 1R5, Canada

The broad-spectrum enzyme-linked immunosorbent assay (ELISA) for *Legionella* antigenuria is an intragenus assay with a specificity that approaches 100% (5). It was introduced as a routine diagnostic test in June 1985. Up to May 1991, a total of 6,873 urine specimens had been tested, with a positive rate of 1.4%. There was a total of 280 cases of legionellosis in that period. The ELISA was positive in 98 of 136 cases of legionellosis for which urine specimens were obtained.

Comparison of ELISA and DFA culture. In 57 cases, both respiratory tract specimens (for direct fluorescent antibody testing [DFA]/culture) and urines (for ELISA) were collected. In 23 cases, both DFA/culture and ELISA were positive, and in 17 cases each, only one test was positive. The sensitivity for both DFA/culture and ELISA was 70% (40 of 57 cases). Of the 17 DFA/culture-positive-only cases, 13 were positive by culture and 4 were positive by DFA. In 10 of these cases, urine specimens were collected at much later dates than were respiratory tract specimens. In the 17 ELISA-positive-only cases, 10 had inadequate follow-up or inappropriate respiratory tract specimens, and thus identification to the species level could not be made.

The discrepancies observed between the tests can be attributed primarily to three factors: (i) the collection of appropriate respiratory tract specimens which, taken on consecutive days, may give variable results; (ii) collection of urine specimens at inappropriate phase of illness; and (iii) the lower sensitivity (below 70%) of the majority of respiratory tract specimens such as sputa and bronchial washes.

Since DFA/culture and ELISA detect different entities, our results may indicate that the two sets of tests complement each other and that both specimen types should be submitted.

Comparison of IFA and ELISA. For indirect fluorescent antibody (IFA) testing, formalized antigens of up to 45 serogroups of 30 species were used in pools initially and tested individually where indicated. Serum and urine samples were received in 96 cases. The IFA sensitivity was 47%, and the ELISA sensitivity was 69%. Of 20 cases that were both IFA and ELISA positive, 18 were initially ELISA positive and IFA negative and then on follow-up reversed to ELISA negative and IFA positive; 2 cases were ELISA and IFA positive simultaneously. In 24 of 27 cases that were IFA positive only, urine samples were taken after seroconversion, when the ELISA would be expected to be negative. In 3 of the 27 cases, the ELISA was negative even during the acute phase of illness. In 43 of the 49 cases that were ELISA positive only, single acute-phase sera were collected; in only 6 cases were follow-up sera collected > 14 and < 30 days after onset. This made it difficult to compare the relative sensitivities of ELISA and IFA because in many cases, specimens were either not collected at proper intervals or not followed up.

The antigen excretion dynamics were assessed in 26 cases for which urine ELISA was initially positive and for which follow-up urine samples were obtained. ELISA became negative in 11 cases within 7 days of the initial test, in 10 cases within 14 days, and in 3 cases within 21 days. In two cases, antigen was detectable for more than 22 days.

Distribution of *Legionella* isolates identified for those cases that were ELISA positive varied among 13 serogroups of nine species, as confirmed by DFA, culture, or IFA (Table 1). Cases were considered IFA positive only when the following criteria were met: (i) at least a fourfold seroconversion, (ii) clear-cut species identification and serogrouping, and (iii) negative results for other legionellae and bacterial or viral pathogens.

Soluble antigens from cell extracts of 32 other *Legionella* serogroups were detectable by ELISA, but the efficacy of the ELISA in clinical cases for these serogroups could not be assessed because of a lack of cases.

Our results were consistent with our previous study and projections (5). They compared well with other studies on urinary antigen detection (1–4). The ELISA has proven to be as sensitive as DFA/culture, has the highest positive rate among all routine tests, and provides rapid results (3 h), and specimens are easily obtained. We conclude

TABLE 1. *Legionella* species detected by ELISA

Species	Serogroup	No. of cases
L. pneumophila	1	19
	3	2
	6	4
	8	2
	12	3
L. bozemanii	1	2
L. cincinnatiensis		1
L. hackeliae	1	1
	2	2
L. maceachernii		3
L. micdadei		1
L. parisiensis[a]		1
L. sainthelensi[a]	1	1

[a] First report of human infection.

that the broad-spectrum ELISA for *Legionella* antigenuria is an excellent screening test for diagnosis of community-acquired and nosocomial acute *Legionella* infections. For optimal sensitivity in the diagnosis of acute legionellosis, we maintain that both ELISA and DFA/culture should be carried out.

REFERENCES

1. **Bibb, W. F., P. M. Arnow, L. Thacker, and R. M. McKinney.** 1984. Detection of *Legionella pneumophila* antigen in serum and urine specimens by enzyme-linked immunosorbent assay with monoclonal and polyclonal antibodies. *J. Clin. Microbiol.* **20:**478–482.
2. **Kohler, R. B.** 1986. Antigen detection for the rapid diagnosis of mycoplasma and *Legionella* pneumonia. *Diagn. Microbiol. Infect. Dis.* **4:**47S–59S.
3. **Kohler, R. B., W. C. Winn, and L. J. Wheat.** 1984. Onset and duration of urinary antigens excretion in Legionnaires disease. *J. Clin. Microbiol.* **20:**605–607.
4. **Kohler, R. B., S. E. Zimmerman, E. Wilson, S. D. Allen, P. H. Edelstein, L. J. Wheat, and A. White.** 1981. Rapid radioimmunoassay diagnosis of Legionnaires' disease. *Ann. Intern. Med.* **94:**601–605.
5. **Tang, P. W., and S. Toma.** 1986. Broad spectrum enzyme-linked immunosorbent assay for detection of *Legionella* soluble antigens. *J. Clin. Microbiol.* **24:**556–558.

Comparative Study of the Bactericidal Activity of Ampicillin/Sulbactam and Erythromycin against Intracellular *Legionella pneumophila*

JULIO A. RAMIREZ, JAMES T. SUMMERSGILL, RICHARD D. MILLER, TRACY L. MEYERS, AND MARTIN J. RAFF

Louisville Veterans Affairs Medical Center and Division of Infectious Diseases, Department of Medicine, and Department of Microbiology and Immunology, University of Louisville School of Medicine, Louisville, Kentucky 40292

The reported incidence of Legionnaires disease as a cause of community-acquired pneumonia ranges from 1 to 30%, suggesting that *L. pneumophila* is one of the most prevalent etiologic pathogens for this disease (5, 7, 12). The high mortality rate is greatest when patients are not initially treated with erythromycin (4).

The pulmonary alveolar macrophage is the lower respiratory tract's first line of defense against *Legionella* infection. After ingestion by coiling phagocytosis, legionellae often resist intraleukocytic killing. Multiplying within the cytoplasm, the organisms rupture and kill the phagocyte, releasing legionellae, which then infect other macrophages (9). Because of this subversion of host defenses, the ideal antibiotic for treatment of Legionnaires disease should enter the phagocyte and kill intracellular organisms. Erythromycin is currently the drug of choice for treatment of Legionnaires disease. It enters macrophages and monocytes but is not bactericidal for legionellae, and treatment failure is well documented (1).

Beta-lactam antibiotics have been shown to have little or no ability to enter phagocytic cells (6, 8) and, in theory, do not reach the area in which legionellae multiply. They are consequently not considered alternatives for treating Legionnaires disease. Numerous treatment failures with penicillins and cephalosporins have been reported (1). In fact, the failure of pneumonia to respond to beta-lactam antibiotics is frequently interpreted as a clue to the presence of Legionnaires disease (3).

The combination of ampicillin and the beta-lactamase inhibitor sulbactam is used as empirical therapy for community-acquired pneumonia (2). Ampicillin/sulbactam has good in vitro activity against pathogens causing community-acquired pneumonia, including *Streptococcus pneumoniae*, *Haemophilus influenzae*, *Moraxella catharralis*, *Klebsiella pneumoniae*, and *Staphylococcus aureus* (10). Susceptibility data for *Legionella pneumophila* are lacking. This study provides data on the activity of ampicillin and sulbactam, alone and in combination, compared with that of erythromycin against intracellular *L. pneumophila* in an in vitro model.

Subcultures of a macrophage-like cell line,

U-937 (ATCC CRL-1593), were maintained in RPMI 1640 (GIBCO, Grand Island, N.Y.) supplemented with 10% fetal bovine serum, L-glutamine, penicillin-streptomycin, and gentamicin and were incubated at 37°C with 5% carbon dioxide. Cells were harvested, washed twice in RPMI 1640 free of additives, and resuspended in RPMI 1640 supplemented with 10% newborn calf serum, L-glutamine, penicillin-streptomycin, and gentamicin to a concentration of 10^6/ml. After addition of phorbol 12-myristate 13-acetate (10 ng/ml) (Sigma, St. Louis, Mo.), 1.0 ml of suspension (10^6 cells) was placed in each of 24 wells of tissue culture plates (Costar, Cambridge, Mass.) and incubated for 24 h at 37°C in 5% carbon dioxide to allow differentiation into adherent cell monolayers. Wells were examined for successful differentiation and washed twice in unsupplemented RPMI 1640.

A clinical isolate of *L. pneumophila* serogroup 1, strain IDL-1V, was used in all assays. The organism was stored at −70°C, subcultured twice onto buffered charcoal-yeast extract agar (Difco, Detroit, Mich.), and incubated for 48 h at 37°C in 5% CO_2. Colonies were then aseptically swabbed from plates and adjusted colorimetrically to a concentration of 10^8 CFU/ml. Bacterial suspensions were washed and resuspended in RPMI 1640 supplemented with 20% normal human serum obtained from donors free of Legionnaires disease, and 0.1 ml was then placed in each well of the monolayers, resulting in a bacterium/cell ratio of 10:1. Opsonization occurred during subsequent incubation for 2 h to allow for sufficient uptake. All monolayers were then washed three times and resuspended in RPMI 1640 without additives. Cell monolayer integrity was monitored with uninfected control wells. Intracellular growth of *L. pneumophila* was allowed to occur during 6 h before the addition of antibiotics.

Dilutions of antibiotics were prepared in RPMI 1640, dispensed at final ampicillin, sulbactam, and erythromycin concentrations of 150, 50, and 10 μg/ml, respectively, and stored at −20°C. Drug concentrations reflected peak serum levels achieved with therapeutic doses of these antibiotics in patients with pneumonia. Appropriate controls were used. At 2-h intervals, the cell suspension medium was removed and cell monolayers were lysed with distilled water; dilutions of lysate were spread immediately onto buffered charcoal-yeast extract plates and incubated at 37°C for 72 h. Viable bacteria were estimated as CFU per milliliter by counting plates containing 30 to 300 colonies.

Changes in intracellular counts of *L. pneumophila* over time were expressed in log CFU per milliliter. Counts of intracellular *L. pneumophila* in the absence of antibiotics were compared with those following incubation with antibiotics. Statistical significance ($P < 0.05$) of differences between results was calculated by analysis of variance with a Newman-Keuls posttest (SPSS,PC+, Chicago, Il.). If increases or decreases in bacterial counts occurred, differences were also expressed in percentages and defined as percentage of growth (PG) or percentage of killing (PK) of intracellular *L. pneumophila*.

Intracellular replication of *L. pneumophila* began 4 h after inoculation of U-937 cell cultures and by 8 h was in the logarithmic growth phase, at which time antibiotics were added. Following 8 h of incubation, the numbers of viable bacteria in untreated cell cultures increased 0.9 log CFU/ml from values measured at the time at which either control solution or antibiotics were added ($P < 0.05$). Addition of erythromycin resulted in a decrease of 0.8 log CFU of viable bacteria per ml from counts at the time of inoculation ($P < 0.05$), also significantly less than the value for the untreated control ($P < 0.05$). With ampicillin/sulbactam, the number of viable bacteria decreased 2.9 log CFU/ml from the baseline counts ($P < 0.05$), significantly less than the value for either the untreated controls or cells treated with erythromycin ($P < 0.05$).

Results comparing ampicillin, sulbactam, and ampicillin/sulbactam combined indicated that ampicillin or sulbactam produced no change in the log CFU per milliliter from the initial counts after 8 h of incubation. These final counts were, however, significantly less than those in untreated controls ($P < 0.05$) and greater than the final counts seen in cells treated with ampicillin/sulbactam ($P < 0.05$).

A summary of PG and PK values, with statistical significances, is presented in Fig. 1. The control PG was 16% ($P < 0.05$). The PKs were 2% for sulbactam (P = not significant), 4% for ampicillin (P = not significant), 16% for erythromycin ($P < 0.05$), and 39% for ampicillin/sulbactam ($P < 0.05$).

From the results of retrospective clinical studies, erythromycin is considered the antibiotic of choice for treatment of Legionnaires disease (1). Its clinical superiority to beta-lactam antibiotics appears related to its ability to penetrate human macrophages. Clinical failures in treatment of Legionnaires disease with erythromycin have been documented and may reflect the lack of bactericidal activity of erythromycin against intracellular *L. pneumophila* (1). Antibiotics capable of entering macrophages and killing intracellular *L. pneumophila* may, in theory, be a better alternative to erythromycin in the treatment of Legionnaires disease.

The results of this in vitro study suggest that the combination of ampicillin and the beta-lactamase inhibitor sulbactam is able to enter the cells of a human macrophage-like cell line (U-937). In addi-

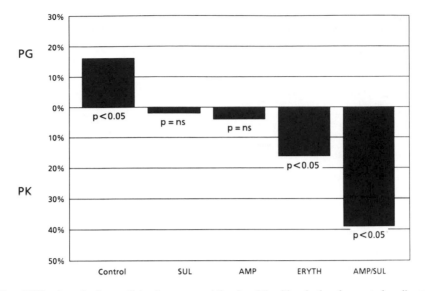

FIG. 1. PG and PK values for intracellular *L. pneumophila* after 8 h of incubation for control, sulbactam (SUL), ampicillin (AMP), erythromycin (ERYTH), and ampicillin/sulbactam (AMP/SUL) samples. ns, not significant.

tion, bactericidal activity of ampicillin/sulbactam against intracellular *L. pneumophila* is significantly superior to erythromycin in this cell model. By 8 h after addition of antibiotics to infected U-937 cells, ampicillin/sulbactam was able to decrease the intracellular *L. pneumophila* concentration (CFU per milliliter) to a statistically greater degree than was erythromycin. The 39% PK with ampicillin/sulbactam was significantly greater than that with erythromycin (PK of 16%). The PKs for sulbactam and ampicillin were 2 and 4%, respectively, suggesting that either sulbactam or ampicillin alone was able to inhibit the growth of intracellular *L. pneumophila*, but decreasing bacterial counts from their initial levels did not reach statistical significance.

One possible explanation for these results is that ampicillin/sulbactam was acting against extracellular rather than intracellular bacteria. After 2 h of incubation, monolayers were washed three times to removed extracellular bacteria, although bacteria attached to macrophages may still remain extracellular. Antibiotics were added to the medium 6 h later, allowing sufficient time for phagocytosis of attached bacteria. The increased bacterial counts seen in the control experiment are a reflection of intracellular growth, since *L. pneumophila* did not multiply in cell-free RPMI 1640 culture medium (data not shown).

It may be theorized that the antibiotic activity was due to multiplication of intracellular *L. pneumophila*, macrophage death, and release of bacteria. Antibiotics then killed extracellular bacteria before they were phagocytosed by other macro-

phages. Light microscopy, however, showed that cell monolayers remained confluent throughout the experiment, with no evidence of cell destruction. This finding agrees with studies indicating that cytopathological effects on U-937 cells by *L. pneumophila* do not occur until 24 h after infection (11).

It is theorized that sulbactam and ampicillin enter the macrophage at concentrations which are inhibitory, but not lethal, for *L. pneumophila*. The ampicillin/sulbactam combination, however, appears to be bactericidal. In addition, the PK of intracellular *L. pneumophila* for ampicillin/sulbactam was significantly greater than expected from the sum of the PKs seen with ampicillin and sulbactam. It is suspected that ampicillin/sulbactam is synergistic in concentrations entering the macrophage, resulting in intracellular killing of *L. pneumophila*.

In view of the superior activity of ampicillin/sulbactam in comparison with erythromycin in this in vitro model, and in comparison with the empirical use of ampicillin/sulbactam in treating community-acquired pneumonia (2), studies are warranted to delineate the clinical significance of these in vitro data.

This work was supported in part by grant 91-S-0579 from Roerig Division, Pfizer Inc.

REFERENCES

1. **Bartlett, C. L. R., A. D. Macrae, and J. T. MacFarlane.** 1986. *Legionella Infections*, p. 56–66. Edward

Arnold, London.

2. **Castellano, M. A.** 1988. Sulbactam/ampicillin in the treatment of lower respiratory infections. *Drugs* **35**:53–56.

3. **Edelstein, P. H., and R. D. Meyer.** 1988. Legionella pneumonias, p. 381–402. *In* J. E. Pennington (ed.), *Respiratory Infections: Diagnosis and Management.* Raven Press, New York.

4. **Falco, V., T. Fernandez de Sevilla, J. Alegre, A. Ferrer, and J. M. M. Vasquez.** 1991. *Legionella pneumophila.* A cause of severe community-acquired pneumonia. *Chest* **100**:1007–1011.

5. **Fang, G. D., M. Fine, J. Orloff, et al.** 1990. New and emerging etiologies for community-acquired pneumonia with implications for therapy. *Medicine* **69**:307–316.

6. **Johnson, J. D., W. L. Hand, J. B. Francis, et al.** 1980. Antibiotic uptake by alveolar macrophages. *J. Lab. Clin. Med.* **95**:429–439.

7. **Macfarlane, J. T., R. G. Finch, M. J. Ward, et al.** 1982. Hospital study of adult community-acquired pneumonia. *Lancet* **i**:255–258.

8. **Mandell, C. L.** 1973. Interaction of intraleukocytic bacteria and antibiotics. *J. Clin. Invest.* **52**:1673–1679.

9. **McCusker, K. T., and D. Low.** 1991. *Legionella pneumophila:* denizen of defenders. *Semin. Respir. Infect.* **6**:58–65.

10. **Neu, H. C.** 1990. Other beta-lactam antibiotics, p. 257–263. *In* G. L. Mandell, R. G. Douglas, Jr., and J. E. Bennet (ed.), *Principles and Practices of Infectious Diseases.* Churchill Livingstone, Inc., New York.

11. **Pearlman, E. A. H. Jiwa, N. C. Engleberg, and B. I. Eisentein.** 1988. Growth of *Legionella pneumophila* in a human macrophagelike (U937) cell line. *Microb. Pathog.* **5**:87–95.

12. **Reingold, A. L.** 1988. Role of Legionellae in acute infections of the lower respiratory tract. *Rev. Infect. Dis.* **10**:1018–1028.

Legionellosis in Ontario, Canada: Laboratory Aspects

P. TANG AND C. KRISHNAN

Central Public Health Laboratory, Ontario Ministry of Health, Toronto, Ontario M5W 1R5, Canada

From May 1978 to April 1991, 492 sporadic cases of legionellosis were identified in our laboratory. The routine methods used were indirect fluorescent antibody, direct fluorescent antibody, culture, and since June 1985, a broad-spectrum enzyme-linked immunosorbent assay for antigenuria (2). All reagents used for these tests were produced in house. The average age of patients was 56.6 years, with 297 (60%) males and 195 (40%) females. The monthly totals of cases for July, August, and September were twice that of any other month of the year. There was a wide distribution of legionellae among 27 serogroups of 17 species (Table 1). Two species, *Legionella bozemanii* serogroup 2 and *L. feeleii* serogroup 1, were first isolated in Ontario (1, 4). *L. oakridgensis* was reported earlier in the first cases of human infection (3). *L. parisiensis, L. santicrucis,* and *L. sainthelensi* serogroup 1 are being reported here for the first time as human pathogens. There were three cases of double infections. *L. pneumophila* serogroup 1 was responsible for 45.7% of positive cases. Limited environmental surveys, mostly in hospitals, yielded *L. pneumophila* and some uncommon species such as *L. anisa* and *L. rubrilucens* (Table 2). Positive cases diagnosed by the four diagnostic tests are listed in Table 3. The numbers of cases in Table 3 were higher than the total of 492 because multiple specimen types were submitted in some instances. In 1981, *L. feeleii* serogroup 1 was responsible for 317 cases of Pontiac fever in an industrial work place in Windsor, Ontario (1). The only other outbreak occurred in a nursing home involving 12 patients. These cases are not included in the 492 cases mentioned above.

TABLE 1. Distribution of *Legionella* species in sporadic cases

Species	No. (%) of cases	
Single infections		
L. pneumophila		
1[a]	225	(45.7)
2	1	(0.2)
3	11	(2.2)
4	6	(1.2)
5	5	(1.0)
6	42	(8.5)
8	10	(2.0)
12	3	(0.6)
L. micdadei	22	(4.5)
L. dumoffii	11	(2.2)
L. gormanii	9	(1.8)
L. bozemanii		
1	15	(3.1)
2	1	(0.2)
L. longbeachae		
1	9	(1.8)
2	3	(0.6)
L. feeleii		
1	4	(2.9)
L. oakridgensis	14	(2.9)
L. jordanis	5	(1.0)
L. maceachernii	16	(3.3)
L. wadsworthii	1	(0.2)
L. hackeliae		
1	1	(0.2)
2	3	(0.6)
L. anisa	1	(0.2)
L. parisiensis	2	(0.4)
L. cincinnatiensis	3	(0.6)
L. santicrucis	3	(0.6)
L. sainthelensi		
1	1	(0.2)
Double infections		
L. pneumophila		
1 and 5	1	(0.2)
1 and 6	1	(0.2)
L. pneumophila 6 and *L. oakridgensis*	1	(0.2)

[a] Numbers indicate serogroups.

TABLE 2. Environmental isolates from 11 institutions (including 9 hospitals)

Location	Source	No. of isolates	Species
Hospital, Bermuda	Water tank	3	*L. pneumophila* 1[a]
		1	*L. bozemanii* 1
Hospital, Toronto	Hot water tank	7	*L. anisa*
		3	*L. pneumophila* 6
	Water tap	10	*L. pneumophila* 6
	Water tank	3	*L. pneumophila* 8
		4	*L. anisa*
College, Toronto	Whirlpool survey	5	*L. pneumophila* 1
		3	*L. pneumophila* 6
		2	*L. pneumophila* 8
Laboratory, Toronto	Water tap	1	*L. pneumophila* 1
Hospital, Hamilton	Hot water tank	3	*L. rubrilucens*
Hospital, London	Water tap	1	*L. pneumophila* 4
	Cooling tower	2	*L. pneumophila* 6
Hospital, Windsor	Shower heads	4	*L. pneumophila* 8
Hospital, Brantford	Water tap	4	*L. anisa*
		2	*L. pneumophila* 8

[a]Numbers indicate serogroups.

TABLE 3. Positive cases by test

Test	Total no. of specimens	No. (%) of positive cases
Indirect FA	44,414	310 (0.70)
Direct FA	12,281	86 (0.70)
Culture	12,317	127 (1.03)
ELISA	6,873	98 (1.43)

Our study, covering a period of 13 years, has shown some unique features: (i) a large variety of species and serogroups, (ii) a low occurrence of outbreaks, and (iii) poor correlation between the serogroups and species from environmental and clinical sources.

REFERENCES

1. **Herwaldt, L. A., et al.** 1984. A new *Legionella* species, *Legionella feeleii* species nova, causes Pontiac fever in an automobile plant. *Ann. Intern. Med.* **100**:333–338.
2. **Tang, P. W., and S. Toma.** 1986. Broad spectrum enzyme-linked immunosorbent assay for detection of *Legionella* soluble antigens. *J. Clin. Microbiol.* **24**:556–558.
3. **Tang, P. W., S. Toma, and L. G. MacMillan.** 1985. *Legionella oakridgensis*: laboratory diagnosis of a human infection. *J. Clin. Microbiol.* **21**:462–463.
4. **Tang, P. W., S. Toma, C. W. Moss, A. G. Steigerwalt, T. G. Cooligan, and D. J. Brenner.** 1984. *Legionella bozemanii* serogroup 2: a new etiological agent. *J. Clin. Microbiol.* **19**:30–33.

Indirect Immunofluorescent Antibody Tests with *Legionella longbeachae* Serogroup 1 Antigen in Confirmed Infections

W. E. WINSLOW AND T. W. STEELE

Institute of Medical and Veterinary Science, Box 14, Rundle Mall Post Office, Adelaide, South Australia 5000, Australia

Evaluation and standardization of indirect immunofluorescent antibody tests (IFAT) using antigens other than *Legionella pneumophila* serogroup 1 have been limited by the paucity of culture-confirmed cases of infection due to other species and the difficulties that most laboratories have in obtaining serum samples from control subjects with pneumonia of known etiology.

Using a heat-killed antigen prepared from a patient isolate of *L. longbeachae* serogroup 1 suspended in 0.5% yolk sac to a density recommended for tests with *L. pneumophila* serogroup 1 antigen (4), we evaluated the serological responses of 12 patients with culture-confirmed *L. longbeachae* serogroup 1 infection, 19 patients with culture-confirmed *L. pneumophila* infection, 1 patient with *L. bozemanii* serogroup 1 infection, and 1 patient with a subcutaneous infection due to *L. anisa*. Adequately spaced paired sera were obtained from the majority of these patients, but samples were collected in convalescence only from two patients with *L. longbeachae* infection and from the patients with *L. bozemanii* and *L. anisa* infections.

TABLE 1. Antibody response and persistence of antibody in patients with confirmed *L. longbeachae* serogroup 1 pneumonia, measured by IFAT

Case no.	Days from onset		Reciprocal titer		Reciprocal titer in sample showing persistence of antibody (mos)	Antibody class
	Sample 1	Sample 2	Sample 1	Sample 2		
1	19	30	512	2,048	256 (39)	IgA/G/M[a]
2	6	12	32	2,048	64 (8)	IgA/G/M
3	12	13	16,384	16,384	8,192 (7)	IgG/M
4	14	41	512	1,024	128 (9)	IgA/G/M
5	10	16	128	512		IgA/G/M
6	8	14	256	2,048	1,024 (13)	IgG
7	16	31	64	512	128 (15)	IgG
8	3	16	32	512	256 (12)	IgG
9	7	11	<32	2,048		IgM
10	12	19	<32	4,096		IgM
11	7	12	32	512		IgM
12	5	30	<8	<8		

[a]IgA/G/M, immunoglobulin A/immunoglobulin G/immunoglobulin M.

Paired serum samples from 40 patients with confirmed bacterial, rickettsial, and viral pneumonias acquired in the community (2) and convalescent sera from 14 patients with Q fever were also examined by IFAT. Finally, the prevalence of antibody to *L. longbeachae* in 115 employees of our institute was determined. The median age of these subjects was 39 years (range, 22 to 64 years).

Since apparent cross-reactions to other *Legionella* species have been documented previously (5) and reactions with confirmed *L. bozemanii* se-rogroup 2 (3) and *L. dumoffii* infections have been reported more recently (1), the pattern of cross-reactions to a wide range of *Legionella* antigens (see Table 2) was determined with the paired serum sets from nine patients with *L. longbeachae* infection and to a more limited range with the single serum samples from the patients with confirmed *L. bozemanii* serogroup 1 and *L. anisa* infections.

Of the 12 patients with *L. longbeachae* infection, 9 developed a fourfold or greater rise in anti-

TABLE 2. Species specificity of the immune response to *L. longbeachae* serogroup 1, measured by IFAT[a]

Species	No. of serum sets showing:	
	Seroconversion[b]	Cross-reaction[c]
L. longbeachae sgp 1	9	NA
L. longbeachae sgp 2	8	7
L. santicrucis	9	9
L. cincinnatiensis	8	8
L. sainthelensi	8	7
L. jordanis	8	6
L. bozemanii sgp 1 and 2	7	4
L. anisa	7	3
L. hackeliae sgp 1 and 2	1	1
L. oakridgensis	1	0
L. pneumophila sgp 1–14	0	
L. dumoffii	0	
L. gormanii	0	
L. micdadei	0	
L. wadsworthii	0	
L. feeleii sgp 1 and 2	0	
L. maceachernii	0	
L. birminghamensis	0	

[a]Data show reactivities of paired serum sets from nine patients with confirmed *L. longbeachae* serogroup (sgp) 1 infection.
[b]Defined as a fourfold or higher titer rise to ≥ 1:128.
[c]A seroconversion was considered to be a cross-reaction if the titers differed from those to *L. longbeachae* sgp 1 by less than fourfold. NA, not applicable.

body titer to 512 or higher, 2 had high stationary titers, and 1 failed to form detectable antibody on IFAT or by Western immunoblotting. Table 1 shows the initial and final titers of the 11 patients who exhibited reactions and the nature and persistence of the antibodies formed by seven patients who survived.

The majority of these patients formed antibody to seven other species or serogroups of *Legionella*, with titers frequently being close to those with the homologous antigen (Table 2). Fourfold rises in antibody to antigenically unrelated species were not detected with eight of these serum sets, but one patient developed a fourfold rise in antibody to *L. hackeliae* to a titer of 128.

Patients with community-acquired pneumonia due to *L. pneumophila* and to a variety of other bacterial, rickettsial, and viral agents, which included psittacosis, Q fever, *Mycoplasma pneumoniae,* tuberculosis, and the most commonly encountered bacterial and viral agents causing pneumonia, did not show a fourfold rise in antibody to *L. longbeachae* antigen on IFAT. The titers of antibody to antigens cross-reacting with *L. longbeachae* serogroup 1-positive sera in patients with confirmed *L. bozemanii* and *L. anisa* infections are shown in Table 3. Of the 115 normal subjects tested, 6 had antibody titers of ≥ 128 to *L. longbeachae* antigen, 2 of whom had titers of 256 and 512.

From these studies, it was concluded that the IFAT when applied to paired serum samples from patients with community-acquired pneumonias had a high specificity and a sensitivity of at least 75%. Patients with *L. longbeachae* infection requiring hospital treatment usually developed titers of 512 or higher. In the immune response to *L. longbeachae*, a single class of antibody did not predominate. This finding highlighted the need to use in the IFAT a fluorescence-labeled conjugate that detects all classes of antibody. High titers of antibody to *L. longbeachae* persisted for more than a year after recovery. This observation, and the finding of elevated titers in 2% of normal subjects, made interpretation of single high titers dif-

TABLE 3. Serological cross-reactions in patients with confirmed infection due to *L. bozemanii* serogroup 1 and *L. anisa*

IFAT antigen	Reciprocal IFAT titers in patients infected with:	
	L. bozemanii sgp[a] 1	*L. anisa*
L. bozemanii sgp 1	2,048	32
L. bozemanii sgp 2	1,024	32
L. anisa	1,024	128
L. longbeachae sgp 1	1,024	128
L. longbeachae sgp 2	1,024	256
L. santicrucis	1,024	128
L. cincinnatiensis	512	128
L. sainthelensi	1,024	128
L. jordanis	2,048	512

[a] sgp, serogroup.

ficult in our community. Extensive cross-reactions seen with antigenically related species during *L. longbeachae* infection were also seen with infections due to *L. bozemanii* and *L. anisa*. It is not known under what circumstances a species-specific response could occur that does not involve a response to antigenically related species.

REFERENCES

1. **Edelstein, P. H., and E. P. Pryor.** 1985. A new biotype of *Legionella dumoffii. J. Clin. Microbiol.* **21:**641–642.
2. **Lim, I., D. R. Shaw, D. P. Stanley, R. Lumb, and G. A. McLennan.** 1989. A prospective hospital study of the aetiology of community acquired pneumonia. *Med. J. Aust.* **151:**87–91.
3. **Tang, P. W., T. Sandu, C. W. Moss, A. G. Steigerwalt, T. G. Cooligan, and D. J. Brenner.** 1984. *Legionella bozemanii* serogroup 2: a new etiological agent. *J. Clin. Microbiol.* **19:**30–33.
4. **Wilkinson, H. W.** 1986. Serodiagnosis of *Legionella pneumophila* disease, p. 395–398. *In* N. R. Rose, H. Friedman, J. L. Fahey (ed.), *Manual of Clinical Laboratory Immunology,* 3rd ed. American Society for Microbiology, Washington, D.C.
5. **Wilkinson, H. W., A. L. Reingold, B. J. Brake, D. L. McGiboney, G. W. Gorman, and C. V. Broome,** 1983. Reactivity of serum from patients with suspected legionellosis against 29 antigens of *Legionellaceae* and *Legionella*-like organisms by indirect immunofluorescence assay. *J. Infect. Dis.* **147:**23–31.

A Rat Model of *Legionella pneumophila* Pneumonia for Efficacy Studies with Beta-Lactam Antibiotics

G. M. SMITH, K. H. ABBOTT, M. J. WILKINSON, AND R. SUTHERLAND

SmithKline Beecham Pharmaceuticals, Brockham Park, Betchworth, Surrey RH3 7AJ, United Kingdom

The β-lactamase inhibitor clavulanic acid displays a low order of antibacterial activity against most bacteria but has been reported to be highly active in vitro against *Legionella pneumophila*, and synergy was noted between amoxicillin plus clavulanic acid (1, 2, 7). β-Lactam antibiotics are usually considered to penetrate mammalian cells only poorly, but amoxicillin plus clavulanic acid and clavulanic acid alone were shown to display pronounced bactericidal effects against intracellular *L. pneumophila* in tissue culture studies (8). To assess the efficacy of these agents in vivo, it was thought necessary to develop a model of *L. pneumophila* pneumonia in the rat, as the conventional guinea pig model of legionellosis is not suitable for testing β-lactams because of the intolerance of this species to these agents.

In initial studies, weanling male rats were infected by nonsurgical intubation and intrabronchial instillation (3) of an inoculum containing 10^7 to 10^8 CFU of *L. pneumophila* 1624 (serogroup 1; clinical isolate). A respiratory infection developed, resulting in counts of 10^5 to 10^6 CFU in the lungs at 48 h, but the numbers of organisms decreased thereafter as the infection resolved naturally upon infiltration of polymorphonuclear leukocytes (PMNs), with very few organisms present in the lungs after 96 h. However, by administration of cyclophosphamide 3 days before and on the day of intubation, numbers of leukocytes were reduced from 6.1×10^3 to 1.8×10^3 cells per mm^3 for the initial 4 days after infection, allowing the infection to persist at between 10^5 and 10^6 CFU in the lungs for at least 96 h, with 10^3 to 10^5 CFU still detectable in the lungs at 7 days, although at this time the infection was again resolving upon the influx of PMNs. By administering a third dose of cyclophosphamide at 96 h, the influx of PMNs was delayed for a further 4 days, resulting in an infection that persisted at around 10^6 CFU in the lungs for at least 10 days (Fig. 1).

At intervals after infection, groups of animals were sacrificed, and their lungs were removed and assessed bacteriologically, histologically, and by transmission electron microscopy. Light microscopy showed that the histological characteristics of the infection were similar to those seen in the conventional guinea pig model of the disease and in humans (5). By 6 h after infection, the majority of the organisms were intracellular, and consolidation of lung tissue was evident by 48 h, with an increase in numbers of PMNs and alveolar macrophages. Transmission electron microscopy using immunogold-silver labeling confirmed that the organisms were intracellular within the alveolar macrophages and PMNs (Fig. 2). By 96 h, there was considerable consolidation and inflammation of lung tissue, with PMNs, macrophages, lymphocytes, and fibrin typifying the inflammatory response of advanced pneumonia.

The majority of therapy studies were carried out on rats receiving cyclophosphamide on day -3 and immediately prior to infection. The model was used to investigate the efficacy of amoxicillin/clavulanic acid in immunocompetent rats (4), and the immunocompromised animal model was used to study the activities of amoxicillin/clavulanic acid (6) and ticarcillin/clavulanic acid (5). Doses of antibiotics were selected to produce areas under the curves in rat plasma similar to those achieved in human serum following stan-

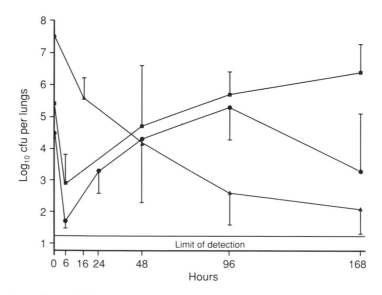

Fig. 1. Comparison of lung viable counts from an *L. pneumophila* respiratory infection in immunocompetent and immunocompromised rats. Symbols: ▲, immunocompetent rats; ●, cyclophosphamide-treated rats (days -3 and 0); ■, cyclophosphamide-treated rats (days -3, 0, and $+3$).

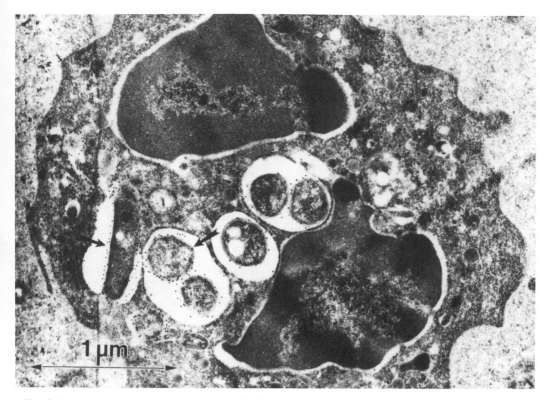

Fig. 2. Transmission electron micrograph of a PMN in rat lung at 12 h postinfection. This section was immunogold labeled and shows several *L. pneumophila* cells with cytoplasmic vesicles (arrows).

dard therapy. Subcutaneous therapy commenced 6 h after infection and continued four times daily up to 86 h (erythromycin was administered three times daily because of its longer half-life). At 96 h, 4 days after infection, groups of six rats were sacrificed, and their lung homogenates were used for viable counts. Therapy with the broad-spectrum β-lactam antibiotics amoxicillin and ticarcillin was ineffective in reducing bacterial numbers, whereas clavulanic acid, amoxicillin/clavulanic acid, and ticarcillin/clavulanic acid compared favorably with the standard agent, erythromycin, in significantly reducing numbers of *L. pneumophila* in the lungs (Fig. 3), thereby reducing inflammation and consolidation.

In addition, a number of β-lactam antibiotics, including ampicillin/sulbactam, cefoxitin, ceftazidime, and cefaclor, have been tested in tissue culture and in this infection model, but the clavulanate formulations remain unique among the β-lactams in their activity against intracellular legionellae. It is of interest that in these studies, clavulanic acid was highly active in its own right, and the activity of amoxicillin/clavulanic acid was no greater than that of clavulanic acid. However, a

significant enhancement in activity has been seen repeatedly in vivo with ticarcillin/clavulanic acid, indicating synergy between the agents (5), although the mechanism is unknown.

In summary, the immunocompromised rat model described here has been developed for research studies to determine the antibacterial activity of β-lactams against *L. pneumophila*. The model has the histological characteristics of the infection in the standard guinea pig model and in humans, although the infection is ethically designed to be nonfatal, so that the lung viable counts achieved in the rat are inevitably lower than those in the guinea pig. Clavulanic acid is unique among the β-lactams for its intracellular activity, and although there is no enhanced activity with amoxicillin/clavulanic acid, a significant improvement in activity has been repeatedly seen with ticarcillin/clavulanic acid, indicating a synergistic interaction. These results suggest that amoxicillin/clavulanic acid and ticarcillin/clavulanic acid may be worthy of clinical trial.

We thank S. A. Smith, M. J. Newman, and M. Digance for excellent technical assistance.

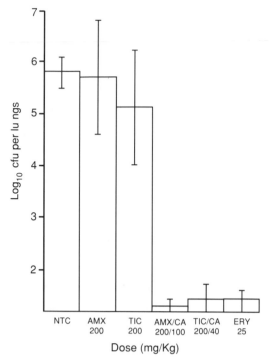

Fig. 3. *L. pneumophila* lung viable counts from immunocompromised rats 96 h after infection: therapy with β-lactam antibiotics in comparison with erythromycin. Abbreviations: NTC, nontreated control; AMX, amoxicillin; TIC, ticarcillin; AMX/CA, amoxicillin/clavulanic acid; TIC/CA, ticarcillin/clavulanic acid; ERY, erythromycin.

REFERENCES

1. **Jones, R. N., and C. Thornsberry.** 1984. Beta-lactamase studies of eight *Legionella* species: antibacterial activity of Augmentin compared to newer cephalosporins, erythromycin and rifampin. *Postgrad. Med.* Sept.–Oct.: 259–262.
2. **Pohlod, D. J., L. D. Saravolatz, E. L. Quinn, and M. M. Somerville.** 1980. Effect of clavulanic acid on minimal inhibitory concentrations of 16 antimicrobial agents tested against *Legionella pneumophila. Antimicrob. Agents Chemother.* **18:**353–354.
3. **Smith, G. M.** 1991. A simple non-surgical method of intrabronchial instillation for the establishment of respiratory infections in the rat. *Lab. Anim.* **25:**46–49.
4. **Smith, G. M., K. H. Abbott, M. J. Wilkinson, A. S. Beale, and R. Sutherland.** 1991. Bactericidal effects of amoxycillin/clavulanic acid against a *Legionella pneumophila* pneumonia in the weanling rat. *J. Antimicrob. Chemother.* **27:**127–136.
5. **Smith, G. M., K. H. Abbott, M. J. Wilkinson, A. S. Beale, and R. Sutherland.** 1991. Bactericidal effects of ticarcillin/clavulanic acid against *Legionella pneumophila* pneumonia in immunocompromised weanling rats. *Antimicrob. Agents Chemother.* **35:**1423–1429.
6. **Smith, G. M., K. H. Abbott, and R. Sutherland.** 1992. Bactericidal effects of co-amoxiclav (amoxicillin/clavulanic acid) against a *Legionella pneumophila* pneumonia in the immunocompromised weanling rat. *J. Antimicrob. Chemother.* **30:**525–534.
7. **Stokes, D. H., B. Slocombe, and R. Sutherland.** 1989. Bactericidal effects of amoxycillin/clavulanic acid against *Legionella pneumophila. J. Antimicrob. Chemother.* **23:**43–51.
8. **Stokes, D. H., M. J. Wilkinson, J. Tyler, B. Slocombe, and R. Sutherland.** 1989. Bactericidal effects of amoxycillin/clavulanic acid against intracellular *Legionella pneumophila* in tissue culture studies. *J. Antimicrob. Chemother.* **23:**547–556.

Application of a Genus-Specific Monoclonal Antibody for the Detection of Legionellae in Clinical Specimens and the Identification from Culture Plates

I. STEINMETZ, C. RHEINHEIMER, and M. FROSCH

Institute for Medical Microbiology, Hannover Medical School, 3000 Hannover 61, Germany

Direct detection of legionellae in clinical specimens by a genus-specific sandwich enzyme-linked immunosorbent assay (ELISA). Many different species and serogroups of *Legionella* which cause disease in humans have been described. In the past, it has not been uncommon for newly named species from environmental sources to later be associated with human illness. It is reasonable to assume that the number of different serogroups and new legionellae of importance in human infections is likely to expand and increase the complexity of the diagnostic procedure.

The identification of legionellae directly in clinical specimens offers the most rapid procedure for the diagnosis of legionellosis. Screening methods beyond the genus level are not available for all species and serogroups and would be clearly impracticable. It is therefore desirable to start a widespread screening for legionellae in clinical specimens on the genus level.

We recently developed a sandwich ELISA which exclusively detects all members of the genus *Legionella* on the basis of recognition by monoclonal antibody (MAb) 2125 of a genus-specific epitope on the 60-kDa heat shock protein (HSP) (2). Since the target molecule is located predominantly in the cytoplasmic, membrane-free fraction of *Legionella* cells, release of the 60-kDa HSP is essential for sensitive detection of this antigen. Detection of the 60-kDa HSP in a sandwich ELISA in which the same MAb is used as both a capture and a developing antibody is most likely due to the existence of this protein in its native form as a homomultimer consisting of 10 to 11 60-kDa subunits. In this way, enough identical epitopes are accessible. The high specificity and sensitivity of this test made us examine the potential use of the ELISA for direct detection of legionellae in respiratory tract specimens. In a pilot series, bronchial washings and tracheal secretions of four patients with culture-confirmed legionellosis (caused by *Legionella pneumophila*) were examined in the sandwich ELISA (Fig. 1). All samples were found to be clearly positive, whereas an equal number of specimens exhibiting no growth of legionellae were negative (Fig. 1). This test might have the potential to be used in a screening of clinical specimens for legionellae on the genus level without cultivation. Obviously, much higher numbers of specimens are needed for critical evaluation of this test. Its sensitivity and specificity must be compared with those of other methods (i.e., immunofluorescence and nucleic acid probes).

Identification of legionellae from culture plates by a genus-specific colony blot assay. Direct examination of clinical specimens should always be accompanied by cultivation. The

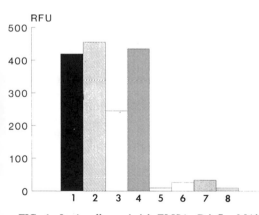

FIG. 1. *Legionella* sandwich ELISA. Briefly, MAb 2125 was used as both a capture antibody and a biotinylated second antibody for detection. The assay was developed with streptavidin–β-galactosidase and 4-methylumbelliferyl-β-D-galactopyranoside as the substrate. The fluorescent product was measured as relative fluorescence units (RFU). Bronchial washings and tracheal secretions were sonicated to release the cytoplasmic 60-kDa HSP of *Legionella* cells. After centrifugation, the supernatant was diluted in bovine serum albumin and tested in the ELISA. Lanes: 1, bronchial washing, patient 1; 2, bronchial washing, patient 2; 3, tracheal secretions, patient 3; 4, bronchial washing, patient 4; 5 through 8, control washings, patients 5 through 8.

different selective media currently used for the cultivation of legionellae are not sufficiently selective and allow many non-*Legionella* organisms to grow. Procedures such as pretreatment of specimens by heat or acid cannot abolish contaminating bacterial flora completely. The different *Legionella* species show a heterogeneous morphology and are not always clearly distinguishable from non-*Legionella* organisms by morphological criteria. The identification of legionellae grown on buffered charcoal-yeast extract agar is long and complex and involves procedures such as confirmation of *Legionella*-specific growth requirements, biochemical characterization, fatty acid analysis, and immunofluorescence methods. Since primary cultures of legionellae from clinical or environmental specimens are often difficult to obtain and may take several days, time-saving methods must be developed to identify legionellae on the genus level as soon as colonies are visible on the agar medium so as to avoid further delay. This rapidity of identification is of special importance for clinical cases in which direct examination of the specimen was negative. We therefore developed a rapid colony blot assay, based on the genus-specific MAb 2125 mentioned above, which makes it possible to screen hundreds of colonies in one test and to identify legionellae in less than 2 h (1).

Briefly, nitrocellulose filters were laid on the surface of an agar plate and allowed to adhere. The filters were then removed, and the adherent bacteria were lysed by a combined treatment with detergent (Triton X-100) and hot steam. Colonies were made visible by the use of biotinylated MAb 2125 and peroxidase-conjugated streptavidin. The filters were developed with 4-chloro-1-naphthol as the substrate.

All different *Legionella* species and serogroups obtained from culture collections that were tested could be visualized as distinct dark blue dots. Bacterial colonies from non-*Legionella* strains showed no reaction. The positive results obtained with primary cultures of legionellae from bronchial washings and tap water demonstrate the usability of this test as a screening method in principle. We think that this immunological confirmation of legionellae growing on agar medium is a highly specific and rapid alternative to the complex and time-consuming identification of legionellae, especially those of species other than *L. pneumophila*.

REFERENCES

1. **Steinmetz, I., C. Rheinheimer, and D. Bitter-Suermann.** 1992. Rapid identification of legionellae by a colony blot assay based on a genus-specific monoclonal antibody. *J. Clin. Microbiol.* **30:**1016–1018.
2. **Steinmetz, I., C. Rheinheimer, I. Hübner, and D. Bitter-Suermann.** 1991. Genus-specific epitope on the 60-kilodalton *Legionella* heat shock protein recognized by a monoclonal antibody. *J. Clin. Microbiol.* **29:**346–354.

Prevalence of Antibodies against *Legionella* Species in Healthy and Patient Populations

C. PASZKO-KOLVA, M. SHAHAMAT, J. KEISER, AND R. R. COLWELL

Advanced Technology Laboratories, Alta Loma, California 91701;
Department of Microbiology, University of Maryland, College Park, Maryland 20742; and
George Washington University Medical Center, Washington, D.C. 20037

Sixteen years after the largest U.S. outbreak of Legionnaires disease in Philadelphia, Pa., in which 34 individuals died, and after the causative agent was isolated and identified, diagnosis of the disease remains difficult. Serological tests such as the immunofluorescence assay, microagglutination test, and enzyme-linked immunosorbent assay (ELISA) may provide only presumptive evidence (6). However, when used in conjunction with other tests, they can provide valuable information. Serological tests used in epidemiological investigations can provide useful retrospective data on the natural prevalence, occurrence, and frequency of disease (1, 2, 4, 12).

Following reports of sporadic cases of putative legionellosis on the University of Maryland campus, a *Legionella* monitoring program was implemented. Direct fluorescent antibody staining of campus environmental samples (air conditioning units, cooling towers, air handling units, steam tunnels, etc.) revealed the presence of *Legionella pneumophila* serogroups 1 through 6 at concentrations of 10^2 to 10^7 cells per ml. However, on buffered charcoal yeast extract (BCYE) agar only *L. pneumophila* serogroups 1, 3, 5, and 6, *Legionella dumoffii*, and *Legionella jordanis* could be cultured. These strains were included in a seroepidemiological survey, together with seven American Type Culture Collection (ATCC) reference strains. The objective of the study presented here was to serve as a retrospective indicator providing evidence suggestive of exposure to *Legionella* spp. and not to detect antibodies for diagnostic purposes.

A total of 378 human serum samples were obtained from the healthy campus population (University of Maryland, College Park) and from patients at a local hospital (George Washington University Hospital) who had suspected respiratory tract infections. We obtained 143 serum samples from apparently healthy campus volunteers (70 male and 73 females) and 235 serum samples from patients (151 males and 84 females).

All antibody titer assays of healthy and patient (both in- and outpatient) sera were done by using an indirect, noncompetitive ELISA. *Legionella* cultures from the ATCC were grown to stationary phase, i.e., 72-h cultures of *L. pneumophila* serogroups 1 to 6 (strains Philadelphia-1, Knoxville-1, Togus-1, Bloomington-2, Los Angeles-1, Dallas-1E, and Chicago-2, respectively). *Le-*

gionella strains representing serogroups 1, 2, 4, and 6 from the ATCC originated from human lung biopsies, while serogroups 3 and 5 were isolated from creek and cooling tower waters, respectively. Additional isolates included in the study were environmental (campus) isolates of *L. pneumophila* serogroups 1, 3, 5, and 6, *L. jordanis*, and *L. dumoffii*. All campus isolates were identified by using biochemical, serological, and nucleic acid techniques as previously described (5). The ELISA was performed by using sterile polystyrene, modified flat-bottom microtiter plates according to the method of Voller et al. (10).

To investigate whether cross-reactions occurred, as reported for direct fluorescent antibody staining (8), the *Legionella*-positive control sera and selected strains used as antigens were used in the ELISA. These strains included *Pseudomonas aeruginosa* ATCC 9721, *Pseudomonas fluorescens* ATCC 13525, *Pseudomonas putida* ATCC 12633, *Xanthomonas maltophilia* ATCC 13637, *Pseudomonas alcaligenes* ATCC 14909, *Flavobacterium* sp. strain ATCC 21044, *Bacillus subtilis* ATCC 6051, *Bacillus licheniformis* ATCC 14580, *P. putida* UMCP 137; *Pseudomonas* sp. strain UMCP 73, and *Pseudomonas* sp. strain UMCP 119. Cross-reactions between control sera and the antigens specified above were uniformly negative.

L. pneumophila is currently believed to be responsible for the majority of *Legionella* infections in the United States, followed by *Legionella micdadei*. A criterion useful for confirming epidemic and sporadic cases of Legionnaires disease, or Pontiac fever, is a fourfold rise in titer to ≥128 for patients with pneumonia. In addition, a single or standing indirect fluorescent antibody titer of ≥256 is often used as presumptive evidence when paired sera are unavailable (11). In this study, corrected sample absorbance values (9) of ≥0.200 at a titer of 128, 256, 512, or 1,024 were analyzed; a corrected absorbance value of >0.200 at a dilution of 256 was considered positive.

Sera from a total of 378 healthy donors and patients were collected and tested against 13 different strains of *Legionella*. Of the three *L. pneumophila* serogroup 1 strains tested, the healthy sera showed a slightly higher percentage of positive reactions (at a titer of ≥256) to the campus isolate UMCP 082 (30.8%) compared with the ATCC strains ATCC 33152 (16.8%) and ATCC

TABLE 1. Positive reactions to *Legionella* antigens obtained by ELISA

Species	Strain	Source[a]	Serogroup	Healthy subjects Total no. of positive samples	Healthy subjects Total no. of samples	Healthy subjects % Positive	Patients Total no. of positive samples	Patients Total no. of samples	Patients % Positive
L. pneumophila	ATCC 33152	H	1	24	143	16.8	64	235	27.2
	ATCC 33153	H	1	39	143	27.3	77	235	32.8
	ATCC 33154	H	2	19	143	13.3	59	235	25.1
	ATCC 33155	E	3	30	143	21.0	81	235	34.5
	ATCC 33156	H	4	60	143	42.0	46	235	19.6
	ATCC 33216	E	5	36	143	25.2	69	235	29.4
	ATCC 33215	H	6	62	143	43.4	59	235	25.1
L. jordanis	UMCP 027	E	1	4	143	2.8	33	235	14.0
L. dumoffii	UMCP 303	E	1	5	143	3.5	36	235	15.3
L. pneumophila	UMCP 082	E	1	44	143	30.8	25	220	11.4
	UMCP 341	E	3	19	143	13.3	13	220	5.91
	UMCP 015	E	5	36	143	25.2	28	220	12.7
	UMCP 351	E	6	48	133	36.1	26	220	11.8

[a]H, human; E, environmental.

33153 (27.3%). Interestingly, this pattern was reversed in the patient group. When reciprocal ELISA antibody titers for the patient group were examined against three *L. pneumophila* serogroup 1 strains, the highest percentages of positive reactions were against the *L. pneumophila* serogroup 1 strains ATCC 33153 Knoxville (38%), ATCC 33152 Philadelphia (27.2%), and UMCP 082 (11.4%) (Table 1). Examination of reciprocal ELISA antibody titers, expressed as percent positive, indicated a range of 2.8 to 43.4% positive for the healthy group and 5.9 to 34.5% for the patient group for the 13 strains tested. Unlike the patient sera, the healthy group sera showed a higher percentage of positive titers to the environmental strains of *L. pneumophila* serogroups 1, 3, 5, and 6 (30.8, 13.3, 25.2, and 31.6%, respectively). Exceptions were *L. jordanis* and *L. dumoffii,* both of which are environmental isolates. They ranked slightly higher in the patient group than in the healthy group, suggesting that these strains may be endogenous to other environments to which the patients had previously been exposed or to the hospital environment of the patients or may be related to the patients' illness. It must be remembered that with increasing age, antibody titer can deteriorate or require a longer time to appear. Also, low titers observed for the patient population against *L. pneumophila* strains may be the result of an immunocompromised state (3, 7). In addition, timing of the seroconversion following exposure or infection, subclinical infection, duration of immunity, and complete lack of seroconversion in culture-positive patients are all factors that must be considered in reviewing serological data.

While the ELISA must be evaluated systematically for specificity, it appears that a significant number of apparently healthy individuals can carry antibodies to legionellae, especially *L. pneumophila* strains isolated on the campus in this study. This is not a surprising finding, given the ubiquity of the organism and a much greater exposure opportunity for the healthy group. What is interesting is that of the two groups, the patient group demonstrated the lowest frequency of positive reactions to the *L. pneumophila* environmental isolates. The ELISA appears to detect strain differences. That a significantly greater proportion of an apparently healthy population harbors antibodies to legionellae than was previously suspected offers a new perspective on the incidence and exposure of *Legionella* spp. in public health considerations.

REFERENCES

1. **Goldman, W. D., and J. S. Marr.** 1980. Are air-conditioning maintenance personnel at increased risk of legionellosis? *Appl. Environ. Microbiol.* **40:**114–116.
2. **Helms, C. M., E. D. Renner, J. P. Viner, W. J. Hierholzer, L. A. Wintermeyer, and W. Johnson.** 1980. Indirect immunofluorescence antibodies to *Legionella pneumophila:* frequency in a rural community. *J. Clin. Microbiol.* **12:**326–328.
3. **James, K.** 1990. Immunoserology of infectious disease. *Clin. Microbiol. Rev.* **3:**132–152.
4. **Muller, H. E.** 1983. Antibodies against Legionellaceae in the population of West Germany and their methodical determination. *Zentralbl Bakteriol. Hyg. A* **255:**84–90.
5. **Shahamat, M., C. Paszko-Kolva, J. Keiser, and R. R. Colwell.** 1991. Sequential culturing method improves recovery of *Legionella* spp. from contaminated environmental samples. *Zentralbl. Bakteriol.* **275:**312–319.
6. **Stanek, G., A. Hirschl, E. Lessy, F. Wewalka, G. Ruckdeschel, and G. Wewalka.** 1983. Indirect immunofluorescence assay (IFA), microagglutination test (MA) and enzyme-linked-immunoabsorbent assay (ELISA) in diagnosis of legionellosis. *Zentralbl. Bakteriol. Hyg. A* **255:**108–114.
7. **Taylor, A. G., and T. G. Harrison.** 1979. Timing of the antibody response in Legionnaires' disease. *Lancet* **ii:**699.
8. **Tenover, F. C., P. H. Edelstein, L. C. Goldstein, J. C. Sturge, and J. J. Plorde.** 1986. Comparison of cross-staining reactions by *Pseudomonas* spp. and fluorescein-

labeled polyclonal and monoclonal antibodies directed against *Legionella pneumophila. J. Clin. Microbiol.* **23:**647–649.

9. **Thompson, T. A, and H. W. Wilkinson.** 1982. Evaluation of a solid-phase immunofluorescence assay for detection of antibodies to *Legionella pneumophila. J. Clin. Microbiol.* **16:**202–204.

10. **Voller, A., D. E. Bidwell, and A. Bartlett.** 1979. The enzyme-linked immunosorbent assay, p. 359–371. *In* N. R. Rose and H. Friedman (ed.), *Manual of Clinical Immunology,* 2nd ed. American Society for Microbiology,

Washington, D.C.

11. **Wilkinson, H. W.** 1986. Serodiagnosis of *Legionella pneumophila* disease, p. 395–398. *In* N. R. Rose and H. Friedman (ed.), *Manual of Clinical Immunology,* 2nd ed. American Society for Microbiology, Washington, D.C.

12. **Wilkinson, H. W., A. L. Reingold, B. J. Brake, D. L. McGiboney, G. W. Gorman, and C. V. Broome.** 1983. Reactivity of serum from patients with suspected legionellosis against 29 antigens of *Legionellaceae* and *Legionella*-like organisms by indirect immunofluorescent assay. *J. Infect. Dis.* **147:**23–31.

Antibody Response to Major Cross-Reactive *Legionella* Antigens during Infection

J. M. BANGSBORG, G. SHAND, AND N. HØIBY

Department of Clinical Microbiology 8223, Rigshospitalet, and Institute of Medical Microbiology, University of Copenhagen, DK-2100 Copenhagen, and Microbiology Department, Dakopatts A/S, DK-2600 Glostrup, Denmark

Despite the development of improved culture methods and direct detection of *Legionella* species involved in human infection, serology remains an important adjunct in diagnosing Legionnaires disease. The generally accepted procedure for antibody detection is the indirect fluorescent antibody test developed and recommended by the Centers for Disease Control (12), but various other methods, such as the microagglutination test (10) or, more rarely, indirect enzyme-linked immunosorbent assays (ELISAs) (6), have been applied. Common to the serological methods in use is the employment of rather crude and undefined antigen preparations and the necessity of establishing a test for each *Legionella* species and serogroup. Taken together with the occurrence of confusing cross-reactions (i.e., with bacteria outside the family *Legionellaceae*) in patient sera (5), the need for defining antigens specific to the *Legionella* genus and at the same time cross-reactive on the serogroup or species level seems obvious.

We have previously investigated cross-reactivity among *Legionella* species and serogroups by means of crossed immunoelectrophoresis (4). As an extension of this work, we applied Western immunoblotting as a simple and sensitive method to investigate the relevance of cross-reactive antigens for a diagnostic test by reacting different *Legionella* antigens with sera from patients with Legionnaires disease in parallel with specific rabbit antisera. Sonic extract antigens (approximately 400 µg per gel) of *Legionella pneumophila* serogroups (SG) 1 and 6 (Lp1 and Lp6 antigens) and *L. micdadei* (Lm antigen) (4) were run in sodium dodecyl sulfate-polyacrylamide gel electrophoresis and transferred to nitrocellulose paper (Schleicher & Schuell, Kassel, Germany) by standard procedures (1). Furthermore, the flagellin subunit from *L. pneumophila* SG 1 (7) and a

whole cell preparation of a recombinant *Escherichia coli* clone expressing the *L. micdadei* macrophage infectivity potentiator (Mip) protein (2) were similarly investigated. Molecular weights were estimated by using a biotinylated marker (Bio-Rad Laboratories, Richmond, Calif.) stained separately with an avidin-horseradish peroxidase conjugate. Nitrocellulose filters carrying the individual antigens were cut into strips and reacted with patient serum or one of the specific rabbit antibodies described below. Patient sera consisted of 13 samples (6 acute, i.e., drawn from 1 to 2 weeks after onset of illness, and 7 convalescent, i.e., drawn after 2 weeks of illness) from seven patients with culture-verified Legionnaires disease caused by *L. pneumophila* SG 1. Furthermore, 18 paired sera from patients with pneumonia and a fourfold rise in titer to *L. micdadei* measured by the indirect fluorescent antibody test were examined. As controls, 16 sera from healthy blood donors were also investigated. Specific antisera were from rabbits immunized with (i) a pooled antigen preparation of sonic extracts from *L. pneumophila* SG 1 to 6 (anti-Lp1-6), (ii) flagellin isolated from *L. pneumophila* SG 1 (antiflagellin), (iii) the *Legionella* 58-kDa (60-kDa) heat shock protein (anti-common antigen) (1), and (iv) the *L. pneumophila* Mip protein (anti-Mip) (3), kindly provided by Nicholas Cianciotto, Northwestern University School of Medicine, Chicago, Ill. Second antibodies were rabbit anti-human immunoglobulin A (IgA)-IgG-IgM, kappa and lambda (P212), and swine anti-rabbit immunoglobulins (P217), both from Dakopatts A/S, Glostrup, Denmark. Blocking, immunostaining, and washing steps were performed as described previously (1). Since no specific precautions were taken to optimize binding of polysaccharides to the nitrocellulose, the antigens visualized by the patient

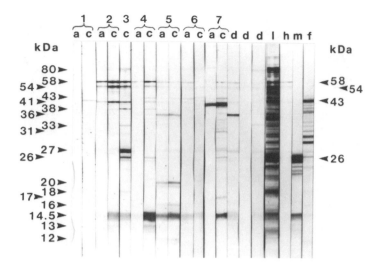

FIG. 1. Lp6 sonic extract antigen reacted with sera from seven patients (designated 1 to 7) with culture-confirmed *L. pneumophila* SG 1 infection in a Western blot. The nitrocellulose strips were incubated with six acute sera (lanes a), seven convalescent sera (lanes c), and three sera from healthy blood donors (lanes d). The remaining strips were incubated with the anti-Lp1-6 (l), anti-common antigen (h), anti-Mip (m), and antiflagellin (f) antibodies. The antigens defined by the monospecific antibodies were the 58-kDa common antigen with a 54-kDa component (lane 1), the 26-kDa Mip protein (lane m), and the flagellin subunit of 43 kDa (lane f). Reactivities of patient sera to the Lp1 and Lp6 antigens were very similar except for a weaker reactivity with the *L. pneumophila* SG 1 than with the *L. pneumophila* SG 6 flagellin.

sera would be expected to be mainly proteins. An indirect ELISA using purified flagellin from *L. pneumophila* SG 1 was performed according to a standard procedure (8).

Both acute and convalescent sera from the seven patients with culture-verified *L. pneumophila* SG 1 pneumonia were reactive with several Lp1 antigens (not shown). None of the antigenic bands were recognized by all patient sera, but in 10 sera (4 acute and 6 convalescent), reactivity with the 58-kDa heat shock protein (9, 11) and a previously described 54-kDa component (1) was found. Sera from healthy blood donors, however, also contained antibodies to this antigen. Apparently specific reactivity was observed with 43-, 41-, 38-, 26-, and 25-kDa antigens, the 26-kDa antigen being identical to the Mip protein, in a few patient sera (two to five). When Lp6 was used as the test antigen, the pattern of reactivity seen was very similar to that obtained with the Lp1 antigen (Fig. 1). In addition to nonspecific reactivity with the 58-kDa common antigen plus the 54-kDa component (nine sera), several patients reacted with the 43-kDa flagellin subunit (two acute and five convalescent sera). This reactivity could be reproduced by using the *L. pneumophila* flagellum as the test antigen. Reactivity with the Mip protein appeared in three sera, all convalescent; the same three sera reacted with the cloned *L. micdadei* Mip antigen (not shown). As for the Lp1 antigen, nonspecific reac-

tivity in patient sera with 80-, 36-, 27-, and 14.5-kDa proteins was observed with the Lp6 antigen.

Immunoblotting of the Lm antigen with serum from the *L. pneumophila* SG 1-infected patients resulted in specific reactivity (five sera) with the flagellin, which in the Lm antigen had a slightly higher molecular mass than did the corresponding Lp6 protein (46 versus 43 kDa), and with the *L. micdadei* Mip protein (five sera, one acute and four convalescent) of 30 kDa. Again, most patients reacted with the 58-kDa common antigen (Fig. 2).

Since these results showed that *L. pneumophila* SG 1-infected patients contained antibodies that reacted with corresponding antigens in *L. pneumophila* SG 6 and *L. micdadei*, it would be reasonable to assume that the opposite phenomenon would also occur, i.e., that sera from patients infected with *L. micdadei* would be reactive with the Lp1 and Lp6 antigens. Since no culture-verified *L. micdadei* infections have been reported in Denmark, this question could be investigated only with serologically confirmed cases. The 18 sera from patients with a fourfold titer rise to *L. micdadei* were used for immunoblotting the Lm, Lp1, and Lp6 antigens (not shown). In general, much weaker reactivity was seen in comparison with the reactions observed in sera from cases of culture-verified *L. pneumophila* infection. Most sera (16 of 18), however, reacted with the 58-kDa protein in all three antigen preparations; reactions with

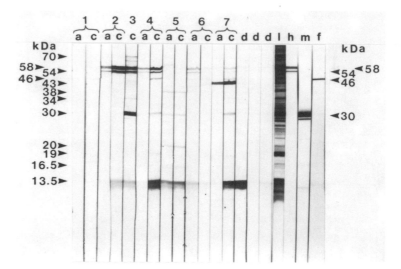

FIG. 2. Immunoblotting of Lm sonic extract antigen with the sera used for Fig. 1. The sera from patients with culture-confirmed *L. pneumophila* SG 1 infection reacted with several Lm antigens, of which the 58-kDa Common antigen (with the 54-kDa component), the Mip protein of 30 kDa, and an antigen of 13.5 kDa were the most prominent. In 5 of the 13 sera, specific reactivity with the 46-kDa *L. micdadei* flagellin was found.

flagellin and the Mip protein were weak and few. Although the antibodies detected in IFA are directed mainly against heat-stable bacterial antigens, including lipopolysaccharide, the reactivity with the present protein or protein-containing antigens in Western blots seemed surprisingly low, granted a true *L. micdadei* infection.

To test whether an antigen preparation based on a single cross-reactive protein would be suitable for a diagnostic test, we developed an indirect ELISA, using purified flagellin as the coating antigen. On the basis of 98% specific cutoff values determined by testing 90 sera from healthy indi-

TABLE 1. Reactivities of sera from culture-verified *L. pneumophila* cases of Legionnaires disease in an indirect flagellin ELISA (98% specific cutoff level)

Patient no.	Serum sample	Reactivity[a]		
		IgG assay	IgA assay	IgM assay
1	Acute	Neg	Neg	Neg
	Convalescent	Pos	Neg	Pos
2	Acute	Neg	Neg	Neg
	Convalescent	Neg	Neg	Pos
3	Convalescent	Neg	Pos	Pos
4	Acute	Neg	Pos	Neg
	Convalescent	Neg	Pos	Neg
5	Acute	Neg	Neg	Neg
	Convalescent	Pos	Neg	Neg
6	Acute	Pos	Neg	Pos
	Convalescent	Pos	Neg	Neg
7	Acute	Neg	Neg	Neg
	Convalescent	Pos	Pos	Pos

[a]Neg, negative; Pos, positive.

viduals, the 13 sera from patients with culture-verified *L. pneumophila* infection were investigated for the presence of IgG, IgA, and IgM antibodies (Table 1). Four out of the seven convalescent sera had a significantly elevated optical density at 492 nm in the IgG assay; for the IgA and IgM tests, three and five samples, respectively, were positive. When results from the three assays were combined, however, all seven convalescent sera and two acute sera were positive.

In summary, with the limited number of sera investigated, both nonspecific and specific reactivities to several cross-reactive antigens were observed. Antibodies to the 58-kDa common antigen (plus the 54-kDa component) were present in both acute and convalescent sera; although the immunogenicity of this antigen has prompted a search for genus-specific epitopes (11), its value for a specific serological test is still unclear. Reactivity with specific cross-reactive antigens such as flagellin and the Mip protein appeared in few sera; however, results from an indirect ELISA with flagellin as the coating antigen suggest that measuring a combination of IgG, IgA, and IgM antibodies to a single antigen could be a useful approach. More sera, preferably also from culture-verified cases of non-*L. pneumophila* SG 1 infections, should be subjected to further evaluation.

REFERENCES

1. Bangsborg, J. M., M. T. Collins, N. Høiby, and P. Hindersson. 1989. The cloning and expression of *Legionella micdadei* common antigen in *E. coli. APMIS* **97**:14–22.
2. Cianciotto, N. P., J. M. Bangsborg, B. I. Eisenstein,

and N. C. Engleberg. 1990. Identification of *mip*-like genes in the genus *Legionella. Infect. Immun.* **58:**2912-2918.

3. **Cianciotto, N. P., B. I. Eisenstein, C. H. Mody, G. B. Toews, and N. C. Engleberg.** 1989. A *Legionella pneumophila* gene encoding a species-specific surface protein potentiates initiation of intracellular infection. *Infect. Immun.* **57:**1255-1262.

4. **Collins, M. T., J. M. Bangsborg, and N. Høiby.** 1987. Antigenic heterogeneity among *Legionella, Fluoribacter,* and *Tatlockia* species analyzed by crossed immunoelectrophoresis. *Int. J. Syst. Bacteriol.* **37:**351-356.

5. **Collins, M. T., J. McDonald, N. Høiby, and O. Aalund.** 1984. Agglutinating antibody titers to members of the family *Legionellaceae* in cystic fibrosis patients as a result of cross-reacting antibodies to *Pseudomonas aeruginosa. J. Clin. Microbiol.* **19:**757-752.

6. **Elder, E. M., A. Brown, J. S. Remington, J. Shonnard, and Y. Naot.** 1983. Microenzyme-linked immunosorbent assay for detection of immunoglobulin G and immunoglobulin M antibodies to *Legionella pneumophila. J. Clin. Microbiol.* **17:**112-121.

7. **Elliott, J. A., and W. Johnson.** 1981. Immunochemical and biochemical relationships among flagella isolated from *Legionella pneumophila* serogroups 1, 2, and 3. *Infect.*

Immun. **33:**602-610.

8. **Hansen, K., P. Hindersson, and N. S. Pedersen.** 1988. Measurement of antibodies to the *Borrelia burgdorferi* flagellum improves serodiagnosis in Lyme disease. *J. Clin. Microbiol.* **26:**338-346.

9. **Hoffman, P. S., L. Houston, and C. A. Butler.** 1990. *Legionella htpAB* heat shock operon: nucleotide sequence and expression of the 60-kilodalton antigen in *L. pneumophila*-infected HeLa cells. *Infect. Immun.* **58:** 3380-3387.

10. **Lind, K., M. T. Collins, and O. Aalund.** 1984. Comparison of a micro-agglutination test and the indirect immunofluorescence test for *Legionella* antibodies in patients. *Acta Pathol Microbiol. Immunol. Scand. Sect. B* **92:** 195-199.

11. **Plikaytis, B. B., G. M. Carlone, C.-P. Pau, and H. Wilkinson.** 1987. Purified 60-kilodalton *Legionella* protein antigen with *Legionella*-specific and nonspecific epitopes. *J. Clin. Microbiol.* **25:**2080-2084.

12. **Wilkinson, H. W., A. L. Reingold, B. J. Brake, D. L. McGiboney, G. W. Gorman, and C. V. Broome.** 1983. Reactivity of serum from patients with suspected legionellosis against 29 antigens of *Legionellaceae* and *Legionella*-like organisms by indirect immunofluorescence assay. *J. Infect. Dis.* **147:**23-31.

B. Epidemiologic Aspects of Legionellosis

STATE OF THE ART LECTURE

Modes of Transmission in Epidemic and Nonepidemic *Legionella* Infection: Directions for Further Study

ROBERT F. BREIMAN

Respiratory Diseases Branch, Division of Bacterial and Mycotic Diseases, National Center for Infectious Diseases, Centers for Disease Control, Atlanta, Georgia 30333

At the international symposium on *Legionella* in Atlanta in 1983, David Fraser discussed a conceptual scheme for focusing on sources and modes of transmission of legionellosis (22). He described a six-link "chain of causation" that must exist to result in human infection. The first link in the chain is an environmental reservoir where legionellae live (Fig. 1); second is one or more amplifying factors that allow legionellae to multiply to high concentrations; third is a mechanism for dissemination of legionellae from the reservoir to a susceptible population; fourth, the strain of disseminated legionellae must be virulent for humans; fifth, the organism must be inoculated at a site on the human host where it is capable of causing infection; and finally, the person exposed must be susceptible to infection.

This chain of causation is helpful for discussing the epidemiology of Legionnaires disease. Interfering with any link in the chain will presumably decrease the occurrence of disease, which from a public health standpoint is our overall goal. While examining what is known about the epidemiology of legionellosis, I will emphasize information available and research needed for the development of efficient and effective strategies for prevention and control of legionellosis.

ENVIRONMENTAL RESERVOIR

Water is the major reservoir for legionellae, and legionellae are frequent inhabitants of most water sources (20, 35). However, *Legionella* organisms may be found occasionally in other sources such as potting soil, as shown during a recent investigation of an outbreak of *Legionella longbeachae* infection in Australia (41). The importance of this finding as a cause of sporadically occurring legionellosis has not been fully explored.

AMPLIFICATION FACTORS

In natural water sources, legionellae are generally present in very low concentrations. However, under certain conditions, usually within manufactured aquatic environments, the concentration of the bacteria may increase markedly (25, 46).

Amoebae appear to have a critical role in the amplification process (19, 40). Biofilms, ubiquitous within plumbing systems, also appear to contribute to the process of supporting the growth of the bacteria (39). Better understanding of this amplification process may lead to methods to limit the multiplication of the bacteria in water and, thus, to interrupt the chain of events leading to transmission.

DISSEMINATION OF THE BACTERIA TO HUMANS

The primary mode of transmission of legionellosis is inhalation of *Legionella* organisms in aerosolized droplets of respirable size (1 to 5

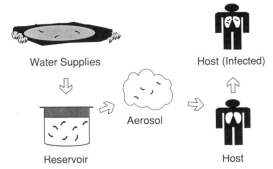

Water Supplies   Host (Infected)

Aerosol

Reservoir   Host

FIG. 1. Chain of causation of legionellosis.

TABLE 1. Known sources for transmission of legionellae via aerosols

Type of water	Transmitting device	Reference(s)
Potable	Showers	6, 9, 25a, 44
	Tap water faucets	11
	Respiratory care equipment	2, 34
Nonpotable	Cooling towers and evaporative condensers	1, 13, 14, 22a, 23, 36a
	Whirlpool baths	24, 31, 40b
	Decorative fountains	18, 40a
	Ultrasonic mist machines	30

μm) (21). Transmission occurs occasionally via other routes, including direct inoculation of surgical wounds with contaminated potable water during placement of surgical dressings and aspiration of contaminated water by persons recovering from head and neck surgery (29). There continues to be no evidence for person-to-person transmission. Known sources for transmission of legionellae via aerosols have been identified during epidemic investigations and are summarized in Table 1.

Numerous epidemic investigations have convincingly demonstrated that cooling towers and evaporative condensers have served as sources of Legionella infection (8, 13, 14, 23). Both are heat rejection devices with reservoirs filled with fairly warm recirculating water. The conditions within cooling tower reservoirs are ideal for the growth of legionellae, and a substantial proportion of reservoirs are contaminated with the bacteria (28). These devices produce aerosols that may be either inhaled directly (13) or passed through an air intake system for a building and then inhaled (8, 14). Transmission via cooling towers and evaporative condensers has been most often documented when cases have been in fairly close proximity (less than 200 m) from contaminated devices (13, 14); however, data from one investigation suggested that legionellosis may be transmitted from cooling tower aerosols that have been carried longer distances (1 to 2 miles [ca. 1.6 to 3.2 km]) (1). While it has been clearly shown that these devices are capable of transmitting disease, it is less certain how often they actually do. Bhopal et al. have suggested that cooling tower aerosols are responsible for a portion of sporadically occurring cases of legionellosis in Scotland (3); others have expressed doubt that they play a major role in disease (36, 43).

Aerosolization of contaminated warm potable water via shower heads or tap water faucets can transmit legionellosis. Potable water has long been suspected to be a potential source of *Legionella* infection (44). Laboratory studies have shown that shower heads and tap faucets can produce aerosols containing legionellae in respirable droplets (1- to 5-μm diameter) (6). An epidemiologic link with showering has been established

recently (9). During investigation in Belgium, exposure to warm water faucets was associated with disease (11). In that study, sponge bathing while standing at sinks within patient rooms was a significant risk factor; being confined to bed was protective, presumably because controls were less likely to come in contact with aerosols from the faucet. Infections caused by *L. pneumophila* serogroups 1 and 6 occurred during the outbreak. These strains were isolated from warm water (temperature of about 40°C) and during air sampling (within respirable droplets) adjacent to the faucets when the faucets were running but not when they were turned off.

Potable water can also serve as the source of legionellosis with respiratory care equipment as the vehicle of transmission (2, 34). In hospitals with contaminated potable water systems, use of tap water to wash jet nebulizers and other equipment used to deliver respiratory care likely represents a substantial risk for patients, many of whom are at increased risk for legionellosis because of chronic lung disease and/or steroid use. Droplets containing the bacteria may be present within equipment set aside for several hours following rinsing (34). Other sources of aerosol that have been shown to transmit disease include whirlpool baths (24, 31), humidifiers (30), and decorative fountains (18).

The value of a careful, systematic epidemiologic approach during investigations of epidemics, often in combination with molecular epidemiologic techniques and air sampling in identifying the source of transmission, has been repeatedly shown. The merit of a methodical approach was highlighted during an investigation of a communitywide epidemic of Legionnaires disease in a small town in Louisiana (30). The setting was an outbreak of pneumonia in over 100 community residents during a 2-month period. Thirty-three of these patients had evidence of Legionnaires disease. There was an industrial plant in the center of town. Devices within the facility produced a huge volume of aerosol visible throughout much of the town. The most obvious initial hypothesis was that the facility was the source. During the subsequent case control study, which systematically focused on exposures and activities throughout the town, infected subjects were shown to be much more likely than controls to shop at a grocery store. Of those who did, infected subjects were more likely to have shopped for at least 30 min and to have bought produce items in one section of the produce display. Adjacent to this display was an ultrasonic mist machine that misted the vegetables. The reservoir of the mist machine contained *L. pneumophila* serogroup 1 with monoclonal antibody subtype matching that of the epidemic strain. Importantly, a strain of the same subtype was isolated from 1 of 200 other water specimens in the town—from a cooling tower at the industrial plant; however, there were no epidemiologic associations between exposure or proximity to the facility and disease. Had the investigation been limited to collection of water from the industrial facility, a cooling tower would have been implicated as the source of infection. The true epidemic source would have remained unidentified, quietly serving as a potential source for additional cases.

VIRULENCE FACTORS

Returning to the chain of causation model, for disease to occur, the bacterium has to be virulent for humans. Since the 1983 symposium, the number of *Legionella* species that have been shown to cause infection has increased dramatically. In 1983, there were just 9 serogroups and 10 species of *Legionella* known. Most of the species represented strains isolated from the environment; few were known to cause disease. Now there are over 25 species and 48 serogroups recognized, and a substantial proportion have been shown to be capable of causing disease. However, when there is an isolate available, *L. pneumophila* accounts for 90% of cases of legionellosis reported to the Centers for Disease Control's surveillance system; 82% of these cases are caused by *L. pneumophila* serogroup 1 (33). *L. micdadei, L. pneumophila* serogroups 6 and 3, and *L. longbeachae* are the organisms isolated next most frequently from patients with legionellosis (33). Many of the species and serogroups appear to be more opportunistic (and presumably less virulent) than *L. pneumophila* serogroup 1, as they cause disease almost exclusively in highly immunosuppressed persons.

Of *L. pneumophila* serogroup 1 strains, certain subtypes, as determined by monoclonal antibody subtyping, are most likely to be associated with epidemics of disease (15, 27, 42). These strains, which react with a specific monoclonal antibody, MAb 2 (26), appear infrequently in environmental specimens. The antigenic determinant reacting with MAb 2 is a lipopolysaccharide (37). The basis for the association of strains bearing this epitope with epidemics is unknown. The epitope

may be a marker for strains with increased virulence or increased survivability during aerosolization. Absence of this marker does not rule out strain virulence; many cases of infection occur with strains of *L. pneumophila* serogroup 1 that are MAb 2 negative. Identifying virulence markers would be useful in efforts to control legionellosis because aggressive primary prevention measures could be targeted to a source with increased potential for transmitting disease. The effect on virulence of a number of other factors, including macrophage infectivity potentiator protein, is actively being studied.

HOST SUSCEPTIBILITY

A key factor in the chain of causation is susceptibility of the host. Persons who have depressed immune systems, such as organ transplant recipients and those on corticosteroids, are at markedly increased risk for infection, although the precise magnitude is not well defined. Early data from the Centers for Disease Control's surveillance system suggested that persons with end-stage renal disease have a 200-fold-greater risk of developing *Legionella* infection than do normal hosts (16). Persons with chronic lung disease and smokers are also at increased risk. Multivariate analyses of risk factor data have not been done to determine whether advancing age and male gender are independent risk factors or are associated with a greater likelihood of development of chronic underlying disease. While pediatric legionellosis has been reported, the disease is extremely rare except among markedly immunosuppressed children (7, 12).

In the laboratory, *Legionella* antigens that produce protective immunity in animal models have been identified (4, 5, 10). While the potential for a successful vaccine appears real, the rationale for vaccine development and use will depend on a better understanding of the incidence of disease and the population at risk.

INCIDENCE OF DISEASE

A number of recent studies indicate that *Legionella* species cause 1 to 5% of community-acquired pneumonias (applying the most stringent case definitions) (17, 32, 38, 45). Preliminary findings of a large, ongoing, population-based prospective study of community-acquired pneumonia requiring hospitalization indicate that the annual rate of non-outbreak-related, community-acquired *Legionella* infection is 6.1/100,000 population per year (Marston et al., this volume). Extrapolation of this rate from this study conducted in Ohio to the adult population in the United States is risky because the incidence of infection may vary by region. However, for a sense of the magnitude of disease, the rate translates to an estimated 11,000 cases of community-acquired *Legionella*-associated pneumonia requiring hospitalization yearly in the United States. This figure may underestimate the true incidence of legionellosis for at least three reasons: a substantial proportion of patients may not be hospitalized; some patients infected with *Legionella* species may not have pneumonia; and serology, urinary antigen detection, and culture are not 100% sensitive.

SPORADICALLY OCCURRING DISEASE

None of the 130 cases of legionellosis identified thus far in the Ohio pneumonia study are part of recognized epidemics or clusters, suggesting that the vast majority of cases sporadically occur. One hypothesis is that sporadic cases are not sporadic at all but rather are unrecognized epidemic or endemic disease resulting from a contaminated source persistently or intermittently releasing aerosols containing *Legionella* organisms. While the epidemiology of sporadically occurring disease needs more elucidation, it is likely to be similar to that for epidemic disease; the chain of causation is a useful template.

Where does transmission of sporadic legionellosis occur? There are a number of possibilities, some of which are shown in Fig. 2. Infection resulting from exposure to aerosols from contaminated warm water in the home is one potentially important consideration. Recent data from a series of patients with sporadically occurring disease in Pittsburgh suggest that such exposure may occur in a limited number of cases and may be a particular concern in multifamily dwellings with larger plumbing systems (43). To sys-

tematically investigate the role of exposures in the home, we and investigators at Ohio State University and Northeastern Ohio Medical School are evaluating case patients with legionellosis identified during the Ohio pneumonia study and matched control patients for exposures to *Legionella* species. The evaluation includes extensive interviews and culture surveys of residences. Data from this study should be available in 1993.

Cooling tower aerosols, carried in the atmosphere for some distance, have been proposed as a cause of sporadically occurring disease. Residences of persons identified with legionellosis during a study in Glasgow, Scotland, were located within close proximity to cooling towers more often than expected in comparison with the distribution of residences in the community (3). Additional systematic studies are needed to confirm these observations.

Travel-related disease appears to account for a substantial proportion of cases in Europe. Exposures while traveling are too numerous to count, making it impossible to identify the exposure responsible for a single case of disease and demonstrating the importance of international surveillance to identify point sources.

The role of the workplace in sporadic or epidemic Legionnaires disease has been the recent focus of a great deal of attention and has raised questions about strategies to prevent transmission of disease in the workplace and to identify workplace settings where the risk of transmission is particularly high. Likewise, the risk of transmission in public places such as shopping areas and public buildings is unknown.

While expensive, epidemiologic studies to identify factors and settings associated with sporadic Legionnaires disease are crucial to focus ef-

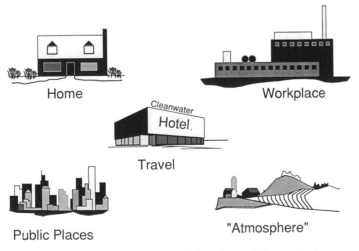

FIG. 2.   Possible sources of transmission of sporadic legionellosis.

forts for prevention and will be well worth the costs. Future studies should evaluate exposures in the community, including public places and work sites.

Wide-ranging policies to minimize the risk of legionellosis are needed, but because eradicating the bacteria from the environment is very difficult, policies are likely to be expensive and of undetermined effectiveness. They are more likely to be effective if they can be targeted to specific types of devices, exposures, or other factors that are associated with an increased risk of disease. On the basis of available data, some settings can now be targeted for policies. Hospitals, in which there is a high concentration of patients at risk for disease and a substantial likelihood that legionellae are present in the water, would be likely targets. However, for other settings, carefully conducted studies are needed to better target and focus prevention strategies.

SUMMARY

Increased understanding of the epidemiology of legionellosis, particularly sporadically occurring disease, will lead to well-targeted, efficient, and practical prevention strategies. The effectiveness and success of these strategies will depend on the development of new technologies to break the chain of causation by one or more of the following approaches: blocking amplification of the bacteria; detecting virulent strains in the environment; developing new, more effective decontamination techniques; decreasing the potential for aerosols to disseminate; and, finally, stimulating protective immunity with vaccines in persons at increased risk for disease.

REFERENCES

1. **Addiss, D. G., J. P. Davis, M. LaVenture, P. J. Wand, M.A. Hutchinson, and R. M. McKinney.** 1989. Community-acquired Legionnaires' disease associated with a cooling tower: evidence for longer distance transport of *Legionella pneumophila. Am. J. Epidemiol.* **130:**557–568.
2. **Arnow, P. M., T. Chou, D. Weil, E. N. Shapiro, and C. Kretzschmar.** 1982. Nosocomial Legionnaires' disease caused by aerosolized tap water from respiratory devices. *J. Infect. Dis.* **146:**460–467.
3. **Bhopal, R. S., R. J. Fallon, E. C. Buist, R. J. Black, and J. D. Urquhart.** 1991. Proximity of the home to a cooling tower and risk of non-outbreak Legionnaires' disease. *Br. Med. J.* **302:**378–383.
4. **Blander, S. J., R. F. Breiman, and M. A. Horwitz.** 1989. A live avirulent mutant *Legionella pneumophila* vaccine induces protective immunity against lethal aerosol challenge. *J. Clin. Invest.* **83:**810–815.
5. **Blander, S. J., and M. A. Horwitz.** 1989. Vaccination with the major secretory protein of *Legionella pneumophila* induces cell-mediated and protective immunity in a guinea pig model of Legionnaires' disease. *J. Exp. Med.* **169:**691–705.
6. **Bollin, G. E., J. F. Plouffe, M. F. Para, and B. Hackman.** 1985. Aerosols containing *Legionella pneumophila* generated by shower heads and hot-water faucets. *Appl. Environ. Microbiol.* **50:**1128–1131.

7. **Brady, M. T.** 1989. Nosocomial Legionnaires disease in a children's hospital. *J. Pediatr.* **115:**46–50.
8. **Breiman, R. F., W. Cozen, B. S. Fields, T. D. Mastro, S. J. Carr, J. S. Spika, and L. Mascola.** 1990. Role of air-sampling in an investigation of an outbreak of Legionnaires' disease associated with exposure to aerosols from an evaporative condenser. *J. Infect. Dis.* **161:**1257–1261.
9. **Breiman, R. F., B. S. Fields, G. N. Sanden, L. Volmer, A. Meier, and J. S. Spika.** 1990. An outbreak of Legionnaires' disease associated with shower use: possible role of amoebae. *JAMA* **263:**2924–2926.
10. **Breiman, R. F., and M. A. Horwitz.** 1987. Guinea pigs sublethally infected with aerosolized *Legionella pneumophila* develop humoral and cell-mediated immune responses and are protected against lethal aerosol challenge. A model for studying host defense against lung infections caused by intracellular pathogens. *J. Exp. Med.* **164:**799–811.
11. **Breiman, R. F., F. L. Van Loock, J. P. Sion, G. N. Sanden, R. F. Benson, W. L. Thacker, R. Colebunders, and S. R. Pattyn.** 1991. Association of "sink-bathing" and Legionnaires' disease, abstr. L-18. In *Abstr. 91st Gen. Meet. Am. Soc. Microbiol. 1991.*
12. **Carlson, N. C., M. R. Kuskie, E. L. Dobyns, M. C. Wheeler, M. H. Roe, and M. J. Abzug.** 1990. Legionellosis in children: an expanding spectrum. *Pediatr. Infect. Dis. J.* **9:**133–137
13. **Cordes, L. G., D. W. Fraser, P. Skaliy, C. A. Perlino, W. R. Elsea, G. F. Mallison, and P. S. Hayes.** 1980. Legionnaires' disease outbreak at an Atlanta, Georgia, country club; evidence for spread from an evaporative condenser. *Am. J. Epidemiol.* **111:**425–431.
14. **Dondero, T. J., R. C. Rentdorff, G. F. Mallison, R. M. Weeks, J. S. Levy, E. W. Wong, and W. Schaffner.** 1980. An outbreak of Legionnaires' disease associated with a contaminated air-conditioning cooling tower. *N. Engl. J. Med.* **302:**365–370.
15. **Dournon, E., W. F. Bibb, P. Rajagopalan, N. Desplaces, and R. M. McKinney.** 1988. Monoclonal antibody reactivity as a virulence marker for *Legionella pneumophila* serogroup 1 strains. *J. Infect. Dis.* **157:**496–501.
16. **England, A. C., D. W. Fraser, B. D. Plikaytis, T. F. Tsai, G. Storch, and C. V. Broome.** 1981. Sporadic legionellosis in the United States: the first thousand cases. *Ann. Intern. Med.* **94:**164–170.
17. **Fang, G. D., M. Fine, J. Orloff, D. Arisumi, V. L. Yu, W. Kapoor, J. T. Grayston, S. P. Wang, R. Kohler, R. R. Muder, Y. C. Yee, J. D. Rihs, and R. M. Vickers.** 1990. New and emerging etiologies for community-acquired pneumonia with implications for therapy—a prospective multicenter study of 359 cases. *Medicine* **69:**307–316.
18. **Fenstersheib, M. D., M. Miller, C. Diggins, S. Liska, L. Detweiler, S. B. Werner, D. Lindquist, W. L. Thacker, and R. F. Benson.** 1990. Outbreak of Pontiac fever due to *Legionella anisa. Lancet* **ii:**35–37.
19. **Fields, B. S., G. N. Sanden, J. M. Barbaree, W. E. Morrill, R. M. Wadowsky, E. W. White, and J. C. Feeley.** 1989. Intracellular multiplication of *Legionella pneumophila* in amoebae isolated from hospital water tanks. *Curr. Microbiol.* **18:**131–137.
20. **Fliermans, C. B., W. B. Cherry, L. H. Orrison, S. J. Smith, D. L. Tison, and D. H. Pope.** 1981. Ecological distribution of *Legionella pneumophila. Appl. Environ. Microbiol.* **41:**9–16.
21. **Fraser, D. W.** 1980. Legionellosis: evidence of airborne transmission. *Ann. N.Y. Acad. Sci.* **353:**61–66.
22. **Fraser, D. W.** 1984. Sources of legionellosis, p. 277–280. *In* C. Thornsberry, A. Balows, J. C. Feeley, and W. Jakubowski (ed.), *Legionella: Proceedings of the 2nd International Symposium.* American Society for Microbiology, Washington, D.C.
22a. **Friedman, S., K. Spitalny, J. Barbaree, Y. Faur, and R. McKinney.** 1987. Pontiac fever outbreak associated

with a cooling tower. *Am. J. Public Health* **77**:568–572.

23. **Garbe, P. L., B. J. Davis, J. S. Weisfeld, L. Markowitz, P. Miner, F. Garrity, J. M. Barbaree, and A. L. Reingold.** 1985. Nosocomial Legionnaires' disease: epidemiologic demonstration of cooling towers as a source. *JAMA* **254**:521–524.

24. **Goldberg, D. J., J. G. Wrench, P. W. Collier, D. J. Fallon, T. M. McKay, T. A. Markwick, J. G. Wrench, J. A. Emslie, G. J. Forbes, A. C. MacPherson, and D. Reid.** 1989. Lochgoilhead fever: outbreak of non-pneumonic legionellosis due to *Legionella micdadei*. *Lancet* **i**:316–318.

25. **Groothuis, D. G., H. R. Veenendaal, and H. L. Dijkstra.** 1985. Influence on temperature on the number of *Legionella pneumophila* in hot water systems. *J. Appl. Bacteriol.* **59**:529–536.

25a. **Hanrahan, J. P., D. L. Morse, V. B. Scharf, et al.** 1987. A community hospital outbreak of legionellosis: transmission by potable hot water. *Am. J. Epidemiol.* **125**:639–649.

26. **Joly, J. R., R. M. McKinney, J. O. Tobin, W. F. Bibb, I. D. Watkins, and D. Ramsay.** 1986. Development of a standarized subgrouping scheme for *Legionella pneumophila* serogroup 1 using monoclonal antibodies. *J. Clin. Microbiol.* **23**:768–771.

27. **Joly J. R., and W. C. Winn.** 1988. *Legionella pneumophila* subgroups, monoclonal antibody reactivity, and strain virulence in Burlington, Vermont. *J. Infect. Dis.* **158**:1412. (Letter.)

28. **Kurtz, J. B., C. L. R. Bartlett, U. A. Newton, R. A. White, and N. L. Jones.** 1982. *Legionella pneumophila* in cooling water systems—report of a survey of cooling towers in London and a pilot trial of selected biocides. *J. Hyg.* (Cambridge) **88**:369–381.

29. **Lowry, P. W., R. J. Blankenship, W. Gridley, R. N. Nancy, N. J. Troup, and L. S. Tompkins.** 1991. A cluster of *Legionella* sternal wound infections due to postoperative topical exposure to contaminated tap water. *N. Engl. J. Med.* **324**:109–113.

30. **Mahoney, F. J., C. W. Hoge, T. A. Farley, J. M. Barbaree, R. F. Benson, R. F. Breiman, and L. M. McFarland.** 1992. Community-wide outbreak of Legionnaires' disease associated with a grocery store mist machine. *J. Infect. Dis.* **165**:736–739.

31. **Mangione, E. J., R. S. Remis, K. A. Tait, W. B. McGee, G. W. Gorman, B. B. Wentworth, P. A. Baron, A. W. Hightower, J. M. Barbaree, and C. V. Broome.** 1982. An outbreak of Pontiac fever related to whirlpool use, Michigan. *JAMA* **253**:535–539.

32. **Marrie, T. J., H. Durant, and L. Yates.** 1989. Community-acquired pneumonia requiring hospitalization: a five year prospective study. *Rev. Infect. Dis.* **11**:586–589.

33. **Marston, B. J., H. Lipman, and R. F. Breiman.** A decade of surveillance for Legionnaires' disease: update on risk factors for morbidity and mortality due to infection with *Legionella*. Submitted for publication.

34. **Mastro, T. D., B. S. Fields, R. F. Breiman, J. Campbell, B. D. Plikaytis, and J. S. Spika.** 1991. Nosocomial

Legionnaires' disease and use of medication nebulizers. *J. Infect. Dis.* **163**:667–670.

35. **Morris, G. K., C. M. Pstton, J. C. Feeley, S. E. Johnson, G. Gorman, W. T. Martin, P. Skaliy, G. F. Mallison, B. D. Politi, and D. C. Mackel.** 1979. Isolation of the Legionnaires' disease bacterium from environmental samples. *Ann. Intern. Med.* **90**:664–666.

36. **Muder, R. R., V. L. Yu, and A. H. Woo.** 1986. Mode of transmission of *Legionella pneumophila*: a critical review. *Arch. Intern. Med.* **146**:1607–1612.

36a. **O'Mahony, M. C., R. E. Stanwell-Smith, H. E. Tillett, et al.** 1990. The Stafford outbreak of Legionnaires' disease. *Epidemiol. Infect.* **104**:361–380.

37. **Petitjean, F., E. Dournon, A. D. Strosberg, and J. Hoebeke.** 1990. Isolation, purification and partial analysis of the lipopolysaccharide antigenic determinant recognized by a nonoclonal antibody to *Legionella pneumophila* serogroup 1. *Res. Microbiol.* **141**:1077–1094.

38. **Research Committee of the British Thoracic Society and the Public Health Laboratory Service.** 1987. Community-acquired pneumonia in adults in British hospitals in 1982–1983: a survey of aetiology, mortality, prognostic factors and outcome. *Q. J. Med.* **62**:195–220.

39. **Rogers, J., and C. W. Keevil.** 1992. Immunogold and fluorescein immunolabelling of *Legionella pneumophila* within an aquatic biofilm visualized by using episcopic differential interference contrast microscopy. *Appl. Environ. Microbiol.* **58**:2326–2330.

40. **Rowbotham, T. J.** 1980. Preliminary report on the pathogenicity of *Legionella pneumophila* for freshwater and soil amoebae. *J. Clin. Pathol.* **33**:1179–1183.

40a. **Schlech, W. F.** 1990. *Legionella* and fountains. *Lancet* **336**:576. (Letter.)

40b. **Spitalny, K. C., R. L. Vogt, L. A. Orciari, et al.** 1984. Pontiac fever associated with a whirlpool spa. *Am. J. Epidemiol.* **120**:809–817.

41. **Steele, T. W., J. Langser, and N. Sangster.** 1990. Isolation of *Legionella longbeachae* serogroup 1 from potting mixes. *Appl. Environ. Microbiol.* **56**:49–53.

42. **Stout, J. E., J. Joly, M. Para, J. Plouffe, C. Ciesielski, M. J. Blaser, and V. L. Yu.** 1988. Comparison of molecular methods for subtyping patients and epidemiologically linked environmental isolates of *Legionella pneumophila*. *J. Infect. Dis.* **157**:486–495.

43. **Stout, J. E., V. L. Yu, P. Muraca, J. Joly, N. Troup, and L. S. Tompkins.** 1992. Potable water as a cause of sporadic cases of community-acquired Legionnaires' disease. *N. Engl. J. Med.* **326**:151–155.

44. **Tobin, J. O., C. L. R. Bartlett, and S. A. Waitkins.** 1981. Legionnaires' disease: further evidence to implicate water storage systems as sources. *Br. Med. J.* **282**:573.

45. **Woodhead, M. A., and J. T. MacFarlane.** 1987. Prospective study of the aetiology and outcome of pneumonia in the community. *Lancet* **146**:671–674.

46. **Yee, R. B., and R. M. Wadowsky.** 1982. Multiplication of *Legionella pneumophila* in unsterilized tap water. *Appl. Environ. Microbiol.* **43**:1330–1334.

Preliminary Findings of a Community-Based Pneumonia Incidence Study

BARBARA J. MARSTON, JOSEPH F. PLOUFFE, ROBERT F. BREIMAN, THOMAS M. FILE, JR., ROBERT F. BENSON, MUNSHI MOYENUDDEN, W. LANIER THACKER, KWEI-HAY WONG, STEVE SKELTON, BARBARA HACKMAN, SARA J. SALSTROM, JAMES M. BARBAREE, AND THE COMMUNITY-BASED PNEUMONIA INCIDENCE STUDY GROUP

Respiratory Diseases Branch, Division of Bacterial and Mycotic Diseases, National Center for Infectious Diseases, Centers for Disease Control, Atlanta, Georgia 30333; Division of Infectious Diseases, Department of Internal Medicine, Ohio State University, Columbus, Ohio 43210; and Division of Infectious Diseases, Department of Internal Medicine, Northeastern Ohio Medical School, Akron, Ohio

Pneumonia is the leading cause of death due to infectious disease in this country. Most studies of the etiology of community-acquired pneumonia (CAP) have been hospital based; thus, the proportion of pneumonias attributable to specific etiologies has been measured, but the incidence of disease has not (2, 5, 6, 8). Population-based data on the incidence of pneumonia caused by specific pathogens are needed in order to set public health priorities and to evaluate the impact of prevention and control measures.

To measure the overall incidence of pneumonia and of pneumonia caused by specific pathogens, all adult residents of Franklin and Summit counties in Ohio who are hospitalized with CAP are enrolled in the Community-Based Pneumonia Incidence Study. The two counties have similar demographic characteristics. Summit County has an adult population of 411,000 and includes the city of Akron; Franklin County has an adult population of 765,000 and includes the city of Columbus.

Since December 1990, all patients with pneumonia or pneumonia-related admission diagnoses have been screened for study enrollment. Study participants must be residents of one of the study counties, 18 years of age or older, and not institutionalized (nursing home residents are excluded). Patients with admission diagnoses of pneumonia are enrolled if a chest radiograph taken within 48 h of admission demonstrates an infiltrate compatible with pneumonia. Patients with admission diagnoses that may be associated with pneumonia (such as exacerbation of chronic lung disease) are enrolled only if radiographic infiltrates are accompanied by cough, fever, or hypothermia.

Basic demographic information is collected for each eligible study patient. A questionnaire addressing exposures and symptoms is administered if the patient consents to participate, and samples of serum, urine, and sputum are obtained. Medical charts are reviewed for all study patients. Final decisions concerning diagnosis and etiology of pneumonia are made following chart review. After 4 weeks, a convalescent-phase blood specimen is collected, along with information about the patient's recovery and return to work.

Paired sera are tested for antibodies to *Legionella pneumophila* with an indirect fluorescent antibody assay (7), to *Mycoplasma pneumoniae* with complement fixation, to *Chlamydia pneumoniae* with a microimmunofluorescence assay (3), and to influenza viruses A and B with complement fixation initially and hemagglutination if complement fixation is positive. Urine samples are tested for the presence of *L. pneumophila* serogroup 1 antigens by radioimmunoassay (4). Respiratory secretions have also been collected and cultured for legionellae since April 1991 (1).

Legionella serologic results are considered positive if there is a fourfold rise in antibody titer or a reciprocal titer of $\geq 1,024$ in either the acute- or convalescent-phase serum specimen. For *M. pneumoniae*, a positive result is defined as a fourfold rise in antibody titer or an acute- or convalescent-phase titer of ≥ 64. For *C. pneumoniae*, a positive result is defined as a fourfold rise in titer of immunoglobulin G (IgG) or IgM antibody or an acute- or convalescent-phase titer of IgG of ≥ 512 or of IgM of ≥ 16. Positive results for influenza virus are defined by a fourfold rise in antibody titer to influenza virus A or B.

Through December 1991, 3,700 patients eligible for the study had been identified. More than 60% responded to the questionnaire and agreed to submit laboratory specimens.

After adjusting for estimates of the proportion of enrolled patients with pneumonia, the annual rate of pneumonia requiring hospitalization in the study counties for 1991 is estimated to be 330/100,000 adults. Extrapolating to the adult U.S. population, 600,000 cases of CAP requiring hospitalization would be expected annually, not including nursing home and other institutionalized adults.

The incidence of pneumonia due to *L. pneumophila* may be estimated from data collected during the first year of the study. A total of 68 cases of legionellosis were identified on the basis of serologic testing, urinary antigen, or culture, for an annual incidence of 6.1 cases of legionellosis requiring hospitalization per 100,000 adults in the study countries. If the incidence of *Legionella* infection is assumed to be geographically constant, the annual number of cases of CAP due to *L. pneumophila* extrapolated to the entire U.S. adult population would be 11,000. This figure is approximately 25-fold higher than the 400 to 500 cases of Legionnaires' disease annually reported (and confirmed) to the passive surveillance system at the Centers for Disease Control. This calculation likely underestimates the incidence of legionellosis, since laboratory tests were performed on only 60% of eligible patients and a substantial number of cases of legionellosis may not require hospitalization.

Two hundred sixty-eight (15.9%) of 1,690 patients tested thus far have evidence of *M. pneumoniae* infection, and 71 (7.9%) of 895 patients tested thus far have evidence of infection with *C. pneumoniae*. During the 1990–91 winter season, influenza virus infection (caused primarily by influenza virus B) was demonstrated serologically in 29 patients.

Overall, 25% of enrollees in the study have evidence of infection with *L. pneumophila*, *M. pneumoniae*, or *Chlamydia pneumoniae*, illustrating the important roles of these pathogens as causes of pneumonia. Because the study is population based and combines data from community and tertiary-care institutions, it provides a unique opportunity to develop accurate estimates of the incidence of CAP and to evaluate the contribution of various respiratory pathogens to the occurrence of this disease in the United States. Because of the large numbers of cases, we will also study the impact of etiology, underlying diseases, and choice and timing of therapy on outcome of pneumonia.

REFERENCES

1. **Buesching, W. J., R. A. Brust, and L. W. Ayerst.** 1983. Enhanced primary isolation of *Legionella pneumophila* from clinical specimens by low pH treatment. *J. Clin. Microbiol.* **17**:1153–1155.
2. **Fang, G. D., M. Fine, J. Orloff, D. Arisumi, V. L. Yu, W. Kapoor, J. T. Grayston, S. P. Wang, R. Kohler, R. R. Muder, Y. C. Yee, J. D. Rihs, and R. M. Vickers.** 1990. New and emerging etiologies for community-acquired pneumonia with implications for therapy—a prospective multicenter study of 359 cases. *Medicine* **69**:307–316.
3. **Grayston, J. T., C. C. Kuo, S. P. Wang, and J. Altman.** 1986. A new Chlamydia psittaci strain, TWAR, isolated in acute respiratory tract infections. *N. Engl. J. Med.* **315**:161–168.
4. **Kohler, R. B., W. C. Winn, Jr., J. C. Girod, and L. J. Wheat.** 1982. Rapid diagnosis of pneumonia due to *Legionella pneumophila* serogroup 1. *J. Infect. Dis.* **146**:444.
5. **Marrie, T. J., H. Durant, and L. Yates.** 1989. Community-acquired pneumonia requiring hospitalization: a five year prospective study. *Rev. Infect. Dis.* **11**:586–589.
6. **Research Committee of the British Thoracic Society and the Public Health Laboratory Service.** 1987. Community-acquired pneumonia in adults in British hospitals in 1982–1983: a survey of aetiology, mortality, prognostic factors and outcome. *Q. J. Med.* **62**:195–220.
7. **Wilkinson, H. W., D. D. Cruce, and C. V. Broome.** 1981. Validation of *Legionella pneumophila* indirect immunofluorescence assay with epidemic sera. *J. Clin. Microbiol.* **13**:139–146.
8. **Woodhead, M. A., and J. T. MacFarlane.** 1987. Prospective study of the aetiology and outcome of pneumonia in the community. *Lancet* **i**:671–674.

Incidence of Legionnaires Disease and Report of *Legionella sainthelensi* Serogroup 1 Infection in Toronto, Canada

M. GARCIA, I. CAMPBELL, P. TANG, AND C. KRISHNAN

The Toronto Hospital, Toronto M5G 2C4, and Central Public Health Laboratory, Toronto, M5W 1R5, Canada

Over a period of 13 years (1978 to 1991), 38 cases of *Legionella* infection were diagnosed at The Toronto Hospital, a large general hospital, by tests performed at the Central Public Health Laboratory. This study was done to examine the incidence of legionellosis in our hospital and to correlate laboratory data with the clinical diagnoses.

Legionellae were distributed among 12 serogroups of eight species, with 25 (66%) of the 38 cases caused by *Legionella pneumophila* (6 serogroups) (Table 1).

Detailed case histories were available for review on 27 of the 38 patients. Six of the 27 cases were nosocomial. The epidemiologic and laboratory data are shown in Tables 2 and 3.

Of special interest was a case of *Legionella sainthelensi* serogroup 1 infection, which occurred in April 1990 in a 58-year-old female with Guillain-Barré syndrome. Three days after admission, the patient, who had been intubated, developed severe, progressive pneumonia with hypotension. The chest X-ray examination demonstrated bilateral infiltrates. When there was no response to penicillin, tobramycin, piperacillin, cloxacillin, and later erythromycin were added. Direct fluorescent antibody testing (DFA) and culture for legionellae were negative on one sputum sample. However, a urine specimen taken 5 days after onset tested positive for broad-spectrum *Le-*

TABLE 1. Summary of *Legionella* spp. isolated from
38 patients, 1978 to 1991

Species	No. (%) of cases
L. pneumophila	
Serogroup 1	19 (50)
Serogroup 3	1
Serogroup 4	2
Serogroup 5	1
Serogroup 8	1
Serogroup 12	1
Subtotal	25 (66)
L. micdadei	1
L. dumoffii	1
L. gormanii	1
L. longbeachae serogroup 1	1
L. oakridgensis	2
L. maceachernii	1
L sainthelensi serogroup 1[a]	1
Unknown[b]	5
Total	38

[a]First case of human infection reported.
[b]Diagnosed only by broad-spectrum ELISA for antigenuria (2).

gionella antigen (2). A routine indirect fluorescent
antibody test (IFA) for legionellae on acute and
convalescent serum samples (3 weeks after onset)
was negative. Testing against additional antigens
demonstrated a titer of less than 1:32 in the acute
serum and 1:256 in the convalescent serum
against *L. sainthelensi* serogroup 1. All 44 other
Legionella antigens and respiratory viruses tested

TABLE 2. Laboratory diagnosis of legionellosis
in 38 patients

Test(s)	No. of patients
Initial diagnosis by:	
DFA	11
Culture	7
Serum antibody test (IFA)[a]	12
Broad-spectrum *Legionella* antigenuria by ELISA[b]	8
Positive test(s) and/or combination of tests	
Culture ± other tests	16
DFA only	3
Antigenuria only[c]	5
Antigenuria with 1 or more tests	5
IFA titer equal or greater than fourfold rise	7
IFA single titer equal or greater than 1:128 and tube agglutination test for specific *Legionella* immunoglobulin M[c]	5

[a]IFA utilized formalinized antigens.
[b]Available since June 1985 (2).
[c]Considered only as possible evidence for current infection unless there was good clinical correlation. See reference 1 for details of the tube agglutination test.

TABLE 3. Demographic features and predisposing
factors for 27 patients

Demographic feature	Value
Males/females	20/7
Mean age (yr)	51
Range of age	26–82
No. of deaths	6
No. of nosocomial cases	6
Location where pneumonia developed	
Hematology and oncology service	2
Medical intensive-care unit	1
Surgical intensive-care unit	1
General medicine	2
Predisposing factor[a]	
Smoking	7
Diabetes	6
Alcoholism	2
Chronic obstructive pulmonary disease	4
Renal failure	8
Organ transplant	2
Collagen vascular disease[a]	2
Immunosuppressed[a]	
Chemotherapy	2
Steroids	8
Hematologic malignancy[a]	8

[a]Some patients have more than one predisposing factor or condition.

produced negative results. The patient recovered
after further erythromycin treatment. This is the
first reported case of human infection that we
know of caused by *L. sainthelensi* serogroup 1.

One case of nosocomial infection was caused
by *L. pneumophila* serogroup 8 in a liver transplant patient in November 1985. A limited environmental study done in July 1985 had yielded *L.
pneumophila* serogroup 8 and *L. anisa* from a
number of shower heads in patient areas.

Retrospective chart reviews of the remaining 25
cases revealed that 22 had a clinical diagnosis consistent with *Legionella* pneumonia and one had
symptoms suggestive of Pontiac fever. In five of
the patients, the laboratory diagnosis was based
solely on broad-spectrum *Legionella* antigenuria.
Two had a clinical diagnosis consistent with
Legionella pneumonia; one had possible Pontiac
fever. Two patients had pneumonia, but the diagnosis of legionellosis could not be confirmed because of the very complicated clinical presentation
and lack of additional laboratory data.

Urinary antigen was positive in association with
other tests in five other patients. In three of these
patients, it was the initial positive diagnostic test;
in the remaining two, DFA became available first.
Three additional patients (not included among
cases of legionellosis) did not have a current clinical infection but tested positive for antigen.
Asymptomatic or past infection could not be ruled
out.

In conclusion, 66% of cases of legionellosis

were caused by *L. pneumophila* (six serogroups). The broad-spectrum enzyme-linked immunosorbent assay (ELISA) for urinary antigen appears to be an excellent screening test, potentially also for other *Legionella* species. It led to the diagnosis of the *L. sainthelensi* serogroup 1 infection reported here.

REFERENCES

1. **Hartigan, D. A.** 1981. Comparison of specific immunoglobulin G, M and agglutinating antibodies against Legionella pneumophila. *Scand. J. Infect. Dis.* **13**:269–272.
2. **Tang, P. W., and S. Toma.** 1986. Broad-spectrum enzyme-linked immunosorbent assay for detection of *Legionella* soluble antigens. *J. Clin. Microbiol.* **24**:556–558.

Occurrence of Nosocomial Legionnaires Disease in Hospitals with Contaminated Potable Water Supply

JEAN R. JOLY AND MICHEL ALARY

Groupe de Recherche en Épidémiologie de l'Université Laval, Hôpital du Saint-Sacrement, 1050 Chemin Sainte-Foy, Quebec G1S 4L8, and Département de Microbiologie and Département de Médecine Sociale et Préventive, Faculté de Médecine, Université Laval, Quebec G1K 7P4, Canada

Legionella pneumophila is a frequent contaminant of hospital water supplies (2, 5). In a previous study, we demonstrated that over two-thirds of hospitals in the province of Quebec were contaminated by members of the family *Legionellaceae* (1), a figure similar to that reported in other areas of the world (6). The presence of *L. pneumophila* in the potable water supply of an institution has frequently been associated with cases of legionellosis (3, 4). Whether or not the presence of legionellae in a hospital environment will eventually be associated with the occurrence of cases is still unknown. The main objective of this study was to assess this possibility.

During a 9-month period, prospective surveillance of nosocomial pneumonia was established in 20 hospitals located in the province of Quebec. Ten of these hospitals were shown to have their potable water supply contaminated by *Legionellaceae,* whereas 10 were not found to have a contaminated potable water supply. One contaminated hospital elected to stop surveillance 2 months after initiation of the study. An additional institution was shown to have its water supply contaminated by *Legionellaceae* 7 months after the beginning of the study. Previously, this hospital was free of these bacteria.

The numbers of admissions and the patient populations were similar in contaminated and uncontaminated institutions. Four cases of Legionnaires disease occurred in 4 of the 10 contaminated institutions, whereas none were diagnosed in the uncontaminated hospitals ($P = 0.054$ by Fisher's exact test).

Hospitals with a water supply contaminated by *Legionellaceae* are more likely to have cases of legionellosis. Specific measures should be taken to avoid further transmission of this infection in contaminated institutions.

This work was supported by research grant 6605-3075-54 from the National Health Research and Development Program (NHRDP) of Health and Welfare Canada. M. Alary was supported by Ph.D. fellowships from the NHRDP (6605-2849-47) and from the Fonds de la Recherche en Santé du Québec (900504). J. R. Joly is a National Health Research Scholar (grant 6605-2693-48) from NHRDP.

REFERENCES

1. **Alary, M., and J. R. Joly.** 1992. Factors contributing to the contamination of hospital water distribution systems by Legionellae. *J. Infect. Dis.* **165**:565–569.
2. **Best, M., V. L. Yu, J. Stout, A. Goetz, R. R. Muder, and F. Taylor.** 1983. *Legionellaceae* in the hospital water-supply. Epidemiological link with disease and evaluation of a method for control of nosocomial Legionnaires' disease and Pittsburgh pneumonia. *Lancet* **ii**:307–310.
3. **Helms, C. M., R. M. Massanari, R. Zeitler, S. Streed, M. J. Gilchrist, N. Hall, W. J. Hausler, Jr., J. Sywassink, W. Johnson, L. Wintermeyer, and J. Hierholzer, Jr.** 1983. Legionnaires' disease associated with a hospital water system: a cluster of 24 nosocomial cases. *Ann. Intern. Med.* **99**:172–178.
4. **Neill, M. A., G. W. Gorman, C. Gibert, A. Roussel, A. W. Hightower, R. M. McKinney, and C. V. Broome.** 1985. Nosocomial legionellosis, Paris, France. Evidence of transmission by potable water. *Am. J. Med.* **78**:581–588.
5. **Tobin, J. O., M. S. Dunnil, M. French, P. J. Morris, J. Beare, S. Fisher-Hock, R. G. Mitchell, and M. F. Muers.** 1980. Legionnaires' disease in a transplant unit: isolation of the causative agent from shower baths. *Lancet* **i**:118–121.
6. **Vickers, R. M., V. L. Yu, and S. S. Hanna.** 1987. Determinants of *Legionella pneumophila* contamination of water distribution systems: 15-hospital prospective study. *Infect. Control* **8**:357–363.

Risk Assessments for Legionnaires Disease Based on Routine Surveillance of Cooling Towers for Legionellae

RICHARD D. MILLER AND KATHY A. KENEPP

Department of Microbiology and Immunology, School of Medicine, University of Louisville, Louisville, Kentucky 40292

The routine surveillance of cooling towers (or other water sources) for purposes of infection control against Legionnaires disease remains a somewhat controversial topic. On the basis of the ubiquitous nature of legionellae in cooling towers in the absence of disease, most public health officials currently recommend against routine testing. Nevertheless, building owners, managers, tenants, and water treatment companies are faced with the ever-present threat of an outbreak of Legionnaires disease originating from their cooling towers. Sincere public health concerns, along with the legal and financial liabilities associated with an outbreak of Legionnaires disease, warrant demands for reliable risk assessments. This issue was addressed recently in a presentation at a meeting of the American Society of Heating, Refrigerating, and Air-Conditioning Engineers, Inc., where suggested guidelines for hazard analysis were introduced (5). These recommendations, based on levels of *Legionella pneumophila* isolated from cooling towers associated with a limited number of outbreaks of disease, propose that immediate remedial action be taken if the level of viable legionellae in a cooling tower exceeds 1,000/ml.

This study represents the results of over 1,100 cooling tower risk assessments made by our laboratory over a 4-year period from 1988 through 1991, using these same criteria. In addition to detecting high levels of legionellae in many of these samples, we noted the frequent absence of any other detectable heterotrophic bacteria, a phenomenon that we first reported in our initial studies (4). Such a situation reflects a selection for legionellae, perhaps as a result of particular chemical biocides. This absence of microbial competition could lead to increased *Legionella* overgrowth in a cooling tower and perhaps should be considered as an additional factor when the risk is evaluated.

Cooling tower samples. All samples used in this study were obtained randomly from cooling towers in the Baltimore–Washington, D.C., area. One-liter samples were obtained by water treatment personnel during normal maintenance activities and were then shipped unrefrigerated to our laboratory for analysis via overnight air express. Previous studies in our laboratory had indicated that the levels of legionellae were not altered significantly during simulated conditions of such shipment, in contrast to refrigeration, which often

led to loss of *Legionella* viability (unpublished data). Information on the specific names and exact schedule of chemical biocide additions was not obtained for individual cooling tower samples in this study. Nevertheless, it was specifically requested that samples not be taken within 24 h after biocide additions.

Isolation and quantitation of legionellae. Legionellae were isolated by using a modification of the low-pH treatment and selective medium protocol first described by Bopp et al. (1). Briefly, a 500-ml sample of each cooling tower was first filtered through a 47-mm-diameter, 0.45-μm-pore-size Nuclepore filter. The filter was then placed in a small plastic jar with 5 ml of sterile distilled water, and the bacteria were removed by mild sonic vibration for 10 min in a bath-type sonicator. A 1-ml portion of the filter-concentrated material was then acidified to pH 2.2 by addition of 1 ml of 0.2 M HCl-KCl buffer. After a 10-min period at room temperature, the sample was neutralized by addition of 1 ml of KOH. Portions (10 and 100 μl) from the acid-treated sample, the filter-concentrated material, and the original sample were spread plated onto both buffered charcoal-yeast extract agar and glycine-vancomycin-polymyxin B selective agar medium and incubated at 37°C. After 3 and 5 days of incubation, typical *Legionella* colonies were counted and confirmed by lack of growth on media without L-cysteine as well as by immunofluorescence microscopy using a monoclonal antibody reagent specific for *L. pneumophila* (Genetics Systems, Inc., Seattle, Wash.). Quantitation of legionellae was calculated from the number of colonies on each agar plate and expressed as CFU per milliliter of original sample (corrected for the dilution or concentration of the sample).

Direct fluorescent antibody (DFA) microscopy. A 10-μl sample of filter-concentrated cooling tower water was placed in a well (7-mm diameter) on a Teflon-coated glass slide, air dried, and heat fixed. The samples were stained with the MERIFLUOR-*Legionella* reagent (Meridian Diagnostics, Cincinnati, Ohio), which recognizes 33 different strains and serogroups of *Legionella*. The number of fluorescing bacteria in the specimen was determined by counting microscopically.

Total bacterial count. The total bacteria count was obtained by plating 10^{-1}, 10^{-2}, 10^{-3}, and 10^{-4} dilutions of the cooling tower samples on buffered charcoal-yeast extract agar and incubat-

TABLE 1. Prevalence of *L. pneumophila* in 1,152 cooling towers sampled during a 4-year period from 1988 through 1991

	No. of towers in each group (%)			
Group	1988	1989	1990	1991
Viable legionellae[a]	107 (51)	72 (28)	103 (32)	60 (17)
Positive only by DFA	51 (24)	131 (50)	157 (49)	166 (46)
Negative	51 (24)	59 (23)	63 (20)	132 (37)
Total	209	262	323	358

[a]Contains all cooling towers that were positive for legionellae by viable cell plate count.

TABLE 3. Quantitation of viable *L. pneumophila* in 342 cooling towers sampled during the 4-year period from 1988 through 1991

Legionellae (CFU/ml)	Risk category[a]	No. of towers in each group			
		1988	1989	1990	1991
>10,000	High	3	0	1	4
1,000–10,000	High	26	10	18	7
100–999	Moderate	35	22	43	26
10–99	Low	29	28	34	20
<10	Very low	14	12	7	3
Total		107	72	103	60

[a]According to the relative risk assessments proposed by Morris and Feeley (5) on the basis of levels of legionellae detected in cooling towers associated with outbreaks of Legionnaires disease.

ing at 37°C. Colonies were counted after 3 and 5 days and expressed as CFU per milliliter of original sample.

Prevalence of legionellae in the cooling towers. As shown in Table 1, a total of 1,152 cooling towers were examined during the 4-year period from 1988 through 1991: 209 in 1988, 262 in 1989, 323 in 1990, and 358 in 1991. The prevalence of legionellae in these towers, as measured by viable cell counts, declined from a high of 51% in 1988 to closer to 30% in 1989 and 1990 (28 and 32%, respectively) and finally to 17% by 1991. All of the isolates from these positive samples were identified as *L. pneumophila*. When levels were measured by immunofluorescence microscopy (living and dead legionellae), numerous additional towers were found to be positive (Table 1). Thus, there was some evidence of *Legionella* colonization in approximately 75 to 80% of the cooling towers during the period from 1988 through 90, which dropped to 63% for 1991.

Quantitation of other bacteria in the cooling towers. The total aerobic bacterial count for each cooling tower sample was also determined to ascertain whether the numbers correlated with the levels of legionellae. As shown in Table 2, the range of numbers for total bacteria in the samples during this 4-year period varied greatly, from <1 to 5,000,000/ml. Although the average cooling

TABLE 2. Quantitation of other bacteria in 1,152 cooling towers sampled during a 4-year period from 1988 through 1991

	Total non-*Legionella* counts in each group (CFU/ml)	
Group	Range	Mean
Viable legionellae[a]	<1–3,000,000	58,000
Positive only by DFA	<1–5,000,000	260,000
Negative	<1–5,000,000	280,000

[a]Contains all cooling towers that were positive for legionellae by viable cell plate count.

tower with viable legionellae had fewer total bacteria than did the towers that were completely negative (or positive only by DFA), the large range of values made it impossible to predict the presence or absence (or the levels) of legionellae solely on the basis of the total bacterial count.

Quantitation of legionellae in the cooling towers. A large range of values was also observed for the numbers of viable legionellae in the samples. For purposes of providing a relative risk assessment of the cooling towers, the towers with viable legionellae were placed in groups according to the criteria of Morris and Feeley (5) (Table 3). A significant number of towers each year were in the high-risk category (greater than 1,000/ml), and several had counts above 10,000/ml. It was observed that 29 of 107 towers (27%) in 1988 were in this high-risk category, followed by 10 of 72 (14%) in 1989, 19 of 103 (18%) in 1990, and 11 of 60 (18%) in 1991. Most of the remainder of the towers fell into the moderate and low categories, with a smaller number that were in the very low category.

Legionella/total bacteria ratios in the cooling towers. The decision to use legionella/total bacteria ratios in the risk assessment of cooling towers was based on two observations. First, Fliermans et al. (3) had reported that legionellae were rarely observed in environmental specimens in excess of 1% of the total bacterial population; second, we had observed that high levels of legionellae were occasionally seen in towers with very few other detectable bacteria. Thus, the legionella/total bacteria ratios (as expressed in Table 4) may reflect relative tendencies to select for legionellae in a tower, perhaps as a result of variations in resistance to the chemical biocides used to treat the water.

While approximately 70% of the towers in this study had ratios of greater than 1% (indicative of some degree of selection), of particular interest were the towers with greater than 50% legionellae

TABLE 4. Legionella/total bacteria ratios in 342 cooling towers sampled during the 4-year period from 1988 through 1991

Legionellae (% of total bacteria)	No. of towers in each group			
	1988	1989	1990	1991
>50	14	4	21	11
11–50	26	13	20	16
1–10	38	26	30	14
<1	29	29	32	19
Total	107	72	103	60

TABLE 5. Levels of legionellae detected in individual cooling towers containing no other culturable bacteria

Total viable legionellae (CFU/ml)			
1988	1989	1990	1991
20,000	20	10,000	30,000
10,000		2,200	15,000
8,000		2,000	7,000
2,000		1,500	2,500
2,000		1,300	1,000
2,000		1,200	500
400		1,000	200
50		500	
		200	
		150	
		10	

(14 of 107 in 1988, 4 of 72 in 1989, 21 of 103 in 1990, and 11 of 60 in 1991). Thus, this selection for legionellae was a common occurrence. Of additional concern was the finding that a few of the towers had 100% legionellae by our culture conditions (Table 5), and the majority of these towers had levels of viable legionellae that were in the high-risk range, suggesting that the loss of a large segment of the microbial competition in the tower water may allow legionellae to proliferate to hazardous levels.

Conclusions. The risk assessment and prevention of disease outbreaks originating from contaminated cooling towers on the basis of routine surveillance of legionellae is complicated by the ubiquitous nature of these bacteria in the aquatic environments as well as the numerous factors involved in the proliferation of legionellae at these sites. These factors include the temperature and pH, availability of nutrients (organic compounds, iron, phosphate, etc.), the numbers and types of other bacteria, the numbers and types of amoebae and other protozoa (2, 6–8), the presence of legionellae in the makeup water, and certainly the nature of the biocide control program.

In addition, while there is general agreement that the persistence of high levels of legionellae in a cooling tower may be undesirable, there is no agreement as to what constitutes a hazardous level. The action guidelines proposed by Morris and Feeley (5) have provided the first real effort to address this issue. However, because of other conditions in the tower at a particular time, the use of a rigid hazard level may occasionally underestimate the relative risk of low to moderate levels of legionellae while overestimating the risk associated with high levels.

From the results of this study, the following conclusions can be drawn.

(i) The prevalence of viable legionellae in this population of cooling towers declined over the 4-year period of study, from 51% in 1988 to 17% in 1991. In each case, all of the isolates were identified as *L. pneumophila* (no serogrouping was performed). The continued disinfection of towers with moderate and high levels of legionellae may account for this decline.

(ii) Risk assessments were based primarily on the number of viable legionellae in each tower sample. Levels in most of the towers were in the low- and moderate-risk ranges (10 to 100 and 100 to 1,000/ml, respectively). Nevertheless, towers in the high-risk category (>1,000/ml) were common and constituted approximately 20% of the samples analyzed. This percentage remained relatively constant over the 4-year period. All towers with moderate or high levels of legionellae were recommended for disinfection.

(iii) Over 70% of the towers with legionellae in this study had levels of legionellae that were greater than 1% of the total bacterial population (suggesting some selection over the other normal aquatic bacteria). Of interest were the towers with few other culturable bacteria (approaching 100% legionellae). The large majority of these towers had levels of legionellae in the high-risk category, suggesting a complete selection for this organism. Recommendations for these towers included immediate disinfection and alterations in the normal biocide treatment program, along with regular follow-up testing.

(iv) In this study, predicting the risk status of a cooling tower solely on the basis of the total bacterial count (i.e., non-*Legionella* bacteria) was totally unreliable because of the wide variation in bacterial numbers in towers with or without legionellae. However, the trend, as judged from the mean values for each group (Table 2), was that the towers with viable legionellae had a lower total bacterial count than did towers that were negative or were positive only by DFA.

More accurate risk assessments of cooling towers will be facilitated by (i) additional data for cooling towers associated with outbreaks of Legionnaires disease, (ii) prospective studies of whether the concentration of legionellae in cooling towers is associated with sporadically occurring disease, (iii) prospective studies correlating *Legionella* numbers with specific types and concentrations of biocides, including the long-term effectiveness of chlorine disinfection, (iv) more specific information on the relationship between *Legionella* proliferation and the types and numbers of amoebae (and other protozoa) in the towers, and (v) a more definitive classification of *Legionella* isolates in terms of overall virulence and survival of aerosolization.

We gratefully acknowledge the support of RO/CO Corp., Aqua Aire Division, Brentwood, Md., for providing financial and technical assistance. In particular, we recognize the significant contributions provided by Matt Mallon and Eric deLaubenfels.

REFERENCES

1. **Bopp, C. A., J. W. Summner, G. K. Morris, and J. G. Wells.** 1981. Isolation of *Legionella* spp. from environmental water samples by low-pH treatment and use of a selective medium. *J. Clin. Microbiol.* **13:**714–719.
2. **Fields, B. S., E. B. Shotts, J. C. Feeley, G. W. Gorman,** and W. T. Martin. 1984. Proliferation of *Legionella pneumophila* as an intracellular parasite of the ciliated protozoan *Tetrahymena pyriformis*. *Appl. Environ. Microbiol.* **47:**467–471.
3. **Fliermans, C. B., W. B. Cherry, L. H. Orrison, S. J. Smith, D. L. Tison, and D. H. Pope.** 1981. Ecological distribution of *Legionella pneumphila*. *Appl. Environ. Microbiol.* **41:**9–16.
4. **Miller, R. D., and K. A. Kenepp.** 1991. Aerobiology 1991, p. 20. *Abstr. Pan-Am. Aerobiol. Assoc. Annu. Meet.*
5. **Morris, G. K., and J. C. Feeley.** 1990. *Abstr. ASHRAE Annu. Meet.*, p. 76.
6. **Newsome, A. L., R. L. Baker, R. D. Miller, and R. R. Arnold.** 1985. Interactions between *Naegleria fowleri* and *Legionella pneumophila*. *Infect. Immun.* **50:**499–452.
7. **Rowbotham, T. J.** 1980. Preliminary report on the pathogenicity of *Legionella pneumophila* for freshwater and soil amoebae. *J. Clin. Pathol.* **33:**1179–1183.
8. **Wadowsky, R. M., L. J. Butler, M. K. Cook, S. M. Verma, M. A. Paul, B. S. Fields, G. Keleti, J. L. Sykora, and R. B. Yee.** 1988. Growth-supporting activity for *Legionella pneumophila* in tap water cultures and implication of hartmannellid amoebae as growth factors. *Appl. Environ. Microbiol.* **54:**2677–2682.

Nosocomial *Legionella pneumophila* Pneumonia in a Hospital with an Instantaneous Hot Water Heater

JOHN A. SELLICK, JR., AND JOSEPH M. MYLOTTE

Division of Infectious Diseases, State University of New York at Buffalo, and Buffalo General Hospital, Buffalo, New York 14203

Legionella pneumophila poses a nosocomial infection risk for patients with compromised T-cell immunity, especially those patients with organ transplants (10). Potable water is an important source for cases of nosocomial legionellosis (3, 4, 7, 12), and *L. pneumophila* is able to grow readily in the warm, stagnant environment of hot water heating or holding tanks (8, 10). Instantaneous hot water heaters (IHWHs) have been suggested as a means to control proliferation of *L. pneumophila* since they are tankless and do not contain stagnant water (8). However, distal plumbing fixtures also have been found to be colonized with *L. pneumophila* (2, 11, 14).

L. pneumophila had not been documented as a cause of nosocomial infection at Buffalo General Hospital since the opening of a new inpatient facility in 1985. Older hospital buildings reportedly harbored *L. pneumophila* in the past, but no environmental sampling had been done since patients were moved to the new building. The occurrence of fatal *L. pneumophila* serogroup 3 pneumonia in a heart transplant recipient in June 1990 prompted this investigation.

Buffalo General Hospital is a 700-bed tertiary-care hospital with active heart and kidney transplantation, medical subspecialty (including oncology), and surgical services. The current inpatient facility is a 16-story tower that opened in 1985.

The hot water supply for most of this building, and for the adjacent older building, which houses offices and outpatient clinics, is an Aerco IHWH system with no heating or holding tanks. The basement through the fourth-floor, north side portion of the tower was completed in 1969, and only the fourth floor houses inpatients. The hot water supply to this area is a conventional heated tank system. There are no shock absorbers or "dead legs" in these systems. New York State Health Department regulations require that heater temperatures be maintained so that user outlet temperature is 110°F (ca. 43°C) or less. All five hospital buildings are in series on a cold water line fed from a city water supply.

No patient rooms in the hospital have windows that open to the outside. All hospital air enters the building from above street level and passes through filters that are rated on the American Society of Heating, Refrigerating, and Air-Conditioning Engineers 52-76 Test Standard at 90 to 95% efficiency. Function of these filters is monitored by computer-linked sensors and visual inspection. Heated and chilled water for air temperature control is transmitted to the main hospital buildings via closed loop systems from a plant and condensing tower building that is located in the next city block and downwind from the patient care building.

Clinical and environmental cultures for *L. pneumophila* were transported to the laboratory rapidly and plated on selective buffered charcoal-yeast extract agar supplemented with cysteine and α-ketoglutarate (BBL, Cockeysville, Md.). When possible, both swabs and 50 ml of water were collected from environmental sites. Positive cultures were confirmed and serogrouped at the Buffalo Department of Veterans Affairs Medical Center by direct fluorescent antibody technique (Zeus, Raritan, N.J.).

L. pneumophila serogroup 3 was cultured from both the anteroom sink and shower fixtures, but not the bathroom sink fixture, in the private room of the index case in June 1990. The patient reportedly had not showered postoperatively and drank only sterile, bottled water. He received aerosolized medications that were administered only with sterile nebulizers and prepared with sterile diluent. A second case of fatal *L. pneumophila* serogroup 3 pneumonia was identified in June 1990 subsequent to a hospitalwide educational program that followed identification of the index case. The latter patient had end-stage multiple myeloma and was being treated with steroids and radiation therapy. The bathroom sink fixtures in his room also grew *L. pneumophila* serogroup 3. Results of initial hospitalwide environmental sampling are summarized in Table 1. Swab cultures of faucet outlets were significantly more sensitive than was culture of "sediment" from 50 ml of the initial water stream.

In retrospect, there had been a precipitous drop in city water pressure as a result of rupture of a main line in February 1990. This drop caused a vacuum to occur in the hospital water lines, and water was discolored for more than 1 week following restoration of water pressure. For this reason, and the potential deleterious effects of hyperchlorination, superheating with distal-site flushing was chosen to attempt to eliminate *L. pneumophila*. In July 1990, the temperature of the hot water heaters was raised to deliver 160°F (ca. 71°C) water at the outlets, and all outlets were opened for 25 min, with monitoring to ensure that the effective temperature was maintained. Faucet aerators were removed when possible and soaked in chlorine bleach during the heat-flush treatment. Subsequent to the heat and flush, multiple distal sites were observed for the presence of *L. pneumophila* on a quarterly basis.

Since the heat treatment in July 1990, scheduled quarterly sampling of previously positive and other randomly selected sites for 18 months revealed no further growth of *L. pneumophila*. However, there have been two isolated occurrences of nosocomial legionellosis. Non-fatal *L. pneumophila* serogroup 1 pneumonia was documented in a patient with steroid-treated rheumatoid arthritis in March 1991. *L. pneumophila* serogroup 1 was cultured from the shower and sink fixtures in his room, which was located on 4 North. All other cultures, including the hot water tank serving that part of the building and most patient bathroom sinks on the involved floor, were negative for *L. pneumophila*. Replacement of the involved fixtures eliminated *L. pneumophila* from the room for the subsequent 11 months.

Following the occurrence of non-fatal *L. pneumophila* serogroup 3 pneumonia in a heart transplant patient in January 1992, the same organism was cultured from the sink in this patient's private room. Positive cultures for *L. pneumophila* serogroup 3 also were obtained from the sink of the activity room located next to this room and from the anteroom and bathroom sinks of a room on another floor. Cultures from 20 other room plumbing fixtures and the hot water return lines were

TABLE 1. Initial positive cultures, July 1990

Site	No. of positive cultures		
	L. pneumophila serogroup 1	*L. pneumophila* serogroup 3	No *L. pneumophila*
Patient rooms			
Water	2[a]	6[b]	25[b]
Swabs	2[a]	14[b]	16[b]
Clinic, old building	1	0	0
Hot water (outlet post-IHWH)	1	0	0
Chilled water loop (from condenser)	0	0	1
Heated water loop (from condenser)	0	0	1
Condenser	0	0	1
City water	0	0	1

[a] Along with *L. pneumophila* serogroup 3.
[b] Positive swab cultures versus positive water cultures (sediment from 50 ml) from same site; corrected $\chi^2 = 3.996$, $P = 0.05$.

negative. The involved fixtures have been changed, and repeat surveillance cultures are being performed.

Our experience with *L. pneumophila* contamination of an IHWH-based hospital hot water system has led to several important observations. Since the individual IHWH units cannot be cultured directly, it cannot be determined whether the units per se were contaminated or whether the problem was primarily in the distribution system and distal sites. In either case, it is apparent that such a system may become contaminated with *L. pneumophila*, particularly if maintained at temperatures that support the growth of *L. pneumophila* (1, 13). Therefore, placing an IHWH in a contaminated hot water system may not control or eliminate *L. pneumophila* colonization (8).

The relationship between the precipitous drop in city and hospital water pressure and contamination of the hospital water system, while speculative, is nonetheless appealing. While we do not have prior *Legionella* surveillance data for either the new or older building, the scenario at our facility is similar to that reported at Wadsworth Veterans Administration Medical Center (12). Additionally, nosocomial *L. pneumophila* serogroup 3 infections have been reported from a suburban community hospital in the Buffalo area (9). Most of the metropolitan Buffalo area is supplied with water from Lake Erie, though the City of Buffalo has a separate water distribution system.

We also have had to develop an effective system for controlling *Legionella* contamination in our hospital water supply. We considered both heat-flush and hyperchlorination control methods, but lingering concerns about water system damage and generation of trichloromethane with hyperchlorination made us favor the former (3, 5, 8). Use of the heat-flush approach resulted in negative routine surveillance cultures for approximately 18 months, but we have had instances of localized *Legionella* contamination, as noted above. The fact that the majority of sites tested have remained negative, and the observation that plumbing fixtures themselves may be colonized (2, 11, 14), has led us to change fixtures in an attempt at local control. Ongoing surveillance of these sites will determine the efficacy of this approach.

Finally, it is difficult to judge the overall efficacy of routine surveillance cultures for legionellae, since we have had positive clinical and environmental cultures in spite of multiple negative routine surveillance cultures. The room housing the most recent case is adjacent to several rooms that have been repeatedly negative on routine surveillance cultures. Routine surveillance may give rise to a false sense of security when cultures are negative but only a portion of sites housing susceptible patients are cultured. It appears that surveillance for legionellosis in compromised hosts may be as reliable as routine surveillance cultures in determining when recolonization of the distal portions of the hot water system has occurred (6).

REFERENCES

1. **Alary, M., and J. R. Joly.** 1992. Factors contributing to the contamination of hospital water distribution systems by Legionellae. *J. Infect. Dis.* **165:**565–569.
2. **Cordes, L. G., A. M. Wiesenthal, G. W. Gorman, J. P. Phair, H. M. Sommers, A. Brown, V. L. Yu, M. H. Magnussen, R. D. Meyer, J. S. Wolf, K. N. Shands, and D. W. Fraser.** 1981. Isolation of *Legionella pneumophila* from hospital shower heads. *Ann. Intern. Med.* **94:**195–197.
3. **Fraser, D. W.** 1985. Potable water as a source for legionellosis. *Environ. Health Perspect.* **62:**337–41.
4. **Helms, C. M., R. M. Massanari, R. Zeitler, S. Streed, M. J. R. Gilchrist, N. Hall, W. J. Hausler, Jr., J. Sywassink, W. Johnson, L. Wintermeyer, and W. J. Hierholtzer, Jr.** 1983. Legionnaires' disease associated with a hospital water system: a cluster of 24 nosocomial cases. *Ann. Intern. Med.* **99:**172–178.
5. **Helms, C. M., R. M. Massanari, R. P. Wenzel, M. A. Pfaller, N. P. Moyer, and N. Hall.** 1988. Legionnaires' disease associated with a hospital water system: a five-year progress report on continuous hyperchlorination. *JAMA* **259:**2423–2427.
6. **Marrie, T. J., S. MacDonald, K. Clarke, and D. Haldane.** 1991. Nosocomial legionnaires' disease: lessons from a four-year prospective study. *Am. J. Infect. Control* **19:**79–85.
7. **Muder, R. R., V. L. Yu, and A. H. Woo.** 1986. Mode of transmission of *Legionella pneumophila*. *Arch. Intern. Med.* **146:**1607–1612.
8. **Muraca, P. W., V. L. Yu, and A. Goetz.** 1990. Disinfection of water distribution systems for *Legionella*: a review of application procedures and methodologies. *Infect. Control Hosp. Epidemiol.* **11:**79–88.
9. **New York State Health Department.** Written communication.
10. **Nguyen, M. H., J. E. Stout, and V. L. Yu.** 1991. Legionellosis. *Infect. Dis. Clin. North Am.* **5:**561–584.
11. **Ribiero, C. D., S. H. Burge, S. R. Palmer, J. O. Tobin, and I. D. Watkins.** 1987. *Legionella pneumophila* in a hospital water system following a nosocomial outbreak: prevalence, monoclonal antibody subgrouping and effect of control measures. *Epidemiol. Infect.* **98:**253–262.
12. **Shands, K. N., J. L. Ho, R. D. Meyer, G. W. Gorman, P. H. Edelstein, G. F. Mallison, S. M. Finegold, and D. W. Fraser.** 1985. Potable water as a source of legionnaires' disease. *JAMA* **253:**1412–1416.
13. **Vickers, R. M., V. L. Yu, S. S. Hanna, P. Muraca, W. Diven, N. Carmen, and F. B. Taylor.** 1987. Determinants of *Legionella pneumophila* contamination of water distribution systems: 15-hospital prospective study. *Infect. Control* **8:**357–63.
14. **Wadowski, R. M., R. B. Yee, L. Mezmar, E. J. Wing, and J. N. Dowling.** 1982. Hot water systems as sources of *Legionella pneumophila* in hospital and nonhospital plumbing fixtures. *Appl. Environ. Microbiol.* **43:**1104–1110.

Community-Acquired Legionnaires Disease: a Reassessment

THOMAS J. MARRIE

Departments of Medicine and Microbiology, Dalhousie University and Victoria General Hospital, 1278 Tower Road, Halifax, Nova Scotia B3H 1V8, Canada

Community-acquired Legionnaires disease accounts for variable percentages of all cases of community-acquired pneumonia (CAP). In general, about 1 to 5% of cases of CAP are caused by *Legionella* spp. We prospectively studied all patients who were admitted to our hospital with CAP from November 1981 to June 1990. This study has allowed us to examine various aspects of community-acquired Legionnaires disease.

A research nurse interviewed all patients who were admitted to the Victoria General Hospital, Halifax, Nova Scotia, Canada, an 800-bed adult acute-care hospital, with a diagnosis of pneumonia as evidenced by acute onset of respiratory symptoms and at least one of the following physical findings: crackles, rhonchi, or consolidation. The details of the investigation of these patients and criteria for etiologic diagnosis of pneumonia have been previously described (1).

During the 8.5-year period of this study, 1,356 patients with CAP were admitted. Twenty-five (1.8%) had definite Legionnaires disease (confirmed by isolation of legionellae or a ≥4-fold rise in antibody titer), while nine (0.6%) had probable Legionnaires disease (evidenced by a high stable titer of ≥1:256). *Legionella* spp. were isolated from 11 patients (33%). *Legionella pneumophila* serogroup 1 was isolated from nine patients, and *L. micdadei* and *L. feelei* were isolated from one patient each. The mortality rate was 26%. A comparison of those who died with those who lived is given in Table 1.

Patients who died were more likely to receive assisted ventilation. Those with definite Legionnaires disease had a significantly higher temperature on admission: $39.1 \pm 0.83°C$ versus $37.33 \pm 1.11°C$ ($P < 0.001$). Microorganisms other than legionellae were isolated from the blood of three patients (*Haemophilus influenzae*, *Neisseria* sp., and *Streptococcus* sp. from one patient each).

TABLE 1. Comparison of 25 patients with community-acquired Legionnaires disease who survived this illness with 9 patients who died

Patient characteristic	Value for patients who:		P
	Lived ($n = 25$)	Died ($n = 9$)	
Mean age $\pm$ SD[a] (yr)	58.4 $\pm$ 19	68 $\pm$ 19	NS[b]
Legionellae were isolated (%)	7 (28)	4 (44)	NS
Received assisted ventilation (%)	4 (16)	8 (89)	<0.001
Did not receive erythromycin, rifampin, or tetracyclines (%)	10 (40)	3 (33)	NS
Mean temp $\pm$ SD (°C)	38.5 $\pm$ 1.2	39.1 $\pm$ 1	NS
Mean respiratory rate/min $\pm$ SD	30.4 $\pm$ 9.8	31.5 $\pm$ 10.8	NS
Mean pulse rate/min $\pm$ SD	101 $\pm$ 23.7	110 $\pm$ 43.8	NS
Mean serum albumin concn $\pm$ SD (g/ml)	26.8 $\pm$ 14.7	29.9 $\pm$ 6.0	NS
Mean leukocyte count $\pm$ SD (10^9/liter)	12.6 $\pm$ 6	9.2 $\pm$ 5	NS
Mean creatinine $\pm$ SD (mmol/liter)	123.5 $\pm$ 49	159.4 $\pm$ 87.5	NS

[a] SD, standard deviation.
[b] NS, not significant.

TABLE 2. Details of seven patients who were exposed to a hospital with endemic nosocomial Legionnaires disease prior to admission to our hospital with community-acquired Legionnaires disease

Patient	No. of days exposed to hospital prior to admission	Methods of diagnosis of *Legionella* infection	Reciprocal titer	
			Acute	Convalescent
1	Therapy in outpatient swimming pool	Isolation of *L. pneumophila*		
2	Discharged from hospital 16 days prior to admission	Serology	1,024	256
3	14	Serology	64	512
4	103	Serology	256	
5	26	Serology	<64	512
6	13	Serology	<64	512
7	13	Serology	64	512

Four patients had serological evidence of concomitant viral infection, one each with influenza A virus, influenza B virus, parainfluenza 1 virus, and respiratory syncytial virus.

Seven patients were exposed to a hospital with endemic nosocomial Legionnaires disease prior to admission to our hospital; however, six of seven were not exposed within 10 days before onset of symptoms (Table 2).

Our data indicate that *Legionella* spp. cause 2.4% of CAP infections and that only one-third of cases are diagnosed by culture. Some cases in our study of apparent community-acquired Legionnaires disease may actually have been nosocomially acquired. Patients who have been discharged from hospital within the past 2 weeks should be excluded from studies of CAP.

This research was supported by a grant from National Health and Welfare Canada.

REFERENCES

1. **Marrie, T. J., H. Durant, and L. Yates.** 1985. Community-acquired pneumonia requiring hospitalization: 5 year prospective study. *Rev. Infect. Dis.* **11**:586–599.

Nosocomial Legionellosis: a One-Year Case Control and Environmental Investigation

STEPHEN P. BLATT, MICHAEL D. PARKINSON, ELIZABETH PACE, PATRICIA HOFFMAN, DONNA DOLAN, PATRICIA LAUDERDALE, ROBERT A. ZAJAC, AND GREGORY P. MELCHER

Departments of Infectious Disease, Infection Control, and Microbiology, Wilford Hall USAF Medical Center, Lackland Air Force Base, Texas 78236-5300, and the Armstrong Laboratory, Epidemiology Division, Brooks Air Force Base, Texas 78235-5301

Since the original description of Legionnaires disease in Philadelphia in 1976 and the subsequent characterization of the etiologic agent, *Legionella pneumophila,* significant progress has been made in defining the epidemiology of infection with this agent (8). Despite this progress, however, nosocomial Legionnaires' disease (NLD) remains a significant problem, with many unresolved questions regarding transmission of the disease to patients (10). Recent studies have implicated aerosolization from showers or respiratory therapy devices, as well as aspiration, as possible mechanisms for disease acquisition (3, 5, 7). An outbreak of NLD associated with the potable water system in our hospital allowed us to study this mechanism in our patient population.

Background. Wilford Hall USAF Medical Center is a 1,000-bed multispecialty military hospital built in 1958 which maintains active programs in solid organ and bone marrow transplantation. During April 1989, two culture-proven cases of NLD occurred in transplant patients on different units. This outbreak prompted increased surveillance for the disease, resulting in the identification of 12 additional cases of NLD by the end of 1989. A case control and environmental investigation was performed to determine risk factors and sources for *Legionella* infection among hospitalized patients.

Case control study. A case of Legionnaires disease was defined as a radiographically documented pneumonia in association with one or more of the following tests: a fourfold or greater rise in titer of indirect fluorescent antibodies to a titer of 1:128 or greater, using a polyvalent antigen battery consisting of *Legionella pneumophila* serogroups 1 to 4 (Zeus Scientific Inc., Raritan, N.J.); a positive direct fluorescent antibody test of respiratory secretions or tissue, using a monoclonal antibody directed against all known serogroups of *L. pneumophila* (Genetic Systems, Seattle, Wash.); or isolation of *L. pneumophila* from respiratory secretions or tissue.

Clinical samples were plated on buffered charcoal-yeast extract and two selective media (Remel Inc., Lenexa, Kans.). Colonies compatible with *Legionella* species were studied with a monoclonal antibody directed against all known serogroups of *L. pneumophila* (Genetic Systems). Serogrouping and monoclonal antibody subtyping of *L. pneumophila* isolates were performed by the Special Pathogens Laboratory at the Pittsburgh Veterans Administration Hospital (Richard M. Vickers and Victor L. Yu) (6). Nonpneumonia control patients were selected and matched by age (±5 years), sex, and date of admission for each case patient in a ratio of 4:1. Attempts to match with respect to duration of hospitalization were not feasible because of the severity of illness and length of stay of case patients. Risk factors for the development of *Legionella* infection were identified by a thorough medical records review of case and control patients performed by Infectious Disease physicians and Infection Control nurses. The past medical history variables present prior to hospitalization and variables associated with hospital

TABLE 1. Univariate analysis of past medical history variables evaluated in the case control study

Risk	No. of cases (%)	No. of controls (%)	Odds ratio	95% Confidence interval
Immunosuppressive use[a]	8 (57)	2 (4)	32.7	4.5–302.6
Steroid use	8 (57)	4 (8)	15.7	2.9–93.1
Chronic renal failure	4 (29)	1 (2)	20.0	1.7–534.8
H_2-blocker use	8 (57)	10 (20)	5.3	1.3–23.3
Diabetes	1 (7)	1 (2)	3.8	0–156.2
Cancer	4 (29)	11 (22)	1.5	0.3–6.6
Dialysis	1 (7)	None	Undefined	Undefined
Cardiovascular disease	5 (36)	16 (31)	1.2	0.3–4.9
Chronic obstructive pulmonary disease	1 (7)	7 (14)	0.5	0–4.7

[a] $P < 0.05$ by sequential bivariate analysis of variables found to be significant in the univariate analysis.

exposure that were studied are shown in Tables 1 and 2. Odds ratios and 95% confidence intervals were calculated by using EPI INFO 5 software (USD, Inc., Stone Mountain, Ga.). Sequential bivariate analysis was performed to identify confounding among those variables that were significant in the univariate analysis.

During calendar year 1989, 14 pneumonia cases met the case definition for NLD. The mean age of case patients was 46.7 years (identical to that for controls), and the sex distribution was equally distributed. The mean duration of hospitalization prior to the onset of disease for case patients was 20.5 days, compared with 5.9 days of hospitalization for control patients. The diagnosis of NLD was confirmed by culture in 3 of the 12 case patients (25%) in whom appropriate cultures were performed, by serology in 4 of 12 cases (33%), and by direct fluorescent antibody test in 11 of 13 cases (85%, mean of 1.7 positive direct fluorescent antibody test specimens per case). All patient isolates were found to be *L. pneumophila* serogroup 1, monoclonal antibody subtype Philadelphia-1 (Ph1). The case fatality rate for patients in this study was 43%. Table 1 shows that in a univariate analysis, use of immunosuppressive therapy, corticosteroids, and H_2 blockers, as well as a history of chronic renal failure, appeared to be significant past medical history variables for the acquisition of NLD in our patients. After analysis for confounding variables, however, only the use of immunosuppressive therapy remained a significant past medical history variable ($P < 0.05$, sequential bivariate analysis). Table 2 demonstrates that of the hospital exposure variables present in the 10 days prior to onset of disease, the presence of a nasogastric (NG) tube, bed bathing, parenteral antibiotic use, nebulizer use, and oxygen use

TABLE 2. Univariate analysis of hospital exposure variables present in the 10 days prior to onset of Legionnaires disease

Exposure	No. of cases (%)	No. of controls (%)	Odds ratio	95% Confidence interval
NG tube[a]	6 (43)	2 (4)	18.4	2.6–166.2
Bed bathing[a]	11 (78)	13 (25)	10.7	2.2–59.0
Antibiotic use[a]	11 (78)	10 (20)	14.6	2.9–84.4
Nebulizer use	4 (29)	1 (2)	20.0	1.7–534.8
Oxygen use	6 (43)	6 (12)	5.6	1.2–27.7
Radiology	8 (57)	14 (27)	3.5	0.8–14.5
Endoscopy	1 (7)	2 (4)	1.8	0–30.7
Bronchoscopy	1 (7)	None	Undefined	Undefined
Pulmonary function tests	1 (7)	1 (2)	3.8	0–156.2
Endotracheal tube	6 (43)	13 (25)	2.2	0.5–8.9
Surgery	5 (36)	24 (47)	0.6	0.1–2.5
Emergency room	1 (7)	6 (12)	0.6	0–5.8
Ambulation	5 (36)	44 (86)	0.1	0–0.4
Showering	5 (36)	27 (53)	0.1	0–0.4

[a] $P < 0.05$ by sequential bivariate analysis of variables found to be significant in the univariate analysis.

appeared to be significant risk factors in a univariate analysis. After analysis for confounding factors, however, only the presence of an NG tube, bed bathing, and antibiotic use appeared to be significant ($P < 0.05$) hospital-associated risk factors for the acquisition of disease. Of note, showering was found to be a negative risk factor for the development of NLD in this study.

Environmental sampling. Air samples were obtained with an Anderson air sampler from four sites around the base of the cooling towers, at 18 air intakes of the hospital, and from the medical air and oxygen systems of the hospital. In addition, water mist samples were obtained from patient bathrooms with a settle plate technique, while the shower was running, in an attempt to isolate aerosolized organisms. We were unable to isolate any *Legionella* species from these air and water mist samples. Water samples were taken from the hospital groundwater, which is supplied by wells on the hospital grounds, from the hospital energy plant, from the two hot water tanks in the hospital, and from 85 patient rooms. *L. pneumophila* was isolated from the groundwater at the well head, from both hot water tanks, and from 24 (28%) of the patient rooms tested.

Serogrouping and monoclonal antibody subtyping revealed that the organisms from the groundwater well, from one of the hot water tanks, and from 13 patient rooms were *L. pneumophila* serogroup 1, Ph1, identical to our patient isolates. The second hot water tank and 11 patient rooms contained *L. pneumophila* serogroup 3. Quantitative analysis for the number of organisms present in potable water revealed 10^4 to 10^6 CFU of *L. pneumophila* per liter in the potable water system.

Conclusions. The case control portion of this study identified the presence of an NG tube, bed bathing, and antibiotic use, in the 10 days prior to the onset of disease, as significant hospital-associated risk factors for the acquisition of NLD. The finding of an association between antibiotic use and *Legionella* infection suggests that NLD may act as a superinfection following the eradication of normal flora by broad-spectrum antibiotics in hospitalized patients. H_2-blocker use, known to put patients at risk for colonization by other hospital-associated organisms (1) and to be associated with the acquisition of nosocomial pneumonia (4), was also found to be a significant univariate medical history risk factor for the acquisition of NLD in this study. Associations with antibiotic and H_2-blocker use would suggest that legionellae may colonize patients prior to causing invasive disease in the nosocomial setting. The presence of an NG tube is well known to predispose to aspiration events. The association noted in this study between NG tube use and NLD supports the concept that NLD may be acquired by aspiration in hospitalized patients. An association with bed bathing

would also be consistent with this hypothesis. Debilitated bed-bound patients who require bed bathing may be more likely to aspirate than are those who are able to get out of bed and take showers. Notably, patients able to take showers were relatively protected from *Legionella* infection in this study.

The isolation of identical strains of *L. pneumophilia* (serogroup 1, Ph1) in the groundwater supply to the hospital, potable water, and case patients implicates the potable water system as the source for legionellae in this outbreak. No *Legionella* organisms were isolated from any air samples, arguing against aerosolization as a mode of transmission of legionellae in this study. Although we did not demonstrate colonization by legionellae in uninfected patients, the risk factors identified in the case control portion of this study suggest that colonization from the potable water supply, followed by aspiration, likely represents the mode of transmission of legionellae in this outbreak. Future studies, directly demonstrating colonization of patients by legionellae, will be important to confirm this epidemiologic observation.

Medication nebulizers rinsed in tap water have recently been associated with an outbreak of NLD (7). Nebulizer use also appeared to be a significant univariate risk factor for NLD in our study, although only four patients (28%) were exposed to this variable. In a blinded survey of our own respiratory therapy personnel, 66% admitted to rinsing nebulizers in tap water. Although not the major mode of disease transmission in this study, nebulizer use may have contributed to the acquisition of NLD in these patients. We concur with the recommendation of Mastro et al. (7) that nebulizers not be rinsed with tap water.

Previous authors have speculated that legionellae gain access to the hospital potable water system from municipal water supplies and reservoirs (11). The discovery of the outbreak-related strain of *L. pneumophila* in the groundwater supply to our hospital provides evidence that external water supplies are the likely source of contamination for hospital water systems. Previous investigations of NLD have revealed *Legionella* concentrations of 10^4 to 10^6 CFU/liter in the potable water systems of affected hospitals (2, 7, 9). An identical burden of organisms found in this outbreak suggests that there may be a critical threshold of *Legionella* contamination that puts susceptible patients at risk for acquiring NLD. Future studies should include quantitative analysis of legionellae in the potable water systems of hospitals with and without cases of NLD.

REFERENCES

1. **Atherton, S. T., and D. J. White.** 1978. Stomach as source of bacteria colonizing respiratory tract during artificial ventilation. *Lancet* **ii:**968–969.

2. **Best, M., V. L. Yu, J. Stout, A. Goetz, R. R. Muder, and F. Taylor.** 1983. Legionellaceae in the hospital water supply: epidemiologic link with disease and evaluation of a method for control of nosocomial Legionnaires' disease and Pittsburgh pneumonia. *Lancet* **ii:**307–310.

3. **Breiman, R. F., B. S. Fields, G. N. Sanden, L. Volmer, A. Meier, and J. S. Spika.** 1990. Association of shower use with Legionnaires' disease: possible role of amoebae. *JAMA* **263:**2924–2926.

4. **Craven, D. E., L. M. Kunches, V. Kilinsky, D. A. Lichtenberg, B. J. Make, and W. R. McCabe.** 1986. Risk factors for pneumonia and fatality in patients receiving continuous mechanical ventilation. *Am. Rev. Respir. Dis.* **133:**792–796.

5. **Johnson, J. T., V. I. Yu, M. G. Best, et al.** 1985. Nosocomial legionellosis in surgical patients with head and neck cancer: implications for epidemiological reservoir and mode of transmission. *Lancet* **ii:**298–300.

6. **Joly, J. R., R. M. McKinney, J. O. Tobin, W. S. Bibb, D. Watkins, and D. Ramsey.** 1986. Development of a standardized subgrouping scheme for *Legionella pneu-* *mophila* serogroup 1 using monoclonal antibodies. *J. Clin. Microbiol.* **23:**768–771.

7. **Mastro, T. D., B. S. Fields, R. F. Breiman, J. Campbell, B. D. Plikaytis, and J. S. Spika.** 1991. Nosocomial Legionnaires' disease and use of medication nebulizers. *J. Infect. Dis.* **163:**667–671.

8. **McDade, J., C. Shepard, D. Fraser, et al.** 1977. Legionnaires' disease: isolation of a bacterium and demonstration of its role in other respiratory diseases. *N. Engl. J. Med.* **297:**1197–1203.

9. **Meenhorst, P. L., A. L. Reingold, D. G. Groothuis, et al.** 1985. Water related nosocomial pneumonia caused by *Legionella pneumophila* serogroups 1 and 10. *J. Infect. Dis.* 152:356–364.

10. **Reingold, A. L.** 1988. Role of legionella in acute infections of the lower respiratory tract. *Rev. Infect. Dis.* **10:**1018–1028.

11. **Stout, J., V. L. Yu, R. M. Vickers, et al.** 1982. Ubiquitousness of *Legionella pneumophila* in the water supply of a hospital with endemic Legionnaires' disease. *N. Engl. J. Med.* **306:**466–468.

Pontiac Fever in Children

RONALD J. FALLON, DAVID J. GOLDBERG, JOHN G. WRENCH, STEPHEN T. GREEN, AND JOHN A. N. EMSLIE

Department of Laboratory Medicine, Communicable Diseases (Scotland) Unit, and Department of Communicable and Tropical Diseases, Ruchill Hospital, Glasgow G20 9NB, and Forth Valley Health Board, Stirling FK8 1DX, Scotland

In the first week of January 1988, a large outbreak of Pontiac fever (Lochgoilhead fever) affected visitors to a hotel and leisure complex in Lochgoilhead, Scotland (6). It was estimated that more than 200 people visited the complex over the New Year holiday period, but only a very small number of these visitors were resident in the hotel and therefore had their names and addresses recorded. As a result of an extensive "snowball survey," 187 of the visitors were contacted and their medical histories were elicited. Among the 187 were 35 children aged under 14 years of age. Because of the way visitors were identified and contacted, this figure of 35 does not provide a firm data base for an exact calculation of the attack rate in children. Of the 187 visitors contacted, 170 had an acute illness characteristic of Pontiac fever (4).

Serological investigation showed that 60 to 72 symptomatic individuals seroconverted to *Legionella micdadei* antigen, and *L. micdadei* was isolated from a whirlpool spa which was the source of infection (2). Legionellosis in children is uncommon, and reports so far have been only of the pneumonic form of the disease, with the majority of persons involved being immunocompromised. In the Lochgoilhead outbreak, all of the children involved were previously healthy, and 31 of the 35 children became ill in the same period as did the rest of the patients.

Details of illness in the children were obtained from one or both parents, and serum was obtained from 12 of the 31 symptomatic and all 4 of the asymptomatic children for tests for antibody to *Legionella* species. Sera were examined for antibodies to all known human-pathogenic *Legionella* species (as of 1988) by the indirect fluorescent antibody test. The test employed was that using formolized yolk sac antigen (FYSA) (7) for *L. micdadei* for comparability of results with those obtained in laboratories in England, which used FYSA in the examination of sera from a small number of the patients domiciled there. Heated antigen (9) was used for examination for antibodies to other *Legionella* species. Tests performed on both antibody-positive and antibody-negative sera were found to give the same results with both FYSA and heated *L. micdadei* antigen. To validate the specificity of the antibody tests, sera from 31 residents of Lochgoilhead who had not visited the hotel and also from 100 healthy travelers were examined and found to be negative for antibodies to *L. micdadei* at a dilution of 16. The children were 2 to 13 years old; 15 were male, and 16 were female. The onset of illness was from 1 to 7 days (median, 3 days) after visiting the leisure complex, and the illness lasted for between 1 and 12 days (median, 2 days). The illness resembled that described in the adults, with headache being most common; the majority of patients reported having tiredness, fever, myalgia, and anorexia. Arthralgia and breathlessness were significantly less evident in children than in adults

(5). Antibody tests on serum samples from all 16 children examined showed a level of at least 64. It is of interest that the asymptomatic children developed antibody, which accords with the finding of antibody in some asymptomatic individuals examined in other outbreaks of Pontiac fever (3, 8). Ten of 13 asymptomatic adults were tested; two were serologically negative and five had elevated or rising titers of antibody to *L. micdadei*. Neither the children nor adults whose sera were examined showed a broad-spectrum antibody response to other *Legionella* species or serogroups, unlike the situation observed in some outbreaks of Legionnaires disease (1). In general, the nature of the illness in children was the same as that in adults and contrasts sharply with the rarity of Legionnaires disease in children compared with adults. This finding suggests that the factors which influence the attack rate of Legionnaires disease in a population may not be operative when one is faced with a microbial challenge leading to Pontiac fever. However, the only outbreak of Pontiac fever involving children has been that described here, which was due to *L. micdadei*, whereas most Legionnaires disease has been caused by *L. pneumophila*, mainly serogroup 1; therefore, direct comparison cannot be made. Nevertheless, the recognition of this difference may lead to investigations that can explain why there are two so very different manifestations of legionellosis and certainly renders the possibility of hypersensitivity due to prior contact as a factor in Pontiac fever most unlikely.

REFERENCES

1. **Fallon, R. J., and R. E. Johnston.** 1987. Heterogeneity of antibody response in infection with *Legionella pneumophila* serogroup 1. *J. Clin. Pathol.* **40:**569–572.
2. **Fallon, R. J., and T. J. Rowbotham.** 1990. Microbiological investigations into an outbreak of Pontiac fever due to *Legionella micdadei* associated with use of a whirlpool. *J. Clin. Pathol.* **43:**479–483.
3. **Friedman, S., K. Spitalny, J. Barbaree, Y. Faur, and R. McKinney.** 1987. Pontiac fever outbreak associated with a cooling tower. *Am. J. Public Health* **77:**568–571.
4. **Glick, T. H., M. B. Gregg, B. Berman, G. Mallison, W. W. Rhodes, Jr., and I. Kassanoff.** 1978. Pontiac fever. An epidemic of unknown etiology in a health department. 1. Clinical aspects. *Am. J. Epidemiol.* **107:**149–160.
5. **Goldberg, D. J., R. J. Fallon, S. T. Green, and J. G. Wrench.** 1992. Pontiac fever in children. *Pediatr. Infect. Dis. J.* **11:**240–241.
6. **Goldberg, D. J., J. G. Wrench, P. W. Collier, J. A. N. Emslie, R. J. Fallon, G. I. Forbes, T. M. McKay, A. C. Macpherson, T. A. Markwick, and D. Reid.** 1989. Lochgoilhead fever: outbreak of non-pneumonic legionellosis due to *Legionella micdadei*. *Lancet* **i:**316–318.
7. **Harrison, T. G., and A. G. Taylor.** 1988. The diagnosis of Legionnaires' disease by estimation of antibody levels, p. 113–135. *In* T. G. Harrison and A. G. Taylor (ed.), *A Laboratory Manual for Legionella*. Wiley, Chichester, England.
8. **Herwaldt, L. A., G. W. Gorman, T. McGrath, S. Toma, B. Brake, A. W. Hightower, J. Jones, A. L. Reingold, P. A. Boxer, P. Tang, C. W. Moss, H. W. Wilkinson, D. J. Brenner, A. G. Steigerwalt, and C. V. Broome.** 1984. A new *Legionella* species, *Legionella feeleii* species nova, causes Pontiac fever in an automobile plant. *Ann Intern. Med.* **100:**333–338.
9. **Wilkinson, H. W., B. J. Fikes, and D. D. Cruce.** 1979. Indirect immunofluorescent test for serodiagnosis of Legionnaires' disease. Evidence for serogroup diversity of Legionnaires' disease bacterial antigens and for multiple specificity of human antibodies *J. Clin. Microbiol.* **9:**379–383.

II. MOLECULAR AND CELL BIOLOGY OF *LEGIONELLA*

Toward an Understanding of Host and Bacterial Molecules Mediating *Legionella pneumophila* Pathogenesis

MARCUS A. HORWITZ

Division of Infectious Diseases, Department of Medicine, University of California, Los Angeles,
Los Angeles, California 90024

By the time of the 1983 International Symposium on *Legionella,* a good general picture of the immunobiology of *Legionella pneumophila* in the mammalian host had been obtained. It was known that the bacterium is an intracellular pathogen of the mononuclear phagocyte, chiefly monocytes and alveolar macrophages (41, 57), that the organism is phagocytized by host cells and resides intracellularly in a specialized phagosome that does not fuse with lysosomes or become highly acidified (35, 36, 38, 40), and that cell-mediated immunity rather than humoral immunity plays a central role in host defense against *L. pneumophila* as it does against other intracellular pathogens (37, 42–44). However, most of the knowledge about the immunobiology of *L. pneumophila* by 1983 was descriptive. What was lacking was an understanding of the molecular basis for the bacterium's interaction with its host cells and the immune system, i.e., of the key host and bacterial molecules that mediate *L. pneumophila* pathogenesis.

Since 1983, substantial progress has been made in understanding the molecular basis for *L. pneumophila* pathogenesis. This review summarizes these advances.

PHAGOCYTOSIS

L. pneumophila is phagocytized frequently but not exclusively by coiling phagocytosis, in which long phagocyte pseudopods coil around the organism as it is internalized (38). Phagocytosis by human monocytes is mediated by a three-component phagocytic system consisting of monocyte complement receptors CR1 and CR3, fragments of complement component C3, and the major outer membrane protein (MOMP) on the surface of *L. pneumophila* (3, 54, 62) (Fig. 1). C3 fixes selectively to MOMP by the alternative pathway of complement activation.

INTRACELLULAR PATHWAY

Inside mononuclear phagocytes, *L. pneumophila* resides in a phagosome that interacts sequentially with host cell smooth vesicles, mitochondria, and ribosomes until a ribosome-lined replicative vacuole is formed (Fig. 2) (35). As already noted, *L. pneumophila* inhibits phagosome-lysosome fusion and phagosome acidification (36, 40).

A mutant *L. pneumophila* that does not inhibit phagosome-lysosome fusion is avirulent for monocytes (39). Complementation of this mutant with wild-type DNA restores its capacity to inhibit phagosome-lysosome fusion, multiply intracellularly in human mononuclear phagocytes, and cause lethal pneumonia in guinea pigs (53).

ROLE OF IRON IN INTRACELLULAR MULTIPLICATION

Virtually all pathogens require iron, but *L. pneumophila* has a relatively high metabolic requirement for this metal ion. *L. pneumophila* acquires iron from the intermediate labile iron pool of the monocyte (17). The iron in this pool is derived from iron-transferrin via transferrin receptors, iron-lactoferrin via lactoferrin receptors, and the iron storage protein ferritin (17, 18, 20).

Agents that reduce the size of the intermediate labile iron pool of the monocyte inhibit *L. pneu-*

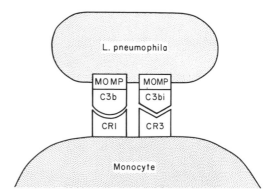

FIG. 1. Diagram illustrating a three-component phagocytic system that mediates phagocytosis of *L. pneumophila* by human monocytes.

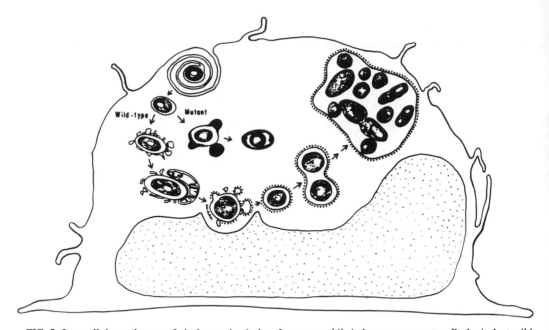

FIG. 2. Intracellular pathways of virulent and avirulent *L. pneumophila* in human monocytes. Both virulent wild-type *L. pneumophila* Philadelphia 1 strain and avirulent mutant 25D derived from it enter phagocytes by coiling phagocytosis. Thereafter, their pathways diverge. Wild-type *L. pneumophila* follows an intraphagosomal pathway in which the phagosome interacts sequentially with host cell smooth vesicles, mitochondria, and ribosomes but does not fuse with lysosomes. Avirulent *L. pneumophila* mutant 25D enters an intraphagolysosomal pathway in which the phagosome does not intereact with the various organelles that surround wild-type phagosomes but does fuse with lysosomes. Wild-type *L. pneumophila* multiplies in the ribosome-lined phagosome until its destroys the monocyte. Mutant 25D remains alive but unable to multiply in the phagolysosome.

mophila intracellular multiplication. Three different types of agents inhibit *L. pneumophila* multiplication in this way. First, the iron chelators, including the nonphysiologic iron chelator deferoxamine and the physiologic iron chelator apolactoferrin, reduce the iron pool by chelating iron within it (17, 20). Second, the weak bases chloroquine and ammonium chloride reduce the iron pool by blocking the pH-dependent release of iron from endocytized iron-transferrin and the pH-dependent proteolysis and release of iron from iron-lactoferrin and ferritin (19). Third, gamma interferon (IFN-γ) reduces iron availability by down-regulating transferrin receptor expression and intracellular ferritin concentration (17, 18).

How *L. pneumophila* internalizes iron remains unknown; possibly, its iron reductase plays a role (48). The iron incorporated into *L. pneumophila* is found in seven major iron-containing proteins, one of which is an iron superoxide dismutase (55). The major iron-containing protein (MICP) of *L. pneumophila* grown on agar has an apparent molecular mass of 210 kDa under nondenaturing conditions and 85 to 90 kDa under denaturing conditions (55). MICP retains iron under mild de-naturing conditions (55). MICP is homologous with *Escherichia coli* aconitase and the human iron responsive element binding protein (54a).

CELL-MEDIATED IMMUNITY

As noted above, the host defends itself against *L. pneumophila* by cell-mediated immune mechanisms. Three different types of cell-mediated immune mechanisms have been studied. First, activated human monocytes and alveolar macrophages, including those activated by IFN-γ, have been shown to inhibit *L. pneumophila* intracellular multiplication (4, 5, 44, 47, 56, 57). Second, polymorphonuclear leukocytes (PMN) activated by IFN-γ and tumor necrosis factor have been found to have an enhanced capacity to kill *L. pneumophila* (7). However, killing was modest and required several days, raising some question as to the significance of this immune mechanism. Third, interleukin-2-activated killer cells from nonimmune subjects have been studied by two groups for their capacity to kill *L. pneumophila*. One group reported positive results, and the other reported negative results (8, 75). Whether antigen-specific cytotoxic lymphocytes capable of lysing infected macrophages are generated in Legionnaires disease remains to be determined.

MECHANISMS OF MACROPHAGE ACTIVATION

Activated mononuclear phagocytes inhibit *L. pneumophila* multiplication in two ways. First, they phagocytize about 50% fewer *L. pneumophila*, thereby restricting access of the bacteria to the intracellular milieu that they require for multiplication (44). The mechanism for this process likely involves IFN-γ-mediated down-regulation of the function of complement receptors that mediate phagocytosis of *L. pneumophila* (62, 69). Second, activated monocytes and macrophages markedly slow the multiplication rate of bacteria that are internalized (44). As noted above, IFN-γ-activated monocytes do so by limiting the availability of iron to intracellular *L. pneumophila*, which occurs as a consequence of IFN-γ-induced coordinate down-regulation of transferrin receptor expression and intracellular ferritin concentration (17, 18, 20a).

PMN-MONOCYTE COOPERATION

PMN are prominent in histological specimens from the lungs of patients with Legionnaires disease, and studies of PMN-depleted guinea pigs challenged with *L. pneumophila* indicate that PMN play an important role in host defense; such guinea pigs have greater susceptibility to infection, higher numbers of *L. pneumophila* in their lungs, and higher mortality than do control animals (31). Yet in in vitro studies, human PMN lack the capacity to kill appreciable numbers of *L. pneumophila*, even in the presence of anti-*L. pneumophila* antibody and complement (42) or when activated with IFN-γ and tumor necrosis factor (7). The finding that apolactoferrin inhibits *L. pneumophila* intracellular multiplication in human monocytes has raised the possibility that PMN play a role in host defense by cooperating with monocytes (20). Apolactoferrin is a major protein in the specific granules of PMN that is released at sites of inflammation, such as occurs in the *L. pneumophila*-infected lung. By providing infected mononuclear phagocytes with apolactoferrin and thereby allowing them to inhibit *L. pneumophila* intracellular multiplication, PMN may play an important indirect role in host defense against *L. pneumophila* (20) (Fig. 3).

IMMUNOPROTECTION

Four different antigenic preparations have been shown to induce strong cell-mediated immune responses, manifest by cutaneous delayed-type hypersensitivity and splenic lymphocyte proliferation, and strong protective immunity in the guinea pig model of Legionnaires disease: the avirulent mutant described above that fails to inhibit phagosome-lysosome fusion; *L. pneumophila* membranes; the 39-kDa major secretory protein (MSP) of *L. pneumophila*; and the major cytoplasmic membrane protein (MCMP) of *L. pneumophila*, a genus-common antigen and member of the Hsp60 family of heat shock proteins (9–12, 12a, 14). The MSP is able to induce protective immunity across serogroups of *L. pneumophila* and in some cases across species of *Legionella* (11). Interestingly, although MSP is a highly potent immunoprotec-

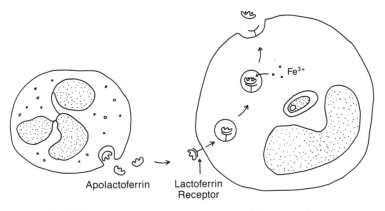

PMN   Monocyte

FIG. 3. Potential PMN-monocyte cooperation in host defense against *L. pneumophila*. Apolactoferrin is released by PMN at sites of inflammation. Apolactoferrin is endocytized by lactoferrin receptors on the surface of monocytes. By chelating iron in the intracellular labile iron pool of the cell, apolactoferrin inhibits *L. pneumophila* intracellular multiplication. Thus, PMN may play an indirect role in host defense by providing monocytes with apolactoferrin in the *L. pneumophila*-infected lung.

TABLE 1. Characteristics of *L. pneumophila* MSP

Characteristic	Reference
Biologic	
Major secretory protein	39
Zinc metalloprotease	27
Weak hemolytic activity	49
Cytotoxic for CHO cells	49
Genetic, immunologic, and cytoxic differences among species	63
Structurally and functionally homologous to *Pseudomonas aeruginosa* elastase	6
Produced intracellularly in monocytes	25
Immunologic	
Protective immunogen	10
Cross-serogroup and variable cross-species protection	12
Virulence	
Not virulence determinant in human mononuclear phagocytes	72
Not virulence determinant in guinea pigs	13
Homologous with zinc metalloprotease and potential virulence determinant of fish pathogen *Vibrio anguillarum*	59

tive molecule, it is not a virulence determinant in the guinea pig model of Legionnaires disease (13). Isogenic MSP$^+$ and MSP$^-$ strains of *L. pneumophila* have the same 50% and 100% lethal doses for guinea pigs, multiply at the same rate in the guinea pig lung, and cause indistinguishable pathologic lesions in the lung.

MSP has been extensively studied. Its major characteristics are summarized in Table 1.

ANTIGEN PROCESSING AND PRESENTATION

The finding that MSP is not a virulence determinant demonstrates that an immunoprotective molecule need not be a virulence determinant. What it presumably must be is a molecule that allows the immune system, especially lymphocytes, to recognize infected host cells and mount an effective antimicrobial defense against them. This assumption lead us to postulate that MSP is released by *L. pneumophila* in infected monocytes and subsequently processed and presented on the surface of the monocytes in association with major histocompatibility complex (MHC) molecules. Consistent with this hypothesis, immunohistochemical and immunoelectron microscopy studies using affinity-purified anti-MSP antibody have demonstrated that *L. pneumophila* produces MSP and releases it into its phagosome in infected human monocytes (25). It is not released by *L. pneumophila* in the presence of erythromycin, which blocks bacterial protein synthesis and inhibits *L. pneumophila* intracellular multiplication (4, 45).

Interestingly, immunoelectron microscopy studies have demonstrated that MHC class I and II molecules are scarce on the membrane of phago-

somes containing *L. pneumophila* (26a). Such molecules are excluded from the phagosome during coiling phagocytosis of *L. pneumophila* (26). This finding suggests that immunogenic epitopes of MSP may not bind to MHC molecules in the phagosome but may bind elsewhere in the cell in an extraphagosomal compartment.

VIRULENCE DETERMINANTS

Only one *L. pneumophila* molecule, the Mip protein, has been rigorously shown to be a virulence determinant. This 24-kDa protein is required for the full expression of virulence of *L. pneumophila* in mononuclear phagocytes and guinea pigs (22, 23). Interestingly, Mip recently has been shown to inhibit protein kinase C activity (46).

Several other molecules of *L. pneumophila* that are potentially important to pathogenesis have been isolated. Biologic and immunologic characteristics of these molecules are summarized in Table 2. In addition, two molecules from *Legionella micdadei* are of potential significance. First, a protein kinase of apparent molecular mass 35 kDa catalyzes phosphorylation of PMN proteins, including tubulin, and phosphatidylinositol (66). Second, an acid phosphatase of apparent molecular mass 68 kDa inhibits superoxide production by human PMN and dephosphorylates phosphatidylinositol biphosphate (64, 65).

CONCLUSION

Substantial strides have been made in understanding key host and bacterial molecules that mediate *L. pneumophila* pathogenesis. However,

TABLE 2. *L. pneumophila* molecules of potential importance to pathogenesis

Molecule	Subunit apparent molecular mass (kDa)	Characteristic(s)	Reference(s)
Flagellin	47	Common antigen in serogroups 1–3	28
Legiolysin	39	Hemolytic activity	73
		Tyrosine-dependent browning and yellow-green fluorescence	73
Lipopolysaccharide	Variable	Weak endotoxin activity in vivo	74
		Predominant molecule recognized by human antiserum	32
		Serogroup-specific antigen	24, 60
		Complex and unusual structure that lacks lipid A moieties essential for maximal endotoxic effects	71
MCMP	58/60/65	Major cytoplasmic membrane protein	33
		Predominant protein recognized by human antiserum	33, 68
		Genus-common antigen	61, 68
		Heat shock protein	50, 51
		Member Hsp60/65 family	70
		Protective immunogen	12a
		Gene cloned and sequenced	34, 67
MICP	85/90	Major iron-containing protein on solid medium	55
		Aconitase activity	54a
		Homologous with *E. coli* aconitase and human iron responsive element binding protein	54a
		Gene cloned and sequenced	54a
Mip	24	Potentiates infection of human mononuclear phagocytes	23
		Virulence determinant in guinea pigs	22
		Protein kinase C-inhibitory activity	46
		Conserved throughout genus	21
		L. pneumophila and *L. micdadei* gene sequenced	2, 29
MOMP	25/29	Cation-selective porin	32
		Genus-specific epitope	16
		Species-specific epitope	58
		C3 acceptor molecule	3
MSP	38/39	See Table 1	
PBP	31	Peptidoglycan-bound protein	15
PAL	19	Peptidoglycan-associated lipoprotein	30, 52
Phospholipase C	50/54	Hydrolyzes phosphatidylcholine	1

large gaps in our knowledge remain. For example, molecules that mediate the selection of the intra-phagosomal pathway, inhibition of phagosome-lysosome fusion, and inhibition of phagosome acidification; molecules that mediate iron uptake; iron-containing molecules; immunoprotective molecules in addition to MSP; and virulence determinants in addition to Mip remain to be identified and characterized.

I am Gordon MacDonald Scholar at UCLA. This work was supported by grants AI22421 and AI28825 from the National Institutes of Health.

REFERENCES

1. **Baine, W. B.** 1988. A phospholipase C from the Dallas 1E strain of *Legionella pneumophila* serogroup 5: purification and characterization of conditions for optimal activity with an artificial substrate. *J. Gen. Microbiol.* **134:**489–498.

2. **Bangsborg, J. M., N. P. Cianciotto, and P. Henderson.** 1991. Nucleotide sequence analysis of the *Legionella micdadei* Mip gene, encoding a 30-kilodalton analog of the *Legionella pneumophila* Mip protein. *Infect. Immun.* **59:**3836–3840.

3. **Bellinger-Kawahara, C., and M. A. Horwitz.** 1990. Complement component C3 fixes selectively to the major outer membrane protein (MOMP) of *Legionella pneumophila* and mediates phagocytosis of liposome-MOMP complexes by human monocytes. *J. Exp. Med.* **172:**1201–1210.

4. **Bhardwaj, N., and M. A. Horwitz.** 1988. Gamma interferon and antibiotics fail to act synergistically to kill *Legionella pneumophila* in human monocytes. *J. Interferon Res.* **8:**283–293.

5. **Bhardwaj, N., T. Nash, and M.A. Horwitz.** 1986. Gamma interferon-activated human monocytes inhibit the intracellular multiplication of *Legionella pneumophila*. *J. Immunol.* **137:**2662–2664.

6. **Black, W. J., F. D. Quinn, and L. S. Tompkins.** 1989. *Legionella pneumophila* zinc metalloprotease is structurally and functionally homologous to *Pseudomonas aeruginosa* elastase. *J. Bacteriol.* **172:**2608–2613.

7. **Blanchard, D. K., H. Friedman, T. W. Klein, and J. Y. Djeu.** 1989. Induction of interferon-gamma and tumor necrosis factor by *Legionella pneumophila*: augmentation of human neutrophil bacteridical activity. *J. Leukocyte Biol.* **45:**538–545.

8. **Blanchard, D. K., W. E. Stewart II, T. W. Klein, H. Friedman, and J. Y. Djeu.** 1987. Cytolytic activity of human peripheral blood leukocytes against *Legionella pneumophila*-infected monocytes: characterization of the effector cell and augmentation by interleukin 2. *J. Immunol.* **139:**551–556.

9. **Blander, S. J., R. F. Breiman, and M. A. Horwitz.** 1989. A live avirulent mutant *Legionella pneumophila* vaccine induces protective immunity against lethal aerosol challenge. *J. Clin. Invest.* **83:**810–815.

10. **Blander, S. J., and M. A. Horwitz.** 1989. Vaccination with the major secretory protein of *Legionella pneumophila* induces cell-mediated and protective immunity in a guinea pig model of Legionnaires' disease. *J. Exp. Med.* **169:**691–705.

11. **Blander, S. J., and M. A. Horwitz.** 1991. Vaccination with *Legionella pneumophila* membranes induces cell mediated and protective immunity in a guinea pig model of Legionnaires' disease. *J. Clin. Invest.* **87:**1054–1059.

12. **Blander, S. J., and M. A. Horwitz.** 1991. Vaccination with the major secretory protein of Legionella induces humoral and cell-mediated immune responses and protective immunity across different serogroups of *Legionella pneumophila* and different species of Legionella. *J. Immunol.* **147:**285–291.

12a. **Blander, S. J., and M. A. Horwitz.** The major cytoplasmic membrane protein of *Legionella pneumophila*, a genus common antigen and member of the hsp 60 family of heat shock proteins, induces protective immunity in a guinea pig model of Legionnaires' disease. *J. Clin. Invest.*, in press.

13. **Blander, S. J., L. Szeto, H. A. Shuman, and M. A. Horwitz.** 1990. An immunoprotective molecule, the major secretory protein of *Legionella pneumophila*, is not a virulence factor in a guinea pig model of Legionnaires' disease. *J. Clin. Invest.* **86:**817–824.

14. **Breiman, R. F., and M. A. Horwitz.** 1987. Guinea pigs sublethally infected with aerosolized *Legionella pneumophila* develop humoral and cell-mediated immune responses and are protected against lethal aerosol challenge. A model for studying host defense against lung infections

caused by intracellular pathogens. *J. Exp. Med.* **164:**799–811.

15. **Butler, C. A., and P. S. Hoffman.** 1990. Characterization of a major 31-kilodalton peptidoglycan-bound protein of *Legionella pneumophila*. *J. Bacteriol.* **172:**2401–2407.

16. **Butler, C. A., E. D. Street, T. P. Hatch, and P. S. Hoffman.** 1985. Disulfide-bonded outer membrane proteins in the genus *Legionella*. *Infect. Immun.* **48:**14–18.

17. **Byrd, T. F., and M. A. Horwitz.** 1989. Interferon gamma-activated human monocytes down-regulate transferrin receptors and inhibit the intracellular multiplication of *Legionella pneumophila* by limiting the availability of iron. *J. Clin. Invest.* **83:**1457–1465.

18. **Byrd, T. F., and M. A. Horwitz.** 1990. Interferon gamma-activated human monocytes downregulate the intracellular concentration of ferritin: a potential new mechanism for limiting iron availability to *Legionella pneumophila* and subsequently inhibiting intracellular multiplication. *Clin. Res.* **38:**481A.

19. **Byrd, T. F., and M. A. Horwitz.** 1991. Chloroquine inhibits the intracellular multiplication of *Legionella pneumophila* by limiting the availability of iron. A potential new mechanism for the therapeutic effect of chloroquine against intracellular pathogens. *J. Clin. Invest.* **88:**351–357.

20. **Byrd, T. F., and M. A. Horwitz.** 1991. Lactoferrin inhibits or promotes *Legionella pneumophila* intracellular multiplication in nonactivated and interferon gamma activated human monocytes depending upon its degree of iron saturation. Iron-lactoferrin and nonphysiologic iron chelates reverse monocyte activation against *Legionella pneumophila*. *J. Clin. Invest.* **88:**1103–1112.

20a. **Byrd, T. F., and M. A. Horwitz.** Regulation of transferrin receptor expression and ferritin content in human mononuclear phagocytes: coordinate upregulation by iron-transferrin and downregulation by interferon gamma. *J. Clin. Invest.*, in press.

21. **Cianciotto, N. P., J. M. Bangsborg, B. I. Eisenstein, and N. C. Engleberg.** 1990. Identification of *mip*-like genes in the genus *Legionella*. *Infect. Immun.* **58:**2912–2918.

22. **Cianciotto, N. P., B. I. Eisenstein, C. H. Mody, and N. C. Engleberg.** 1990. A mutation in the mip gene results in an attenuation of *Legionella pneumophila* virulence. *J. Infect. Dis.* **162:**121–126.

23. **Cianciotto, N. P., B. I. Eisenstein, C. H. Mody, G. B. Toews, and N. C. Engleberg.** 1989. A *Legionella pneumophila* gene encoding a species-specific surface protein potentiates initiation of intracellular infection. *Infect. Immun.* **57:**1255–1262.

24. **Ciesielski, C. A., M. J. Blaser, and W.-L. L. Wong.** 1986. Serogroup specificity of *Legionella pneumophila* is related to lipopolysaccharide characteristics. *Infect. Immun.* **51:**397–404.

25. **Clemens, D. L., and M. A. Horwitz.** 1990. Demonstration that *Legionella pneumophila* produces its major secretory protein in infected human monocytes and localization of the protein by immunocytochemistry and immunoelectron microscopy. *Clin. Res.* **38:**480A.

26. **Clemens, D. L., and M. A. Horwitz.** 1992. Membrane sorting during phagocytosis: selective exclusion of MHC molecules but not complement receptor CR3 during conventional and coiling phagocytosis. *J. Exp. Med.* **175:**1317–1326.

26a. **Clemens, D. L., and M. A. Horwitz.** Unpublished data.

27. **Dreyfus, L. A., and B. H. Iglewski.** 1986. Purification and characterization of an extracellular protease of *Legionella pneumophila*. *Infect. Immun.* **51:**736–743.

28. **Elliott, J. A., and W. Johnson.** 1981. Immunological and biochemical relationships among flagella isolated from *Legionella pneumophila* serogroups 1, 2 and 3. *Infect. Immun.* **33:**602–610.

29. **Engleberg, N. C., C. Carter, D. R. Weber, N. P. Cianciotto, and B. I. Eisenstein.** 1989. DNA sequence of *mip*, a *Legionella pneumophila* gene associated with macro-

phage infectivity. *Infect. Immun.* **57**:1263–1270.

30. **Engleberg, N. C., D. C. Howe, J. E. Rogers, J. Arroyo, and B. I. Eisenstein.** 1991. Characterization of a *Legionella pneumophila* gene encoding a lipoprotein antigen. *Mol. Microbiol.* **5**:2021–2029.

31. **Fitzgeorge, R. B., A. S. R. Featherstone, and A. Baskerville.** 1988. Effects of polymorphonuclear leukocyte depletion on the pathogenesis of experimental Legionnaires' disease. *Br. J. Exp. Pathol.* **69**:105–112.

32. **Gabay, J. E., M. S. Blake, W. Niles, and M. A. Horwitz.** 1985. Purification of the major outer membrane protein of *Legionella pneumophila* and demonstration that it is a porin. *J. Bacteriol.* **162**:85–91.

33. **Gabay, J. E., and M. A. Horwitz.** 1985. Isolation and characterization of the cytoplasmic and outer membranes of the Legionnaires' disease bacterium (*Legionella pneumophila*). *J. Exp. Med.* **161**:409–422.

34. **Hoffman, P. S., L. Houston, and C. A. Butler.** 1990. *Legionella pneumophila htpAB* heat shock operon: nucleotide sequence and expression of the 60-kilodalton antigen in *L. pneumophila*-infected HeLa cells. *Infect. Immun.* **58**:3380–3387.

35. **Horwitz, M. A.** 1983. Formation of a novel phagosome by the Legionnaires' disease bacterium (*Legionella pneumophila*) in human monocytes. *J. Exp. Med.* **158**:1319–1331.

36. **Horwitz, M. A.** 1983. The Legionnaires' disease bacterium (*Legionella pneumophila*) inhibits phagosome-lysosome fusion in human monocytes. *J. Exp. Med.* **158**:2108–2126.

37. **Horwitz, M. A.** 1983. Cell-mediated immunity in Legionnaires' disease. *J. Clin. Invest.* **71**:1686–1697.

38. **Horwitz, M. A.** 1984. Phagocytosis of the Legionnaires' disease bacterium (*Legionella pneumophila*) occurs by a novel mechanism: engulfment within a pseudopod coil. *Cell* **36**:27–33.

39. **Horwitz, M. A.** 1987. Characterization of avirulent mutant *Legionella pneumophila* that survive but do not multiply within human monocytes. *J. Exp. Med.* **166**:1310–1328.

40. **Horwitz, M. A., and F. R. Maxfield.** 1984. *Legionella pneumophila* inhibits acidification of its phagosome in human monocytes. *J. Cell Biol.* **99**:1936–1943.

41. **Horwitz, M. A., and S. C. Silverstein.** 1980. The Legionnaires' disease bacterium (*Legionella pneumophila*) multiplies intracellularly in human monocytes. *J. Clin. Invest.* **66**:441–450.

42. **Horwitz, M. A., and S. C. Silverstein.** 1981. Interaction of the Legionnaires' disease bacterium (*Legionella pneumophila*) with human phagocytes. I. *L. pneumophila* resists killing by polymorphonuclear leukocytes, antibody, and complement. *J. Exp. Med.* **153**:386–397.

43. **Horwitz, M. A., and S. C. Silverstein.** 1981. Interaction of the Legionnaires' disease bacterium (*Legionella pneumophila*) with human phagocytes. II. Antibody promotes binding of *L. pneumophila* to monocytes but does not inhibit intracellar multiplication. *J. Exp. Med.* **153**:398–406.

44. **Horwitz, M. A., and S. C. Silverstein.** 1981. Activated human monocytes inhibit the intracellular multiplication of Legionnaires' disease bacteria. *J. Exp. Med.* **154**:1618–1635.

45. **Horwitz, M. A., and S. C. Silverstein.** 1983. The intracellular multiplication of Legionnaires' disease bacteria (*Legionella pneumophila*) in human monocytes is reversibly inhibited by erythromycin and rifampin. *J. Clin. Invest.* **71**:15–26.

46. **Hurley, M., K. Balazovich, M. Albano, N. C. Engleberg, and B. I. Eisenstein.** 1992. *Legionella pneumophila* Mip inhibits protein kinase C, p. 9, abstr. 6. *Program Abstr. 1992 Int. Symp. Legionella.*

47. **Jensen, W. A., R. M. Rose, A. S. Wasserman, T. H. Kalb, K. Anton, and H. G. Remond.** 1987. *In vitro* activation of the antibacterial activity of human pulmonary macrophages by recombinant gamma interferon. *J. Infect. Dis.* **155**:574–577.

48. **Johnson, W., L. Varner, and M. Poch.** 1991. Acquisition of iron by *Legionella pneumophila:* role of iron reductase. *Infect. Immun.* **59**:2376–2381.

49. **Keen, M. G., and P. S. Hoffman.** 1989. Characterization of a *Legionella pneumophila* extracellular protease exhibiting hemolytic and cytotoxic activities. *Infect. Immun.* **57**:732–738.

50. **Lema, M. W., A. Brown, C. A. Butler, and P. S. Hoffman.** 1988. Heat-shock response in *Legionella pneumophila. Can. J. Microbiol.* **34**:1148–1153.

51. **Lema, M. W., A. Brown, and G. C. C. Chen.** 1986. Altered rate of synthesis of specific peptides in the legionellae in response to growth temperature. *Curr. Microbiol.* **12**:347–352.

52. **Ludwig, B., A. Schmid, R. Marre, and J. Hacker.** 1991. Cloning, genetic analysis, and nucleotide sequence of a determinant coding for a 19-kilodalton peptidoglycan-associated protein (Pp1) of *Legionella pneumophila. Infect. Immun.* **59**:2515–2521.

53. **Marra, A., S. J. Blander, M. A. Horwitz, and H. A. Shuman.** 1992. Identification of a *Legionella pneumophila* locus required for intracellular multiplication in human macrophages. *Proc. Natl. Acad. Sci. USA* **89**:9607–9611.

54. **Marra, A., M. A. Horwitz, and H. A. Shuman.** 1990. The HL-60 model for the interaction of human macrophages with the Legionnaires' disease bacterium. *J. Immunol.* **144**:2738–2744.

54a. **Mengaud, J. M., and M. A. Horwitz.** Unpublished data.

55. **Mengaud, J. M., P. van Schie, T. F. Byrd, and M. A. Horwitz.** 1992. Major iron-binding proteins of *Legionella pneumophila*, p. 14, abstr. I-13. *Program Abstr. Int. Symp. Legionella.*

56. **Nash, T., D. M. Libby, and M. A. Horwitz.** 1988. Gamma interferon activated human alveolar macrophages inhibit the intracellular multiplication of *Legionella pneumophila. J. Immunol.* **140**:3978–3981.

57. **Nash, T. W., D. M. Libby, and M. A. Horwitz.** 1984. Interaction between the Legionnaires' disease bacterium (*Legionella pneumophila*) and human alveolar macrophages. Influence of antibody, lymphokines, and hydrocortisone. *J. Clin. Invest.* **74**:771–782.

58. **Nolte, F. S., and C. A. Conlin.** 1986. Major outer membrane protein of *Legionella pneumophila* carries a species-specific epitope. *J. Clin. Microbiol.* **23**:643–646.

59. **Norquist, A., B. Norrman, and H. Wolf-Watz.** 1990. Identification and characterization of a zinc metalloprotease associated with invasion by the fish pathogen *Vibrio anguillarum. Infect. Immun.* **58**:3731–3736.

60. **Otten, S., S. Lyer, W. Johnson, and R. Montgomery.** 1986. Serospecific antigens of *Legionella pneumophila. J. Bacteriol.* **167**:893–904.

61. **Pau, C.-P., B. B. Plikaytis, G. M. Carlone, and I. M. Warner.** 1988. Purification, partial characterization, and seroreactivity of a genuswide 60-kilodalton *Legionella* protein antigen. *J. Clin. Microbiol.* **26**:67–71.

62. **Payne, N. R., and M. A. Horwitz.** 1987. Phagocytosis of *Legionella pneumophila* is mediated by human monocyte complement receptors. *J. Exp. Med.* **166**:1377–1389.

63. **Quinn, F. D., M. G. Keen, and L. S. Tompkins.** 1989. Genetic, immunological, and cytotoxic comparisons of *Legionella* proteolytic activities. *Infect. Immun.* **57**:2719–2725.

64. **Saha, A. K., J. N. Dowling, K. L. LaMacro, S. Das, A. T. Remaley, N. Olomu, M. T. Pope, and R. H. Glew.** 1985. Properties of an acid phosphatase from *Legionella micdadei* which blocks superoxide anion production by human neutrophils. *Arch. Biochem. Biophys.* **243**:150–160.

65. **Saha, A. K., J. N. Dowling, A. W. Pasculle, and R. H. Glew.** 1988. *Legionella micdadei* phosphatase catalyzes the hydrolysis of phosphatidylinositol 4,5-bisphosphate in human neutrophils. *Arch. Biochem. Biophys.* **265**:94–104.

66. **Saha, A. K., J. W. Dowling, N. K. Mukhopadhyay, and R. H. Glew.** 1989. *Legionella micdadei* protein kinase catalyzes phosphorylation of tubulin and phosphatidylinositol. *J. Bacteriol.* **171**:5103–5110.

67. **Sampson, J. S., S. P. O'Connor, B. P. Holloway, B. B. Plikaytis, G. M. Carlone, and L. W. Mayer.** 1990. Nucleotide sequence of *htpB*, the *Legionella pneumophila* gene encoding the 58-kilodalton (kDa) common antigen, formerly designated the 60-kDa common antigen. *Infect. Immun.* **58:**3380–3387.

68. **Sampson, J. S., B. B. Plikaytis, and H. W. Wilkinson.** 1986. Immunologic response of patients with legionellosis against major protein-containing antigens of *Legionella pneumophila* serogroup 1 as shown by immunoblot analysis. *J. Clin. Microbiol.* **23:**92–99.

69. **Schlesinger, L. S., and M. A. Horwitz.** 1991. Phagocytosis of *Mycobacterium leprae* by human monocyte-derived macrophages is mediated by complement receptors CR1 (CD35), CR3 (CD11b/CD18), and CR4 (CD11c/CD18) and interferon gamma activation inhibits complement receptor function and phagocytosis of this bacterium. *J. Immunol.* **147:**1983–1994.

70. **Shinnick, T. M., M. H. Vodkin, and J. C. Williams.** 1988. The *Mycobacterium tuberculosis* 65-kilodalton antigen is a heat shock protein which corresponds to common antigen and to the *Escherichia coli* GroEL protein. *Infect. Immun.* **56:**446–451.

71. **Sonesson, A., E. Jantzen, K. Bryn, L. Larsson, and J. Eng.** 1989. Chemical composition of a lipopolysaccharide from *Legionella pneumophila*. *Arch. Microbiol.* **153:**72–78.

72. **Szeto, L., and H. A. Shuman.** 1990. The *Legionella pneumophila* major secretory protein, a protease, is not required for intracellular growth or cell killing. *Infect. Immun.* **58:**2585–2593.

73. **Wintermeyer, E., U. Rdest, B. Ludwig, A Debes, and J. Hacker.** 1991. Cloning and characterization of a DNA sequence, termed legiolysin (lly), responsible for hemolytic activity, color production and fluorescence of *Legionella pneumophila*. *Mol. Microbiol.* **5:**1135–1143.

74. **Wong, K. H., C. W. Moss, D. H. Hochstein, R. J. Arko, and W. O. Schalla.** 1979. "Endotoxicity" of the Legionnaires' disease bacterium. *Ann. Intern. Med.* **90:**624–627.

75. **Zychlinsky, A., M. Karim, R. Novacs, and J. D.-E. Young.** 1990. A homogeneous population of lymphokine-activated killer (LAK) cells is incapable of killing virus-, bacteria-, or parasite-infected macrophages. *Cell. Immunol.* **125:**261–267.

Genetic Studies of *Legionella* Pathogenesis

N. CARY ENGLEBERG

Department of Internal Medicine and Department of Microbiology and Immunology, University of Michigan Medical School, Ann Arbor, Michigan 48109-0620

Although we are still quite far from a comprehensive, genetically based view of pathogenesis, it is reasonable to suggest that important discoveries now are just beyond the horizon. The advancement of the field to this point has depended on two critical influences: first, the persistent genetic and phenotypic analysis of *Legionella* species, and second, the emergence in the 1980s of new insights in microbial pathogenesis, largely as a result of the revolution in molecular biology. These insights include the recognition of global regulation of virulence as a common theme in pathogenesis, the molecular exploration of cellular invasion, and the recurring observation that pathogens, once thought to be simple and unidimensional, often turn out to possess redundant and complex mechanisms of virulence. These notions, and others, have colored our view of *Legionella* virulence and have stimulated novel lines of experimentation.

Variations in *Legionella pneumophila* virulence were documented almost as soon as the bacterium was characterized. In the early 1980s, a series of epidemiologic studies suggested that clinical and predominantly environmental variants of *L. pneumophila* could be distinguished by their capacity to bind various monoclonal antibodies (7, 35). A comparison of isolates representing these two types showed that the disease-associated variants were more virulent in guinea pigs (6), more resistant to the bactericidal activity of complement (34), and better able to survive in aerosols (14). It was later suggested that a single monoclonal antibody (MAB2) identifies the more "clinical" subtype, and it is now known that this antibody binds to a specific domain within lipopolysaccharide (LPS) (15).

The phenotypic analyses of these subtypes have always been done by comparing different isolates. As a result, there is always a question of whether the antibodies define a molecular configuration of LPS that is required for virulence or whether they simply identify a stable subpopulation of *L. pneumophila* that also happens to possess certain enhanced virulence attributes, i.e., a virulent cohort or clone. To clarify this issue by eliminating the property of coassociation as a confounder, we have generated an isogenic series of LPS variants. Isolates having a monoclonal antibody binding pattern associated with environmental isolates emerged spontaneously, and at a surprisingly high frequency, from clinical-type strains. By comparing the isogenic pairs, it was made clear that the loss of reactivity with MAB2 was associated with loss of serum resistance, suggesting that a particular configuration of LPS and the property of complement resistance are genetically linked (Rogers et al., this volume).

A second type of virulence variant has been described by numerous groups, i.e., those that have become attenuated or avirulent in association with passage on artificial media. The various bacterial strains reported in these studies are almost certainly a heterogeneous group. In some cases, the avirulent strains are clearly stable mutants; in others, they may be phenotypic or phase variants or mixtures of mutant and wild-type bacteria, since they are readily reversible (9, 19, 28). These avirulent variants and mutants have in common that they fail to grow in macrophages. This recurring observation supports the proposition that intracellular infection is necessary for disease. To date, there have been no reports of virulent infection in intact animals by mutants that cannot grow in vitro in the animal's cells. (Of course, the capacity to grow in cells is not sufficient for virulence.)

Since cellular infection by *L. pneumophila* is readily assayable at the bench, most genetics-oriented investigators have chosen to study this phenomenon to represent virulence. The cellular and immunologic events that accompany intracellular infection have been elegantly described (Horwitz, this volume). Nevertheless, we know very little about the processes that occur within the bacterium during this process. In fact, the adaptation of the bacterium to the intracellular environment is massive and extremely complex. The complexity is apparent when the proteins expressed by *L. pneumophila* growing in chemically defined media are compared with those of the bacterium growing within U937 cells. To do this analysis, the bacteria are labeled with [^{35}S]methionine and then analyzed by two-dimensional gel electrophoresis. The infected U937 cells are treated with cycloheximide prior to the addition of [³⁵S]methionine to prevent labeling of host cell proteins. The analysis shows that intracellular and extracellular *L. pneumophila* isolates are very different bacteria (Abu Kwaik et al., this volume). Some of the proteins detected in intracellular bacteria were not detected at all in broth-grown bacteria, and vice versa. Although some of these changes may be attributable to certain specific stress responses that can be simulated in vitro, no single stimulus or combination of stimuli can reproduce the complete mosaic of changes in protein expression that occurs during intracellular infection.

Because so many proteins are induced during intracellular growth, it is likely that there are many different genes that are necessary for full expression of virulence. For the same reason, it is also likely that there is no bacterial factor (or even a combination of associated factors) that is both necessary and sufficient for virulence or even for intracellular infection. There will be no "smoking gun." The story of *Legionella* pathogenesis is not like a murder mystery in which all of the plot elements and the evidence are derived from and eventually lead back to the one guilty party. Instead, it is like a Russian novel, with too many characters to remember and a dizzying array of interwoven plots and themes.

One can extend this analogy to characterize the progress in the genetic analysis of *Legionella* virulence. To date, the approach has been to identify characters in the story and then to flip through the book, looking to see what they are doing at various points in the sequence of events. Some of the characters seem to be involved in one subplot or another, whereas others cannot be located anywhere in the book. The infection of host cells by legionellae is one chapter of the book, although it may be the most climactic, and it is the one that is usually examined first. The task ahead is to identify more of the characters that appear in that climactic chapter and to determine their importance to the story line.

Actually, it has been forgivingly simple to identify some of the characters by using genetic methods, since so many *Legionella* genes are well expressed in *Escherichia coli*. In fact, virtually all of the genes that have been cloned thus far have been identified by their expression in the cloned state. Table 1 lists the genes that have been cloned by screening genomic libraries for various phenotypes. Of the antigens cloned in 1984 and reported at the Second International Symposium on *Legionella,* the 24-kDa antigen is the protein that we now call Mip (for macrophage infectivity potentiator); the 19-kDa antigen, also cloned by Hindahl and Iglewski (24), is now known to be the peptidoglycan-associated lipoprotein (22). The identity of the 66-kDa protein is still unknown.

TABLE 1. *Legionella* genes cloned by expression in *E. coli*

Gene	Reference
Encoding antigens	
Surface proteins (19, 24, and 66 kDa) ...	22
Common 19-kDa outer membrane antigen	24
58–60-kDa common antigen from:	
L. pneumophila	26
L. micdadei	3
L. micadei Mip analog	2
Encoding extracellular enzymes	
Zinc metalloproteases	
proA	36
mspA	39
Cytolysin	40
Legiolysin (*lly*)	41
Other	
recA	16

The so-called common antigen is now known to be a major heat shock protein, the *Legionella* equivalent of GroEL (26). The Mip analog of *Legionella micdadei* was also cloned by using antisera to screen a library (2).

At least three groups have cloned the major extracellular protease of *L. pneumophila* by screening clones in situ for proteolytic activity. In one case, cloning of the gene enabled the investigators to confirm that all three activities ascribed to this extracellular enzyme (proteolytic, hemolytic, and cytolytic) reside in the same molecule (36). Another group used the gene to make a site-specific mutation in the native gene (39). A third group is using the gene primarily for diagnostic purposes (40). Finally, the *recA* gene of *L. pneumophila* was cloned by selecting for resistance of *E. coli* clones to methyl methanesulfonate and then scoring for resistance to UV light and for the ability to promote homologous recombination (16). The *Legionella* RecA protein substituted quite well for the *E. coli* protein in these functions.

The sequences of several *Legionella* genes have been reported (Table 2). In some cases, the sequences showed significant homology to cognate genes from other bacteria. For example, the *Legionella recA* gene was about 70 and 75% identical to the *E. coli* and *Pseudomonas aeruginosa* genes, respectively (42). The identities of the GroEL and the peptidoglycan-associated lipoproteins were also confirmed by sequence homology (23, 27, 30, 37). Of note, the latter molecule may not have a significant active role in virulence, but lipopeptides that mimic its inferred N-terminus have potent adjuvant activity. We have observed that this molecule is one of the few proteins that reliably elicits a humoral response in guinea pigs after infection by the intratracheal route.

The sequence of the *L. pneumophila* protease

TABLE 2. *Legionella* genes for which DNA sequences
have been determined

Gene	Reference
mip	
L. pneumophila	20
L. micdadei	2
recA	42
proA	42
htpAB (*groEL*)	
L. pneumophila	37
	27
L. micdadei	25
19-kDa lipoprotein genes	
plpAB	30
pal	23

revealed that the enzyme was more than 70% homologous with *Pseudomonas* elastase (4). Subsequent studies using specific protease inhibitors
showed that the two enzymes were also functionally similar. In contrast, the situation with *mip*
was unusual in that it was the first gene of its class
to be entered knowingly into the electronic data
bases (20). As a consequence, it was originally
thought that the gene was unique to the genus;
now we know it to be evolutionarily conserved in
prokaryotic and eukaryotic organisms, including
humans.

Although cloning and sequencing may permit
the identification of characters in the story of *Legionella* pathogenesis, an assessment of their
functional roles depends on the ability to manipu-
late genes in *Legionella* cells. Table 3 lists some
of the landmark contributions in the genetic manipulation of these bacteria. Conjugal transfer has
been the staple method for introducing genes into
Legionella sp. in the absence of transducing phage
or methods for transformation (10, 17). However,
we and others have introduced DNA (even recombinant cosmids of 40 kb) by electroporation. A
Russian group reported the transformation of *Legionella* cells; however, it is not clear whether this
technique is generally applicable (31).

Transposition has been suggested as a means to

TABLE 3. Genetic manipulation of legionellae

Method	Reference
Conjugal transfer of broad-host-range	
plasmids	10
	18
Conjugal transfer of recombinant	
plasmids	21
Plasmid transformation	31
Electroporation of plasmids	Various workers
Transposition of bacteriophage Mu ..	33
Of Tn5	29
Of Tn903dIIlacZ	36a
Site-specific mutagenesis	13

generate random mutations in *L. pneumophila*.
Mu and its derivatives transpose readily and, apparently, randomly in *L. pneumophila* (33). They
have the potential disadvantages of producing
multiple transpositions, deletions, and rearrange-
ments of DNA. Tn5 and its derivatives are also
functional, but at an impractically low frequency
(29).

As in other recombinationally proficient bacteria, site-specific mutagenesis can be performed
readily in *L. pneumophila* by using cloned genes
with mutations first introduced either in vitro or in
vivo, by transpositional inactivation in a separate
background (e.g., *E. coli* [39]). The specific mutation of a designated *L. pneumophila* gene in its
native background is the most direct and definitive
approach to address the role of any specific gene
in pathogenesis. Thus far, only three specific genetic loci have been studied in this way (Table 4).
An insertion in a locus of unknown function, *efa,*
demonstrated that the methods for site-specific
mutagenesis per se do not cause a defect in cellular infection (13). In contrast, a mutation in *mip*
resulted in attenuated virulence in macrophages
and in guinea pigs (11, 12). The possible reasons
for this attenuation have been amply discussed at
this meeting (Dumais et al., this volume; Hurley
et al., this volume).

To the surprise of many, a site-specific mutation
in the gene encoding the extracellular protease
yielded no change in cellular infectivity or in
guinea pig virulence (5, 39). This finding may
mean that the protease has no necessary function
in pathogenesis, or it may be a case of looking for
the significant role of a character in the wrong
chapter of the book. That is, another assay system
may be needed to reveal the pathogenesis-associ-
ated phenotype of the gene. Thus far, the only
report of a mutant with a known phenotype that is
totally unable to grow in cells is the thymidine
auxotroph reported by Mintz et al. (32).

As noted above, all of the studies reported to
date have used genetic techniques to determine
whether specific genes are relevant to virulence,
within our capacity to measure it. Although this is
a perfectly legitimate approach, its application is
limited to proteins that we already know about and
genes that are readily clonable. The challenge now
is to find new genes that may be important for
virulence.

Figure 1 shows four general approaches that are
currently being used to uncover new genes that
affect the growth or survival of *L. pneumophila* in
cells. One approach (Fig. 1A) is to transfer a genomic library to a nonreverting, avirulent *L. pneumophila* mutant. Then, host cells are infected in
order to select an isolate carrying a cosmid (or
plasmid) that complements the mutation. A mutant that fails to evade phagosome-lysosome fusion was complemented by using this approach,

TABLE 4. Genetic studies of *L. pneumophila* pathogenesis and virulence

Genetic locus	Function	Mutant phenotype		Reference
		Intracellular infection	Animal virulence	
	Thymidine synthesis	Avirulent		32
efa	Unknown	None		13
mip	Enhanced survival in cells	Attenuated	Attenuated	12
				11
msp	Extracellular protease	None	None	39
				5

and the responsible genetic locus is now being characterized (31a).

A second approach (Fig. 1B) is to focus on those genes that are expressed in the intracellular environment but not in medium-grown bacteria. One way to do this is to begin with a phenotypic analysis, e.g., using the two-dimensional protein analysis mentioned above to identify proteins that are expressed only in bacteria grown in cells. Once the relevant proteins are identified, their genes can be cloned. A direct, genetic approach to the same problem would employ transposons to create random transcriptional fusions in the *L. pneumophila* chromosome. After generating a large population of bacteria carrying independent transposon insertions, one would then infect cells and either select or screen for the gene product encoded by the transposon. The expression of the fusion product in intracellular bacteria, but not in medium-grown bacteria, would indicate that the fusion had been formed in a gene that is expressed specifically during intracellular infection. Isola-

tion of the relevant gene(s) would be a simple, technical matter.

If the intracellular demise of a bacterium depends on its active growth, then it may be possible to enrich or to select for mutants that fail to grow in cells. For example, since beta-lactam antibiotics kill only growing bacteria, mutants that survive high levels of methicillin after entering cells may be defective in intracellular growth (Fig. 1C). This approach was used to isolate *Listeria monocytogenes* mutants that are defective in intracellular infection (8). Berger and Isberg (3a) reported a conceptually similar approach that uses an avirulent, thymine auxotroph of *L. pneumophila* that fails to survive in cells. Transpositional mutagenesis of this strain followed by sequential infections of U937 cells permitted the investigators to enrich for mutations that arrest growth and thereby protect against intracellular demise. Several classes of avirulent *Legionella* mutants have been identified by this procedure.

Finally, my laboratory has chosen to focus on a

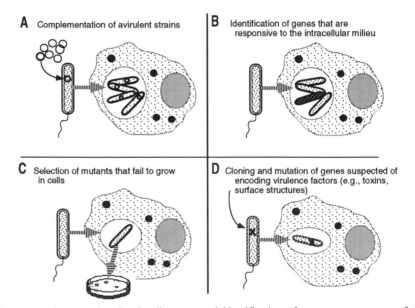

FIG. 1. Four general approaches for the discovery and identification of new genes necessary for *Legionella* pathogenesis (described in the text).

subset of *L. pneumophila* gene products that are likely to be involved in intracellular infection, i.e., proteins that are either exported or localized to the bacterial envelope (Fig. 1D). We are using alkaline phosphatase gene fusions to identify insertion mutations in genes expressing secreted proteins, a more restricted number of proteins that have a greater likelihood of functioning in pathogenesis. Since Tn5 and its derivatives transpose inefficiently in *L. pneumophila*, we use a procedure called shuttle mutagenesis in which the transposition step is performed in the more permissive *E. coli* background. The details of this procedure are reported by Arroyo et al. in this volume. Briefly, a cosmid library of *L. pneumophila* is mutageneized with the fusion-generating transposon, Tn*phoA*. Insertions into cloned *L. pneumophila* genes that create phosphatase-positive fusions are first identified in *E. coli* on indicator media, and then the gene fusions are transferred to *L. pneumophila*. Because the frequency of homologous recombination in *L. pneumophila* is orders of magnitude greater than the frequency of Tn*phoA* transposition, the gene fusion on the cosmid can be readily exchanged for the native chromosomal gene. This results in insertional inactivation of the chromosomal gene and production of secreted product that is a chimera of the native gene and *E. coli* alkaline phosphatase. This mutant strain can then be screened for its capacity to grow in U937 cells.

Limited application of the procedure to date has identified a few, distinct genes that encode secreted proteins needed for intracellular infection (Arroyo et al., this volume). An obvious limitation of the technique is that it depends on the expression of the gene fusions in *E. coli*. It is therefore not possible to isolate fusions in genes that are conditionally expressed in *L. pneumophila*. To address this concern, we also constructed a transposon that is capable of generating phosphatase fusions directly in *L. pneumophila*, i.e., Mud*phoA*(1). Thus far, only a handful of phosphatase-positive *L. pneumophila* strains have been generated with Mud*phoA*. However, two of them tested so far have significant loss of cellular infectivity. Taking the results with Tn*phoA* shuttle mutagenesis and Mud*phoA* transpositional mutagenesis together, we estimate that about 10% of the strains with phosphatase-positive fusions will be attenuated or totally unable to grow in U937 cells. This finding suggests once again that a large number of genes participate in intracellular infection and underscores the complexity of the pathogenic process.

The difficulties encountered in identifying the characters and subplots in the story of *Legionella* pathogenesis can be daunting. Up to now, interest in this aspect of *Legionella* infection has been limited, and progress has been slow. In evidence,

TABLE 5. Published articles on gram-negative intracellular pathogens that employ molecular genetic techniques, 1981 through 1991[a]

Pathogen	No. of articles
Salmonella sp.	1,014
Yersinia sp.	101
Legionella sp.	38

[a]From Medline-Paperchase. Papers concerning each pathogen were searched by using the following keywords: gene; gene library; genomic library; DNA recombinant; DNA mutational analysis; cloning, molecular; chromosomal mapping; gene amplification; base sequence; transformation, genetic; and recombination, genetic.

Table 5 shows the results of a Medline search for published articles during the past 10 years that employ molecular genetic techniques in studies of either *Legionella* sp. or two other gram-negative, intracellular pathogens. A pessimistic view of this obvious disparity in published output might be that all of the important work is being done in other systems and that there will be little of a novel nature to be discovered in *Legionella* spp. Alternatively, the findings may suggest that *Legionella* research is underrepresented in the field relative to its clinical importance and true potential as a model system for study. Whether the data reflect past bankruptcy or future opportunity is a matter of interpretation and opinion. Nevertheless, the recent, exciting contributions reported at this meeting certainly seem to suggest that latter possibility.

I am supported by National Institutes of Health grants AI 26232 and AI 24731.

REFERENCES

1. **Albano, M., J. Arroyo, B. I. Eisenstein, and N. C. Engleberg.** 1992. PhoA gene fusions in *Legionella pneumophila* in vivo using a new transposon, Mud*phoA*. *Mol. Microbiol.* **6:**1829–1839.

2. **Bangsborg, J. M., N. P. Cianciotto, and P. Hindersson.** 1991. Nucleotide sequence analysis of the *Legionella micdadei mip* gene, encoding a 30-kilodalton analog of the *Legionella pneumophila* Mip protein. *Infect. Immun.* **59:**3836–3840.

3. **Bangsborg, J. M., M. T. Collins, N. Høiby, and P. Hindersson.** 1989. Cloning and expression of the *Legionella micdadei* "common antigen" in *Escherichia coli*. *APMIS* **97:**14–22.

3a. **Berger, K. H., and R. R. Isberg.** 1992. p. 9, abstr. 2. *Program Abstr. Int. Symp. Legionella*.

4. **Black, W. J., F. D. Quinn, and L. S. Tompkins.** 1990. *Legionella pneumophila* zinc metalloprotease is structurally and functionally homologous to *Pseudomonas aeruginosa* elastase. *J. Bacteriol.* **172:**2608–2613.

5. **Blander, S. J., L. Szeto, H. A. Shuman, and M. A. Horwitz.** 1990. An immunoprotective molecule, the major secretory protein of *Legionella pneumophila*, is not a virulence factor in a guinea pig model of Legionnaires' disease. *J. Clin. Invest.* **86:**817–824.

6. **Bollin, G. E., J. F. Plouffe, M. F. Para, and R. B. Prior.** 1985. Difference in virulence of environmental isolates of *Legionella pneumophila*. *J. Clin. Microbiol.* **21:**674–677.

7. **Brown, A., R. M. Vickers, E. M. Elder, M. Lema, and**

G. M. Garrity. 1982. Plasmid and surface antigen markers of endemic and epidemic *Legionella pneumophila* strains. *J. Clin. Microbiol.* **16**:230–235.

8. **Camilli, A., C. R. Paynton, and D. A. Portnoy.** 1989. Intracellular methicillin selection of *Listeria monocytogenes* mutants unable to replicate in a macrophage cell line. *Proc. Natl. Acad. Sci. USA* **86**:5522–5526.

9. **Catrenich, C. E., and W. Johnson.** 1988. Virulence conversion of *Legionella pneumophila:* a one-way phenomenon. *Infect. Immun.* **56**:3121–3125.

10. **Chen, G. C., M. Lema, and A. Brown.** 1984. Plasmid transfer into members of the family Legionellaceae. *J. Infect. Dis.* **150**:513–516.

11. **Cianciotto, N. P., B. I. Eisenstein, C. H. Mody, and N. C. Engleberg.** 1990. A mutation in the *mip* gene results in an attenuation of *Legionella pneumophila* virulence. *J. Infect. Dis.* **162**:121–126.

12. **Cianciotto, N. P., B. I. Eisenstein, C. H. Mody, G. B. Toews, and N. C. Engleberg.** 1989. A *Legionella pneumophila* gene encoding a species-specific surface protein potentiates initiation of intracellular infection. *Infect. Immun.* **57**:1255–1262.

13. **Cianciotto, N. P., R. Long, B. I. Eisenstein, and N. C. Engleberg.** 1988. Site-specific mutagenesis in *Legionella pneumophila* by allelic exchange using counterselectable ColE1 vectors. *FEMS Microbiol. Lett.* **56**:203–208.

14. **Dennis, P. J., and J. V. Lee.** 1988. Differences in aerosol survival between pathogenic and non-pathogenic strains of *Legionella pneumophila* serogroup 1. *J. Appl. Bacteriol.* **65**:135–141.

15. **Dournon, E., W. F. Bibb, P. Rajagopalan, N. Desplaces, and R. M. McKinney.** 1988. Monoclonal antibody reactivity as a virulence marker for *Legionella pneumophila* serogroup 1 strains. *J. Infect. Dis.* **157**:496–501.

16. **Dreyfus, L. A.** 1989. Molecular cloning and expression in *Escherichia coli* of the *recA* gene of *Legionella pneumophila. J. Gen. Microbiol.* **135**:3097–3107.

17. **Dreyfus, L. A., and B. H. Iglewski.** 1985. Conjugation-mediated genetic exchange in *Legionella pneumophila. J. Bacteriol.* **161**:80–84.

18. **Dreyfus, L. A., and B. H. Iglewski.** 1986. Purification and characterization of an extracellular protease of *Legionella pneumophila. Infect. Immun.* **51**:736–743.

19. **Elliott, J. A., and W. Johnson.** 1982. Virulence conversion of *Legionella pneumophila* serogroup 1 by passage in guinea pigs and embryonated eggs. *Infect. Immun.* **35**:943–946.

20. **Engleberg, N. C., C. Carter, D. R. Weber, N. P. Cianciotto, and B. I. Eisenstein.** 1989. DNA sequence of *mip,* a *Legionella pneumophila* gene associated with macrophage infectivity. *Infect. Immun.* **57**:1263–1270.

21. **Engleberg, N. C., N. Cianciotto, J. Smith, and B. I. Eisenstein.** 1988. Transfer and maintenance of small, mobilizable plasmids with ColE1 replication origins in *Legionella pneumophila. Plasmid* **20**:83–91.

22. **Engleberg, N. C., D. J. Drutz, and B. I. Eisenstein.** 1984. Cloning and expression of *Legionella pneumophila* antigens in *Escherichia coli. Infect. Immun.* **44**:222–227.

23. **Engleberg, N. C., D. C. Howe, J. E. Rogers, J. Arroyo, and B. I. Eisenstein.** 1991. Characterization of a *Legionella pneumophila* gene encoding a lipoprotein antigen. *Mol. Microbiol.* **5**:2021–2029.

24. **Hindahl, M. S., and B. H. Iglewski.** 1987. Cloning and expression of a common *Legionella* outer membrane antigen in *Escherichia coli. Microb. Pathog.* **2**:91–99.

25. **Hindersson, P., N. Høiby, and J. Bangsborg.** 1990. Sequence analysis of the *Legionella micdadei groELS* operon. *FEMS Microbiol. Lett.* **61**:31–38.

26. **Hoffman, P. S., C. A. Butler, and F. D. Quinn.** 1989. Cloning and temperature-dependent expression in *Escherichia coli* of a *Legionella pneumophila* gene coding for a genus-common 60-kilodalton antigen. *Infect. Immun.* **57**:1731–1739.

27. **Hoffman, P. S., L. Houston, and C. A. Butler.** 1990. *Legionella pneumophila htpAB* heat shock operon: nucleotide sequence and expression of the 60-kilodalton antigen in *L. pneumophila*-infected HeLa cells. *Infect. Immun.* **58**:3380–3387.

28. **Horwitz, M. A.** 1987. Characterization of avirulent mutant *Legionella pneumophila* that survive but do not multiply within human monocytes. *J. Exp. Med.* **166**:1310–1328.

29. **Keen, M. G., E. D. Street, and P. S. Hoffman.** 1985. Broad-host-range plasmid pRK340 delivers Tn*5* into the *Legionella pneumophila* chromosome. *J. Bacteriol.* **162**:1332–1335.

30. **Ludwig, B., A. Schmid, R. Marre, and J. Hacker.** 1991. Cloning, genetic analysis, and nucleotide sequence of a determinant coding for a 19-kilodalton peptidoglycan-associated protein (Ppl) of *Legionella pneumophila. Infect. Immun.* **59**:2515–2521.

31. **Marakusha, B. I., E. Feoktistova, I. S. Tartakovskii, and S. V. Prozorovskii.** 1990. The transformation of legionellae by plasmid DNA. *Zh. Mikrobiol. Epidemiol. Immunobiol.* **3**:20–23.

31a. **Marra, A., S. J. Blander, and M. A. Horwitz.** 1992. p. 9, abstr. 1. *Program Abstr. Int. Symp. Legionella.*

32. **Mintz, C. S., J. X. Chen, and H. A. Shuman.** 1988. Isolation and characterization of auxotrophic mutants of *Legionella pneumophila* that fail to multiply in human monocytes. *Infect. Immun.* **56**:1449–1455.

33. **Mintz, C. S., and H. A. Shuman.** 1987. Transposition of bacteriophage Mu in the Legionnaires disease bacterium. *Proc. Natl. Acad. Sci. USA* **84**:4645–4649.

34. **Plouffe, J. F., M. F. Para, and K. A. Fuller.** 1985. Serum bactericidal activity against *Legionella pneumophila. J. Clin. Microbiol.* **22**:863–864.

35. **Plouffe, J. F., M. F. Para, W. E. Maher, B. Hackman, and L. Webster.** 1983. Subtypes of *Legionella pneumophila* serogroup 1 associated with different attack rates. *Lancet* **ii**:649–650.

36. **Quinn, F. D., and L. S. Tompkins.** 1989. Analysis of a cloned sequence of *Legionella pneumophila* encoding a 38 kD metalloprotease possessing haemolytic and cytotoxic activities. *Mol. Microbiol.* **3**:797–805.

36a. **Sadoski, A. B., L. A. Wiater, and H. A. Shuman.** 1992. p. 13, abstr. I-10. *Program Abstr. Int. Symp. Legionella.*

37. **Sampson, J. S., S. P. O'Connor, B. P. Holloway, B. B. Plikaytis, G. M. Carlone, and L. W. Mayer.** 1990. Nucleotide sequence of *htpB,* the *Legionella pneumophila* gene encoding the 58-kilodalton (kDa) common antigen, formerly designated the 60-kDa common antigen. *Infect. Immun.* **58**:3154–3157.

38. **Selfert, H. S., E. Y. Chen, M. So, and F. Heffron.** 1986. Shuttle mutagenesis: a method of transposon mutagenesis for *Saccharomyces cerevisiae. Proc. Natl. Acad. Sci. USA* **83**:735–739.

39. **Szeto, L., and H. A. Shuman.** 1990. The *Legionella pneumophila* major secretory protein, a protease, is not required for intracellular growth or cell killing. *Infect. Immun.* **58**:2585–2592.

40. **Tartakovskii, I. S., I. G. Nagaev, B. I. Marakusha, N. A. Zigangirova, A. L. Gintsburg, G. B. Smirnov, and S. V. Prozorovskii.** 1990. The use of a molecular DNA probe based on the cloned cytolysin gene for the identification of *Legionella. Zh. Mikrobiol. Epidemiol. Immunobiol.* 20–23.

41. **Wintermeyer, E., U. Rdest, B. Ludwig, A. Debes, and J. Hacker.** 1991. Cloning and characterization of a DNA sequence, termed legiolysin (*lly*), responsible for hemolytic activity, color production and fluorescence of *Legionella pneumophila. Mol. Microbiol.* **5**:1135–1143.

42. **Zhao, X., and L. A. Dreyfus.** 1990. Expression and nucleotide sequence analysis of the *Legionella pneumophila recA* gene. *FEMS Microbiol. Lett.* **58**:227–231.

Legionella pneumophila Mip Inhibits Protein Kinase C

M. C. HURLEY, K. BALAZOVICH, M. ALBANO, N. C. ENGLEBERG, AND B. I. EISENSTEIN

Department of Internal Medicine and Department of Microbiology and Immunology, University of Michigan Medical School, Ann Arbor, Michigan 48109-0620

Mip (macrophage infectivity potentiator) is a surface protein of *Legionella pneumophila* and other *Legionella* species that is required for optimal intracellular infection and for full expression of animal virulence (2, 3). Using in vitro and in vivo genetic manipulations, we constructed a new series of isogenic *L. pneumophila* strains that differ in expression of Mip. A 726-bp deletion of the *mip* coding region was introduced into the wild-type, virulent strain AA100 by a site-specific, homologous recombination technique to yield mutant strain AA108. AA108 is Mip⁻, but it is wild type in all other respects. Strain AA109 was constructed by recombining a copy of the native *mip* gene into the site of the *mip* deletion. This strain is Mip⁺, but it is similar to AA108 in all other respects.

To clarify further the effect of Mip during early infection of phagocytic cells, equivalent inocula of these three strains were incubated with differentiated U937 cell monolayers for 30 min, washed with RPMI culture medium, lysed at various time intervals, and cultured quantitatively (8). At 30 min, there was already a significant difference in recovery of AA100 and AA108 (Fig. 1). However, between 1 and 4 h, there was a 10-fold reduction in recovery of AA108 that was not seen with either AA100 or AA109. After 8 h, recovery of the viable bacteria increased, and viable counts approached those of the parent strain by 22 h. AA109 behaved like the parental strain in this assay. This study shows that the presence of Mip protects against an early loss of viability after *L. pneumophila* infects U937 cells.

A possible clue to the function of Mip came with the discovery that it shares sequence homology with a class of eukaryotic proteins, the FK-binding proteins (FKBPs) (9). FKBPs are known to have two distinct functions: they catalyze folding of proteins at proline residues (*cis-trans* peptidyl-prolyl isomerase activity), and they serve as receptors for the immunosuppressive drug FK506 (6). A recent report suggested identity of FKBP with an endogenous inhibitor of protein kinase C (PKC), fueling speculation that the immunosuppressive effects of FK506 might be explained by this interaction (5, 7). However, this report was retracted after it was shown that recombinant human FKBP had no PKC-inhibitory activity (4). We speculated that inhibition of PKC and inter-

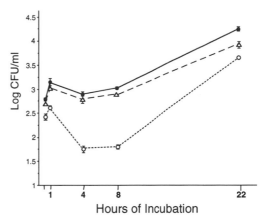

FIG. 1. Infection of differentiated U937 cells with isogenic Mip⁺ and Mip⁻ *L. pneumophila*. Each data point represents the mean and standard deviation of colony counts from eight replicate monolayers. Inoculated strains were AA100 (●), AA108 (○), and AA109 (△).

ruption of host cell signal transduction might explain the phenotype seen with the Mip⁻ mutant (Fig. 1). Therefore, we tested purified Mip for inhibitory activity in an in vitro assay of PKC activity.

To perform this assay, we purified Mip by using a differential ethanol precipitation procedure and two chromatography steps. However, the fraction obtained after the first anion-exchange column was essentially pure, with only trace protein contaminants. PKC was purified from human neutrophils and assayed by established methods (1). All preparations of enzyme were confirmed to have less than 10% kinase activity in the absence of added calcium and phospholipid.

In our inhibition assay, Mip was added to a mixture of 25 mM Tris-HCl (pH 7.5), 10 mM MgCl₂, 0.6 mM CaCl₂, 160 µg of type IIIS histone per ml, 10 µg of phosphatidylserine per ml, and 50 µM ATP, including [γ-³²P]ATP. After a 5-min incubation at 30°C, approximately 200 U of PKC activity was added to the assay mixture for an additional 10 min. (One unit of PKC activity is defined as the amount of enzyme that catalyzes the transfer of phosphate from ATP to histone at a rate of 1 pmol/min.) Finally, radioactivity in trichloroacetic acid-precipitable proteins was quanti-

TABLE 1. Inhibition of human neutrophil PKC by Mip

Mip concn (nM)	% Inhibition of PKC $\pm$ SD
0	0
15	7 $\pm$ 1.0
39	14 $\pm$ 1.6
76	48 $\pm$ 8.1
152	60 $\pm$ 9.1
380	91 + 10.9

tated by liquid scintillation counting. The data points shown in Table 1 represent the mean values from triplicate determinations in three separate experiments, expressed as percent inhibition of PKC activity compared with the activity in control samples with no added Mip. When the results were repeated with a preparation of Mip that had been further purified to homogeneity by gel filtration chromatography, the specific inhibitory activity was slightly increased. Although we do not yet know the mechanism of PKC inhibition, preliminary results suggest that Mip affects the interaction of the enzyme with phospholipids, since the Mip effect can be partially reversed by addition of excess phosphatidylserine to the assay mixture.

In preliminary experiments, we transiently expressed Mip in eukaryotic cells and demonstrated inhibition of two PKC-dependent networks of gene activation. This work supports the notion that Mip may be an active inhibitor of PKC in vivo. To continue to explore the functional relevance of the inhibitory activity, we will determine whether Mip is colocalized with PKC during cellular infection, whether PKC inhibition actually occurs around a forming phagosome, and, if so, whether this inhibition produces the potentiation of infectivity that we have seen in our cellular and animal studies.

Work reported from our laboratories was supported by Public Health Service grants RO1A124731 and AI26232 from the National Institutes of Health. M. Albano is supported by NIH training grant 5T32 AI07360.

REFERENCES

1. **Balazovich, K. J., J. E. Smolen, and L. A. Boxer.** 1986. Endogenous inhibitor of protein kinase C: association with human peripheral blood neutrophils but not with specific granule-deficient neutrophils or cytoplasts. *J. Immunol.* **137:**1665–1673.
2. **Cianciotto, N. P., B. I. Eisenstein, C. H. Mody, and N. C. Engleberg.** 1990. A mutation in the *mip* gene results in an attenuation of *Legionella pneumophila* virulence. *J. Infect. Dis.* **162:**121–126.
3. **Cianciotto, N. P., B. I. Eisenstein, C. H. Mody, G. B. Toews, and N. C. Engleberg.** 1989. A *Legionella pneumophila* gene encoding a species-specific surface protein potentiates initiation of intracellular infection. *Infect. Immun.* **57:**1255–1262.
4. **Cryan, J., S. H. Y. Hung, G. Wiederrecht, N. H. Signal, and J. J. Siekierka.** 1991. FKBP, the binding protein for the immunosuppressive drug, FK-506, is not an inhibitor of protein kinase C activity. *Biochem. Biophys. Res. Commun.* **180:**846–852.
5. **Goebl, M. G.** 1991. The peptidyl-prolyl isomerase, FK506-binding protein, is most likely the 12 kd endogenous inhibitor 2 of protein kinase C. *Cell* **64:**1051–1052.
6. **McKeon, F.** 1991. When worlds collide: immunosuppressants meet protein phosphatases. *Cell* **66:**823–826.
7. **Mosier, N. M., H. A. Zurcher-Neeley, D. M. Guido, W. R. Mathews, R. L. Heinrickson, E. D. Fraser, M. P. Walsh, and D. J. Pearson.** 1990. Amino acid sequence of a 12-kDa inhibitor of protein kinase C. *Eur. J. Biochem.* **194:**19–23.
8. **Pearlman, E., A. H. Jiwa, N. C. Engleberg, and B. I. Eisenstein.** 1988. Growth of Legionella pneumophila in a human macrophage-like (U937) cell line. *Microb. Pathog.* **5:**87–95.
9. **Tropschug, M., E. Wachter, S. Mayer, E. R. Schonbrunner, and F. X. Schmid.** 1990. Isolation and sequence of an FK506-binding protein from N. crassa which catalyses protein folding. *Nature* (London) **346:**674–677.

Distribution and Regulation of the *Legionella mip* Gene

CONSTANCE DUMAIS-POPE, WILLIAM O'CONNELL, AND NICHOLAS P. CIANCIOTTO

Department of Microbiology and Immunology, Northwestern University School of Medicine, Chicago, Illinois 60611

The *Legionella pneumophila mip* gene encodes an antigenic 24-kDa surface protein (Mip) (4, 7). Mip is required for optimal intracellular infection of human macrophages in vitro and for full virulence in a guinea pig model of legionellosis (3, 4). The other species of *Legionella* each contain a *mip*-like gene and generally express a 24- to 30-kDa Mip-like protein (2). Interestingly, *L. pneumophila mip* (Mip⁻) mutants are defective not only in the ability to infect macrophages but also in the capacity to parasitize amoebae, ciliates, and lung epithelial cells (4, 5, 8). These data indicate that Mip is critical for *Legionella* infection of different host cell types and that it must be interacting with a cellular component(s) which is conserved in eukaryotic cells. Furthermore, the phenotype of the *mip* mutant within macrophages and protozoa suggests that Mip is involved in bacterial resistance to intracellular killing (4, 5). We now report that *mip*-related sequences are present and expressed in members of the family *Rickettsiaceae*. In addition, as a first step toward under-

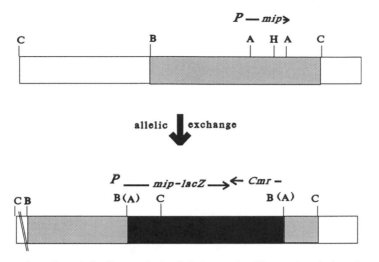

FIG. 1. Construction of a *mip-lacZ* transcriptional fusion strain. The top bar depicts the region of the *L. pneumophila* strain 130b chromosome (hatched box) that contains the *mip* gene (arrow) with its promoter (P). The bottom bar represents the corresponding region of the chromosome within fusion strain NU204. During allelic exchange, an approximately 0.7-kb *Afl*II fragment that contains all of the *mip* coding region was deleted and replaced with a DNA fragment (black box) containing a promoterless *lacZ* gene and an intact chloramphenicol resistance gene (Cmr). Within strain NU204, LacZ (β-galactosidase) expression is controlled by the *mip* promoter. The 5′ *Afl*II site (left "A" on the top bar) is located between sequences corresponding to the start of transcription and to the ribosome binding site, and the 3′ *Afl*II site (right "A" on the top bar) is located at sequences encoding the termination codon (7). Abbreviations for other restriction enzyme sites: C, *Cla*I; B, *Bam*HI; H, *Hin*dIII.

standing Mip regulation, we determined that *mip* transcription changes during *L. pneumophila* extracellular growth.

Given the broad distribution of the *mip* gene among the legionellae and the role of Mip in infection of multiple cell types, we posited that *mip* (Mip) analogs might exist in other prokaryotes. Initially, we focused our attention on those bacteria that are most closely related to the legionellae and are intracellular parasites, e.g., *Coxiella burnetii*, the agent of Q fever and an obligate intracellular parasite (10). To assay for the presence of a *mip* analog, *C. burnetii* DNA was hybridized with a *mip*-specific DNA probe under low-stringency conditions (approximately 25% base pair mismatch allowed) (2). The probe, an approximately 0.7-kb *Afl*II fragment, is internal to the *mip* gene and contains all of its coding region (Fig. 1, top). Interestingly, *Coxiella* DNA hybridized to the *L. pneumophila* probe nearly as well as did DNAs from the other *Legionella* species. Given this result, we assayed for *mip*-related sequences in other members of the family *Rickettsiaceae* (10). Whereas DNAs from *Rickettsia* spp. did not hybridize to the *mip* probe, DNA from *Rochalimaea quintana*, the agent of trench fever, did. These data suggest that *mip*-related sequences are present in non-*Legionellaceae*. To determine whether Mip-related proteins are present in these bacteria, we performed immunoblot analyses using anti-Mip monoclonal and polyclonal anti-

sera (2, 4). Not surprisingly, strains of *C. burnetii* and *R. quintana* contained Mip-like proteins ranging in size from 14 to 20 kDa. However, strains of *Rickettsia* spp. also contained a number of cross-reactive proteins. In addition to these findings, recent computer searches have identified potential Mip analogs in *Chlamydia, Neisseria,* and *Pseudomonas* species (1). Taken together, these data suggest that Mip-related proteins constitute a family of prokaryotic proteins. It is tempting to speculate that the Mip analogs are, like Mip, critical for intracellular infection and/or other host-parasite interactions.

To fully appreciate the significance of the Mip-related proteins in pathogenesis, we have begun studies designed to explore the mechanisms of *mip* (Mip) regulation in *L. pneumophila*. To facilitate these studies, a *mip-lacZ* transcriptional fusion strain was constructed so that *mip* promoter activity could be easily and quantitatively assayed by measuring LacZ (β-galactosidase) activity (9). The fusion strain NU204 was constructed by using modifications of our previously described allelic exchange protocol (Fig. 1) (4–6). Immunoblot analyses using anti-Mip and anti-β-galactosidase antisera confirmed that NU204 was Mip⁻ LacZ⁺. The fusion strain grew in buffered yeast extract (BYE) broth at a rate that was comparable to that of its wild-type parent strain 130b (Fig. 2), confirming that Mip, though required for intracellular growth, is not required for extracellular growth. In

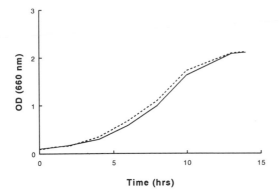

Time (hrs)

FIG. 2. Growth of *L. pneumophila* wild-type strain 130b (———) and its *mip-lacZ* fusion derivative, strain NU204 (- - -), in BYE broth. OD, optical density.

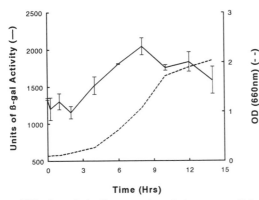

Time (Hrs)

FIG. 3. *mip-lacZ* expression during extracellular growth in BYE broth. The right vertical axis relates to the growth curve for strain NU204 (- - -). The left vertical axis depicts the corresponding levels of β-galactosidase activity, i.e., levels of *mip-lacZ* transcripts. At each time point, an aliquot of the bacterial culture was diluted to an optical density at 660 nm [OD (660nm)] equal to 0.1, lysed, and assayed for enzymatic activity. Each error bar represents the standard deviation of the mean from triplicate cultures.

addition, these data indicate that β-galactosidase expression does not per se alter *Legionella* growth. To determine whether *mip* expression changes during the growth cycle, strain NU204 was grown in BYE broth, and at various times, a constant number of bacteria were assayed for levels of β-galactosidase activity. Enzyme activity

was quantitated as previously described (9). β-Galactosidase activity was lowest during lag phase, increased during log phase, and peaked at late log/early stationary phase (Fig. 3). These data indicate that Mip expression changes during the course of growth and that regulation occurs at the level of transcription. More generally, these studies demonstrate that gene fusion technology is applicable to studying gene expression in legionellae.

We thank Leena Dhand for technical assistance and thank Lou Mallavia and Greg Dasch for providing *Coxiella*, *Rochalimaea*, and *Rickettsia* samples. N.C. acknowledges support from the National Institutes of Health (AI30064-02). C.D.-P. was supported in part by funds from the Cell and Molecular Basis of Disease Training Program (T32-GM0861).

REFERENCES

1. **Bangsborg, J. M., N. P. Cianciotto, and P. Hindersson.** 1991. Nucleotide sequence analysis of the *Legionella micdadei mip* gene, encoding a 30-kilodalton analog of the *Legionella pneumophila* Mip protein. *Infect. Immun.* **59:**3836–3840.
2. **Cianciotto, N. P., J. M. Bangsborg, B. I. Eisenstein, and N. C. Engleberg.** 1990. Identification of *mip*-like genes in the genus *Legionella*. *Infect. Immun.* **58:**2912–2918.
3. **Cianciotto, N. P., B. I. Eisenstein, C. H. Mody, and N. C. Engleberg.** 1990. A mutation in the *mip* gene results in an attenuation of *Legionella pneumophila* virulence. *J. Infect. Dis.* **162:**121–126.
4. **Cianciotto, N. P., B. I. Eisenstein, C. H. Mody, G. B. Toews, and N. C. Engleberg.** 1989. A *Legionella pneumophila* gene encoding a species-specific surface protein potentiates initiation of intracellular infection. *Infect. Immun.* **57:**1255–1262.
5. **Cianciotto, N. P., and B. S. Fields.** 1992. *Legionella pneumophila mip* gene potentiates intracellular infection of both protozoa and human macrophages. *Proc. Natl. Acad. Sci. USA* **89:**5188–5191.
6. **Cianciotto, N. P., R. Long, B. I. Eisenstein, and N. C. Engleberg.** 1988. Site-specific mutagenesis in *Legionella pneumophila* by allelic exchange using counterselectable ColE1 vectors. *FEMS Microbiol. Lett.* **56:**203–208.
7. **Engleberg, N. C., C. Carter, D. R. Weber, N. P. Cianciotto, and B. I. Eisenstein.** 1989. DNA sequence of *mip*, a *Legionella pneumophila* gene associated with macrophage infectivity. *Infect. Immun.* **57:**1263–1270.
8. **Kim, J., D. Kamp, B. Fields, and N. Cianciotto.** 1991. *Program Abstr. 31st Intersci. Conf. Antimicrob. Agents Chemother.*, abstr. 431.
9. **Miller, J. H.** 1972. *Experiments in Molecular Genetics*, p. 398–404. Cold Spring Harbor Laboratory, Cold Spring Harbor, N.Y.
10. **Weisburg, W. G., M. E. Dobson, J. E. Samuel, G. A. Dasch, L. P. Mallavia, O. Baca, L. Mandelco, J. E. Sechrest, E. Weiss, and C. R. Woese.** 1989. Phylogenetic diversity of the rickettsiae. *J. Bacteriol.* **171:**4202–4206.

Spontaneous Changes in Lipopolysaccharide and Monoclonal Antibody Binding in a Single Line of *Legionella pneumophila* Serogroup 1 Cells

J. E. ROGERS, B. I. EISENSTEIN, AND N. C. ENGLEBERG

Department of Microbiology and Immunology and Department of Internal Medicine, University of Michigan Medical School, Ann Arbor, Michigan 48109-0620

The serogroup-specific antigens of *Legionella pneumophila* reside in the lipopolysaccharide (LPS) of the outer membrane. During our study of the role of LPS in intracellular infection, we discovered that a strain of *L. pneumophila* serogroup 1 (SG1) Los Angeles spontaneously lost the ability to bind an SG1-specific monoclonal antibody (MAb). We describe our further investigations of the spontaneous alterations of *L. pneumophila* LPS structure, which include the use of MAbs that are widely used in SG1 subtyping. We also studied the biochemical and structural changes associated with these spontaneous alterations and the effects of these changes on cellular infectivity and serum resistance.

L. pneumophila AA103, a Str^r Nal^r derivative of AA100, was plated on buffered charcoal-yeast extract plates at a density of ~10^3 colonies per plate. Colonies were lifted onto nitrocellulose disks, and an in situ enzyme immunoassay was performed with various MAbs. The MAbs used were 1C5, an SG1-specific MAb cloned in our laboratory, and the SG1-specific subtyping MAbs 4E9 and MAB2 (1). The results of our screen (Table 1) indicate that changes in MAb binding occurred spontaneously and at relatively high frequencies (~10^{-4} to 10^{-3}).

LPS was extracted from various strains and analyzed by sodium dodecyl sulfate (SDS)-polyacrylamide gel electrophoresis (PAGE) and MAb immunoblotting. Samples were also hydrolyzed with trifluoroacetic acid, and component sugars were identified by high-pressure liquid chromatography (HPLC) following hydrolysis. SDS-PAGE showed that 4E9$^+$ variants had altered silver staining and migration patterns, resulting in bands that stained light yellow, in contrast to the parental 4E9$^-$ variants with grey-black bands. These changes suggest alterations in charge (affecting staining) and sugar composition (affecting migration). In contrast, 1C5$^+$ and 1C5$^-$ LPS variants were identical, suggesting that a minor alteration, such as phosphorylation or deletion of a single, small sugar, may have occurred. Our immunoblots showed that all three MAbs bound to the lowest region of LPS stained in SDS-polyacrylamide gels.

HPLC analysis identified glucosamine in the 1C5 epitope and fucose in the MAB2 epitope. We were unable to identify the sugars involved in the MAb 4E9 epitope specifically. Our HPLC results with the MAB2$^-$ variant confirm the findings of Petitjean et al. (5, 6), who reported that a fucosamine-like residue is at least one of the sugars involved in the MAB2 epitope. There are a number of variable, unknown peaks in the elution profiles of the variants strains that remain to be identified.

Environmental isolates have been reported to have increased sensitivity to serum (7) and to be more likely to be MAB2$^-$ (1). Therefore, we tested these isogenic strains for survival in 90% human serum. MAb 4E9$^+$ strains that had also lost the MAB2 epitope were serum sensitive (100% kill of 10^6 CFU after 2 h at 37°C). Since these strains were independently isolated, we conclude that serum resistance of *L. pneumophila* is linked to expression of the MAB2 epitope.

To determine whether the changes in MAb binding affect the virulence of *L. pneumophila* for

TABLE 1. Spontaneous LPS mutants isolated by using an in situ enzyme immunoassay with MAbs 1C5 and 4E9[a]

Strain	Screened for:	Isolation frequency	Other MAb binding phenotype		
			1C5	4E9	MAB2[b]
AA103			+	−	+
A002–A009	1C5$^-$	8/8,900	−	−	+
B001, B004, B005	4E9$^+$	3/30,000	−	+	−
B002	4E9$^+$	1/30,000	+	+	+

[a]MAb 1C5 was isolated in our laboratory; MAb 4E9 was kindly provided by R. Kohler, University of Indiana.
[b]Originally isolated by R. McKinney, Centers for Disease Control, Atlanta, Ga.

TABLE 2. Cytopathic effect of isogenic MAb
4E9-positive and -negative variants of *L. pneumophila*
in a U937 cell assay

Strain	OD of remaining monolayer ± SD[a]	% of monolayer destroyed in 72 h[b]
Uninoculated (control)	0.84 ± 0.09	0
AA103	0.28 ± 0.02	67
B002	0.34 ± 0.08	60
B004	0.28 ± 0.02	67

[a]The monolayer was stained with MTT after 3 days of incubation (4). The mean optical densities (OD) at 550 nm and the
standard deviations (SD) were calculated from measurements
of eight monolayers infected with each strain.
[b](Optical density at 550 nm of the test strain/optical density at
550 nm of uninoculated control wells) × 100.

tissue culture cells, the infectivity of *L. pneumophila* was examined by using the U937 cell
assay (4). The ratio of bacteria to U937 cells was
1:1, and the cells were assayed for cytopathic
effect by using MTT (3-[4,5-dimethylthia-
zol-2yl]-2,5-diphenyltetrazolium bromide) after
72 h. The results (Table 2) suggest that none of the
LPS form variants were attenuated in the capacity
to infect U937 cells.

Our investigation shows that the spontaneous
alterations in *L. pneumophila* LPS can be demonstrated by loss or acquisition of MAb reactivities.
Similar spontaneous alterations in LPS structure
were originally demonstrated in *Salmonella*
strains and termed "form variation" by Kauffmann (2). Later, Mäkelä showed that such
changes in LPS structure are due to the loss or
gain of a sugar transferase activity and that the
changes may be reversible or irreversible (3). In

L. pneumophila, these structural alterations in
LPS occur at relatively high frequencies ($\sim 10^{-4}$
to 10^{-3}). The alterations are not reversible at
these frequencies, although there may be growth
conditions, unknown to us, that are selective for
the original LPS forms. Investigators who use
LPS MAbs for typing and long-range epidemiologic studies need to be aware of the potential
for spontaneous variation in MAb reactivity.

This work was supported by Public Health Service grant
RO1AI26232 from the National Institutes of Health. J. E.
Rogers is supported by NIH training grant 5T32 AI07360.

REFERENCES

1. **Dournon, E., W. F. Bibb, P. Rajagopalan, N. Desplaces,
   and R. M. McKinney.** 1988. Monoclonal antibody reactivity as a virulence marker for *Legionella pneumophila* serogroup 1 strains. *J. Infect. Dis.* **157**:496–501.
2. **Kauffmann, F.** 1941. A typhoid variant and a new serological variation in the *Salmonella. J. Bacteriol.* **41**:127–140.
3. **Mäkelä, P. H.** 1973. Glucosylation of lipopolysaccharide in
   Salmonella: mutants negative for O-antigen factor 12₂. *J.
   Bacteriol.* **116**:847–856.
4. **Pearlman, E., A. H. Jiwa, N. C. Engelberg, and B. I.
   Eisenstein.** 1988. Growth of *Legionella pneumophila* in a
   human macrophage-like (U937) cell line. *Microb. Pathog.*
   5:87–95.
5. **Petitjean, F., E. Dournon, A. D. Strosberg, and J.
   Hoebeke.** 1990. Isolation, purification, and partial analysis
   of the lipopolysaccharide antigenic determinant recognized
   by a monoclonal antibody to *Legionella pneumophila* serogroup 1. *J. Res. Microbiol.* **141**:1077–1094.
6. **Petitjean, F., J. G. Guillet, B. Vray, A. D. Strosberg,
   and J. Hoebeke.** 1987. Partial characterization of a *Legionella pneumophila* serogroup 1 immunodominant antigenic determinant recognized by a monoclonal antibody.
   Comp. Immunol. Microbiol. Infect. Dis. **10**:9–23.
7. **Plouffe, J. F., M. F. Para, and K. A. Fuller.** 1985. Serum
   bactericidal activity against *Legionella pneumophila. J.
   Clin. Microbiol.* **22**:863–864.

Legionella pneumophila Surface Proteins: Gene Regulation and Cellular Immunity

P. S. HOFFMAN, M. RIPLEY, R. WEERATNA, R. FERNANDEZ, G. FAULKNER, D. HOSKIN,
T. J. MARRIE, S. M. LOGAN, AND M. A. TREVORS

*Department of Microbiology and Division of Infectious Diseases, Department of Medicine,
Dalhousie University, Halifax, Nova Scotia B3H 4H7, Canada*

Legionella pneumophila is an invasive facultative intracellular parasite and a cause of acute
pneumonitis in humans. The bacteria reside in
phagosome vacuoles of alveolar macrophages,
where they abrogate phagolysosomal fusion by an
unknown mechanism. Resistance to and survival
from legionellosis requires an active cellular immune response; however, specific cellular immune antigens of *L. pneumophila* have been
extensively studied. Work by Blander and Horwitz
has shown that the metalloprotease and outer
membrane material elicit cellular immune re-

sponses in guinea pigs (1, 2). Two proteins that
we have found associated with the cell surface of
L. pneumophila include a 28-kDa major outer
membrane protein (MOMP or OmpS [5]) and a
60-kDa heat shock protein (HtpB or Hsp60 [4]).
Guinea pigs surviving lethal challenge with virulent *L. pneumophila* exhibit strong cutaneous delayed-type hypersensitivity (DTH) reactions to
both of these proteins. In contrast, strong humoral
immune responses were noted against Hsp60,
whereas no humoral immune responses were observed by enzyme-linked immunosorbent assay

(ELISA) or immunoblot against OmpS. Thus, knowledge of mechanisms associated with processing and presentation of these antigens by macrophages and other antigen-presenting cells is of fundamental importance to our understanding of how the host immune system responds to intracellular parasites.

We have identified a fundamental difference between virulent and avirulent isogenic strains of *L. pneumophila* that may be germane to the early events associated with abrogation of phagolysosomal fusion. Virulent, but not avirulent, strains sense and respond to environmental changes associated with becoming intracellular. The response is characterized by a rapid increase in the synthesis of stress proteins (HtpB or Hsp60) and a concomitant shift in location of Hsp60 from the cytoplasm and periplasm to the cell surface. Since Hsp60 is a molecular chaperone, it is conceivable that the protein interferes with phagosome membrane proteins involved in initiating phagolysosomal fusion. The shift of Hsp60 to the bacterial cell surface is not dependent on de novo protein synthesis, which is consistent with the observation that all of the proteins required for invasion and abrogation of phagolysosomal fusion by virulent strains of *L. pneumophila* are preexisting. Finally, we propose that virulence is not only multifactoral but also rather subtle, i.e., no "smoking gun."

Guinea pigs surviving lethal challenge were skin tested with several pure proteins from *L. pneumophila* at 6 weeks postinfection. We found strong cutaneous DTH responses in these guinea pigs to both 28-kDa MOMP (9 mm at 24 h and 6 mm at 48 h) and the 60-kDa protein (12 mm at 24 h and <4 mm at 48 h), while the response to pure exoprotease was somewhat lower (6 mm at 24 h and 0 mm at 48 h). No response was noted with ovalbumin as a negative control. A homologous antigen (Hsp65) from *Mycobacterium tuberculosis* is recognized as a major T-cell antigen and implicated in various autoimmune diseases. What led us to consider the *L. pneumophila* 60-kDa protein as a possible cellular immune antigen was the fact that the protein appeared on the cell surface of virulent cells during intracellular infection of host cells, as judged by immunofluorescence (4). In collaboration with Paul Edelstein, we tested the hypothesis that vaccination of guinea pigs with pure 60-kDa protein in Freund's complete adjuvant would be protective against lethal challenge. We found that vaccinated guinea pigs did not elicit strong DTH reactions, were not protected from lethal challenge, and developed a strong humoral response against this protein, as demonstrated by ELISA and immunoblot (3). It is evident from these studies that the route of antigen processing may be important for the development of strong cellular immune responses against the Hsp60 protein.

Guinea pigs surviving lethal challenge were divided into three groups (Table 1). Animals were skin tested, and their spleens were removed for measuring mixed lymphocyte responses (MLRs) to these antigens. Animals sublethally infected were generally negative by skin test, while spleen lymphocytes responded to MOMP and Hsp60. In fact, the responses were equal to, if not greater than, those observed with animals surviving more acute illness. In fact, animals challenged with low and high lethal doses appeared to be suppressed relative to animals challenged with sublethal doses. An examination of peripheral blood for antibody responses to MOMP and Hsp60 in these animals revealed that all of the animals surviving lethal infection had titers (ELISA) of 10^4 to 10^5 against Hsp60, whereas responses to MOMP were less than 10^2. Immunoblots confirmed that immune serum reacted with Hsp60 (HtpB), while the response against MOMP appeared to be lipopolysaccharide related and weak (data not shown). Taken together, these data suggest that guinea pigs surviving sublethal as well as lethal challenge mount both cellular and humoral immune responses against Hsp60 and essentially only cellular immune responses against MOMP.

To determine whether guinea pigs develop cellular immune responses when vaccinated with MOMP, 12 guinea pigs were divided into three groups and immunized with either ovalbumin (group 1), 28-kDa MOMP (group 2), or 100-kDa MOMP porin (group 3) in Freund's incomplete adjuvant. We believed that the intact porin might better simulate what happens in the infected animal. MLRs were performed with peripheral blood lymphocytes. The DTH reactions for animals vaccinated with MOMP or 100-kDa porin were generally greater than 1.5 cm. As expected, no DTH reactions were noted with ovalbumin for ovalbumin-vaccinated animals, since complete Freund's adjuvant is required. Both sets of animals vaccinated with MOMP or 100-kDa porin exhibited substantial MLRs relative to controls (stimulation index range, 16 to 56). The results also suggest that the oligomeric porin is more difficult to process and present than is the purified 28-kDa MOMP monomer. This conclusion was also borne out by examination of the antibody responses in these animals. Those animals receiving the 28-kDa protein as immunogen exhibited an ELISA titer of 10^4, compared with a value of <500 (range, 50 to 500) for animals receiving 100-kDa porin. Similarly, immunoblots confirmed antibody responses to 28-kDa MOMP (data not presented).

In L929 cells, both virulent and avirulent strains are internalized, but only virulent strains are able to abrogate phagolysosomal fusion and multiply. Using this model, we have addressed the possibility that selected proteins are preferentially syn-

TABLE 1. Guinea pig DTH (24 h) and spleen MLR[a]

| | Reaction in guinea pigs | | | | | | | | | | | | | | | | | |
| | CG1 | | CG2 | | CG3 | | LD1 | | LD2 | | LD3 | | HD1 | | HD2 | | HD3 | |
Antigen	DTH (mm)	MLR	DTH (mm)	MLR	DTH (mm)	MLR	DTH (mm)	MLR	DTH (mm)	MLR	DTH (mm)	MLR	DTH (mm)	MLR	DTH (mm)	MLR	DTH (mm)	MLR
ConA	0	10.9	4	47.7	0	14.3	0	17.7	0	5.2	0	15.3	0	2.0	0	15.4	0	2.3
PWM	0	15.2		65.6	0	22.4	0	40.3	0	7.1	0	22.5	0	2.6	0	19.3	0	3.2
Ovalbumin	0	1.1	0	0.9	0	1.0	0	1.0	0	1.1	0	0.9	0	1.1	0	1.0	0	1.2
MOMP	0	8.8	3.5	9.4	0	12.4	6.6	16.0	4.0	7.3	6.0	7.3	4.5	5.9	6.5	12.4	10.0	5.1
Hsp60	4	6.1	5	9.6	2	11.8	8.5	13.4	16.0	8.5	9.0	7.2	4.5	5.9	6.5	7.8	8.0	2.9

[a]Guinea pigs surviving sublethal (CG) and lethal (low lethal dose [LD], 10^6 CFU; high lethal dose [HD], 10^7 to 10^8 CFU) *L. pneumophila* challenge were skin tested with 10 µg each of ovalbumin, MOMP, and Hsp60. Seventy-two hours later, spleens were removed and MLRs were determined. Concanavalin A (ConA) and pokeweed mitogen (PWM) were used at 1 µg/ml, while the other antigens were used at 10 µg/ml. The MLR values presented are the means of triplicate determinations. Sublethally infected animals exhibited no DTH reactions to MOMP and weak reactions to Hsp60, while MLRs were equal to if not greater than those observed with animals surviving lethal challenge.

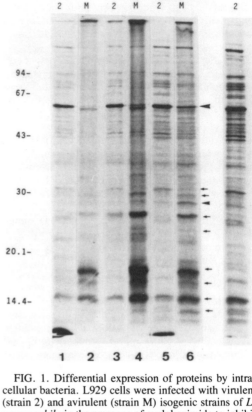

FIG. 1. Differential expression of proteins by intracellular bacteria. L929 cells were infected with virulent (strain 2) and avirulent (strain M) isogenic strains of *L. pneumophila* in the presence of cycloheximide to inhibit host cell protein synthesis. At intervals (0, 30, and 60 min) postinfection, intracellular bacteria were pulse-labeled for 10 min with [^{35}S]methionine in RPMI medium. Equal counts per minute were loaded on each lane of panel A. Panel B shows the results for virulent strain 2; the sodium dodecyl sulfate-polyacrylamide gel was loaded with material equal to that loaded on lane 6. The large arrowhead points to Hsp60.

thesized by virulent organisms. Figure 1 displays the results of a time course experiment comparing protein profiles between virulent (strain 2) and avirulent (strain M) organisms over 1 h. While low-molecular-weight proteins appear to be preferentially synthesized by the avirulent strain, Hsp60 is preferentially synthesized by the virulent strain. The profile in Fig. 1B at 60 min originated from the same number of bacterial cells as did that at the 60-min point for the avirulent M strain. It is striking that virulent cells synthesize much less MOMP than do avirulent cells. A similar result can be obtained by suspending bacteria in Dulbecco modified Eagle medium (DMEM) or RPMI medium (data not shown). Also, it should be noted that when these two isogenic strains are

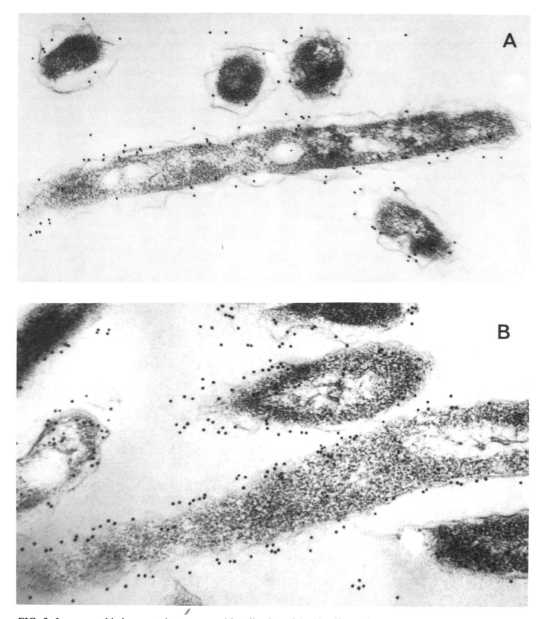

FIG. 2. Immunogold electron microscopy and localization of the Hsp60 protein. *L. pneumophila* SVir was grown in BYE broth at 37°C and subjected to various stresses. Following the stress response, the bacteria were washed in phosphate-buffered saline, fixed, embedded, and sectioned. The sections were treated first with a rabbit polyclonal anti-Hsp60 antibody and then with a 10-nm-gold-conjugated anti-rabbit monoclonal antibody. (A) *L. pneumophila* cells grown at 37°C in BYE broth (unstressed); (B) *L. pneumophila* suspended in DMEM for 30 min at 37°C. In *L. pneumophila*, the protein appears to be associated with the inner and outer membranes, particularly following a stress response. Similar observations regarding location of this protein have been made for other bacterial genera.

grown in buffered yeast extract (BYE) broth, radiolabeling patterns are identical, as are the protein profiles following classical heat shock experiments. In the latter experiments, MOMP is one of the major proteins incorporating radiolabel. We have also examined mRNA synthesis by

Northern (RNA) blot analysis to confirm differential gene expression. An examination of mRNA levels for *htpAB* (stress operon) from the virulent strain suspended in DMEM at 37°C exhibited a twofold difference relative to the avirulent strain over a 30-min period (data not shown). By 1 h, the mRNA levels declined. The MOMP message remained low (probed with *ompS* DNA) in the virulent strain, whereas it remained unaltered (high) in the avirulent strain. Even at zero time, the virulent strain is initiating a stress response, whereas the avirulent strain seems slow to either sense or respond to the environmental change. Whether initiation of a stress response, coordinate with down-regulation of *ompS*, correlates with virulence remains to be established. However, these data are consistent with the hypothesis that regulatory differences distinguish virulent from avirulent strains and that these strains respond differently to environmental signals. We have cloned and sequenced the *L. pneumophila* gene encoding MOMP (*ompS*). The promoter region does not resemble a typical *Escherichia coli*-like promoter, and the mRNA exhibits substantial secondary structure. In contrast, the *htpAB* operon is controlled from a consensus heat shock promoter (4).

Immunogold electron microscopy was used to confirm the observation that Hsp60 is expressed on the cell surface of virulent intracellular organisms or organisms suspended in DMEM. Figure 2A shows the location of Hsp60 in *L. pneumophila* SVir grown in BYE broth at 37°C, and Fig. 2B shows the surface location of Hsp60 following suspension of the bacteria in DMEM for 30 min at 37°C. Immunogold localization of recombinant Hsp60 produced in *E. coli* pSH16 established that the Hsp60 protein is located

exclusively in the cytoplasm. Broader localization studies with other genera of bacteria reveal that periplasmic or surface expression of Hsp60 may be a common feature for pathogenic bacteria, including *Bordetella pertussis*. An aim of this study is to address the question of whether the release of Hsp60, a chaperone protein, in the phagosome vacuole interferes with sensory or regulatory proteins associated with phagolysosomal fusion.

REFERENCES

1. **Blander, S. J., and M. A. Horwitz.** 1989. Vaccination with the major secretory protein of *Legionella pneumophila* induces cell-mediated and protective immunity in a guinea pig model of Legionnaires' disease. *J. Exp. Med.* **169**:691–705.
2. **Blander, S. J., and M. A. Horwitz.** 1991. Vaccination with *Legionella pneumophila* membranes induces cell-mediated and protective immunity in a guinea pig model of Legionnaires' disease. *J. Clin. Invest.* **87**:1054–1059.
3. **Edelstein, P., P. S. Hoffman, M. Edelstein, Z. Chen, and J. Weidenfeld.** 1991. *Legionella pneumophila* 60-kDa heat shock protein in experimental Legionnaires' disease, p. 444. *Program, Abstr. 31st Intersci. Conf. Antimicrob. Agents Chemother.*
4. **Hoffman, P. S., L. Houston, and C. A. Butler.** 1990. *Legionella pneumophila htpAB* heat shock operon: nucleotide sequence and expression of the 60 kilodalton antigen in *L. pneumophila*-infected HeLa cells. *Infect. Immun.* **58**:3380–3387.
5. **Hoffman, P. S., M. Ripley, and R. Weeratna.** 1992. Cloning and nucleotide sequence of a gene (*ompS*) encoding the major outer membrane protein of *Legionella pneumophila*. *J. Bacteriol.* **174**:914–920.

Opsonin-Independent Adherence of *Legionella pneumophila* to MRC-5 and U937 Cells

F. C. GIBSON III, F. G. RODGERS, AND A. O. TZIANABOS

Department of Microbiology, Spaulding Life Science Center, University of New Hampshire, Durham, New Hampshire 03824-3544

Specific recognition of host cells by pathogenic bacteria forms a necessary prelude to the initial stages of the disease state (2). Adherence of bacteria via adhesins is common for pathogens and commensals (5, 7). The most intensely studied form of pathogen attachment to host cells is pili or fimbriae mediated as shown by *Escherichia coli*, *Neisseria gonorrhoeae*, and *Pseudomonas aeruginosa* (4, 9, 11); however, flagella, capsular mucopolysaccharide, lectin-like molecules, and outer membrane proteins have been implicated in bacterial attachment.

Legionella pneumophila is a facultative intracellular pathogen that in infected individuals multiplies in human alveolar macrophages. Attempts to elucidate the manner by which legionellae infect cells have led to investigations of the interac-

tions between the organism and a variety of host cells (1, 8, 10). Such interactions have important clinical as well as environmental implications for the prevention of severe, especially nosocomial, disease. *L. pneumophila* has many potentially adhesive structures, including flagella, fimbriae, and outer membrane evaginations (blebs), which have been identified by electron microscopy (12, 13).

Host cells possess a variety of docking sites or receptors to which intracellular bacteria bind prior to initiating infection. Work on bacterial adherence to host cells as a prelude to infection by *L. pneumophila* has involved both opsonin-dependent and opsonin-independent mechanisms of attachment. Cells that are not professionally phagocytic, such as MRC-5, HEp-2, and Vero cells (10), and professional phagocytes, such as human monocytes (8) and environmental protozoa (1), have been used. Bellinger-Kawahara and Horwitz (3) demonstrated that the CR3 receptor on human monocytes was responsible for host cell recognition of *L. pneumophila* in the presence of opsonins; however, the bacterial adhesive molecule remains undefined.

Organism. *L. pneumophila* Nottingham-7 (N7), a highly virulent clinical isolate from a fatal case of Legionnaires disease, was passed twice on low-sodium-containing *Legionella* blood agar and plated on buffered charcoal-yeast extract agar supplemented with α-ketoglutarate (BCYEα) (Difco, Detroit, Mich.). Virulence was monitored by using fertile hen's eggs (14). Growth on BCYEα plates was harvested 72 h postinoculation and diluted in buffered yeast extract (BCYEα) broth to give approximately 5×10^5 CFU/ml. This batch culture was grown for 24 h at 37°C in a shaking water bath to mid-logarithmic phase and harvested by centrifugation at $5,500 \times g$. Cells were washed three times in Hanks' balanced salt solution, pH 7.2 (HBSS), and the final cell concentration was adjusted to give 5×10^8 CFU/ml in HBSS.

Host cells. MRC-5 cells are semicontinuous, human embryonic lung fibroblasts. The cells were grown in T-75 flasks at 37°C in 5% CO_2, using Eagle's minimum essential medium (pH 7.2) supplemented with 10% bovine calf serum (HyClone, Logan, Utah) and 3 mM L-glutamine in the absence of antibiotics. After three washings in Ca^{2+}/Mg^{2+}-free EDTA, cells were trypsinized, washed, counted, and grown to confluency in 6- or 24-well cell culture plates containing Eagle's minimum essential medium and serum (2×10^5 to 3×10^5 or 1×10^5 to 2×10^5 cells per well respectively).

U937 is a transformed, human histiocytic lymphoma cell line. The cells were grown to 1×10^6 to 2×10^6 cells per ml in RPMI 1640 medium (pH 7.2) supplemented with 10% fetal bovine serum (Sigma, St. Louis, Mo.) and 3 mM L-glutamine. Cells harvested by centrifugation at 200 $\times g$ were resuspended in fresh medium, counted, and treated at 37°C with 10^{-8} M phorbol myristate acetate for 24 h. Adherent cells were washed three times with HBSS, scraped from the flasks with a rubber policeman, and collected by centrifugation at $200 \times g$. The cells were resuspended in fresh medium to give 5×10^5 cells per ml, added to 6- or 24-well cell culture plates, and allowed to readhere for 24 h at 37°C prior to use.

Assays. Monolayers of MRC-5 or U937 cells in 6- and 24-well plates were washed four times with HBSS to remove opsonic serum components from the culture medium, and fresh HBSS was added. All sugar, enzyme, fixative, and chemical degradative treatments were prepared in HBSS at pH 7.2 and filter sterilized prior to use. Eukaryotic cells were inoculated with *L. pneumophila* N7 at a multiplicity of infection of 100 bacteria per host cell. For competitive binding studies, sugars were added to cells in each well 10 min prior to the addition of organisms. Surface modification of either the prokaryotic or eukaryotic cell membranes was done prior to addition of organisms to host cells. Following each treatment regimen, legionellae were allowed to adhere for 1 h, washed three times with HBSS to remove nonadherent bacteria, and assayed by viable bacterial cell colony counts (VBCCC) and indirect immunofluorescent antibody (IFA) assay.

VBCCC. Inoculated monolayers in 24-well cell culture plates were lysed by using 1 ml of sterile distilled water. The resultant lysates were serially 10-fold diluted in 1% peptone and plated in duplicate on BCYEα agar, and *Legionella* colonies were enumerated after 48 to 72 h.

IFA assay. Prior to addition of MRC-5 or U937 cells to the 6-well cell culture plates, 22-mm^2 sterile glass coverslips were added to each well and the cell cultures were allowed to adhere to the coverslips. Following competitive binding as well as prokaryotic and eukaryotic cell surface treatments, monolayers were inoculated with *L. pneumophila* as described for VBCCC.

After 1 h of incubation, host cells were washed three times to remove nonadherent bacteria and fixed in 10% formalin in phosphate-buffered saline, pH 7.2 (PBS), for 1 h at 25°C. After three further washings with PBS, monolayers were treated with rabbit polycolonal anti-*L. pneumophila* N7 serum for 1 h at 37°C. Unbound globulin was removed, and goat anti-rabbit fluorescein isothiocyanate-conjugated antibody (Sigma) was added. After multiple washing with PBS, cells were stained with 0.01% propidium iodide in PBS for 30 min, washed, air dried, and mounted in glycerol containing 1% 1,4-diazobicyclo(2,2,2)octane. A 50% change in adherence data was the criterion used to assess the significance of a particular treatment. IFA results were averages of three trials enumerating the number of adherent bacteria on the first 200 cells per trial counted. VBCCC results were averages of 10 trials, each in duplicate for all treatments.

Adhesins and receptors. Bacterial adherence to eukaryotic cells is a complex interaction. Experimental procedures often lead to contradictory results, and data from studies investigating these interactions are difficult to interpret, making definitive adherence criteria problematic. However, the results of this study suggested that the adhesive structure used by *L. pneumophila* to attach to MRC-5 and U937 cells was protein or carbohydrate in nature, possibly a lectin-like surface structure. Preliminary characterization of the host cell receptor suggested a carbohydrate or glycolipid recognition moiety. In saturation kinetic studies using VBCCC and IFA assays, a bacterial multi-

TABLE 1. Opsonin-independent attachment of *L. pneumophila* to host cells following competitive binding, organism surface treatment, or host cell membrane treatment[a]

	U937 cells			MRC-5 cells	
Competitive binding	Organism treatment	Cell treatment	Competitive binding	Organism treatment	Cell treatment
	Formaldehyde Glutaraldehyde Sodium metaperiodate Protease Trypsin Chymotrypsin β-Galactosidase Lipase	Formaldehyde Glutaraldehyde WGA ConA Sodium metaperiodate Nonidet P-40		Formaldehyde Glutaraldehyde Sodium metaperiodate Protease Trypsin Chymotrypsin	Formaldehyde Glutaraldehyde WGA ConA Sodium metaperiodate Nonidet P-40
(Galactose) (Glucose) (Fucose) (Mannose) (N-Acetylgalactosamine) (N-Acetylglucosamine) (N-Acetylneuraminic acid)	(Neuraminidase)	(Pepsin) (Trypsin) (Protease) (Chymotrypsin) (Lipase) (Neuraminidase) (Cytochalasin B)	(Galactose) (Glucose) (Fucose) (Mannose) (N-Acetylgalactosamine) (N-Acetylglucosamine) (N-Acetylneuraminic acid)	(β-Galactosidase) (Lipase) (Neuraminidase)	(Chymotrypsin) (Trypsin) (Pepsin) (Protease) (Lipase) (Neuraminidase) (Cytochalasin B)

[a] For each cell type, data generated by either VBCCC or IFA, with each treatment regimen, were similar. Treatments in parentheses showed <50% reduction in bacterial adherence to host cells. WGA, wheat germ agglutinin; ConA, concanavalin A.

plicity of infection of 100 approached saturation of host cell receptors on both MRC-5 and U937 cells (data not shown). The influences of binding competition and of organism- or host cell-modifying treatments on adherence are shown in Table 1.

Coincubation of saccharides with legionellae and host cells showed no competitive inhibition of adherence. However, the possibility of complex oligosaccharides or carbohydrates other than those examined cannot be excluded. Modification of host cell surfaces suggested the general chemical class that the Legionnaires disease bacterium utilized to adhere to cells. Indeed, metaperiodate oxidation of carbohydrate moieties strongly indicated a role for saccharides as cell receptors for both MRC-5 and U937 cells. Although lipids may be involved as docking sites for *L. pneumophila*, proteins and neuraminic acid residues were not. Treatment of MRC-5 and U937 cells with the lectins wheat germ agglutinin, which binds *N*-acetylglucosamine residues, and concanavalin A, which binds mannose, disrupted attachment and supported the potential role of lectin-like structures in organism binding. However, these results may have reflected steric phenomena in which masking of the receptors occurred. Such masking of receptors may also occur as a result of the presence on the host cell surfaces of complex oligosaccharides, glycolipids, or proteins which undergo conformational changes during bacterial attachment. The mannose-sensitive, lectin-like molecule described for *E. coli* (9) does not appear to initiate *Legionella* binding. Cleavage or immobilization of proteins located on the bacterial surface by enzymes or fixatives and oxidation of similarly arranged carbohydrate moieties by sodium metaperiodate also supported the role of proteins and carbohydrates in attachment. The present study supported the observation that *L. pneumophila* was incapable of penetrating the membranes of cytochalasin-treated guinea pig alveolar macrophages in vitro (6); however, bacterial attachment was unaffected by cytochalasin treatment of MRC-5 or U937 cells.

MRC-5 and U937 cells, both of human origin, supported the intracellular growth of *L. pneumophila*. Although the U937 cell is a professional phagocyte, it is derived from a histiocytic lymphoma and may differ in surface structure from alveolar macrophages, while MRC-5 cells are fibroblast in origin. That results were essentially similar for these apparently disparate cell types suggested that the organism may utilize a conserved mechanism for adherence to host cells independent of CR3 and opsonin-mediated uptake. It would be of interest to investigate the mechanisms of adherence of this bacterium to environmental protozoa.

After the initial recognition event, attachment of bacterial pathogens to host cell surfaces is a crucial step in the establishment of disease (2, 5). For legionellae (as well as other organisms), a combination of van der Waals interactions, thermodynamic forces, and hydrophobic bonding may act sequentially or concomitantly to initiate the wash-sensitive, loose or weak host cell-microbe attachment. In this study, the subsequent establishment of an opsonin-independent *Legionella* adhesin-host cell receptor complex induced the wash-resistant, firm or strong binding detected. This process eventually led to bacterial uptake and intracellular replication (see Gibson and Rodgers, this volume). Data from these studies offer evidence that *L. pneumophila* adheres to host cells by opsonin-independent binding via a protein- or carbohydrate-containing structure on the bacterial surface which possesses lectin-like properties. Establishing the mechanism of *L. pneumophila* attachment will assist in elucidating those attachment events for other intracellular pathogens and may possibly play a role in the development of vaccine strategies and thereby facilitate the prevention and control of legionellosis.

This study was supported by Public Health Service grant AI 27929 from the National Institutes of Health and by a CURF grant from the Office of Sponsored Research, University of New Hampshire.

REFERENCES

1. **Barbaree, J. M., B. S. Fields, J. C. Feeley, G. W. Gorman, and W. T. Martin.** 1985. Isolation of protozoa from water associated with a legionellosis outbreak and demonstration of intracellular multiplication of *Legionella pneumophila*. *Appl. Environ. Microbiol.* **51:**422–424.
2. **Beachey, E. H.** 1981. Bacterial adherence: adhesin-receptor interactions mediating the attachment of bacteria to mucosal surfaces. *J. Infect. Dis.* **143:**325–345.
3. **Bellinger-Kawahara, C., and M. A. Horwitz.** 1990. Complement component C3 fixes selectively to the major outer membrane (MOMP) of *Legionella pneumophila* and mediates phagocytosis of liposome-MOMP complexes by human monocytes. *J. Exp. Med.* **172:**1201–1210.
4. **Doig, P., T. Todd, T. T. Sastry, K. K. Lee, R. S. Hodges, W. Paranchych, and R. T. Irvin.** 1988. Role of pili in adhesion of *Pseudomonas aeruginosa* to human respiratory epithelial cells. *Infect. Immun.* **56:**1641–1646.
5. **Duguid, J. P.** 1959. Fimbriae and adhesive properties in *Klebsiella* strains. *J. Gen. Microbiol.* **21:**271–286.
6. **Elliot, J. A., and W. C. Winn, Jr.** 1986. Treatment of alveolar macrophages with cytochalasin D inhibits uptake and subsequent growth of *Legionella pneumophila*. *Infect. Immun.* **51:**31–36.
7. **Gibbons, R. J.** 1973. Bacterial adherence in infection and immunity. *Rev. Microbiol.* **4:**48–60.
8. **Horwitz, M. A., and S. C. Silverstein.** 1980. Legionnaires' disease bacterium (*Legionella pneumophila*) multiplies intracellularly in human monocytes. *J. Clin. Invest.* **131:**697–706.
9. **Ofek, I., D. Mirelman, and N. Sharon.** 1977. Adherence of *Escherichia coli* to human mucosal cells is mediated by mannose receptors. *Nature* (London) **265:**623–625.
10. **Oldham, L. J., and F. G. Rodgers.** 1985. Adhesion, penetration and intracellular replication of *Legionella pneumophila*: an in vitro model of infection. *J. Gen. Microbiol.* **131:**697–706.

11. **Punsalang, A. P., and W. D. Sawyer.** 1973. Role of pili in the virulence of *Neisseria gonorrhoeae. Infect. Immun.* **8**:255–263.

12. **Rodgers, F. G.** 1983. The role of structure and invasiveness on the pathogenicity of *Legionella. Zentralbl. Bakteriol. I Abt. Orig. A* **255**:138–144.

13. **Rodgers, F. G., P. W. Greaves, A. D. Macrae, and M.**

J. Lewis. 1980. Electron microscopic evidence of flagella and pili on *Legionella pneumophila. J. Clin. Pathol.* **33**:1184–1188.

14. **Tzianabos, A. O., and F. G. Rodgers.** 1989. Pathogenesis and chemotherapy of experimental *Legionella pneumophila* infection in the chick embryo. *Zentralbl. Bakteriol. I Abt. Orig. A* **271**:293–303.

Detection of Major Iron Proteins of *Legionella pneumophila*

JÉRÔME MENGAUD, PAULA M. van SCHIE, THOMAS F. BYRD, and MARCUS A. HORWITZ

Division of Infectious Diseases, Department of Medicine, School of Medicine, University of California, Los Angeles, Center for the Health Sciences, Los Angeles, California 90024

Iron availability is a key determinant of *Legionella pneumophila* growth both extracellularly and intracellularly. On solid culture medium, *L. pneumophila* is unable to multiply in the absence of iron supplementation (6), and in broth culture medium, *L. pneumophila* is unable to multiply when iron chelators are present (7). In human mononuclear phagocytes, *L. pneumophila* multiplication is dependent on the availability of iron in the intermediate labile iron pool of the cell, which derives its iron from three major iron-binding proteins: transferrin, lactoferrin, and ferritin (2, 3, 5).

Agents that reduce iron availability inhibit *L. pneumophila* intracellular multiplication. Three types of agents inhibit *L. pneumophila* intracellular multiplication in this way. First, iron chelators, such as the nonphysiologic iron chelator deferoxamine and the physiologic iron chelator apolactoferrin, bind iron in the intracellular iron pool (2, 5). Second, the weak bases chloroquine and ammonium chloride raise endocytic and lysosomal pH and consequently inhibit the pH-dependent release of iron from endocytized transferrin as well as the pH-dependent proteolysis of ferritin and subsequent release of iron from this molecule (4). Third, gamma interferon decreases iron availability by down-regulating transferrin receptor expression on the cell surface and consequently reducing iron uptake into the cell and by down-regulating the intracellular concentration of ferritin (2, 3). The inhibitory effect of gamma interferon on *L. pneumophila* multiplication can be reversed by adding high concentrations of iron compounds to the extracellular medium of the cell (2, 5). *L. pneumophila* thus relies on host cell iron transport systems to deliver iron to it in the replicative phagosome.

Iron is required for the synthesis of a large variety of bacterial iron enzymes and proteins, including heme proteins, iron-sulfur proteins, and iron-binding proteins. These proteins are involved in such diverse functions as electron transfer, oxygen metabolism, peroxide and superoxide metabolism, regulation of gene expression, iron storage, and oxygen binding. While much has been learned about the provision of iron to *L. pneumophila* by host cell iron transport systems, little is known about the role of iron in the physiology of *L. pneumophila,* nor is it known why this organism appears to have such a high metabolic requirement for iron. To learn more about this matter, we have developed methods for detecting major iron proteins of *L. pneumophila,* taking advantage of the very high sensitivity of iron detection allowed by the use of the radioisotope ^{59}Fe as a label.

We were able to detect iron proteins by growing bacteria in the presence of radiolabeled iron, subjecting bacterial proteins to polyacrylamide gel electrophoresis under nondenaturing conditions, and visualizing the iron proteins by autoradiography. When grown on charcoal-yeast extract agar medium, *L. pneumophila* incorporated iron into seven major proteins with apparent molecular masses of approximately 500, 450, 250, 210, 150, 130, and 85 kDa under the conditions studied. The 210-kDa protein was the major iron protein. The 150-kDa protein comigrated with superoxide dismutase activity when analyzed by the method of Beauchamp and Fridovich (1). In cellular fractionation studies, all of the iron proteins were detected in the cytoplasmic and periplasmic fractions; none were detected in the membrane fraction. When grown in yeast extract broth, *L. pneumophila* incorporated iron into the same seven proteins, but their relative amounts differed. Iron proteins were not detected in culture supernatants.

This study demonstrates that ^{59}Fe can be used as a label to visualize the major iron proteins of *L. pneumophila,* and it shows that *L. pneumophila* incorporates iron into seven major proteins. One of the *L. pneumophila* iron proteins may be an iron-containing superoxide dismutase. The role of the other major iron proteins remains to be determined.

This methodology for detecting iron proteins of

L. pneumophila can be used to trace *L. pneumophila* iron proteins during different steps in their purification. Additional studies are required to characterize the iron proteins, determine their precise subcellular localization, and determine their role in iron metabolism and virulence.

This work was supported by grant AI28825 from the National Institutes of Health. J. Mengaud is supported by a fellowship from the European Molecular Biology Organization. M. A. Horwitz is Gordon MacDonald Scholar at UCLA.

REFERENCES

1. **Beauchamp, C., and I. Fridovich.** 1971. Superoxide dismutase: improved assays and an assay applicable to acrylamide gels. *Anal. Biochem.* **44**:276–287.
2. **Byrd, T. F., and M. A. Horwitz.** 1989. Interferon gamma-activated human monocytes downregulate transferrin receptors and inhibit the intracellular multiplication of *Legionella pneumophila* by limiting the availability of iron. *J. Clin. Invest.* **83**:1457–1465.
3. **Byrd, T. F., and M. A. Horwitz.** 1990. Interferon gamma-activated human monocytes downregulate the intracellular concentration of ferritin: a potential new mechanism for limiting iron availability to *Legionella pneumophila* and subsequently inhibiting intracellular multiplication. *Clin. Res.* **38**:481A.
4. **Byrd, T. F., and M. A. Horwitz.** 1991. Chloroquine inhibits the intracellular multiplication of *Legionella pneumophila* by limiting the availability of iron: a potential new mechanism for the therapeutic effect of chloroquine. *J. Clin. Invest.* **88**:351–357.
5. **Byrd, T. F., and M. A. Horwitz.** 1991. Lactoferrin inhibits or promotes *Legionella pneumophila* intracellular multiplication in nonactivated and interferon gamma activated human monocytes depending upon its degree of iron saturation. *J. Clin. Invest.* **88**:1103–1112.
6. **Feeley, J. C., G. W. Gorman, R. E. Weaver, D. C. Mackel, and H. W. Smith.** 1978. Primary isolation media for Legionnaires disease bacterium. *J. Clin. Microbiol.* **8**:320–325.
7. **Reeves, M. W., L. Pine, S. H. Hutner, R. J. George, and W. Knox Harrell.** 1981. Metal requirements of *Legionella pneumophila*. *J. Clin. Microbiol.* **13**:688–695.

Isolation of a *Legionella pneumophila* Mutant That Produces Antigenically Altered Lipopolysaccharide

CLIFFORD S. MINTZ AND CHANG HUA ZOU

Department of Microbiology and Immunology, University of Miami School of Medicine, Miami, Florida 33101

Background. *Legionella pneumophila* is a gram-negative intracellular pathogen capable of entering and growing in alveolar macrophages and monocytes (3). Recent evidence (1, 9) suggests that opsonic complement component C3 and corresponding phagocyte complement receptors CR1 and CR3 facilitate the uptake of *L. pneumophila* by monocytes. Although it was demonstrated that incubation of *L. pneumophila* is normal human serum (NHS) results in the activation of complement and the deposition of C3 on the *Legionella* cell surface (1), the bacterial ligand responsible for complement activation remains to be identified. It recently was shown that lipopolysaccharide (LPS) isolated from *L. pneumophila* Philadelphia-1 can activate complement in NHS (6a). This finding suggests that LPS may play a role in the uptake of *L. pneumophila* by mononuclear phagocytes.

The isolation of mutants that produce altered LPS has contributed to the understanding of the role of LPS in the pathogenesis of a variety of gram-negative infections. In general, structural changes in LPS significantly alter the interaction between gram-negative pathogens and target host cells (5). Therefore, to more clearly define the role of LPS in the *L. pneumophila*-monocyte interaction, we sought to isolate LPS mutants from *L. pneumophila*.

Isolation and characterization of mutant LPS. Following mutagenesis with bacteriophage Mu (7), we isolated a mutant from *L. pneumophila* ΛM511 (a restriction-minus derivative of strain Philadelphia-1) that was unable to bind the serogroup 1 LPS-specific monoclonal antibody (MAb) 1E6. The mutant was subsequently designated strain CS280. Sodium dodecyl sulfate (SDS)-polyacrylamide gel electrophoresis analysis of LPS isolated from strain CS280 and from the wild type by the EDTA-Folch method (8) showed that there was no discernible difference in the electrophoretic profiles of the two LPSs (data not shown). Both LPSs exhibited a ladder-like banding pattern characteristic of *L. pneumophila* LPS (8). This finding suggested that there were no obvious structural changes in the LPS produced by the mutant compared with the wild type. Of interest, carbohydrate analysis of isolated LPS by anion-exchange chromatography with pulsed amperometric detection (2) revealed that there was no difference in the sugar contents of the mutant and wild-type LPSs (data not shown).

The results from Western immunoblot experiments revealed that isolated CS280 LPS did not bind MAb 1E6 (Fig. 1A). In contrast, LPS from strain CS280 retained the ability to bind polyclonal serogroup 1 serum (Fig. 1B). Wild-type LPS bound both MAb 1E6 and serogroup 1 serum. These results indicated that CS280 LPS was structurally similar to wild-type LPS but lacked the

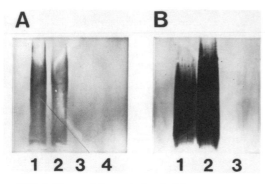

FIG. 1. Western blot analysis of wild-type and mutant LPSs. LPS was electrophoresed in 10% SDS-polyacrylamide gels, transferred to nitrocellulose, and probed with MAb 1E6 (A) or polyclonal serogroup 1 antiserum (B). (A) Lanes: 1, Philadelphia-1 LPS; 2, AM511 LPS; 3, CS280 LPS; 4, Bloomington-2 LPS. (B) Lanes: 1, AM511 LPS; 2, CS280 LPS; 3, Bloomington-2 LPS. Strain Bloomington-2 LPS was included as a negative control. This strain produces serogroup 3 LPS, which does not bind MAb 1E6 or polyclonal serogroup 1 antiserum.

epitope recognized by MAb 1E6.

Strain CS280 does not contain a Mu insertion. Surprisingly, Southern hybridization experiments using a Mu-specific probe (7) revealed that strain CS280 did not contain a chromosomal Mu insertion (data not shown). This finding suggested that the inability of strain CS280 to bind MAb 1E6 may have resulted from a spontaneous mutation in a gene(s) involved in serogroup 1 LPS biosynthesis rather than from an insertion mutation caused by bacteriophage Mu. Alternatively, a DNA rearrangement or deletion within a serogroup 1 LPS gene(s) caused by the imprecise excision of Mu from the CS280 chromosome could explain the inability of the mutant LPS to bind MAb 1E6.

Effect of LPS mutation on the serum resistance of strain CS280. A common pleiotropic effect of LPS mutations is an increased susceptibility of LPS mutants, compared with the wild type, to complement-mediated killing in NHS (5). The results from serum bactericidal experiments showed that there was no significant difference in the ability of strains AM511 and CS280 to resist killing during incubation in 50% NHS. The resistance to serum of strain AM511 was determined to be 65%, whereas that of strain CS280 was 48%. This finding indicated that loss of the MAb 1E6–specific LPS epitope did not significantly alter the serum-resistant phenotype of strain CS280.

Effect of the LPS mutation on the intracellular growth of strain CS280. To determine whether the LPS epitope recognized by MAb 1E6 contributed to the intracellular growth of *L. pneumophila*, we compared strains AM511 and CS280

for the ability to grow in monocyte-like U937 cells and the amoeba *Hartmannella vermiformis* (4). Loss of the MAb 1E6–specific epitope from serogroup 1 LPS did not interfere with the intracellular multiplication of strain CS280 in U937 cells (Fig. 2). Strain CS280 was also unaltered in its ability to grow intracellularly in *H. vermiformis* (data not shown).

It is well documented that enterobacterial LPS mutants with defects in LPS structure (e.g., mutants that do not make O antigen or produce incomplete core structures) are less virulent than wild-type organisms (5). Since the mutant LPS did not contain any obvious structural defects compared with the wild type, it was not surprising that strain CS280 was unaltered in its ability to resist killing by NHS or to multiply in U937 cells and *H. vermiformis*. It is possible that the inability of CS280 LPS to bind MAb 1E6 resulted from a conformational change in the mutant LPS. This explanation seems likely, since carbohydrate analysis of the mutant LPS revealed that there was no difference in the molar ratios of sugars contained within wild-type and mutant LPSs.

Concluding remarks. Recently, recombinant cosmids from libraries containing Philadelphia-1 genomic DNA fragments that restore the ability of the mutant to bind MAb 1E6 were identified (6). This finding demonstrates that strain CS280 may be useful for the identification of genes involved in serogroup 1 LPS biosynthesis and assembly. We are currently attempting to isolate other LPS mutants to facilitate molecular genetic analysis of

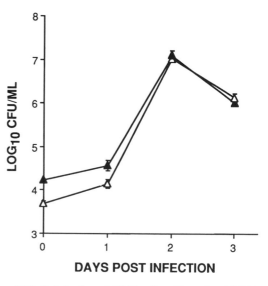

FIG. 2. Infection of U937 cells with strains AM511 and CS280. U937 cell monolayers were infected with strains AM511 (△) and CS280 (▲) as described in the text. Each point represents the mean ± standard error for three separate U937 cell cultures.

L. pneumophila LPS and to gain a better understanding of the role of LPS in the interaction between *L. pneumophila* and mononuclear phagocytes.

We thank William Johnson for helpful discussions concerning *L. pneumophila* LPS and for supplying MAb 1E6. Special thanks to Steven Hull for conducting the carbohydrate analysis of mutant and wild-type LPSs and to Barry Fields for performing the *H. vermiformis* infection experiments. This work was supported by a grant from the American Lung Association of Florida to C. Mintz.

REFERENCES

1. **Bellinger-Kawahara, C., and M. A. Horwitz.** 1990. Complement component C3 fixes selectively to the major outer membrane protein (MOMP) of *Legionella pneumophila* and mediates phagocytosis of liposome-MOMP complexes by human monocytes. *J. Exp. Med.* **172:**1201–1210.
2. **Hardy, M. R., R. R. Townsend, and J. C. Lee.** Monosaccharide analysis of glycoconjugates by anion exchange chromatography with pulsed amperometric detection. *Anal. Biochem.* **170:**54–62.
3. **Horwitz, M. A., and S. C. Silverstein.** 1980. Legionnaires' disease bacterium multiplies intracellularly in human monocytes. *J. Clin. Invest.* **66:**441–450.
4. **King, C. H., B. S. Fields, E. B. Shotts, and E. H. White.** 1991. Effects of cytochalasin D and methylamine on intracellular growth of *Legionella pneumophila* in amoebae and human monocyte-like cells. *Infect. Immun.* **59:**758–763.
5. **Makela, P. K., and B. A. D. Stocker.** 1984. Genetics of lipopolysaccharide, p. 59–119. *In* E. T. Rietschel (ed.), *Handbook of Endotoxin,* vol. 1. *Chemistry of Endotoxin.* Elsevier, Amsterdam.
6. **Mintz, C.** Unpublished data.
6a. **Mintz, C. S., D. R. Schultz, P. J. Arnold, and W. Johnson.** 1992. *Legionella pneumophila* lipopolysaccharide activates the classical complement pathway. *Infect. Immun.* **60:**2769–2776.
7. **Mintz, C. S., and H. A. Shuman.** 1987. Transposition of bacteriophage Mu in the Legionnaires' disease bacterium. *Proc. Natl. Acad. Sci. USA* **84:**4645–4669.
8. **Otten, S., S. Iyer, W. Johnson, and R. Montgomery.** 1986. Serospecific antigens of *Legionella pneumophila. J. Bacteriol.* **167:**893–904.
9. **Payne, N. R., and M. A. Horwitz.** 1987. Phagocytosis of *Legionella pneumophila* is mediated by human monocyte complement receptors. *J. Exp. Med.* **166:**1377–1389.

Construction of *phoA* Gene Fusions in *Legionella pneumophila* That Attenuate Intracellular Infection

J. ARROYO, B. I. EISENSTEIN, AND N. C. ENGLEBERG

Department of Microbiology and Immunology and Department of Internal Medicine, University of Michigan Medical School, Ann Arbor, Michigan 48109–0620

In a continuing effort to understand the interaction between the surface of *Legionella pneumophila* and phagocytic cells, we are identifying and mutating secreted bacterial proteins by generating alkaline phosphatase translational fusions in chromosomal genes. Our initial attempts to generate such fusions were frustrated by (i) the inefficiency of Tn*phoA* transposition in *L. pneumophila* and (ii) difficulties in detecting alkaline phosphatase production in the background of the native neutral phosphatase activity.

To be able to generate phosphatase fusions in the *L. pneumophila* chromosome, we developed a method of shuttle mutagenesis in which phosphatase fusions are first constructed in *L. pneumophila* genes cloned in an *Escherichia coli* cosmid library. The transposon used for this purpose is a derivative of Tn*phoA*, modified by insertion of *oriT* into the streptomycin resistance locus. Transduction is performed by using a modified small-scale version of the procedure previously described (3). Cosmids that carry PhoA⁺ fusions

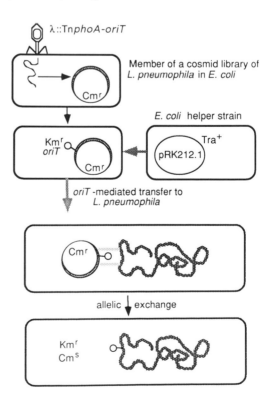

FIG. 1. Schematic representation of the shuttle mutagenesis procedure. Individual *E. coli* clones are transduced in groups of 96 wells in microtiter plates. Only positive cosmid fusions are individually transferred into *L. pneumophila*.

are individually transferred to *L. pneumophila* via *oriT,* and exchange of the gene fusion for the native sequence can be selected. The use of *oriT* to mobilize plasmids into legionellae has been described elsewhere (2). By using the vector pTLP5, counterselection of the plasmid can be obtained at a frequency of 10^{-2}, and loss of the plasmid after allelic exchange can be scored on the basis of chloramphenicol sensitivity. Figure 1 summarizes the steps during shuttle mutagenesis.

Allelic exchanges with wild-type genes in *L. pneumophila* are confirmed on the basis of PhoA activity, kanamycin resistance, and chloramphenicol sensitivity and by Southern hybridizations in some cases. The assay to determine *E. coli* PhoA activity in *L. pneumophila* is described elsewhere (1).

Figure 2 shows two phosphatase-positive (PhoA$^+$) mutants (AA124 and AA125) that were analyzed by Southern hybridization to confirm the

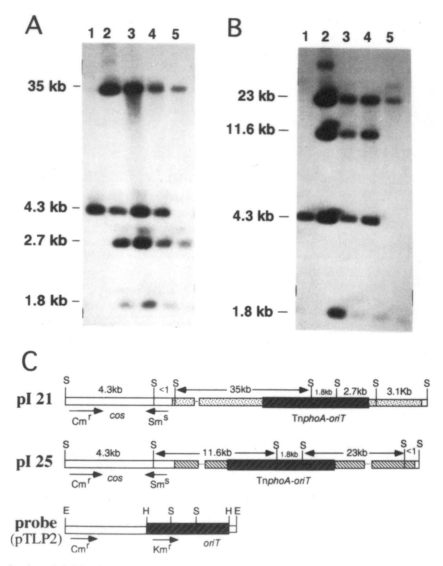

FIG. 2. Southern hybridizations of DNA from *L. pneumophila* strains that have PhoA translational fusions. (A) Lanes 1, cosmid I 21; 2, cosmid I 21::Tn*phoA-oriT;* 3, AA107 (pI21) Cm^r (5 µg/ml); 4, AA107 (pI21) Cm^r (2.5 µg/ml); 5, AA124. (B) Lanes: 1, cosmid I 25; 2, cosmid I 25::Tn*phoA-oriT;* 3, AA107 (pI25) Cm^r (5 µg/ml); 4, AA107 (pI25) Cm^r (2.5 µg/ml); 5, AA125 (all DNA samples were digested with *Sma*I). (C) Linear maps of Tn*phoA-oriT* insertions in cosmids I 21 and I 25. Note that a 4.3–kb band specific to vector pTLP5 is lost after allelic exchange (lanes 5 in panels A and B). A 1.8-kb band is an internal fragment from Tn*phoA-oriT.* Other bands are transposon specific and can shift, depending on the positions of *Sma*I sites (S) in the chromosome.

allelic exchange. A vector pTLP5-specific SmaI fragment of 4.3 kb is lost after the exchange, while a 1.8-kb fragment, internal to the transposon, is retained. Two other transposon bands can be detected, but they vary in relation to the SmaI sites in the cloned Legionella chromosome fragments.

Once constructed, PhoA⁺ L. pneumophila mutants are tested for attenuation, using the U937 cell model of infectivity as described previously (4). Like the majority of PhoA⁺ mutants constructed by this technique, strain AA124 has wild-type cytopathicity. In contrast, strain AA125 is reproducibly at least 50% less cytopathic in U937 cells. The cytopathicity of AA125 has been restored after complementation with the cloned wild-type DNA fragment both in trans and in cis, supporting the conclusion that the TnphoA insertion is responsible for the attenuation in cellular infectivity (data not shown).

At the present time, 126 independent PhoA⁺ fusions have been isolated in L. pneumophila genes cloned in E. coli. Eighty-five of these cosmids have been transferred to L. pneumophila, and in 47, the fusion was exchanged for the native, chromosomal gene. All but one of these exchange mutants were PhoA⁺. Only 32 of these PhoA⁺ Legionella mutants have been tested for loss of cytopathicity in U937 cells so far; 3 mutants have shown significant attenuation.

This shuttle mutagenesis approach has led to the isolation of attenuated Legionella mutants in a relatively short time. The nature of the procedure is such that the intact and mutated genes for any interesting mutation are already cloned in E. coli, and they are available for subcloning, complementation studies, and DNA sequencing. In addition, the collection of PhoA⁺ L. pneumophila strains and cosmids is a potential resource for studying the roles of regulatory genes in the future.

We have simultaneously developed an alternative method for generating phosphatase fusions. Since derivatives of bacteriophage Mu transpose readily in L. pneumophila, we cloned the E. coli alkaline phosphatase gene into MudII4041 in a manner that permits translational gene fusions to be generated through the right end of Mu. We designated this novel transposon MudphoA. Details on the construction of MudphoA and testing of Legionella MudphoA fusion mutants is published elsewhere (1). A major advantage of using MudphoA is that chromosomal insertions can be selected in vivo under different environmental conditions, thereby allowing identification of selectively expressed genes that may be important for virulence but are otherwise difficult to identify by using standard cultivation methods. A few attenuated mutants have already been isolated by using this transposon.

The combined, limited experience with both shuttle mutagenesis and MudphoA transposition suggests that ~10% of the PhoA⁺ mutants isolated will have attenuated phenotypes of various degrees, as determined by the U937 cell model of Legionella infectivity. This finding suggests that a large number of secreted products are probably involved in the survival and growth of L. pneumophila in cells. Moreover, by concentrating on mutations of secreted proteins, we have probably increased the likelihood of identifying products involved in host-parasite interactions. Since the number of different mutants that can be isolated by these techniques is limited to a few hundred, screening them all for virulence attentuation in tissue culture cells is a manageable goal.

This work was supported by Public Health Service grants RO1 AI26232 and AI24731 from the National Institutes of Health.

REFERENCES

1. **Albano, M. A., J. Arroyo, B. I. Eisenstein, and N. C. Engleberg.** 1992. PhoA gene fusions in Legionella pneumophila generated in vivo using a new transposon, MudphoA. Mol. Microbiol. **6:**1829–1839.
2. **Engleberg, N. C., N. P. Cianciotto, J. Smith, and B. I. Eisenstein.** 1988. Transfer and maintenance of small, mobilizable plasmids with ColE1 replication origins in Legionella pneumophila. Plasmid **20:**83–91.
3. **Manoil, C., and J. Beckwith.** 1985. TnphoA: a transposon probe for protein export signals. Proc. Natl. Acad. Sci. USA **82:**8129–8133.
4. **Pearlman, E., A. H. Jiwa, N. C. Engleberg, and B.I. Eisenstein.** 1988. Growth of Legionella pneumophila in a human macrophage-like (U937) cell line. Microb. Pathog. **5:**87–95.

Intracellular Production of *Legionella pneumophila* Tissue-Destructive Protease in Alveolar Macrophages

A. WILLIAMS, C. RECHNITZER, M. S. LEVER, AND R. B. FITZGEORGE

Public Health Laboratory Service Centre for Applied Microbiology and Research,
Porton Down, Salisbury, Wiltshire SP4 0JG, United Kingdom, and
Rigshospitalet, Tagensvej 20, DK-2200 Copenhagen, Denmark

The tissue-destructive protease (TDP) of *Legionella pneumophila* has been proposed as a pathogenic factor in Legionnaires' disease (LD). Purified enzyme has tissue-destructive (1, 6) and cytotoxic (3, 10) properties, inhibits human phagocyte functions (11), is an immunostimulatory molecule (4), and can degrade proteins of possible significance to host defense (8). The in vivo production of protease has been demonstrated and quantified by an enzyme-linked immunosorbent assay (ELISA) in the lungs of guinea pigs with experimental LD in quantities sufficient to cause some of the effects seen in vitro (7). Immunocytochemical labeling for protease in such lungs showed an intracellular location (13), but production of the enzyme by *L. pneumophila* multiplying intracellularly has not been demonstrated. Intracellular growth assays within guinea pig and human alveolar macrophages were developed and used to show that protease is produced intracellularly in such cells.

Immunological detection of TDP does not prove that the enzyme is capable of the activities described in in vitro studies. To determine whether the enzyme detected in vivo was functional, protease was purified from infected guinea pig lung washouts and its enzymatic function was tested.

Intracellular production of TDP in alveolar macrophages. Guinea pig and human alveolar macrophages were maintained in tissue culture and then incubated with *L. pneumophila* suspensions to allow bacterial uptake by the cells. Extracellular bacteria were then removed, and incubation continued for 24 h. Enumeration of bacteria by viable counts was performed in culture supernatants and macrophage lysates immediately following removal of extracellular bacteria and after 24 h of incubation. These samples were also assayed for TDP by using an ELISA based on immunoglobulin from rabbits immunized with purified protease. This assay has been described previously, and its specificity has been validated by Western immunoblotting (7).

In both guinea pig and human macrophages, bacterial counts in cell lysates increased by 2 to 3 orders of magnitude from 0 to 24 h. Washing procedures following infection of monolayers resulted in few or no extracellular bacteria at 0 h, but after 24 h, *Legionella* counts in the supernatants were similar to those in the lysates. Since the

culture media did not support the growth of this strain, multiplication must have occurred intracellularly.

Tissue culture media and a lysing agent had no effect on the ELISA, and no protease was detected in bacterial suspensions incubated with cell-free culture media. There was no TDP at 0 h, but after 24 h of incubation, approximately 0.1 to 0.2 μg of TDP per 10^6 bacteria was measured in culture supernatants and cell lysates. Although these levels are less than those required to exert some of the effects seen in vitro, it is known that much higher quantities are produced in the lungs of guinea pigs with LD. Macrophages are considered to be the principal site of replication of *L. pneumophila* in the lung, so it is likely that local concentrations of TDP are even higher.

Immunogold labeling of TDP. Guinea pig alveolar macrophages that had been incubated with bacteria for 24 h were harvested and processed for transmission electron microscopy as described by Williams et al. (13). Ultrathin sections of infected cells were immunogold labeled, using an indirect method with rabbit anti-TDP followed by gold (10 nm)-conjugated goat anti-rabbit immunoglobulin G. Figure 1 shows a cell containing numerous bacteria, with gold particles distributed throughout the phagosome and the cell cytoplasm. This result confirms the aforementioned finding that TDP is produced intracellularly.

In vivo activity of TDP. Guinea pigs were given a lethal aerosolized dose of *L. pneumophila* as described by Baskerville et al. (2). After 3 days, their lungs were washed out postmortem and cells were disrupted by sonication. Cell debris and bacteria were removed, and the supernatant was applied to a fast protein liquid chromatography (FPLC) Mono Q anion-exchange column. Fractions containing material that eluted off the column with a 0 to 0.5 M NaCl gradient were assayed for TDP by using the ELISA (Fig. 2). TDP-containing fractions were pooled, concentrated, and then added to wells in an agar plate containing 1% sodium caseinate. After several hours of incubation at 37°C, precipitation of the casein occurred (Fig. 3). This result shows that the TDP produced in vivo is functional.

Conclusions. *L. pneumophila* TDP has been widely studied and variously named cytotoxic protease, zinc metalloprotease, and major secretory protein. Several properties of this enzyme impli-

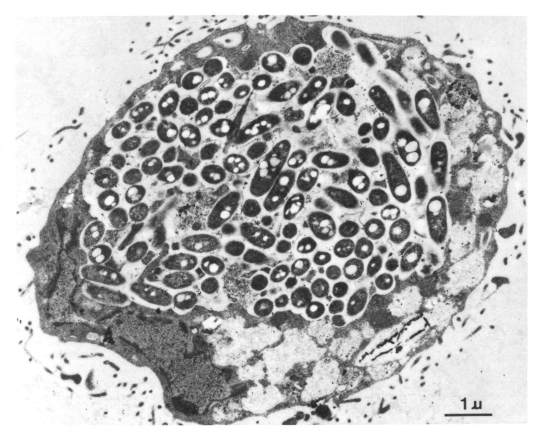

FIG. 1. Immunogold labeling for TDP in guinea pig alveolar macrophages infected in vitro with *L. pneumophila*.

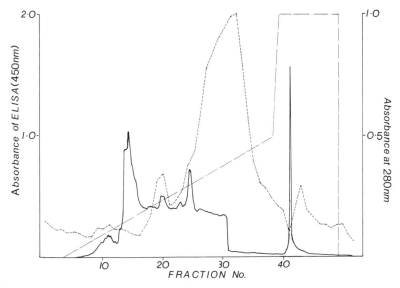

FIG. 2. FPLC anion-exchange chromatography of infected lung lavage supernatant. Lavage supernatant was equilibrated with 25 mM Tris-HCl (pH 7) and loaded onto a Mono Q column. A gradient of 0 to 0.5 M NaCl was applied to elute proteins as shown by A_{280}. Fractions were assayed by ELISA, and the A_{450} due to the substrate color reaction is shown. Symbols: —, A_{280}; – – –, A_{450}; —·—, NaCl gradient.

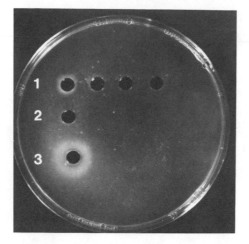

FIG. 3. Casein precipitation assay. Wells were cut into 1% agar containing 1% sodium caseinate. Rows: 1, doubling dilutions of pooled, concentrated ELISA-positive fractions; 2, buffer control; 3, purified TDP (55 μg/ml).

cate it as a pathogenic factor in LD, yet studies of a TDP-deficient mutant of *L. pneumophila* have suggested that it is not required for virulence (5). The same study also proposed that the pathology of disease is the same whether protease is present or not. Against the weight of evidence that supports the role of TDP in producing the lung lesions typical of LD, this finding is surprising. The mutant and its parent strain require large aerosol doses to cause death (5, 9). Since the mutant apparently produces small quantities of TDP (12), it is possible that enough enzyme is produced in vivo to account for the damage seen. Alternatively, during infection with such overwhelming numbers of bacteria, the lung damage could be caused by another factor that may not be significant following challenge with the lower doses of bacteria more typical of experimental LD.

TDP has a broad substrate specificity and is known to degrade structural and functional proteins of importance in the lungs. The fact that large quantities of TDP are produced in vivo and that this protein has enzymatic activity leads to the

assumption that although TDP may not be the only virulence factor, it cannot help but contribute to the pathogenesis of the disease.

REFERENCES

1. **Baskerville, A., J. W. Conlan, L. A. E. Ashworth, and A. B. Dowsett.** 1986. Pulmonary damage caused by a protease from *L. pneumophila*. *Br. J. Exp. Pathol.* **67:**527–536.
2. **Baskerville, A., R. B. Fitzgeorge, M. Broster, P. Hambleton, and P. J. Dennis.** 1981. Experimental transmission of Legionnaires' disease by exposure to aerosols of *Legionella pneumophila*. *Lancet* **ii:**1389–1390.
3. **Belyi, I. F., I. V. Vertiev, I. S. Tartokovskii, I. V. Ezepchuk, and S. V. Prozorovskii.** 1988. Characteristics of the cytolysin of *Legionella pneumophila*. *Zh. Mikrobiol. Epidemiol. Immunobiol.* **2:**4–7.
4. **Blander, S. J., and M. A. Horwitz.** 1989. Vaccination with the major secretory protein of *L. pneumophila* induces cell-mediated and protective immunity in a guinea pig model of Legionnaires' disease. *J. Exp. Med.* **169:**691–705.
5. **Blander, S. J., L. Szeto, H. A. Shuman, and M. A. Horwitz.** 1990. An immunoprotective molecule, the major secretory protein of *Legionella pneumophila*, is not a virulence factor in a guinea pig model of Legionnaires' disease. *J. Clin. Invest.* **86:**817–824.
6. **Conlan, J. W., A. Baskerville, and L. A. E. Ashworth.** 1986. Separation of *L. pneumophila* proteases and purification of a protease which produces lesions like those of Legionnaires' disease in guinea pig lung. *J. Gen. Microbiol.* **132:**1565–1574.
7. **Conlan, J. W., A. Williams, and L. A. E. Ashworth.** 1988. In vivo production of a tissue destructive protease by *L. pneumophila* in the lungs of experimentally infected guinea pigs. *J. Gen. Microbiol.* **134:**143–149.
8. **Conlan, J. W., A. Williams, and L. A. E. Ashworth.** 1988. Inactivation of human α-1–antitrypsin by a tissue destructive protease of *Legionella pneumophila*. *J. Gen. Microbiol.* **134:**481–487.
9. **Fitzgeorge, R. B.** Unpublished data.
10. **Quinn, F. D., M. G. Keen, and L. S. Tompkins.** 1989. Genetic, immunological, and cytotoxic comparisons of *Legionella* proteolytic activities. *Infect. Immun.* **57:**2719–2729.
11. **Rechnitzer, C., and A. Kharazmi.** 1992. Effect of *Legionella pneumophila* cytotoxic protease on human neutrophil and monocyte function. *Microb. Pathog.* **12:**115–125.
12. **Szeto, L., and H. A. Shuman.** 1990. The *Legionella pneumophila* major secretory protein, a protease, is not required for intracellular growth or cell killing. *Infect. Immun.* **58:**2585–2592.
13. **Williams, A., A. Baskerville, A. B. Dowsett, and J. W. Conlan.** 1987. Immunocytochemical demonstration of the association between *L. pneumophila*, its tissue destructive protease and pulmonary lesions in experimental Legionnaires' disease. *J. Pathol.* **153:**257–264.

Phenotypic Modulation by *Legionella pneumophila* upon Infection of Macrophages

YOUSEF ABU KWAIK, N. CARY ENGLEBERG, AND BARRY I. EISENSTEIN

Department of Microbiology and Immunology and Department of Internal Medicine, University of Michigan Medical School, Ann Arbor, Michigan 48109–0620

Legionella pneumophila survives in the environment as an intracellular parasite of freshwater protozoa and is also a human pathogen. The capacity of this pathogen to cause pneumonia is dependent on its ability to invade host cells and to multiply within membrane-bound vesicles. The factors that enable this intracellular organism to manifest these characteristics are not known.

Other intracellular pathogens manifest a regulated expression of genes in response to environmental stimuli. Upon infection of macrophages, *Salmonella typhimurium* responds to the intracellular environment by inducing the synthesis of over 30 proteins and repressing the synthesis of 136 proteins (2). Some of the *Salmonella* proteins that were induced by macrophages are well-known virulence factors (1, 3). The response by the organism to the intracellular environment allows it to adapt, survive, and multiply in macrophages.

In this report, we demonstrate that *L. pneumophila* responds during infection of macrophages by alteration of gene expression. Upon infection of macrophages, the expression of at least 70 proteins, which we designated macrophage-induced proteins (MINs), was induced. Some of the MINs were also induced by different stress conditions in vitro. Our data showed that the response by *L. pneumophila* to the intracellular environment of the macrophage is complex and may involve multiple regulons.

L. pneumophila AA100, the strain used for the study, is a clinical isolate originally named Wadsworth 130b. For radiolabeling of bacterial proteins in vitro, the organism was grown in a complete defined medium in order to limit the amount of nonradioactive methionine, which would allow more efficient incorporation of the radioactive methionine. The growth of strain AA100 in our complete defined medium was comparable to that in the CAA semidefined medium described by Mintz et al. (4).

For radiolabeling of bacterial proteins in the U937 macrophage-like cell line, a monolayer of differentiated U937 cells was infected with *L. pneumophila* AA100. After the infection, the flasks were incubated in a methionine-free tissue culture medium in the presence of [^{35}S]methionine. To inhibit growth of extracellular bacteria and to prevent protein synthesis by macrophages, gentamicin and cycloheximide, respectively, were added. After 20 h of incubation, the infected monolayer was lysed and the intracellular bacteria were harvested by centrifugation. The radiolabeled bacterial proteins were subjected to equilibrium two-dimensional gel electrophoresis as described by O'Farrell (5) and then subjected to autoradiography.

Upon infection of macrophages with *L. pneumophila* AA100, expression of at least 70 bacterial proteins was induced; 39 of these proteins were not detected in organisms grown in complete defined medium. The expression of these newly synthesized proteins may be required only during in vivo infection and may be necessary for the survival of *L. pneumophila* in the host cells. The MINs that were synthesized at low levels in vitro may be essential under a variety of conditions but needed at higher levels in the intracellular environment. In salmonellae, the known MINs that were expressed in vitro at low levels included the heat shock protein GroEL and DnaK (2).

The expression of some of the MINs has also been induced in vitro after exposure of *L. pneumophila* to several stress conditions, such as anaerobiosis, H_2O_2, heat shock, osmotic shock, acidic shock, and iron chelation. Some of the proteins were induced by more than one stress condition. These data suggest the presence of multiple regulons in *L. pneumophila* that are involved in the adaptation of the organisms to the intracellular environment. Similarly, salmonellae respond to the intracellular environment by the induction of many proteins that are contained in multiple regulons, and some of the proteins were also induced by stress conditions in vitro (2). It is possible that some of the MINs of salmonellae and legionellae have similar functions that allow these organisms to survive the macrophage environment.

The expression of at least 35 proteins was repressed upon infection of macrophages, and 12 of these proteins were undetectable in intracellularly grown organisms. The phenotypic modulation by *L. pneumophila* in response to the intracellular environment of the macrophage may reflect the organism's remarkable ability to respond to various intracellular stimuli and may be a necessary adaptation for the establishment of an intracellular infection.

L. pneumophila does not grow in RPMI 1640 tissue culture medium. To exclude the possibility that the phenotypic changes after infection of the macrophages were induced by the tissue culture medium prior to invasion of the macrophages, the protein profile of radiolabeled organisms incubated in RPMI 1640 was examined. The macrophage-induced phenotypic changes were not induced by the tissue culture medium. When U937 cells were incubated under same conditions but without infection by the bacteria, there was no incorporation of radioactivity. Since cycloheximide completely inhibited protein synthesis by the macrophages, all of the radiolabeled proteins were bacterial in origin.

Thus, *L. pneumophila* manifested a global response to the intracellular environment of the macrophage, and that response may be necessary for survival of the organisms in host cells. The response by the organisms to the intracellular environment is rather complex and may involve multiple regulons. These data will allow us to study the pathogenesis of *L. pneumophila* intracellularly and to investigate the factors that enable the organisms to survive and to multiply efficiently in what would otherwise be a hostile environment for bacteria. The techniques that we used may shed light on possible virulence factors that are expressed only in vivo.

REFERENCES

1. **Buchmeier, N. A., and F. Heffron.** 1989. Intracellular survival of wild-type *Salmonella typhimurium* and macrophage-sensitive mutants in diverse populations of macrophages. *Infect. Immun.* **57:**1–7.
2. **Buchmeier, N. A., and F. Heffron.** 1990. Induction of *Salmonella* stress proteins upon infection of macrophages. *Science* **248:**730–732.
3. **Miller, S. I., and J. J. Mekalanos.** 1990. Constitutive expression of the PhoP regulon attenuates *Salmonella* virulence and survival within macrophages. *Infect. Immun.* **172:**2485–2490.
4. **Mintz, C. S., J. Chen, and H. Shuman.** 1988. Isolation and characterization of auxotrophic mutants of *Legionella pneumophila* that fail to multiply in human monocytes. *Infect. Immun.* **56:**1449–1455.
5. **O'Farrell, P. H.** 1975. High resolution two dimensional electrophoresis of proteins. *J. Biol. Chem.* **250:**4007–4021.

The Role of Lymphocyte Activation in Resistance to *Legionella pneumophila* Infection

YOSHIMASA YAMAMOTO, THOMAS W. KLEIN, CATHERINE NEWTON, AND HERMAN FRIEDMAN

Department of Medical Microbiology and Immunology, University of South Florida College of Medicine, Tampa, Florida 33612-4799

Legionella pneumophila causes pneumonia in humans, especially immunocompromised subjects (4, 11). However, the bacteria grow in cultures of human and guinea pig mononuclear phagocytes, and infection appears to be regulated with the cellular immune defense system (5). In this regard, the importance of mononuclear phagocytes in legionellosis has been suggested by a number of investigators, including ourselves (9, 16, 19). Guinea pigs are known to be highly susceptible to *L. pneumophila* infection and therefore have been the preferred animal model for studies of legionellosis. In contrast, mice appear to be resistant to *L. pneumophila* infection, and mouse macrophages were believed to restrict the growth of legionellae (16, 19). Recently, however, we reported that macrophages from the A/J mouse strain support intracellular growth of legionellae (17), but mortality following infection with the bacteria is only slightly greater than that of other inbred mouse strains. The reason why A/J mice are moderately susceptible to *Legionella* infection, even though the macrophages are permissive for the intracellular growth of the bacteria, is not clear. In this study, we examined possible mechanisms for such differences of resistance to *Legionella* infection in susceptible guinea pigs, resistant BDF1 mice, and susceptible A/J mice. It seemed likely that the resistance of mice to *L.* *pneumophila* infection results from nonpermissive macrophages coupled with the responsiveness of lymphocytes. The susceptibility of guinea pigs, on the other hand, may result from both the permissive macrophages and the relative nonresponsiveness of lymphocytes to these bacteria.

Experimental conditions. Female strain 2 guinea pigs (300 to 500 g) and A/J and BDF1 female mice (6 to 8 weeks old) were obtained from the National Cancer Institute, Frederick, Md., and Jackson Laboratory, Bar Harbor, Maine, respectively.

A virulent strain of *L. pneumophila* serogroup 1 was obtained at autopsy from a case of fatal legionellosis at Tampa General Hospital, Tampa, Fla., and cultured on buffered charcoal-yeast extract medium as described previously (16).

Elicited peritoneal macrophages were obtained 4 days after intraperitoneal (i.p.) injection of thioglycolate broth as described previously (16). Elicited macrophages were suspended in RPMI 1640 medium supplemented with 15% heat-inactivated fetal calf serum and then allowed to adhere to tissue culture plates (24 wells) for 2 h in 5% CO_2 at 37°C. The resulting cell monolayers were washed to remove nonadherent cells.

Splenocytes were obtained from guinea pigs or mice. Culture supernatants (lymphokine enriched) were obtained from suspensions of 5×10^6 splenocytes stimulated with concanavalin A (ConA) at a final concentration of 4 μg/ml or formalin-killed *Legionella* vaccine (7) at a final concentration of 10^8 bacteria per ml for 24 h. Murine monoclonal antibody to gamma interferon (IFN-γ) was prepared from R4-6A2 hybridoma cells obtained from the American Type Culture Collection (Rockville, Md.). The neutralizing level for the purified monoclonal antibody was 4,749 U/mg of protein.

For in vitro experiments, the macrophage monolayers (approximately 10^6 cells per well) were infected with 2×10^5 bacteria for 30 min at 37°C, washed to remove nonphagocytized bacteria, and then incubated for various time periods. The number of viable bacteria in the macrophage lysates was obtained by lysis with sterile distilled water, and CFU was determined by standard plate count (16). For the cyclosporin A (CyA) experiments, mice were injected i.p. with CyA (50 mg/kg/day) 24 and 48 h before, simultaneously with, and 24 h after intravenous infection with *L. pneumophila* (2.5×10^6 bacteria per mouse). At 48 h after infection, the liver was removed from each mouse and homogenized in distilled water, and the number of viable bacteria in the homogenates was determined by standard plate count.

For the IFN assay, mouse spleen cells were added at a concentration of 10^7 cells per ml to 24-well tissue culture plates in 1.0 ml of RPMI 1640 medium supplemented with 10% fetal calf serum, antibiotics, and 2×10^{-5} M 2-mercaptoethanol. To each cell preparation was added killed *L. pneumophila* vaccine (10^8 bacteria per ml), and the cultures were then incubated for 24 h at 37°C in 5% CO_2. Cell-free culture supernatants were assayed for IFN activity by using vesicular stomatitis virus and L929 cells (3).

Spleen lymphocyte blastogenic transformation (LBT) was measured by the standard [^{3}H]TdR uptake method, using lymphocytes stimulated with either mitogen (ConA) or formalin-killed *L. pneumophila* vaccine as described previously (8).

Susceptibility of animals to *Legionella* infection. It is now widely accepted that guinea pigs are highly susceptible to infection with *L. pneu-*

mophila, and they have been widely used as an animal model for legionellosis (10). Mice appear to be relatively resistant to this opportunistic bacterium. Such differences in susceptibility to *Legionella* infection may be due to permissiveness of the growth of the bacteria in macrophages (16). Recently, we observed that A/J mouse macrophages, similar to macrophages from guinea pigs, are permissive for *Legionella* growth (17). However, A/J mice are still more resistant than guinea pigs to *Legionella* infection, although more susceptible than other mouse strains. Table 1 summarizes the susceptibilities of guinea pigs and mice to *Legionella* infection. The A/J mouse strain was approximately 10-fold more susceptible to *Legionella* infection than were the other mouse strains tested (BALB/c, DBA/2, C3H/HeN, C57BL/6, and BDF1). Nevertheless, even this susceptibility was lower than the extreme susceptibility of guinea pigs to *Legionella* infection.

***Legionella* growth in macrophages.** Figure 1 shows the multiplication of legionellae in peritoneal elicited macrophages from guinea pigs and mice, both A/J and BDF1. The number of viable bacteria (CFU) increased markedly in cultures from A/J mice as well as guinea pigs. In contrast, BDF1 mouse macrophages did not permit similar growth of the bacteria. From these data, it is apparent that guinea pig and A/J mouse macrophages are permissive for the growth of *L. pneumophila* but BDF1 mouse macrophages are nonpermissive. Our previous data had shown that other mouse macrophages, such as those from BALB/c, DBA/2, C57BL/6, and C3H/HeN mice, are nonpermissive (17). That is, among the inbred mouse strains tested, only A/J mouse macrophages are permissive.

Response of lymphocytes to *L. pneumophila*. It has been reported that normal human peripheral leukocytes respond to *Legionella* antigens to produce IFN-γ and tumor necrosis factor (1, 2). In other words, human lymphocytes respond to *Legionella* antigens even when nonsensitized lymphocytes are used. However, there are no reports of cytokine production by nonsensitized guinea pig lymphocytes in response to *Legionella* anti-

TABLE 1. Comparison of susceptibilities to *Legionella* infection

Animal	Body wt (g)	MLD[a]	Lethality index[b]	MLD/g of body wt	Lethality index
Mouse strains					
A/J	23	5×10^6	5	2.1×10^5	70
BDF1	23	5×10^7	50	2.1×10^6	700
DBA/2	23	5×10^7	50	2.1×10^6	700
BALB/c	23	5×10^7	50	2.1×10^6	700
Guinea pig strain 2	300	1×10^6	1	3×10^3	1

[a]MLD, minimum lethal doses when animals were infected i.p. with *L. pneumophila*.
[b]Normalized to guinea pig value of 1.

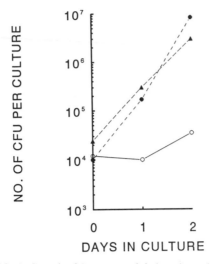

FIG. 1. Growth of *L. pneumophila* in guinea pig and mouse macrophage cultures. Macrophage monolayers were infected with *L. pneumophila* (10 bacteria per macrophage) for 30 min, washed, and then incubated for 2 days. The number of viable bacteria in macrophage lysates was determined by the plate count method. Data represent the means of triplicate macrophage cultures (standard deviation, <20%). Symbols: ○, BDF1 mouse cells; ●, A/J mouse cells; ▲, guinea pig cells.

gens. Figure 2 shows the responses of guinea pig and mouse lymphocytes to *L. pneumophila* antigens in terms of LBT and production of macrophage-activating factors (MAFs). When A/J or BDF1 mouse lymphocytes were stimulated with formalin-killed *Legionella* vaccine, both responded well in terms of [³H]TdR uptake. Figure 2 shows the stimulation index (SI) calculated by the following formula: SI = cpm of *Legionella*-stimulated lymphocytes/cpm of nonstimulated control lymphocytes. The blastogenic responsiveness of the guinea pig lymphocytes was minimal compared with the marked responsiveness of mouse splenocytes stimulated with *Legionella* vaccine. However, guinea pig splenocytes responded well to the mitogen ConA, similar to mouse splenocytes (data not shown).

Furthermore, culture supernatants from splenocytes of guinea pigs were markedly different from supernatants from splenocytes of mice after stimulation with *Legionella* vaccine with respect to macrophage-activating ability. Thus, it is apparent that guinea pig lymphocytes did not respond to *Legionella* antigens in terms of production of MAF, as assayed by inducing inhibition of *Legionella* growth in macrophages. In contrast, supernatants of splenocytes from both guinea pigs and mice, after stimulation with ConA, markedly inhibited *Legionella* growth when added to macrophages (data not shown). Taken together, these observations indicate that

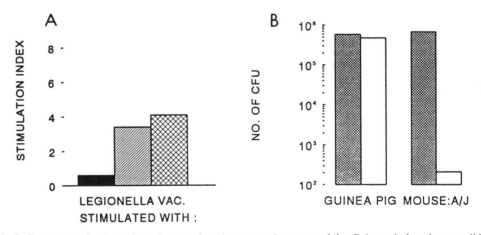

FIG. 2. Responses of guinea pig and mouse lymphocytes to *L. pneumophila*. Guinea pig lymphocytes did not respond to *L. pneumophila* in terms of LBT (A) and MAF (B) production. Lymphocytes obtained from spleens of either guinea pigs or mice were stimulated with *Legionella* vaccine (VAC.) for 2 days and then pulsed with [³H]TdR. Blastogenic response of lymphocytes was expressed as stimulation index. Data represent the means of triplicate cultures (standard deviation, <15%). MAF production from lymphocytes stimulated with *Legionella* vaccine was measured by the following method. Macrophage monolayers were preincubated with or without 10% splenocyte culture supernatants obtained from normal splenocyte cultures stimulated with *Legionella* vaccine for 24 h, incubated for 24 h, and then infected with bacteria. The number of viable bacteria in macrophage lysates was determined 48 h after infection. Data represent the means of triplicate macrophage cultures (standard deviation, <25%). (A) LBT. Solid bar, guinea pig; hatched bar, A/J mouse; cross-hatched bar, BDF1 mouse. (B) MAF production. Cross-hatched bar, control; open bar, plus culture supernatant.

normal guinea pig lymphocytes can respond to a stimulus such as ConA to produce MAF but cannot respond to *L. pneumophila*. In contrast, normal mice, both A/J and BDF1, can produce anti-*Legionella* MAF.

The major MAF is IFN-γ. The major MAF activity observed in splenocyte culture supernatants stimulated by the *Legionella* vaccine appeared to be due to IFN-γ, as demonstrated by experiments in which the supernatants from the *Legionella* vaccine-stimulated splenocytes were neutralized by monoclonal anti-IFN-γ antibody. Furthermore, addition of recombinant murine IFN-γ induced anti-*Legionella* activity in the macrophage cultures. For these experiments, the A/J mouse macrophage monolayers were treated with 10% culture supernatants of A/J mouse splenocytes stimulated with *L. pneumophila* vaccine. Other cultures were treated with 100 U of recombinant IFN-γ per ml or with IFN-γ along with 100 neutralizing units of anti-IFN-γ antibody. The macrophages were infected 24 h later with *L. pneumophila*. As is apparent in Fig. 3, much of the macrophage-activating activity in the supernatants of A/J mouse splenocytes stimulated with

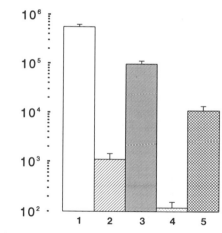

FIG. 3. Effect of monoclonal anti-IFN-γ antibody on MAF activity of *Legionella* vaccine-induced supernatant. MAF activity was neutralized by anti-IFN-γ antibody. Furthermore, recombinant murine IFN-γ induced anti-*Legionella* activity in macrophages. A/J mouse macrophage monolayers were treated with 10% culture supernatant from A/J mouse splenocytes stimulated with *Legionella* vaccine or 100 U of recombinant IFN-γ per ml along with 100 neutralizing units of anti-IFN-γ antibody for 24 h. Macrophages were infected 24 h later with *L. pneumophila*. The number of viable bacteria in macrophage lysates was measured 48 h after infection. Each bar represents the mean ± standard deviation of triplicate macrophage cultures. Bars: 1, control; 2, plus supernatant; 3, plus supernatant and anti-IFN-γ antibody; 4, plus IFN-γ; 5, plus IFN-γ and anti-IFN-γ antibody.

legionellae was diminished with monoclonal anti-IFN-γ antibody. When the recombinant IFN-γ was used as a reference, anti-*Legionella* activity induced by recombinant IFN-γ was also neutralized with monoclonal antibody. Induction of IFNs from murine spleen cells by legionellae has been reported (3), but activity was measured by its antiviral activity in a cytopathic inhibition assay, not by its anti-*Legionella* activity. Here, we identified the production of IFN-γ from *Legionella*-stimulated lymphocytes as an MAF.

How lymphocytes work in *Legionella* infection in vivo: use of CyA as a T-cell inhibitor. Up to now, there has been no direct evidence that lymphocytes and their products can regulate *Legionella* growth in vivo. To study this possibility, we evaluated the role of lymphocytes, especially T lymphocytes, in resistance of animals to *Legionella* infection by using a selective immunosuppressant such as CyA. CyA is a well-known immunosuppressant that causes a selective depletion in function T lymphocytes (13). As is apparent in Fig. 4, treatment of either A/J or BDF1 mice with CyA markedly suppressed the ability of their spleen cells to respond to a T-cell-dependent mitogen. Stimulation of the spleen cells from these mice with ConA resulted in markedly reduced blastogenic responses. The same spleen cells, when stimulated in vitro with a B-cell mitogen, i.e., lipopolysaccharide (LPS), evinced as good a response to this mitogen as did spleen cells from normal control mice not treated with CyA. Furthermore, splenocytes from the CyA-treated A/J mice produced less IFN activity when stimulated in vitro with *Legionella* antigens. These results indicate that CyA treatment of mice under the conditions used induced a selective depletion of T-cell functions, including IFN production, in response to *Legionella* infection.

***Legionella* infection in CyA-treated mice.** Effects of lymphocytes and their products on the resistance of mice to *Legionella* infection were evaluated by using CyA-treated mice that were selectively depleted of T-cell functions. In these experiments, either A/J or BDF1 mice were injected i.p. with CyA four times (i.e., 48 and 24 h before, simultaneously with, and 24 h after infection) and infected intravenously with *L. pneumophila*. At 48 h after infection, the liver was removed from mice and the number of viable bacteria in liver homogenates was determined. As shown in Table 2, legionellae grew much more readily in the livers of A/J mice after immunosuppressive treatment with CyA. In contrast, there was little difference in the recovery of bacteria in the livers of BDF1 mice, either treated with CyA or nontreated. These results might be explained by the following mechanisms. Since BDF1 mouse macrophages are nonpermissive for *Legionella* growth, T-lymphocyte dysfunction in BDF1 mice

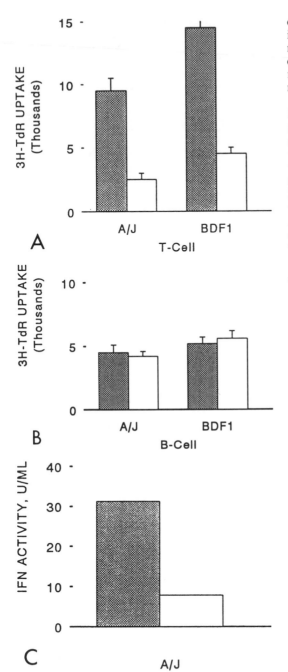

FIG. 4. Effects of CyA treatment on the LBT (A and B) and IFN production (C) of lymphocytes. CyA treatment induced the suppression of T-cell but not B-cell function. Mice, either A/J or BDF1, were injected i.p. with CyA (50 mg/kg/day for 4 days), and their spleens were removed 24 h after the final injection. LBT was measured by using ConA and LPS as mitogens for T and B cells, respectively. The production of IFNs in A/J mouse splenocyte cultures stimulated with *Legionella* vaccine for 24 h was assayed by using vesicular stomatitis virus and L929 cells. Bars: cross-hatched, control; open, plus CyA.

does not induce an increase of *Legionella* growth in nonpermissive macrophages. However, in A/J mice, T-lymphocyte dysfunction induces a serious disturbance of macrophage regulation, so there is nonrestricted growth of legionellae in permissive macrophages.

Restoration of the resistance by lymphokines in T-cell-depleted mice. In additional experiments, the effect of injection of lymphokine-rich culture supernatants into CyA-treated A/J mice was studied. For these experiments, A/J mice were given four injections of CyA, following exactly the protocol described above. A lymphokine-rich culture supernatant from splenocytes from A/J mice stimulated in vitro with ConA was administered i.p. to CyA-treated mice two times a day on the day of infection and 1 day after infection. There was a significant restoration in the ability of the mice to restrict the growth of *L. pneumophila*, as shown by the recovery of bacteria in the livers of these mice compared with the number of bacteria in the livers of CyA-treated mice (Table 2). These findings suggest that lymphokine production after lymphocyte activation with *Legionella* infection may serve a critical role in resistance to *Legionella* infection.

Summary. Figure 5 summarizes the results reported here on the possible roles of both lymphocytes and macrophages in the resistance of animals to *Legionella* infection. Macrophages in permissive guinea pigs readily replicated these bacteria. However, lymphocytes from guinea pigs do not respond well to *Legionella* antigens and are not readily activated to produce MAF, which reduces the susceptibility of macrophages to *Legionella* infection. In contrast, mice, including A/J mice, are somewhat more resistant than guinea pigs to *Legionella* infection. A/J mice, however, are somewhat more susceptible than other mouse strains but much more resistant than guinea pigs. A/J mouse lymphocytes can respond to *Legionella* antigens to produce MAFs, mainly IFN-γ, which can convert susceptible (i.e., permissive) macrophages to resistance (nonpermissive). This process appears to be similar to what may occur in humans, who have lymphocytes that can respond to *Legionella* antigens by producing lymphokines even though their monocytes are susceptible to infection with these bacteria (1, 2). On the other hand, most other mouse strains, such as BALB/c, DBA/2, C57BL/6, and C3H/HeN, have nonpermissive macrophages which innately resist replication of legionellae (17). Furthermore, lymphocytes from these resistant mouse strains, similar to lymphocytes from the more susceptible A/J mice, respond to *Legionella* antigens by producing IFNs and other cytokines that can activate permissive or even nonpermissive macrophages to resist *Legionella* growth. Thus, it is apparent that lymphocytes serve as an important cell type in

TABLE 2. Effects of treatment with CyA and/or lymphokine-rich culture
supernatant on the number of viable *L. pneumophila* in the livers of
A/J and BDF1 mice

Mouse strain	No. of viable bacteria (10^4)/liver[a]		Treatment with CyA and culture supernatant[c]
	Treatment with CyA[b]		
	No	Yes	
A/J	7.0 ± 4.0	95.0 ± 30.0	7.5 ± 2.5
BDF1	1.3 ± 0.7	2.1 ± 0.6	ND

[a]Results determined 48 h after infection. Each value represents the mean ± standard deviation for five mice.
[b]Mice were given four i.p. injections of CyA (50 mg/kg/day for 4 days) and then infected intravenously with *L. pneumophila* (2.5×10^6 bacteria per mouse).
[c]Lymphokine-rich culture supernatant (1.0 ml per mouse each time) was administered i.p. to CyA-treated mice two times a day on the day of infection and 1 day after infection. ND, not done.

responding to *Legionella* antigens, even when macrophages or phagocytic monocytes of a host are genetically susceptible to growth of these opportunistic bacteria (14, 15, 18). Furthermore, the importance of lymphocytes in *L. pneumophila* infection demonstrated here coincides with previous reports which showed that dysfunction of cellular immunity is a high-risk factor for *Legionella* infection in humans (12).

This work was supported by grant AI 16618 from the National Institute of Allergy and Infectious Diseases.

REFERENCES

1. **Blanchard, D. K., J. Y. Djeu, T. W. Klein, H. Friedman, and W. E. Stewart II.** 1987. Induction of tumor necrosis factor by *Legionella pneumophila*. *Infect. Immun.* **55:**433–437.

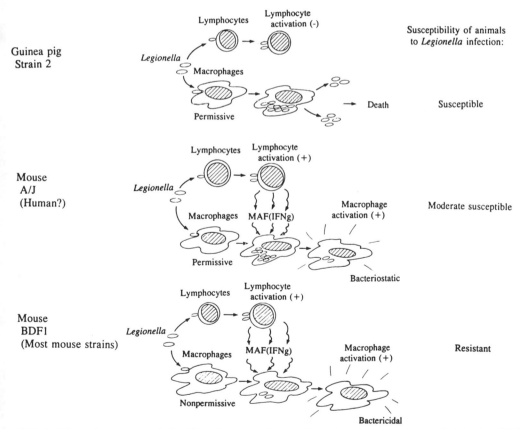

FIG. 5. Schematic summary of role of lymphocytes and macrophages in resistance to *Legionella* infection. IFNg, IFN-γ.

2. **Blanchard, D. K., H. Friedman, T. W. Klein, and J. Y. Djeu.** 1989. Induction of interferon-gamma and tumor necrosis factor by *Legionella pneumophila*: augmentation of human neutrophil bactericidal activity. *J. Leukocyte Biol.* **45:**538–545.

3. **Blanchard, D. K., T. W. Klein, H. Friedman, and W. E. Stewart II.** 1985. Kinetics and characterization of interferon production by murine spleen cells stimulated with *Legionella pneumophila* antigens. *Infect. Immun.* **49:**719–723.

4. **Cordonnier, C., J. P. Farcet, and L. Desforges.** 1984. Legionnaires' disease and hairy-cell leukemia. *Arch. Intern. Med.* **144:**2373–2375.

5. **Eisenstein, T. K., and H. Friedman.** 1985. Immunity to legionella, p. 159–176. *In* S. M. Katz (ed.), *Legionellosis.* CRC Press, Boca Raton, Fla.

6. **Elliot, J. A., W. Johnson, and C. M. Helms.** 1981. Ultrastructural localization and protective activity of a high-molecular-weight antigen isolated from *Legionella pneumophila. Infect. Immun.* **31:**822–824.

7. **Friedman, F., R. Widen, T. Klein, and H. Friedman.** 1984. Lymphoid cell blastogenesis as an in vitro indicator of cellular immunity to *Legionella pneumophila* antigens. *J. Clin. Microbiol.* **19:**834–837.

8. **Friedman, H., R. Widen, T. Klein, L. Searls, and K. Cabrian.** 1984. *Legionella pneumophila*-induced blastogenesis of murine lymphoid cells in vitro. *Infect. Immun.* **43:**314–319.

9. **Horwitz, M. A., and S. C. Silverstein.** 1980. The Legionnaires' disease bacterium (*Legionella pneumophila*) multiplies intracellularly in human monocytes. *J. Clin. Invest.* **66:**441–450.

10. **Katz, S. M., and J. P. Matus.** 1985. Animal models of legionellosis, p. 119–132. *In* S. M. Katz (ed.), *Le-*

gionellosis, vol. II. CRC Press, Boca Raton, Fla.

11. **Korvick, J., and V. L. Yu.** 1988. Simultaneous infection with *Cryptococcus neoformans* and *Legionella pneumophila: in vivo* expression of common defects in immunity. *Respiration* **53:**132–136.

12. **Nguyen, M. H., J. E. Stout, and V. L. Yu.** 1991. Legionellosis. *Infect. Dis. Clin. North Am.* **5:**561–584.

13. **Shevach, E. M.** 1985. The effects of cyclosporin A on the immune system. *Annu. Rev. Immunol.* **3:**397–404.

14. **Yamamoto, Y., T. W. Klein, and H. Friedman.** 1991. *Legionella pneumophila* growth in macrophages from susceptible mice is genetically controlled. *Proc. Soc. Exp. Biol. Med.* **196:**405–409.

15. **Yamamoto, Y., T. W. Klein, and H. Friedman.** 1992. Genetic control of macrophage susceptibility to infection by *Legionella pneumophila. FEMS Microbiol. Immunol.* **89:**137–146.

16. **Yamamoto, Y., T. W. Klein, C. A. Newton, R. Widen, and H. Friedman.** 1987. Differential growth of *Legionella pneumophila* in guinea pig versus mouse macrophage cultures. *Infect. Immun.* **55:**1369–1374.

17. **Yamamoto, Y., T. W. Klein, C. A. Newton, R. Widen, and H. Friedman.** 1988. Growth of *Legionella pneumophila* in thioglycolate-elicited peritoneal macrophages from A/J mice. *Infect. Immun.* **56:**370–375.

18. **Yoshida, S., Y. Gotoi, Y. Mizuguchi, K. Nomoto, and E. Skamene.** 1991. Genetic control of natural resistance in mouse macrophages regulating intracellular *Legionella pneumophila* multiplication in vitro. *Infect. Immun.* **59:**428–432.

19. **Yoshida, S., and Y. Mizuguchi.** 1986. Multiplication of *Legionella pneumophila* Philadelphia-1 in cultural peritoneal macrophages and its correlation to susceptibility of animals. *Can. J. Microbiol.* **32:**438–442.

Activation of Macrophages with Bacterial Protein-Lipopolysaccharide Complexes for Killing Ingested *Legionella pneumophila*

K. NIXDORFF, S. ARATA, C. NEWTON, T. W. KLEIN, AND H. FRIEDMAN

Institut für Mikrobiologie, Technical University, Darmstadt, Germany; Department of Microbial Chemistry, School of Pharmaceutical Science, Showa University, Tokyo, Japan; and Department of Medical Microbiology and Immunology, University of South Florida, Tampa, Florida 33612-4799

Macrophages may be activated by many immune stimulators, and such activated cells can reduce the growth of intracellular opportunistic bacteria. Previous studies in this laboratory showed that peritoneal macrophages from A/J mice are permissive for the growth of *Legionella pneumophila* (10). Furthermore, stimulation of macrophages from A/J mice with immunoadjuvants such as bacterial lipopolysaccharide (LPS) activates the cells so that they resist growth of legionellae (1–3). We have shown previously that LPS from *Proteus mirabilis* stimulates macrophages to produce oxygen radicals, interleukin-1 (IL-1), and tumor necrosis factor (TNF) (7, 8). A protein-rich component (39-kDa protein) extracted from purified cell walls of *P. mirabilis*, when complexed with LPS through sonication and added to macrophages in vitro, suppressed the ability of LPS to induce the production of oxygen

radicals and IL-1 but greatly enhanced the production of TNF (7, 8). It was therefore of interest to determine whether the 39-kDa protein could modulate the LPS-induced killing of a facultative intracellular bacterial pathogen. In this study, it was found that LPS from *P. mirabilis* also has the ability to activate macrophages from A/J mice to resist *Legionella* growth. This resistance was not affected by treatment of macrophages with the LPS-protein complex, indicating that modulation of cytokine production by the 39-kDa protein had little, if any, effect on intracellular killing of legionellae by LPS-activated macrophages.

A/J mice were obtained from Jackson Laboratory, Bar Harbor, Maine. They were 6 to 8 weeks of age at the initiation of an experiment and weighed approximately 18 g. They were fed Purina mouse food and water ad libitum.

L. pneumophila serogroup 1 was obtained from

a case of fatal legionellosis. It was cultured on buffered charcoal-yeast extract agar (GIBCO Laboratories, Grand Island, N.Y.) for 72 h, and the bacteria were harvested from plates by scraping into saline with a sterile swab. A suspension of 10^8 bacteria per ml in RPMI 1640 culture medium (GIBCO) supplemented with 10% fetal calf serum (FCS; HyClone Laboratories, Logan, Utah) but without antibiotics was prepared after washing in Hanks' balanced salt solution and then subjected to centrifugation.

LPS I from *P. mirabilis* 19 was extracted from whole cells by the phenol-water method (9), purified further by treatment with RNase and DNase, and then washed with distilled water in an ultracentrifuge (4). LPS was reextracted with phenol-water to remove contaminating protein as described previously (5, 8). After extensive dialysis, the LPS was lyophilized. For use in the test system, LPS was sonicated in Tris buffer for 2 min in an ice bath with the microtip at maximum power level and diluted to the desired concentrations in RPMI 1640 medium supplemented with 10% FCS but without antibiotics.

The 39-kDa protein was isolated from purified cell walls of *P. mirabilis* 19 by a method described previously (6). Briefly, cell walls free of cytoplasmic membranes and cell contents were extracted with 1% sodium deoxycholate in a Tris buffer at pH 8.0 for 45 min at 37°C. This procedure was followed by gel filtration on Sephacryl S-300 (Pharmacia, Uppsala, Sweden) in a Tris buffer containing 0.25% sodium deoxycholate. The fractions containing the 39-kDa protein were collected, and after extensive dialysis to remove detergent and buffer (6), the product was lyophilized. The extracted protein contained 16% LPS. To obtain a clear solution of the protein in aqueous buffer, 1 mg of protein was first dissolved in 1 part NaOH at pH 9.0 and immediately neutralized with 1 part buffer.

LPS and the 39-kDa protein were mixed together in the ratios to be used in the test system. The protein was first dissolved as described above, and LPS was added. The mixture was then sonicated for 2 min in an ice bath with the microtip at maximum power level and diluted to the desired concentrations in RPMI 1640 medium supplemented with 10% FCS but without antibiotics.

Peritoneal exudate macrophages were obtained from individual mice 3 days after intraperitoneal injection of 3 ml of thioglycolate medium (Difco Laboratories, Detroit, Mich.) as described previously (1–3, 10). The peritoneum was aspirated several times with Hanks' balanced salt solution, and the resulting cells were resuspended to a concentration of 10^6 viable nucleated cells per ml of RPMI 1640 medium supplemented with 10% FCS but without antibiotics.

For in vitro infection, suspensions of macrophages in RPMI medium were placed in 96-well culture plates (Costar, Cambridge, Mass.) at a density of 10^5 cells per well (100 μl per well) and incubated at 37°C in a humidified atmosphere containing 5% CO_2 for 2 h. Thereafter, the cultures were washed, fresh medium was added, and the plates were incubated overnight. On the next day, the supernatants were removed from the cultures, LPS, the 39-kDa protein, or mixtures of LPS with the protein were added, and the plates were incubated again overnight. After overnight incubation, the supernatants were removed and *L. pneumophila* was added to each culture at a concentration of 10^5 bacteria per ml. The plates were incubated for 30 min, and the nonphagocytized bacteria were removed by two washes with Hanks' balanced salt solution. Finally, fresh RPMI medium was added, and the cultures were incubated for 48 h under the conditions described above.

For harvesting of *L. pneumophila*, supernatants were removed from macrophage cultures containing bacteria; 100 μl of 0.1% sterile saponin was added, and the plates were incubated for 10 min. Thereafter, the liquid in each well was aspirated vigorously several times and then collected for dilution and plating on buffered charcoal-yeast extract agar. The agar plates were incubated for 3 to 4 days at 37°C in a humidified atmosphere, and *Legionella* colonies were counted.

As is apparent in Table 1, LPS I from *P. mirabilis* activated peritoneal macrophages from A/J mice to restrict the growth of legionellae. Graded doses of the LPS induced increasing resistance, as shown by the lower numbers of *Legionella* CFU

TABLE 1. Effects of LPS and mixtures of LPS plus the 39-kDa protein from *P. mirabilis* on the growth of *L. pneumophila* in thioglycolate-elicited peritoneal macrophages from A/J mice[a]

Stimulant (ng/ml)	CFU (10^6)/ macrophage culture[b]
None	1.391 ± 0.24
LPS (1)	1.063 ± 0.47
LPS (10)	0.473 ± 0.12
LPS (100)	0.147 ± 0.02
LPS (1,000)	0.054 ± 0.02
LPS (1) + 39-kDa protein (0.5)	1.258 ± 0.24
LPS (10) + 39-kDa protein (5)	0.406 ± 0.10
LPS (100) + 39-kDa protein (50)	0.138 ± 0.01
LPS (1,000) + 39-kDa protein (500)	0.096 ± 0.01

[a]Mixtures of LPS and the 39-kDa protein were prepared by sonication of both components together for 2 min in an ice bath, using the microtip at the maximum power level.

[b]Values represent geometrical means $\pm$ standard errors measured in two to four separate experiments.

TABLE 2. Effects of *P. mirabilis* LPS, the 39-kDa protein, and various mixtures on the growth of *L. pneumophila* in thioglycolate-elicited peritoneal macrophages from A/J mice[a]

Stimulant (ng/ml)	CFU (10^6)/ macrophage culture[b]
None	1.308 ± 0.66
LPS (·100)	0.157 ± 0.01
39-kDa protein (50)	0.339 ± 0.02
39-kDa protein (100)	0.306 ± 0.12
39-kDa protein (200)	0.203 ± 0.02
LPS (100) + 39-kDa protein (50)	0.143 ± 0.01
LPS (100) + 39-kDa protein (100)	0.092 ± 0.01
LPS (100) + 39-kDa protein (200)	0.076 ± 0.01

[a]Mixtures of LPS and the 39-kDa protein were prepared by sonication for 2 min in an ice bath, using the microtip at the maximum power level.
[b]Values represent geometrical means ± standard errors measured in two to three separate experiments.

recovered from LPS-treated cultures than from untreated macrophages. Complexing the 39-kDa protein with LPS in a ratio of 2:1 had little effect on the ability of macrophages to kill ingested bacteria. In this combination, the protein had a profound effect in modulating cytokine production of LPS-activated macrophages. For example, when LPS I from *P. mirabilis* was mixed with the 39-kDa protein in the same ratio or 2:1 (10 μg of LPS plus 5 μg of the 39-kDa protein), we observed a 60% reduction in LPS-induced IL-1 production by macrophages compared with IL-1 production by macrophages stimulated with LPS (10 μg/ml) alone; on the other hand, TNF production was increased 10-fold (7).

Increasing the amount of the 39-kDa protein in the mixture also had little effect in modulating LPS-induced intracellular killing of legionellae (Table 2). The lower numbers of *Legionella* CFU with increasing amounts of the 39-kDa protein added in combination with LPS may simply be due to contamination of the protein preparation with LPS. Indeed, the protein alone was able to activate macrophages (Table 2), approximately in proportion to the amount of LPS contaminating the sample. Binding of LPS to the 39-kDa protein is extremely tight and can be removed only by such drastic methods as phenol-water extraction

(5). Further studies with purified preparations of the 39-kDa protein are warranted.

Nevertheless, the relatively weak activity of the protein in affecting LPS-induced resistance of macrophages to in vitro *Legionella* infection suggests that the strong capacity of the protein to modulate IL-1 or TNF production by macrophages has little effect on intracellular killing processes. This finding is also in agreement with earlier studies which indicated that production of these cytokines does not correlate with the ability of macrophages to kill legionellae (10).

REFERENCES

1. **Arata, S., T. W. Klein, C. Newton, and H. Friedman.** 1991. Tetrahydrocannabinol treatment suppresses growth restriction of *Legionella pneumophila* in murine macrophage cultures. *Life Sci.* **49**:473–479.
2. **Arata, S., C. Newton, T. Klein, and H. Friedman.** 1992. Enhanced growth of *Legionella pneumophila* in tetrahydrocannabinol-treated macrophages. *Proc. Soc. Exp. Biol. Med.* **199**:65–67.
3. **Egawa, K., T. W. Klein, Y. Yamamoto, C. A. Newton, and H. Friedman.** 1992. Enhanced growth restriction of *Legionella pneumophila* in endotoxin treated macrophages. *Proc. Soc. Exp. Biol. Med.* **200**:338–342.
4. **Gmeiner, J.** 1975. The isolation of two different lipopolysaccharide fractions from various *Proteus mirabilis* strains. *Eur. J. Biochem.* **58**:621–626.
5. **Karch, H., J. Gmeiner, and K. Nixdorff.** 1983. Alteration of the immunoglobulin G subclass responses in mice to lipopolysaccharide: effects of nonbacterial proteins and bacterial membrane phospholipids or outer membrane proteins of *Proteus mirabilis*. *Infect. Immun.* **40**:157–165.
6. **Nixdorff, K., H. Fitzer, J. Gmeiner, and H. H. Martin.** 1977. Reconstitution of model membranes from phospholipid and outer membrane proteins of *Proteus mirabilis*. Role of proteins in the formation of hydrophilic pores and protection of membranes against detergent. *Eur. J. Biochem.* **81**:63–69.
7. **Nixdorff, K., G. Weber, K. Kaniecki, W. Ruiner, and S. Schell.** 1992. Bacterial protein-LPS complexes and immunomodulation, p. 49–61. *In* H. Friedman, T. W. Klein, and Y. Yamaguchi (ed.), *Microbial Infections: Role of Biological Response Modifiers*. Plenum Publishing Corp., New York.
8. **Weber, G., D. Heck, R. R. Bartlett, and K. Nixdorff.** 1992. Modulation of effects of lipopolysaccharide on macrophages by a major outer membrane protein of *Proteus mirabilis* as measured in a chemiluminescence assay. *Infect. Immun.* **60**:1069–1075.
9. **Westphal, O., O. Lüderitz, and F. Bister.** 1952. Über die Extraktion von Bakterien mit Phenol/Wasser. *Z. Naturforsch. Teil B* **7**:147–155
10. **Yamamoto, Y., T. W. Klein, C. A. Newton, R. Widen, and H. Friedman.** 1988. Growth of *Legionella pneumophila* in thioglycolate-elicited peritoneal macrophages from A/J mice. *Infect. Immun.* **56**:370–375.

Inhibition by 2-Deoxy-D-Glucose of Intracellular *Legionella pneumophila* Multiplication in A/J Mouse Macrophages

MIDORI OGAWA, SHIN-ICHI YOSHIDA, AND YASUO MIZUGUCHI

Department of Microbiology, School of Medicine, University of Occupational and Environmental Health, Kitakyushu 807, Japan

Legionella pneumophila is a facultative intracellular parasite that can grow in phagosomes of human monocytes (1) and in macrophages of guinea pigs (5) and A/J mice (3, 4). Although intracellular bacterial growth is easily assayed in vitro by using macrophage cultures, the source of nutrition and its metabolism during intracellular growth are not well understood. In an attempt to find agents that inhibit intracellular growth in A/J macrophages, we found that 2-deoxy-D-glucose (2-dG) could do so when added to a macrophage culture. We describe below some effects of 2-dG on intracellular bacterial growth.

L. pneumophila Philadelphia-1 was cultured in buffered yeast extract (BYE) broth or on charcoal-yeast extract agar plates. Multiplication of the bacteria in peritoneal macrophages was measured as described previously (4), with minor modification. In brief, peritoneal exudate cells were obtained from A/J mice 4 days after intraperitoneal injection of 3% thioglycolate medium. A total of 10^6 peritoneal exudate cells was placed in each well of a 24-well tissue culture plate; after incubation for 1.5 h, nonadherent cells were washed out. The peritoneal macrophage monolayers were then infected with approximately 10^6 bacterial cells for 1.5 h, and nonphagocytosed bacteria were also washed out. After 2.5 h of cultivation in RPMI 1640 medium containing 10% newborn calf serum, 2-dG (Nakalai Tesque, Kyoto, Japan) was added at concentrations of 1, 10, and 50 mM. After 0, 24, and 48 h of incubation, the number of bacteria in each well was determined by plating on charcoal-yeast extract agar plates.

The effects of 2-dG on the in vitro growth of *L. pneumophila* in BYE broth were examined. 2-dG at concentrations of 1, 10, and 100 mM neither suppressed nor promoted bacterial growth in BYE broth. As *L. pneumophila* utilizes glucose only minimally, this result shows that the bacterium does not utilize 2-dG.

2-dG was cytotoxic to mouse peritoneal macrophages at concentrations above 1 mM when glucose-deficient RPMI 1640 medium was used for culture. But when glucose (15 mM)-containing RPMI 1640 medium was used, cytotoxicity was not observed at 1 or 10 mM 2-dG. We used glucose-containing medium for the macrophage culture.

When 2-dG was added to the macrophage culture, it suppressed intracellular bacterial growth in a dose-dependent manner (Fig. 1). Because the

suppressive effect was apparent from day 1 of culture, it is not likely that suppression of the phagocytosis of bacteria released from other infected macrophages resulted in the suppression of intracellular growth.

To determine whether the inhibitory effect of 2-dG is reversible, 2-dG was washed out 16 h after in vitro phagocytosis. Intracellular bacterial growth resumed thereafter at the same rate as in the control culture. Thus, the inhibitory effect of 2-dG was reversible.

Next, we examined whether addition of glucose represses the inhibitory action of 2-dG. Addition of glucose at 10 mM was not effective, but 50 mM

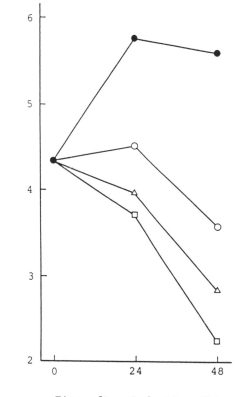

FIG. 1. Inhibitory effects of 2-dG on the intracellular growth of *L. pneumophila* Philadelphia-1 in thioglycolate-elicited A/J mouse peritoneal macrophages. Symbols: ●, no. 2-dG; ○, 1 mM 2-dG; △, 10 mM 2-dG; □, 50 mM 2-dG.

glucose could restore the suppression caused by 1 mM 2-dG.

It has been reported that 2-dG inhibits phagocytosis by mouse peritoneal macrophages (2). To avoid the influence of the inhibition of phagocytosis, we cultured the macrophage monolayer for 2.5 h after in vitro phagocytosis and before the addition of 2-dG. Furthermore, the suppression described here is not due to the suppression of phagocytosis of the bacteria released from the macrophages because the inhibition was clear at 16 h after in vitro phagocytosis. These results indicate that 2-dG suppressed the intracellular growth of the bacteria.

2-dG inhibits glycosylation and protein synthesis and lowers the ATP level (2). In a preliminary examination, we added tunicamycin (a glycosylation inhibitor) to the culture at concentrations of 1, 2, and 5 μg/ml, but tunicamycin could not suppress intracellular bacterial growth. The protein synthesis inhibitor cycloheximide was cytotoxic to the macrophages, but when used at 0.1 μg/ml, cycloheximide could not suppress intracellular bacterial growth.

Although the mechanism by which 2-dG inhibits intracellular bacterial growth is not clear, it appears that 2-dG inhibits intracellular bacterial growth by affecting the glucose metabolism of A/J macrophages.

2-dG will be a useful tool in studies of (i) the mechanism by which *L. pneumophila* grows in macrophages and (ii) how macrophages from A/J and C57BL/6 mice differ such that they permit and suppress, respectively, intracellular bacterial growth (4).

This study was supported by Grant-in-Aid for Scientific Research 03670229 from the Ministry of Education, Science and Culture, Japan.

REFERENCES

1. **Horwitz, M. A., and S. C. Silverstein.** 1980. Legionnaires' bacterium (*Legionella pneumophila*) multiplies intracellularly in human monocytes. *J. Clin. Invest.* **66:**441–450.
2. **Sung, S.S. J., and S. C. Silverstein.** 1985. Role of 2-deoxy-D-glucose in the inhibition of phagocytosis by mouse peritoneal macrophage. *Biochim. Biophys. Acta* **845:**204–215.
3. **Yamamoto, Y., T. W. Klein, C. A. Newton, R. Widen, and H. Friedman.** 1988. Growth of *Legionella pneumophila* in thioglycolate-elicited peritoneal macrophages from A/J mice. *Infect. Immun.* **56:**370–375.
4. **Yoshida, S., Y. Goto, Y. Mizuguchi, K. Nomoto, and E. Skamene.** 1991. Genetic control of natural resistance in mouse macrophages regulating intracellular *Legionella pneumophila* multiplication in vitro. *Infect. Immun.* **59:**428–432.
5. **Yoshida, S., Y. Mizuguchi, Y. Nikaido, M. Mitsuyama, and K. Nomoto.** 1987. Fate of *Legionella pneumophila* Philadelphia-1 strain in resident, elicited, activated, and immune peritoneal macrophages of guinea pigs. *Infect. Immun.* **55:**2477-2482.

Alteration in Lymphocyte Subsets following Infection of Mice with *Legionella pneumophila*

CATHERINE NEWTON, RAYMOND WIDEN, THOMAS W. KLEIN, JUDY SMITH,
AND HERMAN FRIEDMAN

Department of Medical Microbiology and Immunology, University of South Florida College of Medicine, Tampa, Florida 33612-4799

Legionella pneumophila, the etiologic agent of legionellosis, is an intracellular gram-negative opportunistic pathogen that causes pneumonia, mainly in immunocompromised individuals. BALB/c and BDF1 mice have been reported to display signs of immunoalteration following *Legionella* infection (1, 2, 6). In an effort to understand the cellular basis of this immunity, we examined by flow cytometry the changes in spleen and blood lymphocyte subsets following primary infection with legionellae. We found there was a marked increase in the percentages of selected T lymphocytes, especially helper T cells, in the spleen and blood very early after infection, followed by a decrease within a week after infection and then a return to normal. There were also marked changes in other cell types (e.g., B lymphocytes and memory cells) in the spleen and blood of the animals. The results obtained indicate that enhanced immunity following *Legionella* infection is associated first with initial expansion and subsequent disappearance of specific cells from the spleen and blood of the animals, followed by expansion and mobilization of memory immune cells.

Female BALB/c mice (Harlan, Indianapolis, Ind.), 7 to 8 weeks of age, were infected with *L. pneumophila* serogroup 1, which was originally isolated from a case of legionellosis at Tampa General Hospital. The infections were done by intraperitoneal injection with 0.8×10^7 to 1×10^7 bacteria per mouse (5% lethal dose).

At various days after infection, animals were sacrificed by CO_2 asphyxiation, blood was collected by cardiac puncture into heparinized syringes, and spleens were removed. Single-cell suspensions of the spleens were prepared with a Stomacher 80 laboratory blender (Tekmar, Cincinnati, Ohio), and erythrocytes were lysed by quick exposure to a solution of ammonium chloride.

Splenocytes ($10^6/100$ μl) or whole blood (100 μl) was mixed with monoclonal antibodies against various surface markers (4 μl) labeled with either fluorescein isothiocyanate (FITC), R-phycoerythrin (R-PE), Cy-Chrome (Pharmingen, San Diego, Calif.), or Red 613 (Life Technologies, Grand Island, N.Y.) for 30 min at 4°C. By using FITC, R-PE, and either Cy-Chrome or Red 613, cells were analyzed by two- or three-color analysis. The surface markers examined were CD3, B220 (clone RA3-6B2), L3T4, Ly 2, LFA, CD45R (clone 23G2), and Pgp-1. The cells were washed in phosphate-buffered saline (PBS), and the splenocytes were fixed to 1% paraformaldehyde–PBS. The erythrocytes were removed from the peripheral blood leukocytes (PBLs) with Coulter's Whole Blood Lysing Kit (Coulter, Hialeah, Fla.), and then the PBLs were washed and fixed in 1% paraformaldehyde–PBS. The splenocytes and PBLs were analyzed with a FACScan (Becton Dickinson, Mountain View, Calif.). The lymphocyte population was identified and selected (gated) for flow cytometry analysis by forward versus side (90°) light scatter.

Following infection of the mice with a sublethal amount of legionellae (0.8×10^7 to 1×10^7 bacteria), the lymphocyte subsets in both the spleen and peripheral blood underwent marked changes. As is evident in Fig. 1 and 2, the percentage of $CD3^+$ cells (T cells) 1 day after infection increased, then decreased from 4 to 6 days, and returned to normal by day 8 in both the spleen and blood. Among the T-cell subsets, it was the helper cells ($L3T4^+$) that accounted for most of

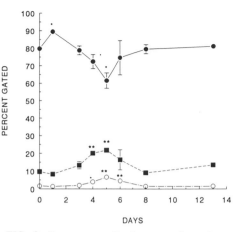

FIG. 2. Percentages of splenocytes from *L. pneumophila*-infected mice positive for T (CD3-FITC; ●) and B (B220-R-PE; ■) markers, or both (○). Cells were analyzed by two-color analysis on a FACScan. Data are expressed as means ± standard errors for 4 to 16 animals. *, $P < 0.05$; **, $P < 0.01$.

the overall T-cell increase and decrease (Fig. 3 and 4). Another T-cell subset, Ly 2 (suppressor/cytotoxic) cells, did not change in the spleen; however, in the blood, the percentage of these cells decreased between day 4 and 6 and then increased on day 8.

The B-cell ($B220^+$) population in the spleen and blood also changed rapidly after infection, in a manner opposite that of the T cells (Fig. 1 and 2). In the spleen, B220 cells showed an increase in percentage between days 4 and 6, while in the

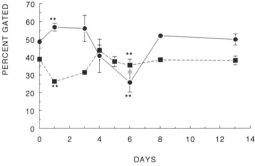

FIG. 1. Percentages of PBLs from *L. pneumophila*-infected mice positive for T (CD3-FITC; ●) and B (B220-R-PE; ■) markers. Cells were analyzed by two-color analysis on a FACScan. Data are expressed as means ± standard errors for 4 to 16 animals. **, $P < 0.01$.

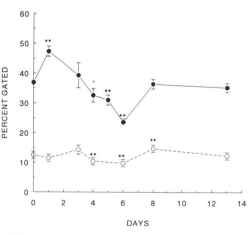

FIG. 3. Percentages of PBLs positive for helper T cells (L3T4-R-PE; ●) or suppressor/cytotoxic T cells (Ly 2-FITC; ○). Cells were analyzed by two-color analysis on a FACScan. Data represent means ± standard errors for 4 to 16 animals. *, $P < 0.05$; **, $P < 0.01$.

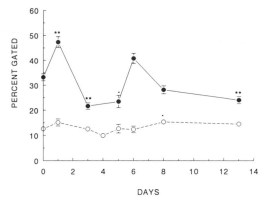

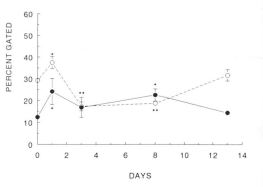

FIG. 4. Percentages of splenocytes positive for helper T cells (L3T4–R-PE; ●) or suppressor/cytotoxic T cells (Ly 2-FITC; ○). Cells were analyzed by two-color analysis on a FACScan. Data represent means ± standard errors for 4 to 16 animals. *, $P < 0.05$; **, P 0.01.

FIG. 6. Percentages of splenocytes positive for the memory marker CD45R (○) or LFA (●). Data are expressed as means ± standard errors for 4 to 16 animals. *, $P < 0.05$; **, $P < 0.01$.

blood, there was a significant decrease 1 day after infection. Although the B220 clone RA3-6B2 is reported to be unique to B cells (5), a B220⁺ CD3 cell population appeared in the spleen between days 4 and 6 (Fig. 2). The function or significance of this unique population is being studied further.

Cells with memory surface markers such as LFA and CD45R (4, 9) also showed changes in the spleen and blood (Fig. 5 and 6). LFA⁺ cells increased by day 8 in the spleen and by day 13 in the blood. Splenocytes positive for CD45R fell below normal on days 3 to 8 in the spleen and then returned to normal levels by day 13, while in the blood, they increased significantly on day 8. The low level of CD45R is consistent with its involvement in memory. Another marker associated with memory is Pgp-1, although its significance in BALB/c mice has been questioned because of its

high levels in comparison with those in C57BL/6 mice (3, 7, 8). In our studies, we found high levels with little fluctuation in the spleen (data not shown). However, the levels in PBL increased following infection (Fig. 5), implying that Pgp-1 may have some memory function in BALB/c mice.

Thus, it is apparent that during the first 2 weeks after infection of BALB/c mice with *L. pneumophila,* there are marked changes in the percentage of lymphoid subpopulations in both the spleen and peripheral blood in comparison with levels in noninfected control animals. These results suggest important changes in the lymphocyte subsets which might account for previously reported alteration in immune function observed in infected mice.

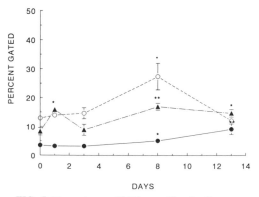

FIG. 5. Percentages of PBLs positive for the memory marker CD45R (○), LFA (●), or Pgp-1 (▲). Data are expressed as means ± standard errors for 4 to 16 animals. *, $P < 0.05$; **, $P < 0.01$.

REFERENCES

1. **Blanchard, D. K., J. Y. Djeu, T. W. Klein, H. Friedman, and W. E. Stewart II.** 1987. Induction of tumor necrosis factor by *Legionella pneumophila. Infect. Immun.* **55:**433–437.
2. **Blanchard, D. K., H. Friedman, W. E. Stewart II, T. W. Klein, and J. Y. Djeu.** 1988. Role of gamma interferon in induction of natural killer activity by *Legionella pneumophila* in vitro and in an experimental murine infection. *Infect. Immun.* **56:**1187–1193.
3. **Budd, R. C., J.C. Cerottini, C. Horvath, C. Brom, T. Pedrazzini, R. C. Howe, and H. R. MacDonald.** 1987. Distinction of virgin and memory T lymphocytes. Stable aquisition of Pgp-1 glycoprotein concomitant with antigenic stimulation. *J. Immunol.* **138:**3120–3129.
4. **Cerottini, J.C., and H. R. MacDonald.** 1989. The cellular basis of T-cell memory. *Annu. Rev. Immunol.* **7:**77–89.
5. **Coffman, R. L.** 1982. Surface antigen expression and immunogloblin gene rearrangement during mouse pre-B cell development. *Immunol. Rev.* **69:**5–23.
6. **Klein, T. W., D. K. Blanchard, Y. Yamamoto, C. Newton, R. Widen, and H. Friedman.** 1988. Role of cytokines in resistance to infection with *Legionella pneumophila. Adv. Biosci.* **68:**259–265.
7. **Lynch, F., and R. Ceredig.** 1988. Ly-24 (Pgp-1) expression by thymocytes and peripheral T cells. *Immunol. Today* **9:**7–10.

8. **MacDonald, H. R., R. C. Budd, and J.C. Cerottini.** 1990. Pgp-1 (Ly 24) as a marker of murine memory T lymphocytes. *Curr. Top. Microbiol. Immunol.* **159:**97–109.

9. **Vitetta, E. S., M. T. Berton, Burger, M. Kepron, W. T. Lee, and X. M. Yin.** 1991. Memory B and T cells. *Annu. Rev. Immunol.* **9:**193–217.

Tumor Necrosis Factor and Lipopolysaccharide Potentiate Gamma Interferon-Induced Resistance of Alveolar Macrophages to *Legionella pneumophila*

SHAWN J. SKERRETT AND THOMAS R. MARTIN

Medical Research Service, Seattle Veterans Affairs Medical Center, Seattle, Washington 98108

Legionella pneumophila is an intracellular parasite of alveolar macrophages, and recovery from legionellosis is associated with activation of alveolar macrophages to resist the intracellular replication of this pathogen (6). The T-lymphokine gamma interferon (IFN-γ) has been shown to activate alveolar macrophages in vitro to inhibit the intracellular growth of *L. pneumophila* (3, 5, 7), and IFN-γ is induced in vivo in experimental legionellosis (1), suggesting that this lymphokine may play an important role in augmenting the resistance of alveolar macrophages to *L. pneumophila*. Macrophage-derived cytokines also may contribute to cellular defense against intracellular pathogens. Tumor necrosis factor (TNF) has been shown to activate mononuclear phagocytes to inhibit intracellular parasites (2) and to potentiate the antimicrobial action of IFN-γ (4). *L. pneumophila* induces TNF in vitro and in vivo (1), indicating a potential role of this monokine in host defense against legionellosis.

To test the hypothesis that macrophage-derived mediators such as TNF contribute to the resistance of alveolar macrophages to *L. pneumophila*, we incubated adherent rat alveolar macrophages with recombinant murine TNF (1 to 10,000 U/ml) or *Escherichia coli* lipopolysaccharide (LPS; 10 μg/ml), in the presence or absence of submaximal recombinant murine IFN-γ (10 U/ml), for 6 h before challenge with *L. pneumophila*. The effect of LPS also was studied in the presence of polyclonal anti-TNF. Monolayers were sonicated and quantitatively cultured on sequential days.

As shown in Table 1, pretreatment of alveolar macrophages with TNF or LPS inhibited the intracellular replication of *L. pneumophila*, and the effect of LPS was blocked by coincubation with anti-TNF. Both TNF and LPS also induced net bacterial killing when combined with IFN-γ, and the coactivating effect of LPS was partially inhibited by anti-TNF. TNF, LPS, and IFN-γ had no direct effect on the viability of *L. pneumophila* or alveolar macrophages.

These data suggest that the induction of monokines such as TNF by parasitized alveolar macrophages may be an important autocrine defense mechanism against *L. pneumophila*, serving to partially protect alveolar macrophages from intracellular parasitism and to potentiate the antimicrobial mechanisms induced by IFN-γ.

TABLE 1. Effects of preincubation of alveolar macrophages with TNF, LPS, and IFN-γ on intracellular growth of *L. pneumophila*

Alveolar macrophage stimulus	Growth of *L. pneumophila* at 48 h ($\log_{10}$ change in CFU/ml)[a]
None	1.58 ± 0.11
TNF	
100 U/ml	1.49 ± 0.13
1,000 U/ml	1.36 ± 0.09
10,000 U/ml	1.00 ± 0.04
LPS	
10 μg/ml	0.49 ± 0.15
10 μg/ml + anti-TNF	1.01 ± 0.03
IFN	
10 U/ml	0.31 ± 0.12
10 U/ml + TNF (100 U/ml)	0.05 ± 0.12
10 U/ml + TNF (1,000 U/ml)	-0.93 ± 0.10
10 U/ml + TNF (10,000 U/ml)	-1.52 ± 0.49
10 U/ml + LPS (10 μg/ml)	-1.08 ± 0.21
10 U/ml + LPS (10 μg/ml) + anti-TNF	-0.22 ± 0.09

[a] Mean $\pm$ standard error of the mean for three to nine monolayers.

REFERENCES

1. **Blanchard, D. K., J. Y. Djeu, T. W. Klein, H. Friedman, and W. E. Stewart II.** 1987. Induction of tumor necrosis factor by *Legionella pneumophila. Infect. Immun.* **55:**433–437.

2. **deTitto, E. H., J. R. Catterall, and J. S. Remington.** 1986. Activity of recombinant tumor necrosis factor on *Toxoplasma gondii* and *Trypanosoma cruzi. J. Immunol.* **137:**1342–1345.

3. **Jensen, W. A., R. M. Rose, A. S. Wasserman, T. H.**

Kalb, and H. G. Remold. 1987. In vitro activation of the antibacterial activity of human alveolar macrophages by recombinant gamma interferon. *J. Infect. Dis.* **155**:574–577.

4. Liew, F. Y., Y. Li, and S. Millott. 1990. Tumor necrosis factor-α synergizes with IFN-γ in mediating killing of *Leishmania major* through the induction of nitric oxide. *J. Immunol.* **145**:4306–4310.

5. Nash, T. W., D. M. Libby, and M. A. Horwitz. 1988. IFN-γ-activated human alveolar macrophages inhibit the intracellular multiplication of *Legionella pneumophila. J. Immunol.* **140**:3978–3981.

6. Skerrett, S. J., and T. R. Martin. 1991. Alveolar macrophage activation in experimental legionellosis. *J. Immunol.* **147**:337–345.

7. Skerrett, S. J., and T. R. Martin. 1992. Recombinant murine interferon-γ reversibly activates rat alveolar macrophages to kill *Legionella pneumophila. J. Infect. Dis.* **166**:1354–1361.

Alpha and Beta Interferons Modulate Macrophage Cytokine Production in *Legionella pneumophila*-Infected Macrophages

YOSHIMASA YAMAMOTO, THOMAS W. KLEIN, AND HERMAN FRIEDMAN

Department of Medical Microbiology and Immunology, University of South Florida College of Medicine, Tampa, Florida 33612-4799

It is now widely recognized that interferons (IFNs) of the three major types, α, β, and γ, can influence immune responses and modify macrophage (MP) functions, especially cytokine production (11). IFN-γ, especially, has a major role in the course of infection to intracellular pathogens, mainly because this IFN has been recognized as one of the main MP-activating factors (12). However, the role of IFN-α and -β in bacterial infections is much less clear. The mechanism of regulation of MP functions against *Legionella* infection by IFNs is important in understanding the role of MPs in *Legionella* immunity in the host. In the studies reported here, we examined the effects of IFNs on cytokine production by MPs infected with *Legionella pneumophila*.

Female A/J mice, 8 to 12 weeks of age, were purchased from Jackson Laboratory, Bar Harbor, Maine. A virulent strain of *L. pneumophila* serogroup 1 was used. *Legionella* suspensions in pyrogen-free saline were prepared as described previously (16).

Recombinant murine IFN-γ and -β were kindly provided by Shionogi Co., Osaka, Japan, and Toray Industries, Inc., Tokyo, Japan, respectively. Recombinant murine IFN-α was purchased from Lee Biomolecular Research, Inc., San Diego, Calif. All reagents were diluted to appropriate concentrations before use with medium.

Thioglycolate-elicited peritoneal MP monolayers were prepared as described previously (16). The MP monolayers in 24-well plates (approximately 10^6 cells per well) were infected with *L. pneumophila* for 30 min at 37°C at an infectivity ratio of 20 bacteria:1 MP. The IFNs were added to the *Legionella*-infected MP monolayers, which were incubated for 2 h and then washed to remove nonbinding IFNs from the MPs. The cultures were then incubated in RPMI 1640 medium containing 10% heat-inactivated fetal calf serum for an additional 6 to 48 h. At the end of incubation, the culture supernatants from the MP monolayers

were collected and assayed for interleukin-1 (IL-1) and colony-stimulating factor (CSF) activities. The MPs were then lysed with 0.1% saponin, and the number of viable bacteria in the lysates was determined by standard colony count on buffered charcoal-yeast extract agar as described previously (16).

The IL-1 content of the culture supernatants was measured by the standard thymocyte proliferation assay, using thymus cells from C3H/HeJ mice (8). The amount of IL-1 activity was expressed as [³H]thymidine incorporation (counts per minute) into the thymocytes. The IFNs had no direct effect on proliferation of the thymocytes. The CSF activity in the culture supernatants of the MP monolayers was measured by using the CSF-dependent cell proliferation assay with FDCP-1 cells, kindly provided by Edward J. Wing, University of Pittsburgh, Pittsburgh, Pa. The amount of CSF activity was expressed as [³H]thymidine incorporation (counts per minute) by the FDCP-1 cells (5).

In our previous study, all three types of IFNs tested, IFN-α, -β, and -γ, were found to suppress production of IL-1 activity in cultures of thioglycolate-induced mouse MPs after stimulation in vitro with lipopolysaccharide (LPS) (data not shown). This down-regulation of IL-1 production by IFN-treated MPs was found to be dose related (1 to 1,000 U/ml). The finding that IFNs suppressed rather than stimulated IL-1 production differs from results of previous studies (2, 4, 6), which showed that IFNs augment IL-1 production. This difference may be related to the source and population of MPs used, i.e., human monocyte/MPs versus mouse peritoneal MPs. In this regard, Brandwein (3) has reported that IFN-γ inhibits IL-1 production by thioglycolate-induced mouse MPs, similar to our observations. In contrast to the down-regulation of IL-1 by IFNs, there was a marked up-regulation of CSF production of LPS-stimulated MPs. CSF production, especially granulocyte-macrophage CSF (GM-CSF), from LPS-stimulated MPs has been reported by several groups (13, 14). In our study, MPs stimulated with LPS also evinced CSF production in a dose-dependent manner; when IFN-α or -β was simultaneously added to the cultures, there was a greater stimulation of CSF production, especially with 1,000 U of IFN per ml (data not shown). However, IFN-γ had little effect on CSF production.

IFN-γ is well known to induce anti-*Legionella* activity in cultured MPs (1, 7, 9, 10). However, induction of anti-*Legionella* activity requires 12 h or more of preincubation with IFN-γ (unpublished data). On the other hand, the role of IFNs in the immune responses to bacterial infections aside from antimicrobial activity is poorly understood. In the study reported here, we evaluated the role of IFNs in the immune responses to *Legionella* infection, especially the effect on MP functions aside from anti-*Legionella* activity. Pulse treatment (2 h) with IFNs was chosen rather than pretreatment such as 24-h preincubation. The purpose

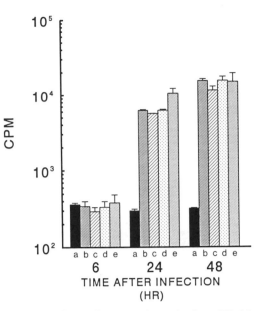

FIG. 2. Effects of IFNs on the production of IL-1 in *Legionella*-infected MPs. Bars: a, no infection; b, infected; c, plus IFN-α; d, plus IFN-β; e, plus IFN-γ.

of pulse treatment is to investigate how IFNs modulate the function of *Legionella*-infected MPs without the suppressive effect on intracellular multiplication of legionellae.

As shown in Fig. 1, there was essentially equivalent growth of *L. pneumophila* at 48 h in the permissive A/J mouse MPs treated with IFN-α or -β for 2 h after infection. IFN-γ treatment of the cultures inhibited replication slightly at 48 h. Thus, the results of this study showed the 2-h pulse treatment did not significantly affect multiplication of legionellae in MPs, even when IFN-γ was used. The IL-1 content in the culture supernatants of such *Legionella*-infected MPs was measured. Figure 2 shows the production of IL-1 in *Legionella*-infected MP cultures. Induction of IL-1 from MPs by stimulation with killed *Legionella* vaccine or *Legionella* antigens has already been reported (8, 15). The data presented here showed that IL-1 production also occurred in *Legionella*-infected MP cultures. However, treatment with the IFNs did not induce any further alteration in IL-1 production. CSF production in the culture supernatants of *Legionella*-infected MPs was measured by using the CSF-dependent cell line FDCP-1. The growth of FDCP-1 is dependent on the presence of IL-3 and GM-CSF (5). In contrast to IL-1 production, infection of the MPs with *L. pneumophila* only minimally increased CSF activity in the supernatants of the MPs, even 48 h after infection (Fig. 3). However, treatment of the cultures with IFN-α or -β increased production of CSF activ-

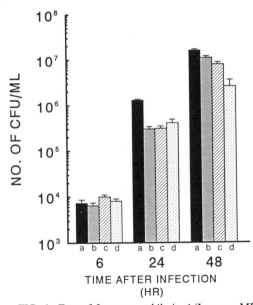

FIG. 1. Fate of *L. pneumophila* in A/J mouse MPs that received a 2-h pulse treatment with IFNs. MP monolayers were infected with *L. pneumophila* for 30 min at 37°C, washed to remove nonphagocytized bacteria, treated with IFNs (100 U/ml) for 2 h, washed to remove IFNs, and then incubated with medium for an additional 6 to 48 h. At the indicated time periods after incubation, the culture supernatant was collected and the IL-1 content and CSF activity were measured. The number of viable bacteria in the MP lysates was determined on buffered charcoal-yeast extract agar. Each bar represents the mean number of CFU ± standard deviation for triplicate MP cultures. Bars: a, control; b, plus IFN-α; c, plus IFN-β; d, plus IFN-γ.

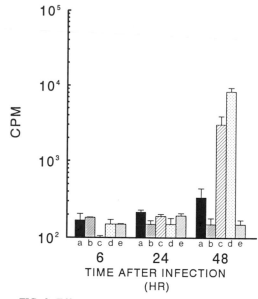

FIG. 3. Effects of IFNs on the production of CSF in *Legionella*-infected MPs. Bars: a, no infection; b, infected; c, plus IFN-α; d, plus IFN-β; e, plus IFN-γ.

ity, although treatment with IFN-γ did not. IFN-α and -β up-regulated production of CSF activity in the infected MPs in a dose-related manner (data not shown). Neutralization with polyclonal anti-GM-CSF antibody showed that the majority of the CSF activity was GM-CSF (data not shown).

It is apparent from this study that both IFN-α and IFN-β do not induce strong anti-*Legionella* activity in *Legionella*-infected MPs but do markedly alter production of cytokines. However, this activity appears to be selective in regard to the type of cytokines involved.

In summary, we found that IFN-α, -β, and γ affect differently production of IL-1 and CSF in elicited peritoneal MPs infected with *L. pneumophila*. The IL-1 activity was measured by using a thymocyte comitogenic assay, and the CSF assay was performed with the CSF-dependent cell line. Multiplication of legionellae in permissive A/J mouse MPs did not appear to be significantly affected by the pulse treatment (2 h) with IFNs. *Legionella* infection induced a large amount of IL-1 in culture supernatants of the MPs. This increased IL-1 activity in *Legionella*-infected MP cultures was not influenced by cotreatment with IFNs, but IFN-α and -β both increased CSF production in cultures infected with *L. pneumophila* which by itself caused only moderate production of CSF. Thus, it appears that IFNs may modulate production of cytokines in LPS-activated MPs, as well as in *Legionella*-infected cultures, and that IFNs may be important during *Legionella* infec-

tion by regulating the production of inflammatory cytokines.

This work was supported by grant AI 16618 from the National Institute of Allergy and Infectious Diseases.

REFERENCES

1. **Bhardwaj, N., T. Nash, and M. A. Horwitz.** 1986. Interferon-gamma-activated human monocytes inhibit intracellular multiplication of *L. pneumophila*. *J. Immunol.* **137:**2662–2669.
2. **Boraschi, O., S. Censini, and A. Tagliabue.** 1984. Interferon-gamma reduces macrophage-suppressive activity by inhibiting prostaglandin E$_2$ release and inducing interleukin 1 production. *J. Immunol.* **133:**764–768.
3. **Brandwein, S. R.** 1986. Regulation of interleukin production by mouse peritoneal macrophages. *J. Biol. Chem.* **261:**8624–8632.
4. **Candler, R. V., B. T. Rouse, and R. T. Moore.** 1985. Regulation of interleukin 1 production by alpha and beta interferons: evidence for both direct and indirect enhancement. *J. Interferon Res.* **5:**179–189.
5. **Dexter, T. M., J. G. D. Scott, E. Scolnick, and D. Metcalf.** 1980. Growth of factor-dependent hemopoietic precursor cell lines. *J. Exp. Med.* **152:**1036–1047.
6. **Haq, A. U., J. J. Rinehart, and R. D. Maca.** 1985. The effect of gamma interferon on IL-1 secretion of in vitro differentiated human macrophages. *J. Leukocyte Biol.* **38:**735–746.
7. **Jensen, W. A., R. M. Rose, A. S. Wasserman, T. H. Kalb, K. Anton, and H. G. Remold.** 1987. In vitro activation of the antibacterial activity of human pulmonary macrophages by recombinant gamma interferon. *J. Infect. Dis.* **155:**574–577.
8. **Klein, T. W., C. A. Newton, D. K. Blanchard, R. Wide, and H. Friedman.** 1987. Induction of interleukin 1 by *Legionella pneumophila* antigens in mouse macrophage and human mononuclear leukocyte cultures. *Zentralbl. Bakteriol. Hyg. A* **265:**462–471.
9. **Klein, T. W., Y. Yamamoto, H. K. Brown, and H. Friedman.** 1991. Interferon-gamma induced resistance to *Legionella pneumophila* in susceptible A/J mouse macrophages. *J. Leukocyte Biol.* **49:**98–103.
10. **Nash, T. W., D. M. Libby, and M. A. Horwitz.** 1988. IFN-gamma-activated human alveolar macrophages inhibit the intracellular multiplication of *Legionella pneumophila*. *J. Immunol.* **140:**3978–3981.
11. **Sonnenfeld, G.** 1980. Modulation of immunity by interferon, p. 113. *In* E. Pick (ed.), *Lymphokine Reports*, vol. 1. Academic Press, New York.
12. **Svedersky, L. P., C. V. Benton, W. H. Berger, E. Rinderknecht, R. N. Harkins, and M. S. Palladino.** 1984. Biological and antigenic similarities of murine interferon-gamma and macrophage-activating factor. *J. Exp. Med.* **159:**812–827.
13. **Sullivan, R., P. J. Gans, and L. A. McCarroll.** 1983. The synthesis and secretion of granulocyte-monocyte colony-stimulating activity (CSA) by isolated human monocytes: kinetics of the response to bacterial endotoxin. *J. Immunol.* **130:**800–807.
14. **Thorens, B., J. Mermod, and P. Vassalli.** 1987. Phagocytosis and inflammatory stimuli induce GM-CSF in macrophages through posttranscription regulation. *Cell* **48:**671–679.
15. **Widen, R., T. W. Klein, C. A. Newton, and H. Friedman.** 1989. Induction of interleukin 1 by *Legionella pneumophila* in murine peritoneal macrophage cultures. *Proc. Soc. Exp. Biol. Med.* **191:**304–308.
16. **Yamamoto, Y., T. W. Klein, C. A. Newton, R. Widen, and H. Friedman.** 1987. Differential growth of *Legionella pneumophila* in guinea pig versus mouse macrophage cultures. *Infect. Immun.* **55:**1369–1374.

Role of Nitric Oxide in Killing of *Legionella pneumophila* in Gamma Interferon-Activated Macrophages

BRAD L. BUSTER, LORI A. POWELL, RICHARD D. MILLER, JULIO A. RAMIREZ, AND JAMES T. SUMMERSGILL

Department of Microbiology and Immunology and Division of Infectious Diseases, Department of Medicine, University of Louisville School of Medicine, Louisville, Kentucky 40292

Legionella pneumophila is a facultative intracellular bacterium, capable of replicating within the phagosomes of human macrophages and monocytes. Gamma interferon (IFN)-activated macrophages, however, are capable of inhibiting this intracellular replication (1). This ability appears to correlate with a combination of downregulating transferrin receptors on the macrophage surface (1) and decreasing expression of intracellular ferritin (2). This process would result in a net decrease in the concentration of intracellular iron (1), an element which *L. pneumophila* must have in abundance in order to replicate.

In murine macrophages, IFN induces the expression of nitric oxide (NO) synthase, a cytosolic enzyme catalyzing the intracellular generation of short-lived NO radicals from L-arginine, the exclusive substrate of this enzyme (6). NO has been identified as the effector molecule in the microbicidal effects of murine macrophages against a variety of intracellular pathogens, including *Toxoplasma gondii*, *Leishmania* spp., *Mycobacterium tuberculosis,* and *Francisella tularensis.* Involvement of NO in the killing of extracellular *Cryptococcus neoformans* and *Schistosoma mansoni* has also been described (reviewed in reference 5). The precise mechanism for this activity is unknown, although a direct killing effect of NO on the organism, one similar to that described for toxic oxygen-containing radicals, has been postulated (5). It has been shown that NO radicals complex with iron to form intracellular iron-nitrosyl complexes, which are subsequently lost from the macrophage (7), and NO may also mediate the direct release of iron molecules from ferritin (8). These effects may complement the down-regulation of transferrin receptors and ferritin in IFN-activated macrophages (1, 2) and contribute to limiting the availability of intracellular iron.

In view of the known toxic effects of NO radicals on other intracellular microorganisms, coupled with the known interactions of NO with intracellular iron, it seemed possible that NO may likewise participate in the intracellular killing of *L. pneumophila*. This activity might occur via a direct killing effect of NO on the bacterium, via a role in the further limitation of intracellular iron, or by a combination of both. This study was designed to determine what role NO might play in altering the intracellular replication of *L. pneumophila* in IFN-activated murine macrophages compared with human macrophages.

RAW 264.7 cells, a murine macrophage cell line, and HL-60 cells, a human promyelocytic leukemia cell line permissive for *L. pneumophila* replication, were maintained in RPMI 1640 supplemented with L-glutamine, 10% fetal calf serum, penicillin, streptomycin, and gentamicin at 37°C in 5% CO_2. Prior to use, cells were harvested and washed once in RPMI 1640 (containing no antibiotics) and suspended to a concentration of 2.0×10^6/ml in RPMI 1640. One milliliter was delivered to each well of 24-well tissue culture plates (Costar, Cambridge, Mass.). HL-60 cells were treated with phorbol myristate acetate (10 ng/ml; Sigma, St. Louis, Mo.) for 24 h to transform them into an adherent macrophage-like monolayer. Each adherent monolayer was washed and overlaid with a suspension of *L. pneumophila* (serogroup 1) at a 1:1 bacterium-to-cell ratio and incubated for 2 h at 37°C. Monolayers were washed three times in RPMI 1640, and the medium was replaced with 1.0 ml of RPMI 1640. Murine recombinant IFN (rIFN) and human rIFN (Genzyme, Cambridge, Mass.) were added to the appropriate wells at a final concentration of 100 U/ml, and N^G-monomethyl-L-arginine (N^GMMA; Calbiochem, San Diego, Calif.), a specific inhibitor of NO synthase, was added to the appropriate wells at a final concentration of 2.0 mM. Control wells, with no rIFN or N^GMMA, were included. All plates were incubated at 37°C, and bacterial viability counts were determined by aspirating the supernatant from each well (saved for nitrite determination; see below) and adding 1.0 ml of sterile distilled water to lyse the monolayer. CFU per milliliter was determined by the standard dilution and plating technique onto buffered charcoal-yeast extract agar.

NO produced by macrophages is rapidly converted to nitrite and is detectable in the supernatant of activated macrophage cultures. Nitrite production by RAW 264.7 and HL-60 cell monolayers was quantitated by using the Griess reaction (4). Briefly, 1.0 ml of supernatant was combined with 1.0 ml of Griess reagent (1% sulfanilimide, 0.1% naphthylethylenediamine dihydrochloride, 2.5% H_3PO_4) and allowed to stand at room temperature for 10 min. A_{550} was measured, and nitrite concentrations (micromolar) were determined by using $NaNO_2$ as a standard.

To determine the effects of rIFN treatment on the concentration of intracellular iron in RAW 264.7 cells, a modification of the assay described by Carter (3) was used. Briefly, 10^7 macrophages were plated in each well of six-well tissue culture plates (Costar, Cambridge, Mass.). Murine rIFN (100 U/ml) and murine rIFN–N^GMMA (2.0 μM) were added to the appropriate wells; control wells containing no rIFN or N^GMMA were also tested. Plates were incubated at 37°C, and intracellular iron was measured in each well following 24 h of incubation as follows. Supernatants were removed, and monolayers were washed three times in RPMI without serum or other additives. Monolayers were lysed in 1.0 ml of distilled water, the supernatant was aspirated, and an equal volume of 6 N HNO_3 was added. Samples were heated at 80°C in a water bath overnight to release protein-associated iron. All iron was reduced to Fe^{2+} with 0.1 ml of 0.1% ascorbic acid, and samples receive 0.1 ml of 56.5% trichloroacetic acid and 0.6 ml of 2.0 M acetate buffer (pH 5.0). Ferrous iron concentration was measured spectrophotometrically (562 nm) after being complexed with 0.1 ml of a 3-mg/ml solution of ferrozine (Sigma). The iron concentration (nanograms per milliliter) was determined against a ferrous ammonium sulfate standard curve and expressed as percentage of the control value. Student's t test was used in all statistical calculations. A P value of <0.05 was considered significant.

rIFN treatment of RAW 264.7 cells significantly increased their bactericidal activity against intracellular *L. pneumophila*, resulting in a decrease from 3.8 log CFU of viable bacteria per ml to 0.7 log CFU/ml by 24 h of incubation ($P < 0.05$). Untreated cells were unable to significantly kill intracellular *L. pneumophila* (3.4 log CFU/ml at 24 h). rIFN-activated RAW 264.7 cells, incubated in the presence of 2.0 μM N^GMMA, were significantly less effective in killing *L. pneumophila* than were rIFN-treated cells, allowing for a 1.5-fold decrease in viable bacteria after 24 h (2.2 log CFU/ml). The increased killing ability of rIFN-treated cells correlated with an increased production of NO via NO synthase activity (58.7 μM) ($P < 0.05$). Control cells and N^GMMA-treated cells had negligible nitrite production (1.38 and 5.65 μM, respectively).

rIFN-activated RAW 264.7 cells (10^7) had significantly decreased levels of intracellular iron after 24 h of incubation in comparison with untreated cells. Total iron levels dropped to below detectable levels in these cells ($P < 0.05$). This decrease correlated with nitrite production of 62.3 μM. rIFN-activated RAW 264.7 cells incubated in the presence of 2.0 μM N^GMMA, which blocks NO production, had intracellular iron levels equal to 72% ($P < 0.05$) of the level in control cells. Neither control cells nor N^GMMA-treated cells

had appreciable levels of nitrite production (4.1 or 5.0 μM, respectively).

Human rIFN-activated HL-60 cells, as expected, demonstrated only bacteriostatic activity against intracellular *L. pneumophila*, allowing no increase in viable bacteria after 72 h of incubation. Untreated HL-60 cells allowed a 2-log increase in viable *L. pneumophila* in this same time period ($P < 0.05$). The bacteriostatic ability of rIFN-treated cells were not altered in the presence of 2.0 mM N^GMMA. Nitrite was not detectable above background in any HL-60 cell culture supernatant, regardless of treatment.

These data suggest that induced NO synthase activity in RAW 264.7 cells is involved in killing of *L. pneumophila*, and this effect correlates with a depletion of intracellular iron. N^GMMA treatment restores intracellular iron levels to approximately 72% of the level in untreated cells, indicating a role for NO in this effect, possibly by acting in concert with the down-regulation of transferrin receptors and ferritin (1, 2). It seems unlikely, however, that iron depletion could be totally responsible for the bactericidal activity of RAW 264.7 cells. One would suspect only an enhanced bacteriostatic effect. These data, therefore, suggest a crucial role for the NO radical itself in the direct killing of *L. pneumophila*, although this remains to be determined. Such a role would not be surprising in view of the known effects of NO on other microorganisms (4).

In contrast to RAW 264.7 cells, NO production appears to have no detectable role in altering the intracellular fate of *L. pneumophila* in HL-60 cells in vitro. Others have reported NO production in HL-60 cells (9); however, we were unable to detect any appreciable nitrite production under any incubation condition. Indeed, there are conflicting reports in the literature on the expression of NO synthase in human macrophages. This is obviously a pertinent question to be answered with respect to the relevance of the role of the NO pathway in the control of legionellosis.

In view of the contrasting results for involvement of the NO pathway between murine and human cells obtained thus far, investigators using murine or other nonhuman models for Legionnaires disease should interpret their data appropriately.

REFERENCES

1. **Byrd, T. F., and M. A. Horwitz.** 1989. Interferon gamma-activated human monocytes down-regulate transferrin receptor and inhibit the intracellular multiplication of *Legionella pneumophila* by limiting the availability of iron. *J. Clin. Invest.* **83:**1457–1465.
2. **Byrd, T. F., and M. A. Horwitz.** 1990. Interferon-gamma activated human monocytes downregulate the intracellular concentration of ferritin: a potential new mechanism for limiting iron availability to *Legionella pneumophila* and subsequently inhibiting intracellular multiplication. *Clin. Res.* **38:**481A.

3. **Carter, P.** 1971. Spectrophotometric determination of serum iron at the submicrogram level with a new reagent (ferrozine). *Anal. Biochem.* **40**:450–458.

4. **Green, L. C., D. A. Wagner, et al.** 1982. Analysis of nitrite, nitrate and [^{15}N]-nitrite in biological fluids. *Anal. Biochem.* **126**:131–138.

5. **Green, S. J., C. A. Nacy, and M. S. Meltzer.** 1991. Cytokine-induced synthesis of nitrogen oxides in macrophages: a protective host response to *Leishmania* and other intracellular pathogens. *J. Leukocyte Biol.* **50**:93–103.

6. **Hibbs, J. B., Z. Vavrin, and R. R. Taintor.** 1987. L-Arginine is required by expression of the activated macrophage effector mechanism causing selective metabolic inhibition of target cells. *J. Immunol.* **138**:550–565.

7. **Lancaster, J. R., and J. B. Hibbs.** 1990. EPR demonstration of iron-nitrosyl complex formation by cytotoxic activated macrophages. *Proc. Natl. Acad. Sci. USA* **87**:1223–1227.

8. **Reif, D. W., and R. D. Simmons.** 1990. Nitric oxide mediates iron release from ferritin. *Arch. Biochem. Biophys.* **283**:537–541.

9. **Schmidt, H. H. H. W., R. Seifert, and E. Bohme.** 1989. Formation and release of nitric oxide from human neutrophils and HL-60 cells induced by a chemotactic peptide, platelet activating factor and leukotriene B$_4$. *FEBS Lett.* **244**:357–360.

Inhibition of Oxidative Burst and Chemotaxis in Human Phagocytes by *Legionella pneumophila* Protease

NAREN N. SAHNEY, JAMES T. SUMMERSGILL, AND RICHARD D. MILLER

Department of Microbiology and Immunology and Division of Infectious Diseases, Department of Medicine, School of Medicine, University of Louisville, Louisville, Kentucky 40292

Legionella pneumophila produces several extracellular enzymes and toxins, but their role in the pathogenesis of Legionnaires disease (LD) is unclear. The major secretory protein, a 38-kDa zinc metalloprotease, has been cloned and sequenced (5), and it has been found to exhibit hemolytic and cytotoxic properties (4, 5). The protease has been shown not to be required for intracellular growth or cell killing (9) and is not a required virulence factor in a guinea pig model of LD (1). However, its role in infections of humans remains to be examined. The protein is detected in vivo in lungs of guinea pigs with experimental LD (10) and within human monocytes in vitro (2). Protease has also been demonstrated to inactivate human alpha-1-antitrypsin (3) and can inhibit human natural killer cell activity (6). More recently, we demonstrated that total exoproducts from a protease-deficient mutant of *L. pneumophila* were unable to inhibit polymorphonuclear leukocytes (PMN) superoxide anion generation and chemotaxis, in contrast to the activity demonstrated by total exoproducts from wild-type strains (8). In the present study, we examined the effects of purified protease on the oxidative burst and chemotaxis of human phagocytes.

PMN and monocytes were isolated from healthy volunteers and treated with sublethal concentrations of protease that had been purified by the method of Rechnitzer et al. (7). Cells were stimulated by (i) receptor-mediated stimuli (formylmethionylleucylphenylalanine [fMLP] and zymosan-activated particles [ZAP]) and (ii) non-receptor-mediated phorbol myristate acetate (PMA), a direct activator of protein kinase C, and then assayed for superoxide anion production, chemiluminescence (CL), and nitroblue tetrazolium dye reduction. Under-agarose chemotaxis was performed with PMN in response to fMLP as a chemoattractant. All results were expressed as a percentage of the control value. Viability of cells was checked by the trypan blue dye exclusion test ($>95\%$).

Superoxide anion generation by PMN stimulated by the three stimuli showed a dose-dependent inhibition when cells were exposed to increasing concentrations of the protease. Significant inhibition of superoxide anion production was achieved with 100 U/ml (47, 64, and 37% of the control value in response to ZAP, fMLP, and PMA, respectively), with complete inhibition observed with 1,200 U of protease per ml. Complete suppression of superoxide anion production in adherent monocytes was achieved at slightly lower concentrations of protease (1,000 U/ml) with all stimuli.

In the second assay of oxidative burst, PMN were stimulated with fMLP and PMA, and then their nitroblue tetrazolium dye-reducing ability was measured. Cells exposed to increasing concentrations of protease showed a dose-dependent loss in dye reduction, and a substantial decrease occurred in PMN treated with 1,000 U of protease per ml (8 and 18% of the control value with fMLP and PMA, respectively).

The third assay of oxidative burst, lucigenin-enhanced CL, gave slightly different results. Cumulative CL response was measured in PMN treated with protease and stimulated with ZAP or PMA over a 2-h period. Cells showed a statistically significant but incomplete inhibition of the CL response (57% of the control value; $P < 0.05$) when cells were exposed to 1,500 U of protease per ml and exposed to ZAP. To achieve virtually complete inhibition, cells were preincubated with 3,000 U of protease per ml for 1 h (6% of the control value). The CL response in monocytes stimulated with ZAP gave similar results except that inhibition (45% of the control value) was observed at slightly lower concentrations of protease (1,000 U/ml). Treatment with 3,000 U of protease per ml resulted in a further loss of CL response (14% of the control value). On the other hand, both PMN and monocytes were able to respond completely normally to PMA even when exposed to high levels (i.e., 3,000 U) of protease. The differences seen with the CL assay may be due to the fact that the CL response is an amplified response and may involve different reaction products.

The second functional parameter examined was the under-agarose chemotaxis of PMN in response to fMLP. Cells were exposed to increasing amounts of protease, and the chemotactic differential was measured and compared with that of untreated controls. A dose-dependent decrease in PMN chemotactic ability was seen, with a significant reduction in chemotaxis demonstrated with 500 and 1,200 U of protease per ml (37 and 11%, respectively, of the control value).

To determine whether the inhibitory effects of protease on phagocyte oxidative burst and chemotaxis were reversible, cells were preincubated with protease and washed. Superoxide anion generation and chemotaxis were measured as described above. PMN that were preincubated for 2 h with protease and washed maintained a substantial loss of superoxide anion production when stimulated with fMLP but were able to respond normally to PMA. This result suggested that the inhibitory effect of protease on PMN stimulated by the receptor-mediated stimulus fMLP was irreversible after 2 h of preincubation, whereas the non-receptor-mediated event was reversible. Cells preincubated with protease for 1 h and washed free of protease showed a normal chemotactic response to fMLP, suggesting that the effect of protease on PMN chemotaxis was completely reversible.

In conclusion, this study showed that *L. pneumophila* protease inhibited the oxidative burst, as measured by three different assays. This inhibition was seen in response to both receptor- and non-receptor-mediated stimuli, suggesting different mechanisms of action. The protease also inhibited PMN chemotaxis in a dose-dependent manner. These results suggest that *L. pneumophila* pro-

tease has inhibitory effects on human phagocyte functions, which may enhance the survival of the organism in the extracellular milieu during the early stages of disease. Sufficient amounts of protease produced in the alveolus could possibly prevent PMN from entering the site of infection and also diminish their oxidative killing ability. In addition, protease could degrade cytokines and thus alter the activation of macrophages. Future studies will be required to establish the concentrations of protease present in the lungs during human infections and to examine the mechanisms by which protease alters these phagocyte functions.

REFERENCES

1. **Blander, S. J., L. Szeto, H. A. Shuman, and M. A. Horwitz.** 1990. An immunoprotective molecule, the major secretory protein of *Legionella pneumophila*, is not a virulence factor in a guinea pig model of Legionnaires' disease. *J. Clin. Invest.* **86:**817–824.

2. **Clemens, D. L., and M. A. Horwitz.** 1990. Demonstration that *Legionella pneumophila* produces its major secretory protein in infected human monocytes and localization of the protein by immunocytochemistry and immunoelectron microscopy. *Clin. Res.* **38:**480A.

3. **Conlan, J. W., A. Williams, and L. A. E. Ashworth.** 1988. Inactivation of human alpha-1 antitrypsin by a tissue-destructive protease of *Legionella pneumophila*. *J. Gen. Microbiol.* **134:**481–487.

4. **Keen, M. G., and P. S. Hoffman.** 1989. Characterization of a *Legionella pneumophila* extracellular protease exhibiting hemolytic and cytotoxic activities. *Infect. Immun.* **57:**732–738.

5. **Quinn, F. D., and L. S. Tompkins.** 1989. Analysis of a cloned sequence of *Legionella pneumophila* encoding a 38 Kd metalloprotease possessing haemolytic and cytotoxic properties. *Mol. Microbiol.* **3:**797–805.

6. **Rechnitzer, C., M. Diamant, and B. K. Pedersen.** 1989. Inhibition of human natural killer cell activity by *Legionella pneumophila* protease. *Eur. J. Clin. Microbiol. Infect. Dis.* **8:**989–992.

7. **Rechnitzer, C., M. Tvede, and G. Doring.** 1989. A rapid method for purification of homogenous *Legionella pneumophila* cytotoxic protease using fast protein liquid chromatography. *FEMS Microbiol. Lett.* **59:**39–44.

8. **Sahney, N. N., B. C. Lambe, J. T. Summersgill, and R. D. Miller.** 1990. Inhibition of polymorphonuclear leukocyte function by *Legionella pneumophila* exoproducts. *Microb. Pathog.* **9:**117–125.

9. **Szeto, L., and H. A. Shuman.** 1990. The *Legionella pneumophila* major secretory protein, a protease, is not required for intracellular growth or cell killing. *Infect. Immun.* **58:**2585–2592.

10. **Williams, A., A. Baskerville, A. B. Dowsett, and J. W. Conlan.** 1987. Immunocytochemical demonstration of the association between *Legionella pneumophila*, its tissue-destructive protease, and pulmonary lesions in experimental Legionnaires' disease. *J. Pathol.* **153:**257–264.

Role of Endogenous Gamma Interferon in Natural Resistance of Mice to *Legionella pneumophila* Infection

HIRONOBU FUJIO, SHIN-ICHI YOSHIDA, HIROSHI MIYAMOTO, AND YASUO MIZUGUCHI

Department of Microbiology, School of Medicine, University of Occupational and Environmental Health, Kitakyushu 807, Japan

It has been shown that *Legionella pneumophila* can grow in human monocytes and human alveolar macrophages and that gamma interferon (IFN-γ) activates these macrophages to inhibit the intracellular growth of the bacteria (2, 4). Among rodents, there is an interspecies difference in susceptibility to *L. pneumophila* infection. Guinea pigs are highly susceptible, the 50% lethal dose (LD$_{50}$) being 7.6×10^4 CFU per animal by intraperitoneal injection. On the other hand, many strains of mice are highly resistant to *L. pneumophila*; for example, the LD$_{50}$ for BALB/c mice was found to be 6.7×10^7 CFU per animal (10). The bacteria could proliferate in macrophages of guinea pigs but not in macrophages of many strains of mice (10). It was suggested that the difference in abilities of macrophages to suppress intracellular bacterial growth resulted in the difference in susceptibility between guinea pigs and mice. Recently, Yamamoto et al. reported that *L. pneumophila* could proliferate well in thioglycolate-elicited peritoneal macrophages of A/J mice (9) and that IFN-γ activated the macrophages to inhibit intracellular bacterial growth (8).

In this study, we investigated the role of endogenous IFN-γ in natural resistance of A/J mice against *L. pneumophila* infection.

First, the LD$_{50}$ was determined by injecting A/J mice (five animals per group) intravenously (i.v.) with different doses of *L. pneumophila* Philadelphia-1 (ATCC 33152; donated by the Centers for Disease Control). The LD$_{50}$ for A/J mice was 2.7×10^7 CFU, greater than the LD$_{50}$ for guinea pigs (7.6×10^4 CFU).

To examine the ability of A/J mice to produce IFN-γ, spleen cell cultures of nonimmunized mice were stimulated in vitro with formalin-killed *L. pneumophila* for 18 h, and IFN-γ activity in the culture supernatant fluids was assayed by enzyme immunoassay. The amount of IFN-γ produced by splenocytes of A/J mice was 467.9 ± 169.1 IU/ml (mean $\pm$ standard deviation for four animals), whereas the value for C57BL/6 mice was 655.5 ± 63.0 IU/ml; the difference in titers of IFN-γ production between the two strains was not significant ($P = 0.067$). Thus, splenocytes of normal A/J mice could produce a large amount of IFN-γ within 18 h of stimulation in vitro with formalin-killed *L. pneumophila*.

To investigate the role of endogenous IFN-γ in *L. pneumophila* infection, mice were injected i.v.

with 30 μg of rat anti-mouse IFN-γ monoclonal antibody (MAb) or normal rat globulin (30 μg) 2 h before injection i.v. with a sublethal dose (10^7 CFU) of *L. pneumophila*. The number of *L. pneumophila* cells in livers, spleens, and lungs of treated mice was determined on days 0, 1, and 2 of infection, (Fig. 1). Bacterial counts in the organs of A/J mice pretreated with anti-IFN-γ MAb increased significantly compared with those in control mice. Data from the preliminary experiment indicate that the LD$_{50}$ for A/J mice pretreated with anti-IFN-γ MAb before infection would be far below 5.3×10^6 CFU per mouse; we are investigating this possibility further. Results obtained so far show that IFN-γ plays a critical role in resistance of A/J mice to *L. pneumophila* infection.

The natural resistance of A/J mice to *L. pneumophila* will be better understood by comparing it with that of guinea pigs. Despite the evidence that macrophages of both A/J mice and guinea pigs permitted intracellular growth of *L. pneumophila*, the LD$_{50}$ of *L. pneumophila* for A/J mice was 2.7×10^7 CFU, much higher than that for guinea pigs (7.6×10^4 CFU) (10). After several hours of culture with *Legionella* antigen, A/J splenocytes could produce IFN-γ in vitro, while macrophage-activating factor (IFN-γ) could not be produced by normal guinea pig splenocytes upon in vitro antigen stimulation (6, 8). In addition, we have reported that in guinea pigs, the enhancement of resistance to *L. pneumophila* occurs 4 days after infection; i.e., this factor is not produced until day 4 of infection (6). From the comparison presented above, prompt IFN-γ production is thought to be one of the reasons why A/J mice are very resistant to *Legionella* infection.

It was suggested that mouse natural killer cells are responsible for in vitro production of IFN-γ in response to antigens of several intracellular bacteria, including *L. pneumophila* (1) and *Listeria monocytogenes* (7). Dunn and North showed in vivo studies that early elimination of natural killer cells by treatment with rabbit antiserum to asialo GM1 resulted in exacerbation of listerial infection (3). Nauciel and Espinassa-Maes reported that cells other than T lymphocytes, possibly natural killer cells, participated in the rapid IFN-γ production in response to *Salmonella* infection (5). On the other hand, Yamamoto et al. suggested that some interaction between functional T cells

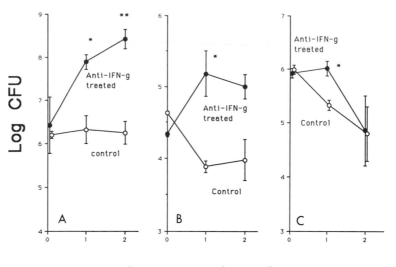

Days after infection

FIG. 1. Effect of anti-IFN-γ MAb administration on the resistance of A/J mice injected i.v. with a sublethal dose (10^7 CFU) of *L. pneumophila*. Bacterial growth in the organs was determined at intervals. The data are means ± standard deviations for three animals. * and ** indicate $P < 0.05$ and $P < 0.01$, respectively, with respect to control mice. IFN-g, IFN-γ. (A) Liver; (B) lungs; (C) spleen.

and B cells was required for mouse IFN-γ production in response to *Legionella* vaccine stimulation (8). In our laboratory, however, the administration of antiserum to asialo GM1, anti-L3T4 (CD4) MAb, or anti-Lyt2.2 (CD8) MAb, or combined administration of these three antibodies, did not affect the resistance of mice to *L. pneumophila* (unpublished data). The cell population responsible for the production of IFN-γ in the course of infection remains to be determined.

This study was supported by Grant-in-Aid for Scientific Research 03670229 from the Ministry of Education, Science and Culture, Japan.

REFERENCES

1. **Blanchard, D. K., H. Friedman, W. E. Stewart II, T. W. Klein, and J. Y. Djeu.** 1988. Role of gamma interferon in induction of natural killer activity by *Legionella pneumophila* in vitro and in an experimental murine infection model. *Infect. Immun.* **56**:1187–1193.
2. **Byrd, T. F., and M. A. Horwitz.** 1989. Interferon gamma-activated human monocytes downregulate transferrin receptors and inhibit the intracellular multiplication of *Legionella pneumophila* by limiting the availability of iron. *J. Clin. Invest.* **83**:1457–1465.
3. **Dunn, P. L., and R. J. North.** 1991. Early gamma interferon production by natural killer cells is important in defense against murine listeriosis. *Infect. Immun.* **59**:2892–2900.
4. **Nash, T. W., D. M. Libby, and M. A. Horwitz.** 1988. IFN-γ activated human alveolar macrophages inhibit the intracellular multiplication of *Legionella pneumophila*. *J. Immunol.* **140**:3978–3981.
5. **Nauciel, C., and F. Espinassa-Maes.** 1992. Role of gamma interferon and tumor necrosis factor alpha in resistance to *Salmonella typhimurium* infection. *Infect. Immun.* **60**:450–454.
6. **Nikaido, Y., S. Yoshida, Y. Goto, Y. Mizuguchi, and A. Kuroiwa.** 1989. Macrophage-activating T-cell factor(s) produced in an early phase of *Legionella pneumophila* infection in guinea pigs. *Infect. Immun.* **57**:3458–3465.
7. **Wherry, J. C., R. D. Schreiber, and E. R. Unanue.** 1991. Regulation of gamma interferon production by natural killer cells in *scid* mice: roles of tumor necrosis factor and bacterial stimuli. *Infect. Immun.* **59**:1709–1715.
8. **Yamamoto, Y., T. W. Klein, C. Newton, and H. Friedman.** 1992. Differing macrophage and lymphocyte roles in resistance to *Legionella pneumophila* infection. *J. Immunol.* **148**:584–589.
9. **Yamamoto, Y., T. W. Klein, C. A. Newton, R. Widen, and H. Friedman.** 1988. Growth of *Legionella pneumophila* in thioglycolate-elicited peritoneal macrophages from A/J mice. *Infect. Immun.* **56**:370–375.
10. **Yoshida, S., and Y. Mizuguchi.** 1986. Multiplication of *Legionella pneumophila* Philadelphia-1 in cultured peritoneal macrophages and its correlation to susceptibility of animals. *Can. J. Microbiol.* **33**:438–442.

Ultrastructure of the Adherence and Intracellular Replication of *Legionella pneumophila* in Macrophage-Like U937 Cells

F. C. GIBSON III AND F. G. RODGERS

Department of Microbiology, Spaulding Life Science Center, University of New Hampshire, Durham, New Hampshire 03824-3544

Legionella pneumophila is a facultative intracellular bacterial pathogen that multiplies within many eukaryotic cells, including human alveolar macrophages and monocytes, as well as a variety of human and animal epithelial and fibroblast cells, primary explants, and protozoa of environmental origin (1, 4–7). *L. pneumophila* adheres to host cell membranes prior to uptake and intracellular replication. The initial attachment mechanisms and thus the nature of the adhesive structure employed by *L. pneumophila* to attach to host cells, a prerequisite for intracellular infection, is unknown. However, putative *Legionella* adhesins have been proposed as well as visualized by electron microscopy (EM) (9, 10). Following cellular infection, *L. pneumophila* survives in the inhospitable environment of the macrophage phagosome by preventing phagosome-lysosome fusion (2), eventually leading to cell destruction.

Ultrastructural studies using eukaryotic cells have been used to document the course of intracellular infection. Using a variety of cell types, Oldham and Rodgers (7) investigated the cellular and subcellular aspects of *Legionella* intracellular replication. Cellular infection occurred rapidly with uptake of bacteria within banded inclusions. Cell death and lysis were complete by 6 days postinfection. Horwitz (3) demonstrated that human monocytes took up Legionnaires disease bacteria through a novel mechanism termed coiling phagocytosis.

U937 cells are transformed, human histiocytic lymphoma cells that are monocyte- or macrophage-like in nature (11, 12). Pearlman et al. (8) showed that these cells supported *L. pneumophila* multiplication and that they constituted an appropriate model for *Legionella*-macrophage interactions. The purpose of this study was to further characterize *Legionella*-U937 cell interactions at the cellular and subcellular levels and so determine the attachment event, intracellular replication, and cytopathic changes in these cells, using transmission EM, scanning EM, and viable bacterial cell colony counts (VBCCC) over a 72-h period. Such studies would augment the data base on the interaction between *L. pneumophila* and U937 cells.

L. pneumophila Nottingham-7, a fully virulent clinical isolate, was passed twice and stored at −70°C in 1% serum–sorbitol. After thawing, bacterial suspensions were plated on buffered charcoal-yeast extract agar supplemented with α-ketoglutarate (BCYE-α) (pH 6.9). After 72 h, cultures were harvested and suspended in buffered yeast extract broth with α-ketoglutarate to 52 Klett units. Multiple broth aliquots of 5 ml were inoculated with 100 μl of culture grown for 24 h. Organisms were washed three times in Hanks' balanced salt solution (HBSS) and resuspended to give 5×10^8 CFU/ml.

U937 cells were cultured in RPMI 1640 medium (pH 7.2) (Sigma, St. Louis, Mo.) supplemented with 10% fetal bovine serum (Sigma) and 3 mM L-glutamine in T-75 flasks (Costar, Cambridge, Mass.). Cells were grown to a density of 1×10^6 to 2×10^6/ml, harvested by centrifugation at $200 \times g$, resuspended in fresh medium, counted, and treated with 10^{-8} M phorbol myristate acetate (Sigma) for 24 h. Adherent cells were washed three times with HBSS, scraped from flasks with a rubber policeman, and collected by centrifugation at $200 \times g$. The cells were resuspended in fresh medium, counted, and distributed at a density of 5×10^5/ml into T-75 flasks for transmission EM, into 6-well culture plates for scanning EM, or into 24-well culture plates for VBCCC. Cells were allowed to readhere for 24 h at 37°C.

Cultures were inoculated at a multiplicity of infection of 100 *Legionella* organisms per host cell and incubated for 1 h. At 6, 12, 24, 48, and 72 h after inoculation, duplicate cultures were washed three times to remove nonadherent bacteria; one sample was fixed with 10% glutaraldehyde in cacodylate buffer containing 10 mM $MgSO_4$ (CB) (pH 7.0) for 24 h for EM, while the other was lysed with sterile distilled water and together with wash supernatants was prepared for VBCCC. Volumes of 100 μl of lysate plus supernatants at each time were diluted 10 times in HBSS, and 25-μl samples of each dilution were plated in duplicate on BCYEα agar.

Fixed cultures were washed 10 times with CB, scraped from the culture flask surface, collected by centrifugation at $200 \times g$, and postfixed in 1% osmium tetroxide for 18 h. Samples were washed five times in CB, dehydrated in a graded ethanol series, and embedded in Epon-aryldite resin. After polymerization at 60°C, samples were thin sectioned, stained with 1% uranyl acetate for 60 s and 0.4% lead citrate for 30 s, and examined in a Hitachi H-600 scanning-transmission electron microscope at 75 kV.

Fixed cultures on coverslips were washed un-

disturbed 10 times with CB, dehydrated in an ethanol series followed by ice-cold hexamethyldisal-
azane, and dried on ice. Samples were mounted on
stubs, sputter coated with 5-nm gold-palladium,
and observed with an AMR scanning electron
microscope.

Receptor-mediated attachment is one of the first
events to occur prior to establishment of disease
by intracellular pathogens. *Legionella* organisms

were attached to U937 cell membranes within 1 h
(Fig. 1a and b), and approximately one bacterium
was found per U937 cell by VBCCC (Fig. 2).
Coiling phagocytosis and banded inclusions were
not observed. Internalized bacteria were evident
and by 6 h were contained within tight phagosomes that were ribosome lined and in close proximity to mitochondria (Fig. 1c). Cellular change
was minimal at this stage of infection. *L. pneu-*

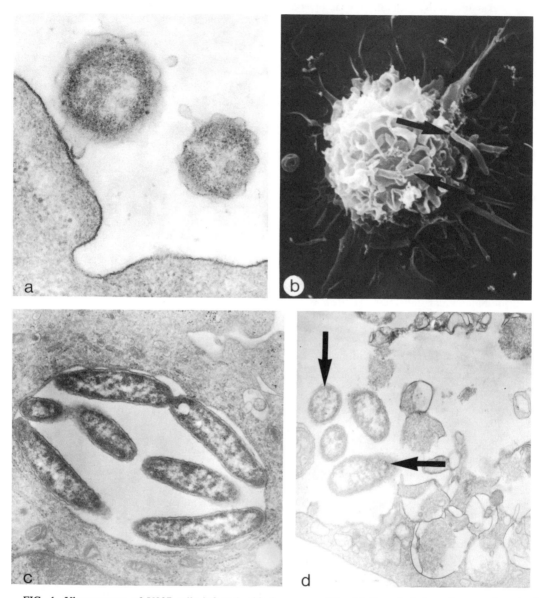

FIG. 1. Ultrastructure of U937 cells infected with *L. pneumophila*. (a) Opsonin-independent attachment of
organisms to host cells occurred within 1 h and appeared to be facilitated by contact between the bacterial outer
membrane and the eukaryotic plasma membrane ($\times 53,760$). (b) Scanning EM of a U937 cell 1 h postinfection. Note
numerous microvilli and adherent legionellae (arrows) ($\times 4,200$). (c) Intracellular multiplication of the organism at
12 h of incubation within a ribosome-lined, membrane-bound vacuole in close association with mitochondria
($\times 18,560$). (d) By 48 h postinoculation, cell lysis and released bacteria (arrows) abound ($\times 21,420$).

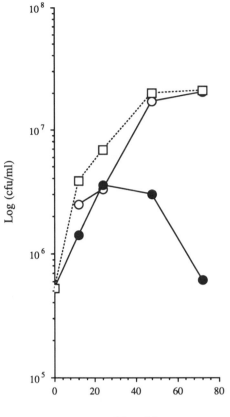

Log (cfu/ml)

Time (h)

FIG. 2. Multiplication of *L. pneumophila* in U937 cells. Symbols: ●, intracellular replication; ○, organism release; □, total numbers of intracellular and extracellular organisms present during the infectious cycle. No bacterial growth occurred in cell-free RPMI 1640 culture medium.

mophila adhered to and replicated within phorbol myristate acetate-treated U937 cells. After uptake, intracellular bacterial multiplication continued unabated and achieved maximal numbers by 24 h postinfection (Fig. 2). Cellular and subcellular changes occurred; these included progressive blunting of microvilli, distention and smoothing of phagosomes, and an increase in numbers and size of intracellular lipid pools. By 48 h, numbers of intracellular legionellae appeared to have stabilized, and they declined thereafter. At this time, extracellular bacterial numbers increased. Extensive U937 cell cytopathic changes included cellular lysis (Fig. 1d), margination of chromatin, and distortion of the nuclear envelope. By 72 h, the numbers of intracellular *L. pneumophila* approached a minimum, while extracellular bacterial numbers stabilized. At this time, >90% of the eukaryotic cell population had detached from the culture surface or were lysed. Ultrastructurally, intact cells contained numerous vacuoles, with large amounts of cellular debris and lytic material predominating.

The macrophage-like U937 cell has been suggested as a model for *Legionella*-macrophage interactions (8). The present study involved the characterization of the cellular and subcellular events following *L. pneumophila* infection of U937 cells, and the results further supported this suggestion. *L. pneumophila* was found to be capable of multiplying within and destroying U937 cells, with the most active multiplication between 12 and 30 h. Between 48 and 72 h, intracellular multiplication gradually declined; however, as a result of bacterially induced host cell destruction, there was a reduction in the numbers of viable U937 cells available for infection. By this stage, there was a sharp increase in the number of extracellular bacteria, indicating that the release phase of the infectious process had commenced (Fig. 2). The mechanism of release is unknown but may be the result of physical disruption of the cells due to massive numbers of intracellular bacteria; however, a role for bacterial protease, the major secretory protein of *L. pneumophila*, cannot be discounted.

The objectives of this study were to delineate the intracellular multiplication of *L. pneumophila* and to define the ultrastructural changes that occurred within U937 cells following infection. Attachment to host cell membranes, the initial infectious event for intracellular pathogens, occurred with *L. pneumophila* by an opsonin-independent mechanism within 1 h and involved a membrane-to-membrane interaction. These ultrastructural findings were in broad agreement with those of other studies which used professional phagocytes as well as a variety of different cell types (4, 5, 7). These and other data (see Gibson et al., this volume) further support the use of the readily available U937 cell line as a model for adherence and intracellular replication of this pathogen. With a better understanding of the events leading to cellular infection as well as the mechanisms involved in intracellular bacterial survival and replication, strategies for prevention and control of Legionnaires disease will be forthcoming.

This study was supported by Public Health Service grant AI 27929 from the National Institutes of Health and by a CURF grant from the Office of Sponsored Research, University of New Hampshire.

REFERENCES

1. **Barbaree, J. M., B. S. Fields, J. C. Feeley, G. W. Gorman, and W. T. Martin.** 1986. Isolation of protozoa from water associated with a legionellosis outbreak and demonstration of intracellular multiplication of *Legionella pneumophila. Appl. Environ. Microbiol.* **51:**422–424.
2. **Horwitz, M. A.** 1983. The Legionnaires' disease bacte-

rium (*Legionella pneumophila*) inhibits phagosome-lyso-some fusion in human monocytes. *J. Exp. Med.* **158**:2108–2126.

3. **Horwitz, M. A.** 1984. Phagocytosis of the Legionnaires' disease bacterium (*Legionella pneumophila*) occurs by a novel mechanism: engulfment within a pseudopod coil. *Cell* **36**:27–33.
4. **Horwitz, M. A., and S. C. Silverstein.** 1980. Legionnaires' disease bacterium (*Legionella pneumophila*) multiplies intracellularly in human monocytes. *J. Clin. Invest.* **131**:697–706.
5. **Marra, A., M. A. Horwitz, and H. A. Shuman.** 1990. The HL-60 model for the interaction of human macrophage with the Legionnaires' disease bacterium. *J. Immunol.* **144**:2738–2744.
6. **Nash, T. W., D. M. Libby, and M. A. Horwitz.** 1984. Interaction between the Legionnaires' disease bacterium (*Legionella pneumophila*) and human alveolar macrophages: influence of antibody, lymphokines and hydrocortisone. *J. Clin. Invest.* **74**:771–782.
7. **Oldham, L. J., and F. G. Rodgers.** 1985. Adhesion,

penetration, and intracellular replication of *Legionella pneumophila*: an *in vitro* model of pathogenesis. *J. Gen. Microbiol.* **131**:697–706.

8. **Pearlman, E., A. H. Jiwa, N. C. Engleberg, and B. I. Eisenstein.** 1988. Growth of *Legionella pneumophila* in a human macrophage-like (U-937) cell line. *Microb. Pathog.* **5**:87–95.
9. **Rodgers, F. G.** 1983. The role of structure and invasiveness on the pathogenicity of *Legionella*. *Zentralbl. Bakteriol. I Abt. Orig. A* **255**:138–144.
10. **Rodgers, F. G., P. W. Greaves, A. D. Macrae, and M. J. Lewis.** 1980. Electron microscopic evidence for flagella and pili on *Legionella pneumophila*. *J. Clin. Pathol.* **33**:1184–1188.
11. **Rovera, G., D. Santoli, and C. Damsky.** 1979. Human promyelocytic leukemia cells in culture differentiate into macrophage-like cells when treated with a phorbol diester. *Proc. Natl. Acad. Sci. USA* **76**:2779.
12. **Sundstrom, C., and K. Nilsson.** 1976. Establishment and characterization of a human histiocytic lymphoma cell line (U-937). *Int. J. Cancer* **17**:565–577.

Cloning and Mapping of pLPG36, a Mobilizable *Legionella pneumophila* Serogroup 1 Plasmid

FÉLIX LÓPEZ DE FELIPE AND JOAQUÍN V. MARTÍNEZ-SUÁREZ

Centro de Investigaciones Biológicas, Consejo Superior de Investigaciones Científicas, Velázquez 144, 28006 Madrid, and Servicio de Bacteriología, Centro Nacional de Microbiología, Madrid, Spain

At present, a genetic system suitable for studies of the structure and expression of *Legionella pneumophila* genes in both native and heterologous hosts is not available. Moreover, techniques for transferring genetic material into *L. pneumophila* need to be developed.

The genetic manipulation of bacteria depends to a large extent on plasmids. However, no large or small plasmid from *L. pneumophila* has been isolated and characterized to date; thus, the techniques of recombinant DNA cannot be applied in studies of this microorganism. Likewise, no relationship between the presence of plasmids and easily selectable phenotypes in *L. pneumophila* has been demonstrated.

We have previously screened plasmids in 78 selected clinical and environmental Spanish strains of *L. pneumophila* serogroup 1. A widely distributed plasmid of 36 MDa, called pLPG36, was chosen for further molecular studies (1).

pLPG36 was isolated from *L. pneumophila* serogroup 1 strain 53048 and purified by CsCl-ethidium bromide density gradient centrifugation as described by Rosenberg et al. (5), with several modifications for the strain used in this work. We selected a method for megaplasmid purification in gram-negative bacteria in order to ensure gentle lysis, thus preventing degradation or loss of plasmid DNA.

Purified pLPG36 was mapped with restriction endonucleases *Sma*I, *Sal*I, *Xho*I, *Sac*I, *Bam*HI,

and *Eco*RI. Single cuts and combinations of double and triple digests of purified pLPG36 DNA were arranged to generate a physical map of this 58-kb *L. pneumophila* plasmid (Fig. 1).

The four *Bam*HI fragments from pLPG36 were separately purified, using the Gene Clean kit (Bio 101, Inc.). Cloning procedures were essentially those described by Maniatis et al. (3). Purified *Bam*HI fragments of 25.7 kb (fragment A), 16.4 kb (fragment B), 10.9 kb (fragment C), and 5.0 kb (fragment D) were cloned from pLPG36 into the unique *Bam*HI site of the cloning vector pUC18, yielding four recombinant plasmids called pFLJ1, pFLJ2, pFLJ3, and pFLJ4, respectively. These four recombinants along with control pUC18 were assayed for plasmid functions in *Escherichia coli*.

All of the recombinant plasmids were incapable of transfer among *Escherichia coli* strains (transfer frequencies of $<10^{-8}$). For the conjugative mobilization of pLPG36 derivatives, donor strains were created by transforming each of the test plasmids into *E. coli* HB101 containing either R702, RP4, pRK231, pN3, R16, R40a, pSa, or R387 as the mobilizing plasmid. The recipient was a rifampin- and nalidixic acid-resistant HB101 strain.

To rule out mobilization as a result of homologous recombination between the mobilized and helper plasmids, a *recA* strain of *E. coli* was used. The broad-host-range IncP plasmid RP4 or the helper plasmid pRK231 did not mobilize pUC18, pFLJ1, pFLJ3, or pFLJ4 but did mobilize pFLJ2

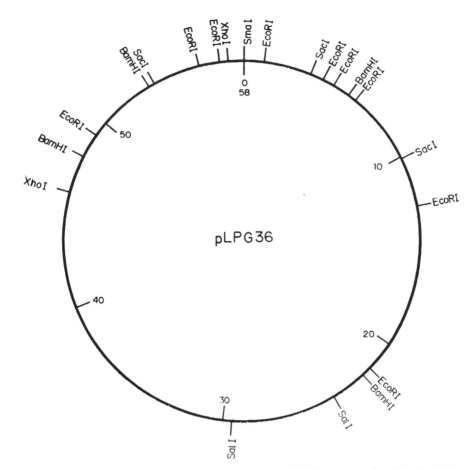

FIG. 1. Restriction map of pLPG36. Restriction sites are oriented with respect to the single *Sma*I site, and the distances (in kilobases) from this site are shown. The *Eco*RI sites are mapped on cloned *Bam*HI fragments B (16.4 kb), C (10.9 kb), and D (5.0 kb). The precise location of five *Eco*RI sites of the 25.7-kb *Bam*HI-A fragment (coordinates 22.2 to 47.2 kb) is not known.

at a frequency of 1.1×10^{-5}. However, the highest mobilization frequency (2×10^{-4}) was obtained for pFLJ2 with the IncP plasmid R702 as the helper. The broad-host-range plasmids pSa (IncW), R40a (IncC), R387 (IncK), pN3 (IncN), and R16 (IncB) did not mobilize any of the pLPG36 recombinant plasmids or pUC18.

Cointegrate formation due to *recA*-independent transposition of insertion elements was excluded by the data obtained from analysis of plasmids present in transconjugants (R702 and pFLJ2 in an unaltered form). This analysis demonstrated that pFLJ2 was mobilized by the IncPα plasmid R702 through a donation mechanism.

The identification of the mobilization function in a cloned region of pLPG36 probably explains the wide distribution of the plasmid that we had previously reported. The ability of pLPG36 DNA to transfer among *E. coli* strains does not support the previous suggestion that *Legionella* plasmids are nontransmissible (4). The widespread distribu-tion of certain *Legionella* plasmids (2) could be due to processes similar to those determined for pLPG36.

The ability of *Legionella* plasmids to transfer may play a role in the spread of antibiotic resis-tance or other selective advantages conferred by plasmids to this microorganism. Recently a conju-gative 36-MDa plasmid of *L. pneumophila* has been demonstrated to confer UV resistance to the strain in which it resides (6). Unfortunately, no restriction pattern analysis of this plasmid was performed, precluding comparison with pLPG36. Nonetheless, the identification of an *oriT* gene function in pLPG36 should facilitate the construc-tion of vectors consisting exclusively of *Le-gionella* DNA.

REFERENCES

1. **López de Felipe, F., and J. V. Martínez-Suárez.** 1991. Wide distribution of a 36 MDal plasmid among clinical and environmental Spanish isolates of *Legionella pneumophila* serogroup 1. *Curr. Microbiol.* **23:**233–236.

2. **Maher, W. E., J. F. Plouffe, M. F. Para.** 1983. Plasmid profiles of clinical and environmental isolates of *Legionella pneumophila* serogroup 1. *J. Clin. Microbiol.* **18:**1422–1423.

3. **Maniatis, T., E. F. Fritsch, and J. Sambrook.** 1989. *Molecular Cloning: a Laboratory Manual*, 2nd ed. Cold Spring Harbor Laboratory, Cold Spring Harbor, N.Y.

4. **Mintz, C. S., and H. A. Shuman.** 1988. Genetics of *Le-*

gionella pneumophila. Microbiol. Sci. **5:**292–295.

5. **Rosenberg, C., F. Casse-Delebart, I. Dusha, M. David, and C. Boucher.** 1982. Megaplasmids in the plant-associated bacteria *Rhizobium meliloti* and *Pseudomonas solanaraceum. J. Bacteriol.* **150:**402–406.

6. **Tully, M.** 1991. A plasmid from a virulent strain of *Legionella pneumophila* is conjugative and confers resistance to ultraviolet light. *FEMS Microbiol. Lett.* **90:**43–48.

A *Legionella* Plasmid Mediates Resistance to UV Light but Not to Solar Radiation

MICHAEL TULLY

Legionella Research Group, Division of Pathology, Public Health Laboratory Service Centre for Applied Microbiology and Research, Porton Down, Salisbury, Wiltshire SP1 3YD, England

Several reports indicate that plasmids are detected only occasionally in clinical and outbreak-related environmental isolates of *Legionella* strains but are commonly demonstrated in isolates from natural environments or from artificial water systems not associated with disease (3, 12, 13). The plasmids vary in size from 12 to >120 kb, are found in most serogroups, replicate stably, and

are cryptic (10). One report (2) suggested that a plasmid-free *Legionella* strain was less likely to cause disease than was a plasmid-bearing strain present in the same hospital. Another possibility, not necessarily in conflict with the foregoing observations, is that *Legionella* plasmids have a role in survival within the natural habitats, surface waters, from which the artificial water systems, the

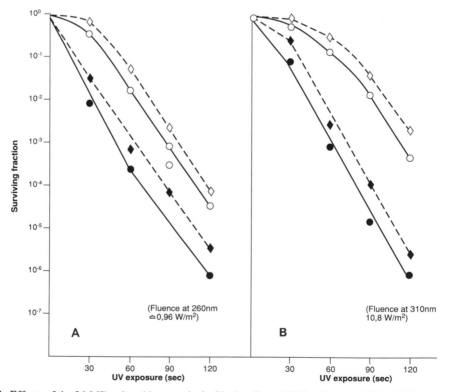

FIG. 1. Effects of the 36-MDa plasmid on survival of legionellae to UV irradiation at 260 and 302 nm. (A) 1002 (Corby derivative, plasmid free) without (●) and with (♦) photoreactivation; (B) D4/1002 (Corby derivative, plasmid containing) without (○) and with (◇) photoreactivation.

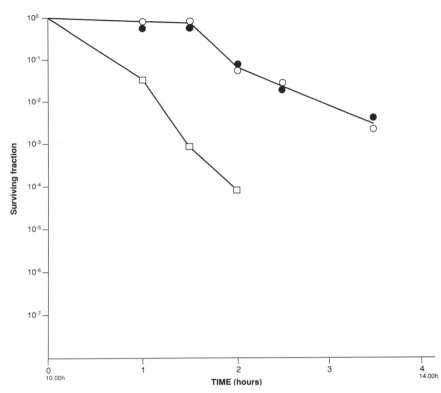

FIG. 2. Survival of legionellae in sunlight. Data presented are from one representative experiment. Replicate experiments show appreciable variation in survival against time; when solar fluence (measured at 310 and 366 nm) was measured, however, results were remarkably reproducible (9). Symbols: ●, 1002; ○, D4/1002; □, D4.

proximal source of infection inoculum, are presumably seeded.

I have shown recently that a 36-MDa conjugative plasmid detected in a clinical isolate of *Legionella pneumophila* (the Dodge strain) confers low-level, error-prone resistance to UV light at 260 nm (15). There is good evidence that the predominant factor in reducing bacterial survival in surface waters is solar radiation (4, 8). Much of the lethal activity of sunlight has been presumed to be mediated by UV radiation at wavelengths of 290 to 320 nm as these wavelengths have the greatest biological effect and wavelengths shorter than these do not penetrate the atmosphere (9). Visible wavelengths (>380 nm) also decrease survival of most bacteria but have little effect on *L. pneumophila* (5). Legionellae, however, like other aquatic bacteria, are very sensitive to UV light at 260 nm (11); indeed, UV light has been used to treat the water in water distribution systems to prevent outbreaks of disease (6).

The studies reported here were designed to assess the effect of the plasmid-coded repair system or the susceptibility of *L. pneumophila* to solar radiation. The construction of otherwise isogenic strains differing in plasmid content has been de-

scribed previously (15), as have all other methods with the exception of photoreactivation, which was induced by exposing inoculated plates to indirect northern sunlight plus irradiation from six Osram daylight fluorescent lamps for 90 min at room temperature before incubation.

Initial experiments compared the inactivation of plasmid-containing and plasmid-free strains of *L. pneumophila* by UV light at wavelengths of 260 and 302 nm (emitted by a UVP TM20 transilluminator; the fluence was measured with a UVX31 detector with a midpoint of 310 nm). The data (Fig. 1) indicate that the plasmid does indeed repair to similar degrees the damage caused at equivalent levels of inactivation at both wavelengths. Equivalent inactivation in these experiments is obtained by fluences of 302-nm radiation more than 10-fold those of 260-nm radiation. This observation is reasonably consistent with previous data (9). These data also indicate that the inactivation caused at both wavelengths is reversible to similar extents by photoreactivation. This finding implies that inactivation is caused at both wavelengths via the same mechanism, the induction of thymine dimers (9). The presence of a photoreactivation repair system in legionellae has been pre-

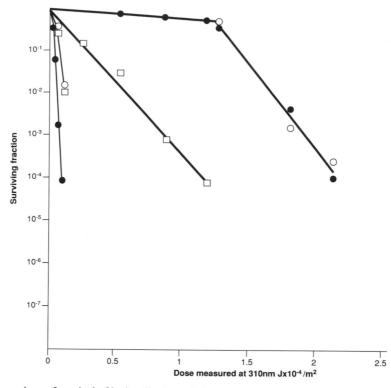

FIG. 3. Comparison of survival of legionellae in sunlight (thick lines; fluence $\simeq$ 1.3–2.1 J/m²) and in UV light (thin lines; illuminator irradiation fluence $\simeq$ 1.05–1.6 J/m²) at 302 nm.

viously documented (11), though the extent of photoreactivation observed in the present work was much less (3-fold rather than 100-fold). Some of the methodological differences between the two studies (fluences, bacterial strains, irradiation of cell suspensions rather than plated cells, conditions of photoreactivation) have been examined unsuccessfully in experiments to identify this discrepancy.

Inactivation by natural sunlight was tested in experiments carried out in the open air on several days in September and October 1991. Initial experiments showed that transport and plating of the irradiated suspensions in the dark did not alter survival in comparison with parallel experiments in which samples were held and manipulated in light, nor was photoreactivation in the laboratory effective. This observation implies that the principal lethal effect of solar radiation on legionellae may not be mediated via formation of thymine dimers. The data indicate that the plasmid has no detectable effect in reducing the lethal effect of solar radiation (Fig. 2).

Unexpectedly, strain D4, whose resistance to UV light at 260 and 302 nm is identical to that of D4/1002, is more susceptible to sunlight than is the Corby strain with or without the D4 plasmid.

The original Dodge strain (lacking the transposon) is also more susceptible to sunlight (data not shown). By comparing solar irradiation data plotted as survival/fluence with data from transilluminator experiments with UV light at 302 nm (Fig. 3) and 366 nm (from a UVP TL33 transilluminator) (Fig. 4), in which photoreactivation was induced during as well as after irradiation, it is evident that the susceptibility of the Dodge strain to sunlight is paralleled by sensitivity to 366-nm light.

As in the previous experiments, there are marked quantitative differences in the fluences required to give a particular level of survival by artificial sources and natural solar radiation. These discrepancies are frequent in such work (9); those observed in Fig. 3 may be explained by the simultaneous photoreactivation of 302-nm-induced damage occurring during solar irradiation being more effective than that obtained in laboratory experiments, and those in Fig. 4 may reflect the effect of solar radiation components of wavelengths shorter than 366 nm.

Plasmid-borne UV repair systems are common in natural isolates of aquatic bacteria, and they have been proposed to be ecologically important (7, 14). The lack of effect of carriage of this plas-

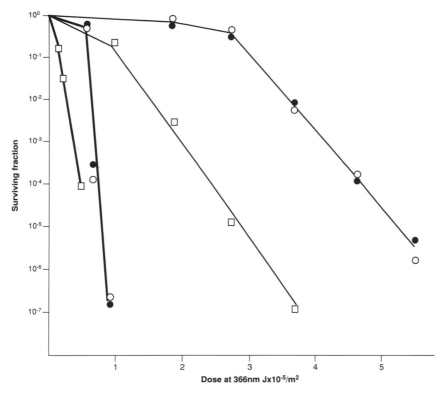

FIG. 4. Comparison of survival of legionellae in sunlight (thick lines; fluence ≃ 5.0–8.5 J/m²) and in UV light (thin lines; illuminator irradiation fluence ≃ 5.0–8.5 J/m², performed in daylight) at 366 nm. Symbols: ●, 1002; ○, D4/1002; □, D4.

mid upon repair of solar radiation-induced lethality in legionellae argues against this possibility. However, since plasmid-borne repair systems apparently vary greatly in their efficiency of repair of UV-induced damage (14, 16), this conclusion may not be general.

The observation that clinical and infection-related environmental strains of *L. pneumophila* generally do not contain plasmids, whereas environmental isolates frequently do, requires further study. Suppression of virulence by plasmids has been documented for other pathogens, including the waterborne gram-negative rods *Pseudomonas aeruginosa* (17) and *Vibrio cholerae* (1), but other more indirect mechanisms, such as interaction of legionellae with other components of the biofilm (in particular amoebae) or incorporation into (or survival within) aerosols, may operate. These possibilities and correlation with plasmid size or structure are all amenable to experimental analysis.

Jon White (medical illustrator, Central Public Health Laboratories, Colindale) provided prompt and willing drafting of the graphs.

REFERENCES

1. **Bartowsky, E. J., S. R. Attridge, C. J. Thomas, G. Mayrhoffer, and P. A. Manning.** 1990. Role of the P plasmid in attenuation of *Vibrio cholerae* O1. *Infect. Immun.* **58:**3129–3134.
2. **Brown, A., R. M. Vickers, E. M. Elder, M. Lema, and G. M. Garrity.** 1982. Plasmid and surface antigen markers of endemic and epidemic *Legionella pneumophila. J. Clin. Microbiol.* **16:**230–235.
3. **Castellani-Pastoris, M., M. G. Mingrone, and C. Passi.** 1987. Plasmid profiles of *Legionella* spp. isolates Italy. *Eur. J. Epidemiol.* **3:**261–264.
4. **Chamberlin, C. E., and R. Mitchell.** 1988. A decay model for enteric bacteria in natural waters, p. 325–348. *In* R. Mitchell (ed.), *Water Pollution Microbiology.* Wiley, New York.
5. **Dutka, B. J.** 1984. Sensitivity of *Legionella pneumophila* to sunlight in fresh and marine waters. *Appl. Environ. Microbiol.* **48:**970–974.
6. **Farr, B. M., J. C. Tartaglino, J. C. Gratz, S. I. Getchell-White, and D. H. M. Groschell.** 1988. Evaluation of ultraviolet light for disinfection of hospital water contaminated with *Legionella. Lancet* **ii:**669–672.
7. **Fry, J. C., and M. J. Day.** 1990. Plasmid transfer in the epilithon, p. 55–80. *In* J. C. Fry and M. J. Day (ed.), *Bacterial Genetics in Natural Environments.* Chapman & Hall, London.
8. **Gameson, A. L. H., and D. J. Gould.** 1975. Effects of solar radiation on the mortality of some terrestrial bacteria in sea water, p. 209–217. *In* A. L. H. Gameson (ed.), *Proceedings of the International Symposium on Discharge*

of Sewage from Sea Outfalls. Pergamon Press, Oxford.
9. **Harm, W.** 1980. *Biological Effects of Ultraviolet Radiation.* Cambridge University Press, Cambridge.
10. **Johnson, S. R., and W. O. Schalla.** 1982. Plasmids of serogroup 1 strains of *Legionella pneumophila. Curr. Microbiol.* **7:**143–146.
11. **Knudson, G. B.** 1985. Photoreactivation of UV-irradiated *Legionella pneumophila* and other *Legionella* species. *Appl. Environ. Microbiol.* **49:**975–980.
12. **Maher, W. E., J. F. Plouffe, and M. F. Para.** 1983. Plasmid profiles of clinical and environmental isolates of *Legionella pneumophila* serogroup 1. *J. Clin. Microbiol.* **18:**1422–1423.
13. **Mellado, A., J. Aguero, A. Seoane, and L. M. Rodriguez-Solorzano.** 1986. Plasmid profiles of *Le-*

gionella pneumophila isolated in Spain. *Eur. J. Epidemiol.* **2:**63–66.
14. **Simonson, C. S., T. A. Kokjohn, and R. V. Miller.** 1990. Inducible UV repair potential of *Pseudomonas aeruginosa* PAO. *J. Gen. Microbiol.* **136:**1241–1249.
15. **Tully, M.** 1991. A plasmid from a virulent strain of *Legionella pneumophila* is conjugative and confers resistance to ultraviolet light. *FEMS Microbiol. Lett.* **90:**43–48.
16. **Upton, C., and R. J. Pinney.** 1983. Expression of eight unrelated Muc+ plasmids in eleven DNA repair-deficient *E. coli* strains. *Mutat. Res.* **112:**261–273.
17. **Wretlind, B., K. Becker, and D. Haas.** 1985. IncP-1 R plasmids decrease the serum resistance and the virulence of *Pseudomonas aeruginosa. J. Gen. Microbiol.* **131:**2701–2704.

Characterization of ADP-Ribosyltransferase Produced by *Legionella pneumophila*

Y. F. BELYI, I. S. TARTAKOVSKII, Y. V. VERTIEV, AND S. V. PROSOROVSKII

Gamaleya Institute of Epidemiology and Microbiology, Moscow 123098, Russia

Investigations into the pathogenesis of legionellosis have led to the characterization of various *Legionella* products that appear to play a significant role in infection: metalloproteinase (5), low-molecular-mass toxin (9, 10), and phosphatases and protein kinases (12, 13). It was shown that these bacterial proteins can inhibit oxidative metabolism, thus allowing intracellular multiplication of legionellae (9, 10), influence regulatory reactions in eukaryotic cells (2), and produce necrotic lesions in lungs (7). However, the pathogenesis of different clinical symptoms (gastrointestinal mulfunctions, disorders of the central nervous system, etc.) has not been studied. Little is known of the molecular mechanisms involved in the intraphagocytic parasitism of legionellae.

It is known that the biological action of most active bacterial products, particularly toxins, depends on ADP ribosylation, i.e., enzymatic splitting of NAD followed by transfer of the ADP-ribose moiety to specific eukaryotic proteins (8). Considering the importance of ADP-ribosylating bacterial enzymes, our group began a survey of similar substances in legionellae.

We succeeded in detecting ADP-ribosyltransferase (ADP-RT) activity in ultrasonic lysates of *Legionella pneumophila* cells. The reaction resulted in intensive endogenous modification of *Legionella* components with molecular masses of 70, 54, and 30 kDa after the addition of [^{32}P]NAD. We speculated that the 54-kDa protein was an ADP-RT, auto-ADP ribosylated under the conditions used. The 70- and 30-kDa components may have been the precursor and product, respectively, of the enzyme's degradation. It was shown that the reaction was not influenced by the addition of guinea pig spleen cell and lung cell lysates

but was considerably increased in the presence of guinea pig peritoneal macrophage lysates (3). Macrophages and other phagocytes are known to be the main target cells for virulent legionellae. From this point of view, the increased ADP-RT activity could be considered a regulatory mechanism that has some role in the process of infection.

To elucidate the precise role of the activity that we detected, a fast protein liquid chromatography-based scheme for purification of *Legionella* ADP-RT was developed. The protocol consisted of Superose 6 preparative-grade gel chromatography, Mono Q ion-exchange chromatography, alkyl-Superose hydrophobic interaction chromatography, and Mono P chromatofocusing (4).

Extremely low production of the protein by *Legionella* cells considerably complicated purification of the enzyme. As a result, the material obtained was not homogeneous. The putative ADP-RT (54-kDa protein) was contaminated by a component with a molecular mass of 38 kDa as well as by some minor components with molecular masses of 53 and 27 kDa.

It has been shown that eukaryotic proteins are the main substrates for bacterial ADP-RTs (8). For this reason, we directed our attention to detection of eukaryotic proteins that could be ADP ribosylated by a partially purified *L. pneumophila* product. In these experiments, we detected modification of eukaryotic acceptors with molecular masses of 20 to 25 kDa present in rabbit pulmonary cell cytosol. Addition of bivalent cations as well as ATP was necessary for ADP ribosylation. Nicotinamide and NAD inhibited incorporation of ADP-ribose into acceptor proteins. Another set of experiments indicated that the modified proteins belonged to the family of G proteins (4).

It is known that bacterial ADP-RTs such as the C3 of *Clostridium botulinum* (1) and exotoxin S of *Pseudomonas aeruginosa* (6) can modify G proteins with similar molecular masses. In contrast to the C3 of *C. botulinum* (a generous gift from A. Efimenko, Laboratory of Botulism, Gamaleya Institute), the ADP-RT of *L. pneumophila* was thermolabile. Exotoxin S produced by *P. aeruginosa*, unlike the *Legionella* enzyme, possessed broad substrate specificity and has been shown to ADP ribosylate a considerable number of proteins as well as 20- to 25-kDa components (6).

The fact that very different microorganisms can produce substances that modify very similar if not identical substrates is quite intriguing. The important role that exotoxin S of *P. aeruginosa* plays in the virulence of the bacterium is well established (11). Therefore, our information may be useful in understanding the mechanisms involved in the virulence of the bacterium responsible for Legionnaires disease.

REFERENCES

1. **Aktories, K., U. Weller, and G. S. Chhatwal.** 1987. *Clostridium botulinum* type C produces a novel ADP-ribosyltransferase distinct from botulinum C2 toxin. *FEBS Lett.* **212:**109–113.
2. **Belyi, Y. F.** 1990. Action of *Legionella* cytolysin on components of the phosphokinase system of eukaryotic cells. *Biomed. Sci.* **1:**494–498.
3. **Belyi, Y. F., I. S. Tartakovskii, Y. V. Vertiev, and S. V. Prosorovskii.** 1991. ADP-ribosyltransferase activity of *Legionella pneumophila* is stimulated by the presence of macrophage lysates. *Biomed Sci.* **2:**94–96.
4. **Belyi, Y. F., I. S. Tartakovskii, Y. V. Vertiev, and S. V. Prosorovskii.** 1991. Partial purification and characterization of ADP-ribosyltransferase produced by *Legionella pneumophila. Biomed. Sci.* **2:**169–174.
5. **Belyi, Y. F., Y. V. Vertiev, I. S. Tartakovskii, and Y. V. Ezepchuk.** 1985. Partial purification and characterization of thermolabile cytotoxin produced by *Legionella pneumophila,* p. 1. *In* Y. V. Ezepchuk (ed.), *Proceedings of the 1st National Conference "Molecular Structure of Bacterial Toxins and Genetic Control of Their Biosynthesis."* Moscow, Russia.
6. **Coburn, J., R. T. Wyatt, B. H. Iglewski, and D. M. Gill.** 1989. Several GTP-binding proteins, including c-H-ras p21, are preferred substrates of *Pseudomonas aeruginosa* exoenzyme S. *J. Biol. Chem.* **264:**9004–9008.
7. **Conlan, J. W., A. Baskerville, and L. A. E. Ashworth.** 1986. Separation of *Legionella pneumophila* proteases and purification of a protease which produces lesions like those of Legionnaires' disease in guinea pig lungs. *J. Gen. Microbiol* **132:**1565–1574.
8. **Foster, J. W., and D. M. Kinney.** 1985. ADP-ribosylating microbial toxins. *Crit. Rev. Microbiol.* **11:**273–298.
9. **Hedlund, K. W.** 1981. *Legionella* toxin. *Pharmacol. Ther.* **15:**123–130.
10. **Lochner, J. E., R. H. Bigley, and B. H. Iglewski.** 1985. Defective triggering of polymorphonuclear leukocyte oxidative metabolism by *Legionella pneumophila* toxin. *J. Infect. Dis.* **151:**42–46.
11. **Nicas, T. Y. and B. H. Iglewski.** 1985. The contribution of exoproducts to virulence of *Pseudomonas aeruginosa. Can. J. Microbiol.* **31:**387–392.
12. **Saha, A. K., J. N. Dowling, K. L. LaMarco, S. Das, A. T. Remaley, N. Olomu, M. T. Pope, and R. H. Glew.** 1985. Properties of an acid phosphatase from *Legionella micdadei* which blocks superoxide anion production by human neutrophils. *Arch. Biochem. Biophys.* **243:**150–160.
13. **Saha, A. K., J. N. Dowling, N. K. Mukhopadhyay, and R. H. Glew.** 1988. Demonstration of two protein kinases in extracts of *Legionella micdadei. J. Gen. Microbiol.* **134:**1275–1281.

III. *LEGIONELLA*-PROTOZOA INTERRELATIONSHIPS

STATE OF THE ART LECTURE

Legionella and Protozoa: Interaction of a Pathogen and Its Natural Host

BARRY S. FIELDS

*Division of Bacterial and Mycotic Diseases, National Center for Infectious Diseases,
Centers for Disease Control, Atlanta, Georgia 30333*

Understanding the unique natural history of legionellae has been a relatively slow process. Eleven years have passed since Rowbotham's initial report on the pathogenicity of *Legionella pneumophila* for free-living amoebae (32). During this time, several studies confirmed the intracellular growth of legionellae in various protozoa (2, 12, 29, 38). Growth of legionellae in the environment in the absence of protozoa has not been documented, and it is believed that protozoa are their primary means of proliferation in nature (11, 33, 39). A few studies established a relationship between legionellae and protozoa present in aquatic environments identified as potential or actual reservoirs of disease-causing strains (3, 15, 16). These studies have presented evidence that protozoa naturally present in their environments can support intracellular growth of legionellae in vitro. Information on the nature of the interaction of these organisms at a cellular level has been limited. We hope to develop strategies to inhibit the growth of legionellae in the environment on the basis of our understanding of this infective process. Certainly, a better understanding of these relationships will improve our capability to prevent and control legionellosis.

The ability of legionellae to survive as intracellular parasites of both protozoan and mammalian cells may be unprecedented. However, a number of bacteria have been reported to survive as parasites or endosymbionts of free-living protozoa, and some of these bacteria are also potential pathogens of vertebrates. Mycobacteria and *Listeria* species are known human pathogens that have been reported to multiply intracellularly in protozoa (24, 25); however, these reports are preliminary and lack confirmation. *Sarcobium lyticum* is an obligate intracellular parasite of acanthamoebae and exhibits some similarities to legionellae (6). There is no known vertebrate host for *S. lyticum*. Five genera of bacteria, all obligate endosymbionts of species of paramecia, have been described by Preer et al. (31). These bacteria multiply in paramecia at lower temperatures, and the existence of a vertebrate host seems unlikely.

We have theorized that some intracellular pathogens of higher vertebrates may have acquired the ability to infect these organisms by first adapting to intracellular life in protozoa. Predation by free-living protozoa appears to be an ideal selective pressure for the evolution of these intracellular bacteria. It is tempting to imagine that they subsequently acquired mechanisms for infecting higher eukaryotic cells. However, this theory contradicts a central doctrine of evolution, that more highly evolved organisms tend to become more specialized.

This matter can be examined further by considering the host range of legionellae. At the time of this publication, five genera of amoebae and one genus of ciliated protozoa (*Tetrahymena*) have been shown to support the intracellular growth of *L. pneumophila* (Table 1). Only one species, *L. pneumophila*, has been reported to infect all of these hosts. In addition, *L. pneumophila* is implicated in the majority of cases of legionellosis and infects all animal and tissue culture models used to study the virulence of the genus. Other species of

TABLE 1. Protozoa supporting the growth of legionellae

Category	Organism
Amoeba	*Acanthamoeba castellanii*
	A. polyphaga
	A. palestinensis
	A. royreba
	A. culbertsoni
	Naegleria gruberi
	N. fowleri
	N. lovaniensis
	N. jadini
	Hartmannella vermiformis
	H. cantabrigiensis
	Vahlkampfia jugosa
	Echinamoeba exudans
Ciliated protozoan	*Tetrahymena pyriformis*
	T. vorax

legionellae exhibit a more restricted host range (33, 40). A strain of *L. anisa* implicated in an outbreak of Pontiac fever, for example, could not infect guinea pigs, human lymphoma (U937) cells, or *Tetrahymena pyriformis* (8). However, these bacteria could multiply intracellularly in the amoeba *Hartmannella vermiformis*. From an evolutionary standpoint, one would consider *L. anisa* more highly evolved, that is, more specialized in its host range. Therefore, *L. pneumophila* would represent a more primitive species of legionellae exhibiting a broad host range. These two theories, adaptation in protozoa to broaden a host range and specialization resulting in a more restricted host range, are, of course, contradictory. Studies of the evolution of legionellae may have implications concerning the origins of intracellular bacteria.

CYCLE OF INFECTION IN AMOEBAE

An overview of the events that result from the addition of virulent *L. pneumophila* to an *Acanthamoeba* culture was described by Rowbotham in the proceedings of the 1983 symposium on *Legionella*. Rowbotham's representation outlines many of the complex events that can result from the interaction of these organisms. These events include changes in bacterial motility during different phases of infection and survival of *L. pneumophila* within amoeba cysts. Nine years later, few, if any, of these events have been characterized at a molecular level.

The remainder of this report addresses the cellular mechanisms of infection of a free-living amoeba, *H. vermiformis*, by *L. pneumophila*. Our laboratory developed an *H. vermiformis*-based model to study the infection of amoebae by *Legionella* spp. Although other protozoan models are undoubtedly useful, the decision to use *H. vermiformis* was not arbitrary. *Hartmannella* spp. appear to be the predominate amoebae in potable water supplies in the United States (35). *H. vermiformis* CDC-19 (ATCC 50237) was isolated from a water sample obtained during an investigation of nosocomial legionellosis (3). The epidemic strain of *L. pneumophila* was associated with the presence of amoebae in potable water samples from this hospital. Potable water sites containing amoebae were much more likely to contain the epidemic strain of *L. pneumophila* than were other potable water sites not containing amoebae. More specifically, the presence of the epidemic strain correlated with the presence of *H. vermiformis*. This strain has been cloned and maintained in axenic culture (10). The amoebae are grown in tissue culture flasks in culture medium 1034 (American Type Culture Collection), resulting in a monolayer of trophozoites analogous to tissue culture.

The bacterium used in these studies was *L. pneumophila* serogroup 1 strain RI-243, initially isolated from a cooling tower implicated in an outbreak of legionellosis. A subclone of this strain that had been passaged fewer than four times on buffered charcoal-yeast extract agar served as the source of virulent *L. pneumophila*. An avirulent subclone (RI-243A) of this strain was derived by passage on Mueller-Hinton IsoVitaleX-hemoglobin (MHIH) agar. After a single passage on MHIH agar, the mutant failed to multiply when coincubated with amoebae or a mammalian cell line (U937) (30). Mutants of *L. pneumophila* derived by passage on MHIH agar are known to be avirulent for guinea pigs and incapable of intracellular growth in several cell culture models (9, 27).

CLASSIFICATION OF ENDOCYTOSIS OF *L. PNEUMOPHILA* BY *H. VERMIFORMIS*

Cytoskeletal and metabolic inhibitors have been useful in describing bacterial invasion of different host cells. The growth of *L. pneumophila* in *H. vermiformis* and in a human monocyte-like cell line (U937) has been investigated by using the inhibitors cytochalasin D and methylamine (23).

Cytochalasin D is an inhibitor of actin filament polymerization involved in plasma membrane invagination during phagocytosis (4). Cytochalasins have been used extensively in describing microfilament-dependent phagocytosis of bacterial pathogens in professional and nonprofessional phagocytic cell models (7, 14). Methylamine is an inhibitor of transglutaminase, a plasma membrane enzyme involved in aggregation of ligand-receptor complexes required for receptor-mediated pinocytosis in fibroblasts and macrophages (20, 37). This compound has been used to inhibit adsorptive pinocytosis of Semliki Forest virus in BHK-21 cells and infection of McCoy cells by *Chlamydia trachomatis* (26, 36).

Cytochalasin D (0.5 or 1.0 μg/ml) inhibited intracellular multiplication of *L. pneumophila* in U937 cells. This finding supports those of an earlier study which demonstrated that cytochalasin D inhibited *L. pneumophila* infection of guinea pig alveolar macrophages (7). In contrast, these concentrations of cytochalasin D had no effect on the intracellular multiplication of *L. pneumophila* in *H. vermiformis*. A recent study has indicated that the infection of *Acanthamoeba castellanii* by *L. pneumophila* is also insensitive to cytochalasin D (28).

Methylamine (10 to 100 mM) inhibited replication of *L. pneumophila* in the amoebae in a dose-dependent manner. All doses of methylamine (10 to 50 mM) inhibited growth of *L. pneumophila* in U937 monocytes. Cytochalasin D and methylamine had no effect on the multiplication of *L. pneumophila* in culture media or on the viability of amoebae or U937 cells.

These findings indicate that the intracellular multiplication L. pneumophila occurs in part by a microfilament-independent process. However, intracellular multiplication in U937 monocytes appears to require an additional microfilament-dependent mechanism. Axenically cultured H. vermiformis does not readily initiate phagocytosis, and this fact may partially explain the insensitivity of these cells to cytochalasin D. Nevertheless, L. pneumophila is still capable of infecting the amoebae by a microfilament-independent process. Whether or not this process represents a form of phagocytosis, receptor-mediated endocytosis, or an undescribed mode of entry is unclear. The terminology used to describe these events is the subject of intense debate among cell biologists. The text Molecular Biology of the Cell (1) states that there are two types of endocytosis: pinocytosis and phagocytosis. It also states that receptor-mediated endocytosis is a form of pinocytosis. Phagocytosis is defined, in part, as a process by which cells ingest large particles such as bacteria. There appears to be an absence of terminology required to describe bacterial uptake by a microfilament-independent process. With increased understanding of the variety of mechanisms used by bacteria to infect host cells, these semantic issues should be resolved.

ATTACHMENT TO H. VERMIFORMIS

The possibility that L. pneumophila cells bind or enter H. vermiformis via specific receptors offers potential insight into the pathogenicity of these bacteria. In addition, interfering with such events could represent a means of controlling the multiplication of legionellae in certain environments. The binding of L. pneumophila to H. vermiformis has been characterized by time course analysis (13). Establishing a monolayer of H. vermiformis over a 3-day period prevented nonspecific attachment of the bacteria to flasks and allowed the monolayer to be washed to remove unbound bacteria. L. pneumophila was harvested from agar plates, washed, and inoculated onto a monolayer of H. vermiformis cells. The suspension was incubated at 4°C to prevent uptake of the bacteria by the amoebae. At the appropriate times, the monolayers were washed, the plates were tapped sharply to suspend the amoebae, and the number of amoeba-associated bacteria was determined by culturing the suspension on buffered charcoal-yeast extract agar.

These experiments showed that L. pneumophila is inefficient in attachment to H. vermiformis under the experimental conditions used. Modifications such as removing fetal bovine serum from the medium, varying the number of bacteria in the inoculum, and using broth-grown versus plate-grown bacteria did not increase the efficiency of attachment. After 1 h of incubation, 2.8×10^4 virulent L. pneumophila cells per ml (0.01%) attached to the monolayer of 1.59×10^6 H. vermiformis cells per ml (Table 2). The number of bound bacteria increased 10- to 20-fold over the next 11 h. A similar number of avirulent L. pneumophila (5.45×10^3 bacteria per ml) attached to the amoebae after 1 h of incubation (Table 2). The number of attached avirulent L. pneumophila increased to 6.60×10^5 in the next 11 h.

These studies suggest that the presence of a specific receptor for binding is unlikely. The possibility of induced synthesis of a specific receptor later in the infection process is not addressed in these studies. Scanning electron micrographs indicated that attachment of L. pneumophila to amoebae frequently occurred at the ends of small processes termed filopodia (Fig. 1). Filopodia are used by the amoebae to adhere to surfaces. Binding to filopodia suggests that attachment is a fortuitous event, requiring that the bacteria encounter a surface that the amoeba commonly uses to anchor itself. The inefficient attachment of L. pneumophila to a natural host such as H. vermiformis appears to be unique among bacterial intracellular pathogens (14). Legionellae do not require colonization of host epithelial surfaces as a prerequisite to invasion as do other pathogens such as salmonellae and shigellae. L. pneumophila appears to survive as a component of biofilms in aquatic environments, thereby ensuring occasional contact with amoebae (21).

TABLE 2. Attachment of L. pneumophila to H. vermiformis at 4°C

Time (h)	Virulent L. pneumophila		Avirulent L. pneumophila	
	Bound bacteria (CFU/ml ± SE)	% Attachment	Bound bacteria (CFU/ml ± SE)	% Attachment
0	2.96×10^7[a]		2.57×10^7[a]	
1	$2.80 \times 10^4 \pm 3.98 \times 10^3$	0.09	$5.45 \times 10^3 \pm 5.73 \times 10^2$	0.02
4	$1.42 \times 10^5 \pm 1.02 \times 10^4$	0.48	$1.08 \times 10^5 \pm 1.21 \times 10^4$	0.42
8	$3.67 \times 10^5 \pm 1.94 \times 10^4$	1.24	$3.14 \times 10^5 \pm 2.59 \times 10^4$	1.22
12	$6.60 \times 10^5 \pm 1.13 \times 10^4$	2.56	$4.60 \times 10^5 \pm 3.79 \times 10^4$	1.55

[a] Total inoculum.

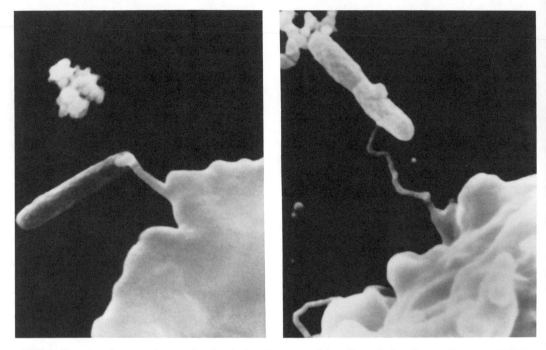

FIG. 1. Scanning electron micrographs of a virulent *L. pneumophila* cell attached to *H. vermiformis* (×20,000). Bacteria were frequently seen attached to the ends of amoeba processes (filopodia). The micrographs were taken from *H. vermiformis* cultures that had been coincubated with *L. pneumophila* for 8 h.

UPTAKE BY *H. VERMIFORMIS*

Transmission electron microscopy was used to quantitate the internalization of *L. pneumophila* by *H. vermiformis*. A total of 200 amoebae representing two separate experiments were counted for each sample time. Virulent *L. pneumophila* began to enter the amoebae soon after attachment. An average of 7.5 bacteria per 100 amoebae were detected intracellularly after 1 h coincubation (Table 3). There appeared to be a lag period of approximately 4 h before the bacteria began to increase logarithmically inside the amoebae. This logarithmic increase probably reflects bacterial replication and not increased uptake, since the

number of infected amoebae increased at only a linear rate. Virulent cells were rarely observed entering the amoeba cells by scanning electron microscopy. Those cells that were observed, however, appeared to enter the amoeba cell one at a time (Fig. 2). Avirulent *L. pneumophila* cells were rarely observed intracellularly in the amoebae throughout the 12-h coincubation (Table 3). Previous studies have documented the uptake of avirulent *L. pneumophila* in mammalian cells via phagocytosis (19). The fact that avirulent *L. pneumophila* cells are not taken up by axenically grown *H. vermiformis* supports the observation that these amoebae are less phagocytic under these conditions. These findings indicate that virulent *L.*

TABLE 3. Time course analysis of the number of intracellular *L. pneumophila*

Time (h)	Virulent *L. pneumophila*		Avirulent *L. pneumophila*	
	LP/HV[b] ± SE	Infected HV[c] ± SE	LP/HV	Infected HV
1	0.07 ± 0.0325	5 ± 1.4	0.05	5
4	0.25 ± 0.43	21.5 ± 3.2	0.03	10.5
8	1.49 ± 0.2125	49 ± 3.5	0.025	2.5
12	8.5 ± 0.995	73.5 ± 0.35	0.01	1

[a] No standard errors are shown because of the low numbers of intracellular bacteria and infected amoebae.
[b] Mean number of intracellular *L. pneumophila* per amoeba cell.
[c] Mean number of *H. vermiformis* containing intracellular *L. pneumophila*.

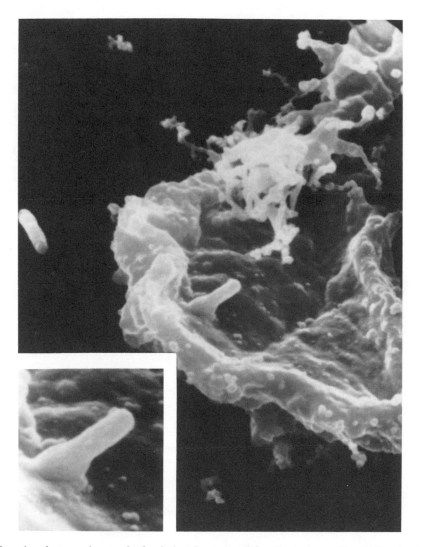

FIG. 2. Scanning electron micrograph of a virulent *L. pneumophila* cell entering an *H. vermiformis* cell (×6,600; insert, ×20,000). Pseudopodia were not observed in the uptake of the bacteria. The micrograph was taken from an *H. vermiformis* culture that had been coincubated with *L. pneumophila* for 12 h.

pneumophila cells enter the amoebae by a micro-filament-independent process such as receptor-mediated endocytosis, while avirulent cells lack some factor necessary for this type of invasion. This form of entry may be fundamental in the infection of amoebae by virulent *L. pneumophila*.

ENDOSOME FUSION WITH THE ENDOPLASMIC RETICULUM

Although subsequent intracellular events have not been characterized in amoebae, *L. pneumophila* is known to survive intracellularly in human monocytes by escaping phagosome-lysosome fusion (18). Receptor-mediated endocytosis has been described as a means of avoiding phago-some-lysosome fusion for other intracellular bacterial parasites (17). Such mechanisms are suspected of directing the infecting agent into vesicles that are destined not to fuse with lysosomes, thereby providing the organism with an opportunity to survive and proliferate. We believe that the mechanism for escaping phagosome-lysosome fusion may be related to the entry of the *L. pneumophila* into the host amoeba.

Ultrastructural examination of infected amoebae shows that immediately after entry, single *L. pneumophila* cells are present in endosomes. These endosomes are frequently surrounded by either smooth or ribosome-studded vesicles structurally identical to smooth or rough endoplasmic reticulum (Fig. 3). We believe that the endosome

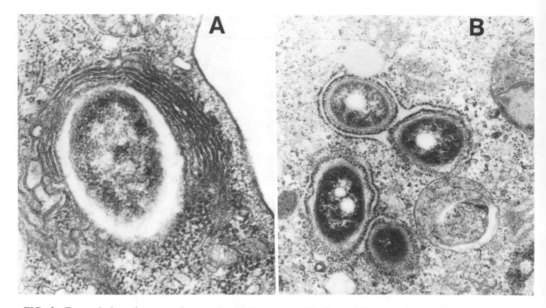

FIG. 3. Transmission electron micrographs of *L. pneumophila* in vesicles associated with smooth or rough organelles of *H. vermiformis*. (A) A single *Legionella* cell in an endosome closely associated with stacks of smooth vesicles (8 h of incubation; ×120,000). (B) *L. pneumophila* within ribosome-studded vesicles, presumably the endoplasmic reticulum of *H. vermiformis* (12 h of incubation; ×60,000). The significance of the double membranes is unknown.

containing the *Legionella* cell fuses with the host cell's endoplasmic reticulum, and this becomes the site of bacterial multiplication. There is both biologic plausibility and precedence for multiplication in the endoplasmic reticulum. The endoplasmic reticulum is rich in nutrients and would prevent exposure to lysosomes. A recent study of the infection of Vero cells by *Brucella* spp. concluded that these facultative intracellular bacteria multiply within the endoplasmic reticulum (5). In addition, the *Brucella* cells entered the host cells in a manner similar to that of legionellae. Further studies are needed to confirm that multiplication of *L. pneumophila* takes place in the endoplasmic reticulum.

CONCLUSIONS AND FUTURE NEEDS

These studies characterize the infection of *H. vermiformis* by *L. pneumophila* in a system analo-

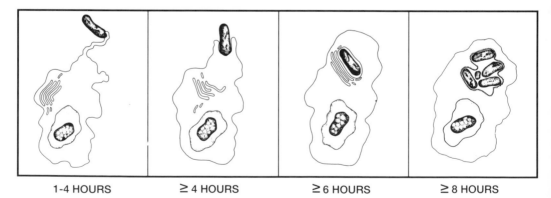

| 1-4 HOURS | ≥ 4 HOURS | ≥ 6 HOURS | ≥ 8 HOURS |

FIG. 4. Schematic representation of the infection of axenically grown *H. vermiformis* by *L. pneumophila*. At 1 to 4 h, *L. pneumophila* cells nonspecifically bind to the ends of amoeba filopodia; at ≥ 4 h, single *L. pneumophila* cells enter the amoebae by a microfilament-independent process; at ≥ 6 h, single *L. pneumophila* cells within endosomes associate with smooth vesicles of the amoebae; at ≥ 8 h, *L. pneumophila* cells initiate multiplication within ribosome-studded vesicles, presumably the endoplasmic reticulum of the amoebae.

gous to tissue culture models of bacterial invasion. In this model, it appears that virulent *L. pneumophila* cells are inefficient in attachment to the amoebae, but once attached, they are proficient at entering the amoeba cells and initiating multiplication. These events are represented chronologically in Fig. 4. The *H. vermiformis* model characterizes an alternative means of bacterial invasion; however, the interaction of these organisms in nature may be very different. In vivo, the amoebae would be actively seeking nutrients and, presumably, have increased phagocytic activity. Legionellae would be physiologically different in an aquatic environment and possibly more prepared to encounter a potential host cell. Other models may be more appropriate for the study of different aspects of the interaction of legionellae and protozoa. For example, we have been unable to detect legionellae within *H. vermiformis* cysts. This intriguing relationship would allow the bacteria to withstand a variety of adverse conditions. However, this phenomenon has been observed only for *Acanthamoeba* species (22, 34). The survival of legionellae within protozoan cysts is a subject that merits further study.

A receptor involved in the uptake of *L. pneumophila* has yet to be established or characterized. Because many of the reservoirs for legionellosis are man-made aquatic environments, it may be ecologically plausible to inhibit the interaction of these organisms in vivo by inactivating such a receptor.

A direct role for protozoa in the transmission of legionellosis has yet to be established. Several investigators have theorized that susceptible individuals might inhale infected amoebae or vesicles of amoebae that contain large numbers of legionellae. If true, such information would influence the calculation of acceptable levels of legionellae in the environment, since these particles would represent a single CFU by culture.

Finally, which protozoan best represents the potential host for amplification of legionellae in the environment? It is doubtful that any single genus or species will suffice. There are, most likely, a multitude of protozoa capable of supporting the intracellular growth of these bacteria. In addition, legionellae may exhibit in situ adaptation to protozoa present in a particular environment. These issues provide a common challenge to environmental microbiologists, molecular biologists, and epidemiologists.

REFERENCES

1. **Alberts, B., D. Bray, J. Lewis, M. Raff, K. Roberts, and J. D. Watson (ed.).** 1989. *Molecular Biology of the Cell*, 2nd ed. Garland Publishing Inc., New York.
2. **Anand, C., A. Skinner, A. Malic, and J. Kurtz.** 1983. Interaction of *Legionella pneumophila* and a free-living amoeba (*Acanthamoeba palenstinensis*). *J. Hyg.* (Cambridge) **91:**167–178.
3. **Breiman, R. F., B. S. Fields, G. N. Sanden, L. Volmer, A. Meier, and J. S. Spika.** 1990. Association of shower use with Legionnaires' disease: possible role of amoebae. *JAMA* **263:**2924–2926.
4. **Cooper, J. A.** 1987. Effects of cytochalasin and phalloidin on actin. *J. Cell Biol.* **105:**1473–1478.
5. **Detilleux, P. G., B. L. Deyoe, and N. F. Cheville.** 1990. Entry and intracellular localization of *Brucella* spp. in Vero cells: fluorescence and electron microscopy. *Vet. Pathol.* **27:**317–328.
6. **Drozański, W. J.** 1991. *Sacrobium lyticum* gen. nov., sp. nov., an obligate intracellular bacterial parasite of small free-living amoebae. *Int. J. Syst. Bacteriol.* **41:**82–87.
7. **Elliot, J. A., and W. C. Winn.** 1986. Treatment of alveolar macrophages with cytochalasin D inhibits uptake and subsequent growth of *Legionella pneumophila. Infect. Immun.* **51:**31–36.
8. **Fields, B. S., J. M. Barbaree, G. N. Sanden, and W. E. Morrill.** 1990. Virulence of a *Legionella anisa* strain associated with Pontiac fever: an evaluation using protozoan, cell culture, and guinea pig models. *Infect. Immun.* **58:**3139–3142.
9. **Fields, B. S., J. M. Barbaree, E. B. Shotts, J. C. Feeley, W. E. Morrill, G. N. Sanden, and M. J. Dykstra.** 1986. Comparison of guinea pig and protozoan models for determining virulence of *Legionella* species. *Infect. Immun.* **53:**553–559.
10. **Fields, B. S., T. A. Nerad, T. K. Sawyer, H. King, J. M. Barbaree, W. T. Martin, W. E. Morrill, and G. N. Sanden.** 1990. Characterization of an axenic strain of *Hartmannella vermiformis* obtained from an investigation of nosocomial legionellosis. *J. Protozool.* **37:**581–583.
11. **Fields, B. S., G. N. Sanden, J. M. Barbaree, W. E. Morrill, R. M. Wadowsky, E. H. White, and J. C. Feeley.** 1989. Intracellular multiplication of *Legionella pneumophila* in amoebae isolated from hospital hot water tanks. *Curr. Microbiol.* **18:**131–137.
12. **Fields, B. S., E. B. Shotts, Jr., J. C. Feeley, G. W. Gorman, and W. T. Martin.** 1984. Proliferation of *Legionella pneumophila* as an intracellular parasite of the ciliated protozoan *Tetrahymena pyriformis. Appl. Environ. Microbiol.* **47:**467–471.
13. **Fields, B. S., S. R. Utley, J. N. Chin Loy, E. H. White, W. L. Steffens, and E. B. Shotts.** Attachment and entry of *Legionella pneumophila* in *Hartmannella vermiformis. J. Infect. Dis.*, in press.
14. **Finlay, B. B., and S. Falkow.** 1989. Common themes in microbial pathogenicity. *Microbiol. Rev.* **53:**210–230.
15. **Harf, C., M. Monteil, and M. T. Vetter.** 1987. Relations amibes libres *Legionella* dans l'environnement. *Colloque Legionella.* Faculte de Medecine Alexis Carrel, Lyon, France.
16. **Henke, M., and K. M. Seidel.** 1986. Association between *Legionella pneumophila* and amoebae in water. *Isr. J. Med. Sci.* **22:**690–695.
17. **Hodinka, R. L., and P. B. Wyrick.** 1986. Ultrastructural study of mode of entry of *Chlamydia psittaci* into L-929 cells. *Infect. Immun.* **54:**855–863.
18. **Horwitz, M. A.** 1983. The Legionnaires' disease bacterium (*Legionella pneumophila*) inhibits phagosome-lysosome fusion in human monocytes. *J. Exp. Med.* **158:**2108–2126.
19. **Horwitz, M. A.** 1987. Characterization of avirulent mutant *Legionella pneumophila* that survive but do not multiply within human monocytes. *J. Exp. Med.* **166:**1310–1328.
20. **Kaplan, J., and E. A. Keogh.** 1981. Analysis of the effect of amines on inhibition of receptor-mediated and fluid-phase pinocytosis in rabbit alveolar macrophages. *Cell* **24:**925–932.
21. **Keevil, C. W.** 1991. *Legionella* biofilms. *Proc. 6th Meet. Eur. Working Group Legionella Infect.*
22. **Kilvington, S., and J. Price.** 1990. Survival of *Legionella pneumophila* within cysts of *Acanthamoeba polyphaga* following chlorine exposure. *J. Appl. Bacteriol.* **68:**519–525.

23. **King, C. H., B. S. Fields, E. B. Shotts, and E. H. White.** 1991. Effects of cytochalasin D and methylamine on the intracellular growth of *Legionella pneumophila* in amoebae and human monocyte-like cells. *Infect. Immun.* **59:**758–763.

24. **Krishna Prasad, B. N., and S. K. Gupta.** 1978. Preliminary report on the engulfment and retention of mycobacteria by trophozoites of axenically grown *Acanthamoeba castellanii* Douglas, 1930. *Curr. Sci.* **47:**245–247.

25. **Ly, T. M. C., and H. E. Muller.** 1990. Interactions of *Listeria monocytogenes, Listeria seeligeri,* and *Listeria innocua* with protozoans. *J. Gen. Appl. Microbiol.* **36:**143–150.

26. **Marsh, M., and A. Helenius.** 1980. Adsorptive endocytosis of Semliki Forest virus. *J. Mol. Biol.* **142:**439–454.

27. **McDade, J. E., and C. C. Shepard.** 1979. Virulent to avirulent conversion of Legionnaires' disease bacterium (*Legionella pneumophila*)—its effect on isolation techniques. *J. Infect. Dis.* **139:**707–711.

28. **Moffat, J. F., and L. S. Tompkins.** 1992. A quantitative model of intracellular growth of *Legionella pneumophila* in *Acanthamoeba castellanii. Infect. Immun.* **60:**296–301.

29. **Newsome, A. L., R. L. Baker, R. D. Miller, and R. R. Arnold.** 1985. Interactions between *Naegleria fowleri* and *Legionella pneumophila. Infect. Immun.* **50:**449–452.

30. **Pearlman, E., H. Jiwa, N. C. Engleberg, and B. I. Eisenstein.** 1988. Growth of *Legionella pneumophila* in a human macrophage-like (U-937) cell line. *Microb. Pathog.* **5:**87–95.

31. **Preer, J. R., L. B. Preer, and A. Jurand.** 1974. Kappa and other endosymbionts in *Paramecium aurelia. Bacteriol. Rev.* **38:**113–163.

32. **Rowbotham, T. J.** 1980. Preliminary report on the pathogenicity of *Legionella pneumophila* for freshwater and soil amoebae. *J. Clin. Pathol.* **33:**1179–1183.

33. **Rowbotham, T. J.** 1986. Current views on the relationships between amoebae, legionellae, and man. *Isr. J. Med. Sci.* **22:**678–689.

34. **Rowbotham, T. J.** Personal communication.

35. **Sawyer, T. K. (RESCON Associates, Inc.).** Personal communication.

36. **Soderlund, G., and E. Kihlstrom.** 1983. Effect of methylamine and monodansylcadaverine on the susceptibility of McCoy cells to *Chlamydia trachomatis* infection. *Infect. Immun.* **40:**534–541.

37. **Teshigawara, K., R. Kannagi, N. Noro, and T. Masuda.** 1985. Possible involvement of transglutaminase in endocytosis and antigen presentation. *Microbiol. Immunol.* **29:**737–750.

38. **Tyndall, R. L., and E. L. Dominique.** 1982. Cocultivation of *Legionella pneumophila* and free-living amoebae. *Appl. Environ. Microbiol.* **44:**954–959.

39. **Wadowsky, R. M., L. J. Butler, M. K. Cook, S. M. Verma, M. A. Paul, B. S. Fields, G. Keleti, J. L. Sykora, and R. B. Yee.** 1988. Growth-supporting activity for *Legionella pneumophila* in tap water cultures and implication of hartmannellid amoebae as growth factors. *Appl. Environ. Microbiol.* **54:**2677–2682.

40. **Wadowsky, R. M., T. W. Wilson, N. J. Kapp, A. J. West, J. M. Kuchta, S. J. States, J. N. Dowling, and R. B. Yee.** 1991. Multiplication of *Legionella* spp. in tap water containing *Hartmannella vermiformis. Appl. Environ. Microbiol.* **57:**1950–1955.

Legionella-Like Amoebal Pathogens

TIMOTHY J. ROWBOTHAM

Leeds Public Health Laboratory, Bridle Path, York Road, Leeds LS15 7TR, England

Legionellae are protozoonotic; that is, they naturally infect protozoa and some sometimes infect humans (11). *Legionella*-like amoebal pathogens (LLAPs) are bacilli that infect and multiply in the cytoplasm of amoebae but do not grow on routine legionella media, such as BCYE [*N*-(2-acetamido)-2-aminoethanesulfonic acid (ACES)-buffered charcoal-yeast extract agar (pH 6.9) with α-ketoglutarate], incubated at 30 or 35°C, in air, or in air plus 2 to 5% (vol/vol) CO_2 (11). The oldest known extant strain of an LLAP is *Sarcobium lyticum* L2 (PCM 2298) (3), isolated from Polish soil by Drożański in 1954 (4). In Leeds, LLAPs have been isolated since 1981 from a variety of sources (Table 1). LLAP-3 was isolated

from a case of persistent pneumonia in 1986, and there is serological evidence for further cases, but more culture-positive cases are needed to validate LLAP serology.

Human LLAP infection (first case). In August 1986, a serum sample from a woman of 82 with persistent pneumonia was examined by the indirect immunofluorescent antibody technique for antibody to *Legionella pneumophila* serogroups 1 through 8. The serum had some activity to the yolk sac-grown, formalin-killed serogroup 1 antigen issued by the Division of Microbiological Reagents and Quality Control at the Central Public Health Laboratory, London (DMRQC), but the activity was of very poor quality. Better activity

TABLE 1. LLAPs isolated or partially purified[a]

Strain	Host amoeba(e)	Source
X	*Vannella platypodia*	Biofilm from overflow channel of an outdoor swimming pool in Majorca. Host amoebae mainly feeding on the green freshwater alga *Oocystis solitaria*.
LLAP-1	*Acanthamoeba polyphaga* and *A. palestinensis*	Deposit from the bottom of a tank of well water. Tank supplied cold water for drinking and washing.
LLAP-2	*Acanthamoeba* sp.	Deposit from the bottom of a garage steam-cleaning pit.
LLAP-3	*A. polyphaga*	Amoebal enrichment of sputum from a patient with persistent pneumonia.
LLAP-4	*A. polyphaga*	Material from the nozzle of a hospital whirlpool bath.
LLAP-5	*A. polyphaga*	Biofilm and deposit from inside a plastic spray gun used for watering indoor plants.
LLAP-6	*A. polyphaga*	Water and sludge from an industrial liquefier tower.
LLAP-7	*A. palestinensis*	Biofilm from tidemark area of a hotel whirlpool spa. LLAP and *L. pneumophila* serogroup 1 isolated from overflow channel biofilm. Two patients with serologically confirmed Legionnaires disease associated with the hotel; both men had used the whirlpool.
LLAP-8	*Hartmannella vermiformis*	Biofilm in hospital shower. Shower associated with a fatal case of nosocomial Legionnaires disease. Similar *L. pneumophila* serogroup 4 strains isolated from postmortem lung and shower. *H. vermiformis* grew at room temperature and at 30, 35, and 37°C but not 42 or 45°C and was a host for *L. pneumophila* serogroup 4 and LLAP-8. Patient had high antibody titer to her own *L. pneumophila* serogroup 4 but no antibody to LLAP-8.
"LLAP"	*A. polyphaga*	Deposit from a pond of a large, natural-updraft power station cooling tower. *Pseudomonas alcaligenes* (API 20 NE profile no. 1000445). Grew on blood agar at 41°C. Grew on BCYE but not on BCYE + MWY Selective Supplement (Unipath Ltd.). Isolated via micromanipulation from a single infected amoeba full of motile bacilli. Readily infected *A. polyphaga*. *Legionella* sp. (*L. feeleii*?) and host amoeba *Vahlkampfia jugosa* also isolated from the same sample.

[a]All of the environmental sources contained more than one species of amoeba, and other protozoa as well, except the source for LLAP-8, which contained only *H. vermiformis*; however, this sample was only tested for amoebae and LLAPs following two disinfections.

TABLE 2. Antibody titers of the original LLAP-3 patient[a]

	Indirect fluorescent antibody titer on given date		
Formalin-killed antigen	9/8/86	19/8/86	20/10/86
L. pneumophila			
Serogroup 1 Pontiac-1	16	32–64	64
Serogroup 1 Bellingham[b]	<8	32	64
Serogroup 2–7	<8	<8	<8
Serogroup 8 Concord-3	32	64	32
Serogroup 10 York-1[c]	16	64	64
LLAPs			
LLAP-1 (grown on BCYE+Se)	<8	<8	<8
LLAP-3 (grown in amoebae)	8[d]	16[d]	32[d], 64

[a]Onset was thought to be about 10 days before the first serum sample was taken.
[b]Bellingham subgroup isolate from steelworks pinch roller water.
[c]Isolate from hospital shower, originally thought to be serogroup 7 and now considered serogroup 10.
[d]Crude antigen.

was found to BCYE agar-grown (multiplicative phase), formalin-killed antigens (Table 2).

A sputum sample taken 10 days after the first serum sample, was negative by immunofluorescence for *L. pneumophila* serogroups 1 through 6, and no legionellae were isolated by direct plating on selective BCYE medium. Cocultivation (11) with *Acanthamoeba polyphaga* AST Ap-1, an LLAP-1 host isolated from the same sample as was LLAP-1 (11), resulted in numerous infected amoebae, but attempts to recover legionellae on BCYE medium from the infected amoebae failed. The patient had rising levels of antibody to several strains of *L. pneumophila* and to the bacilli released from infected amoebae (Table 2); her treatment was changed to include antibiotics suitable for a legionella infection, and she subsequently made an uneventful recovery. The patient had not recently been abroad.

Serological evidence for further cases of LLAP infection. Since 1989, all sera received at Leeds for legionella antibody tests (>5,000) have been screened at a dilution of 1/32 for activity to LLAP-3. The antigen used was produced by infecting washed *A. polyphaga* Linc Ap-1 trophozoites with LLAP-3, incubating them at 35°C until they ruptured, and washing the released bacilli (active infective and passive infective phases) three times in phosphate-buffered saline, pH 7.3 (PBS), before dilution in PBS plus 1% (vol/vol) formalin and 1% (vol/vol) semisolid agar. More than 10 cases of pneumonic illness with appropriately timed rising titers to LLAP-3 and several others with high-titer convalescent-phase sera have been found. Some patients had recently been abroad. Sera of most of the patients had little activity to *L. pneumophila* antigens, but some high-titer LLAP-3 sera had some activity to *L. longbeachae* serogroup 2, and it was not unusual for sera with high titers to LLAP-3 to have some activity to LLAP-1 (Table 3). A few cases of chest infection with rising titers to LLAP-1 but little activity to LLAP-3 have also been found. For example, the LLAP-1 titers of a 60-year-old man

TABLE 3. Three examples of patients with probable LLAP-3 pneumonia

Patient		Days after onset	Indirect fluorescent antibody titer[a] with conjugate to immunoglobulins:			
			LLAP-1		LLAP-3	
Sex	Age (yr)		G, A, and M	M only	G, A, and M	M only
Male	74	5	<8	<8	<8	<8
		17	32	32	128	128
		23	16	16	64	64
Female	64	10	8	<8	8	8
		19	16	16	128	64
		25	32	32	256	256
		26	32	32	512	512
Female	61	1	32	<16	4	4
		11	256	64	256	256

[a]Titers of all sera to the DMRQC *L. pneumophila* serogroup 1 antigen were <16.

with a chest infection and jaundice rose from 8 at 4 days after onset to 512 at 14 days after onset, while his LLAP-3 titers remained < 8.

Ten sera with activity to LLAP-3 had similar activity to *S. lyticum*. Antibodies to legionellae are common in patients with cystic fibrosis, in whom they result from cross-reacting antibodies to *Pseudomonas aeruginosa* (1). Adolescent and young adult patients with cystic fibrosis commonly have titers of 16, 32, or 64 to LLAP-3, presumably due to the same cause. Care is now taken to exclude pseudomonas infection as a possible cause of rising titers in suspected LLAP infections.

A. polyphaga AST Ap-1, an original host amoeba for LLAP-1 and the amoeba used to isolate LLAP-3, contains small numbers of a very tiny, curved, sometimes horseshoe-shaped, nonmotile bacillus. This endosymbiont was required for growth in peptone-yeast extract-glucose broth and for growth on UV-killed *Klebsiella aerogenes*, but the amoeba could grow on live *K. aerogenes* without the endosymbiont. Some human sera, but not those of the patient from whom LLAP-3 was isolated, had antibody to the endosymbiont.

A. polyphaga Linc Ap-1, which is currently used to produce the LLAP-3 antigen, does not contain endosymbionts; it was isolated along with *L. pneumophila* serogroup 1 from the sediment in an outbreak-associated cooling tower (10).

Microbiology. At the end of their development, LLAP-3 are released from infected amoebae as single motile bacilli. When flagellate, legionellae usually have a single subpolar or polar flagellum. Electron microscopy revealed that like legionellae, most LLAP-3 bacilli had a single sub-

polar flagellum. Rare bacilli with a subpolar flagellum at each end were also seen. *S. lyticum* has a bundle of three to five polar flagellae (3), but when strain L2 was reisolated by micromanipulation from a single acid-decontaminated, washed (three times) amoeba full of motile bacilli and then grown in *A. polyphaga* Linc Ap-1, the flagellation was the same as that on LLAP-3 (9). When freshly released, unwashed LLAP-3 was used as the antigen, some human sera (not from cystic fibrosis patients) had antibody to the flagellum as well as to the body of the bacillus. Perhaps activity to LLAP-3 flagellae can distinguish between antibody to a LLAP infection and antibody to a pseudomonas infection.

LLAP-3 did not react significantly with antisera raised against any of the 50 described species and serogroups of *Legionella* except *L. sainthelensi* serogroup 1. LLAP-3, however, appears to be serologically distinct from the type strain of *L. sainthelensi* serogroup 1, since unlike the latter, it fails to react with antisera raised against *L. cincinnatiensis*, *L. oakridgensis*, and *L. santicrucis*. Weak reactions were also noted between LLAP-3 and some *L. longbeachae* serogroup 1 and serogroup 2 antisera (6).

LLAP-1 through LLAP-3 and *S. lyticum* did not grow on BCYE agar at 30 or 35°C. On BCYE agar supplemented with 10 mg of sodium selenate per liter (BCYE + Se) (12), LLAP-1 produced colonies at 30 and 33°C that were indistinguishable from *L. pneumophila*. The colonies did not fluoresce under long-wave UV light, and no growth occurred at 35°C. On BCYE+Se, LLAP-1 had a gas-liquid chromatography fatty acid profile (principal peak, anteiso $C_{15:0}$) consistent with that of the non-pneumophila species

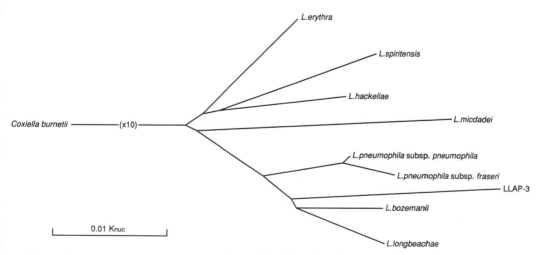

FIG. 1. Phylogenetic tree showing the position of LLAP-3 within the *Legionellaceae*. The tree is rooted by reference to *Coxiella burnetii*. (Reproduced from reference 5 with permission.)

group. Neither LLAP-2, LLAP-3, nor *S. lyticum* grew on BCYE+Se at 30 or 35°C.

Molecular taxonomy. The Gen-Probe genus-specific DNA probe for *Legionella* RNA reacts well with LLAP-3 (7), indicating that LLAP-3 belongs to the genus *Legionella*. Fry et al. (5), using the polymerase chain reaction and primers specific for eubacteria (8), amplified the DNA coding for the 16S rRNA of LLAP-3 directly from amoebae lysed by LLAP-3. The amplified DNA was sequenced (EMBL accession number X60080) and compared with published 16S rRNA sequences. The analysis (Fig. 1) showed that LLAP-3 is a member of the genus *Legionella*, as it is currently described, and that it is different from species, including *L. pneumophila* and *L. longbeachae,* for which 16S rRNA sequence data are available (5). Preliminary data for *S. lyticum* rRNA indicate that it is closely allied to the legionellae but perhaps belongs to a separate group (4). It will be interesting to determine how closely related LLAP-3 and *S. lyticum* are. *Legionella* is a genus of convenience, and if it were split, LLAPs could become sarcobia.

Concluding remarks. LLAPs are common and infect a variety of amoebae. They appear to be a new group of legionellae, one of which can infect humans. The group does not grow on current legionella media. LLAPs may explain the occurrence of Gen-Probe-positive specimens from patients with pneumonic illnesses for whom conventional isolation and serological tests for legionella are negative (2, 8). When probes for rRNA or DNA are used to detect legionellae in environmental samples, there is the danger that true-positive results may be regarded as falsely positive if there is a lack of confirmation by immunofluorescence and conventional culture.

I thank David Johnstone, Department of Microbiology, Scarborough General Hospital, for information concerning the original LLAP-3 case.

REFERENCES

1. **Collins, M. T., J. McDonald, N. Høiby, and O. Aalund.** 1984. Agglutinating antibody titres to members of the family *Legionellaceae* in cystic fibrosis patients as a result of cross-reacting antibodies to *Pseudomonas aeruginosa. J. Clin. Microbiol.* **19**:757–762.
2. **Doebbeling, B. N., M. J. Bale, F. P. Koontz, C. M. Helms, R. P. Wenzel, and M. A. Pfaller.** 1988. Prospective evaluation of the Gen-Probe assay for detection of legionellae in respiratory specimens. *Eur. J. Clin. Microbiol. Infect. Dis.* **7**:748–752.
3. **Drożański, W. J.** 1991. *Sarcobium lyticum* gen. nov., sp. nov., an obligate intracellular bacterial parasite of small free-living amoebae. *Int. J. Syst. Bacteriol.* **41**:82–87.
4. **Drożański, W. J.** Personal communication.
5. **Fry, N. K., T. J. Rowbotham, N. A. Saunders, and T. M. Embley.** 1991. Direct amplification and sequencing of the 16S ribosomal DNA of an intracellular *Legionella* species recovered by amoebal enrichment from the sputum of a patient with pneumonia. *FEMS Microbiol. Lett.* **83**:165–168.
6. **Harrison, T. G. (Legionella Reference Unit, DMRQC).** Personal communication.
7. **Kohne, D. E. (Gen-Probe Inc., San Diego, Calif.).** Personal communication.
8. **Laussucq, S., D. Schuster, W. J. Alexander, W. L. Thacker, H. W. Wilkinson, and J. S. Spika.** 1988. False-positive DNA probe test for *Legionella* species associated with a cluster of respiratory illnesses. *J. Clin. Microbiol.* **26**:1442–1444.
9. **Lewis, D. C. (Leeds Public Health Laboratory).** Personal communication.
10. **O'Mahony, M., A. Lakhani, A. Stephens, J. G. Wallace, E. R. Youngs, and D. Harper.** 1989. Legionnaires' disease and the sick-building syndrome. *Epidemiol. Infect.* **103**:285–292.
11. **Rowbotham, T. J.** 1983. Isolation of *Legionella pneumophila* from clinical specimens via amoebae, and the interactions of those and other isolates with amoebae. *J. Clin. Pathol.* **36**:978–986.
12. **Smalley, D. L., P. A. Jaquess, and J. S. Layne.** 1980. Selenium-enriched medium for *Legionella pneumophila. J. Clin. Microbiol.* **12**:32–34.

Interactions between Soil Amoebae and Soil Legionellae

TREVOR W. STEELE

Institute of Medical and Veterinary Science, Box 14, Rundle Mall Post Office, Adelaide, South Australia 5000, Australia

Since 1987, the prevalence of *Legionella longbeachae* serogroup 1 pneumonia has increased in South Australia (5), and *L. longbeachae* is now the predominant species causing lung infection in this community. Similar changes are occurring in other Australian states. Before 1989, the environmental habitat of *L. longbeachae* serogroup 1 was unknown. Since then, potting mixes made from composted wood products such as sawdust and shredded pine bark in Australia have been found to contain *L. longbeachae* serogroup 1. Blue-white fluorescent species such as *L. bozemanii* and *L. dumoffii* and several other species are also common in some potting mixes (6, 7). Soil legionellae survived for as long as 20 months in some dry mixes and can survive up to 10 months in moistened mixes held at −20 to 35°C. However, they die off when mixes are incubated at 43°C or if the water content of the mix is reduced to 13% by drying at 37°C (6). Examination of potting mixes showed that all contained free-living amoebae. *Acanthamoeba, Naegleria,*

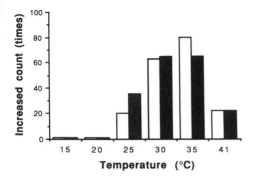

FIG. 1. Effect of temperature on the multiplication of *L. longbeachae* serogroup 1 present in a filtered soil suspension in *Naegleria* trophozoites. Increased count (times) is calculated by subtracting the initial count from final counts and dividing by the initial count. Open bars, at 3 days; hatched bars, at 7 days.

Vahlkampfia, and *Hartmannella* species were common, and more than one genus was present in many potting mixes.

Since free-living amoebae have been shown to be important in the ecology of *L. pneumophila* (1–4, 8), this study was performed to determine whether *L. longbeachae* serogroup 1 and blue-white fluorescent species survived in a free state in dried potting mixes, whether free-living soil amoebae amplified these legionellae in cocultivation, and whether amoebae were important for the multiplication of legionellae in potting mixes.

To determine whether legionellae in a dry potting mix (sample 318, acquired June 1989) were lying free or were within amoebic cysts, a suspension of this mix in sterile water was filtered through cellulose acetate filters with pore sizes of 0.8, 5, and 8 μm. Filtration removed all amoebic cysts but allowed legionellae to pass through. The highest reduction (90%) in count was observed during filtration of *L. longbeachae* serogroup 1,

while the count of *L. bozemanii* and *L. dumoffii* fell by 61% when the suspension was passed through a 0.8-μm-pore-size filter. These results showed that legionellae surviving in dry potting mix for 20 months were lying free and were not within amoebic cysts. They agreed with previous observations (6) that legionellae in potting mixes were killed by conditions that would not affect the viability of amoebic cysts.

The ability of soil legionellae to multiply in two species of commonly encountered soil amoebae, those of the genera *Naegleria* and *Vahlkampfia*, was determined by incubating samples of filtered (5-μm-pore-size filter) wash from potting mix 318 with 5×10^4 trophozoites of the two genera at various temperatures. The results obtained for *Naegleria* trophozoites and *L. longbeachae* serogroup 1 in the wash are shown in Fig. 1; similar results were obtained for *L. longbeachae* and *Vahlkampfia* trophozoites. The blue-white fluorescent species in this wash also infected both amoebae between 25 and 41°C. Amoebae in this experiment were found to encyst at 3 days, but occasional trophozoites persisted. Sustained multiplication of legionellae after this time did not usually occur. *L. dumoffii* grew very slowly at 20°C on laboratory medium, the two other *Legionella* species in this mix did not grow on buffered charcoal-yeast extract medium at 20 or at 43°C, but all grew poorly at 41°C. *L. longbeachae* serogroup 1 also multiplied in *Acanthamoeba* species when cocultivated at 25 to 35°C but not at 41°C.

Since soil legionellae were shown to multiply in soil amoebae in cocultivation experiments, the ability of these amoebae to permit multiplication of legionellae in potting mix was determined. Portions of a sterilized potting mix were seeded with 5×10^5 *Vahlkampfia* or *Naegleria* trophozoites and between 10^4 and 10^5 legionellae were added to each portion (Table 1). Controls without legionellae and without amoebae were included. Seeded soils were incubated at 25°C and were

TABLE 1. Total numbers of legionellae recovered from seeded potting mixes

| Organism recovered | No. of legionellae (CFU) | | Times increased |
	Added initially	Recovered by 4 wk	
Vahlkampfia trophozoites			
L. longbeachae serogroup 1	9.6×10^4	3.18×10^6	32
Blue-white fluorescent species	4.32×10^5	5.2×10^6	11
Naegleria trophozoites			
L. longbeachae serogroup 1	4.4×10^4	6.7×10^5	14
Blue-white fluorescent species	6.4×10^4	6.8×10^6	105
Controls			
No amoebae	As above[a]	$< 10^4$	< 1
No legionellae	None	None	

[a]Legionellae were added as mixed suspension of *L. longbeachae* and blue-white species in each experiment.

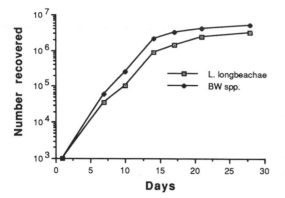

FIG. 2. Cumulative recovery of legionellae from washes of sterile potting mixes seeded with plate-grown suspensions of soil legionellae and *Vahlkampfia* trophozoites. BW, blue-white fluorescent.

gionellae to grow in soil amoebae. Multiplication of legionellae occurred only between 25 and 41°C, the temperature range for growth of soil legionellae on laboratory media. In these experiments, a proportion of amoebae escaped infection and survived in cocultivation.

Seeding of sterilized potting mix with *Vahlkampfia* or *Naegleria* trophozoites facilitated the multiplication of legionellae at 25°C. These results are consistent with the view that multiplication of legionellae in potting mixes occurs through infection of amoebae and release of organisms.

washed by passing a small volume of sterile water through each sample at intervals of up to 30 days. The wash was decontaminated by dilution in HCl-KCl acid buffer (pH 2.2) and legionellae were quantitated on charcoal yeast-extract agar medium containing polymyxin, vancomycin, and natamycin. The results of tests with *Vahlkampfia* trophozoites are shown in Fig. 2; similar results were obtained for *Naegleria* trophozoites and soil legionellae, but more blue-white fluorescent organisms were recovered with *Naegleria* trophozoites (Table 1).

In summary, these studies indicate that *L. longbeachae* serogroup 1 and other soil legionellae survived in a free state in dry potting mix and that survival was independent of amoebic cysts.

Temperature influenced the ability of le-

REFERENCES

1. **Anand, C. M., A. R. Skinner, A. Malik, and J. B. Kurtz.** 1983. Interaction of *Legionella pneumophila* and a free-living amoeba (*Acanthamoeba palestinensis*). *J. Hyg.* (Cambridge) **91:**167–178.
2. **Barbaree, J. M., B. S. Fields, J. C. Feeley, G. W. Gorman, and W. T. Martin.** 1986. Isolation of protozoa from water associated with a legionellosis outbreak and demonstration of intracellular multiplication of *Legionella pneumophila. Appl. Environ. Microbiol.* **51:**422–424.
3. **Fields, B. S., G. N. Sanden, J. M. Barbaree, W. E. Morrill, R. M. Wadowsky, E. H. White, and J. C. Feeley.** 1989. Intracellular multiplication of *Legionella pneumophila* in amoebae isolated from hospital hot water tanks. *Curr. Microbiol.* **18:**131–137.
4. **Rowbotham, T. J.** 1980. Preliminary report on the pathogenicity of *Legionella pneumophila* for freshwater and soil amoebae. *J. Clin. Pathol.* **33:**1179–1183.
5. **Steele, T. W.** 1989. Legionnaires' disease in South Australia 1979–1988. *Med. J. Aust.* **151:**322–326.
6. **Steele, T. W., J. Lanser, and N. Sangster.** 1990. Isolation of *Legionella longbeachae* serogroup 1 from potting mixes. *Appl. Environ. Microbiol.* **56:**49–53.
7. **Steele, T. W., C. V. Moore, and N. Sangster.** 1990. Distribution of *Legionella longbeachae* serogroup 1 and other legionellae in potting soils in Australia. *Appl. Environ. Microbiol.* **56:**2984–2988.
8. **Tyndall, R. L., and E. L. Domingue.** 1982. Cocultivation of *Legionella pneumophila* and free-living amoebae. *Appl. Environ. Microbiol.* **44:**954–959.

Mixed Bacterial Populations Derived from *Legionella*-Infected Free-Living Amoebae

R. L. TYNDALL, A. A. VASS, AND C. B. FLIERMANS

Oak Ridge National Laboratory, Oak Ridge, Tennessee 37831, and Savannah River Laboratory, Aiken, South Carolina 29801

Free-living amoebae and other protozoa interact with a variety of bacteria (1–7, 10, 12). In the case of amoebae, this interaction ranges from bacteria that serve as food sources or are sequestered as endosymbionts within amoebae to bacterial species that are amplified by amoebae.

In recent studies of the microbial flora from home humidifiers (11), we isolated free-living amoebic populations to analyze their associated

bacterial flora. Difficulties were encountered in using classical techniques to purify the bacterial populations associated with some of the amoebae. Since free-living amoebae can destroy some bacterial genera and not others, attempts were made to purify the mixed bacterial cultures by inoculating them into *Acanthamoeba royreba*. Paradoxically, the result was opposite that intended in that the bacterial populations resulting from exposure to the amoebae were more complex than the original mixtures. Consequently, experiments were undertaken to explore the ramifications of this observation.

Amoebae were grown in 5 ml of 712 medium in 25-cm² tissue culture flasks at 37°C for 3 to 4 days until heavy growth occurred. The culture flasks were then placed at room temperature (22°C) for 2 days. An isolated colony of *Legionella* or *Pseudomonas* species in log growth phase was harvested and placed in 712 medium. The *Legionella pneumophila* serogroup 1 cultures originated from either clinical or environmental samples. The environmentally derived isolates have been cocultured with *Naegleria* amoebae for the past 8 years. The *Pseudomonas* cultures were isolated directly from the environment or from amoebae isolated from groundwater aquifers (12). *Legionella* or *Pseudomonas* cells (10⁵) were added to each amoeba culture flask. The caps were securely fastened, and the cultures were left at room temperature for 5 days. Additionally, the *Legionella* and *Pseudomonas* suspensions were streaked on buffered charcoal-yeast extract (BCYE) and Trypticase soy agar media and placed at 37°C to check the purity of the suspensions. After 5 days at room temperature, the culture flasks were opened and the contents were thoroughly mixed at least 10 times with a sterile pipette, concomitantly dislodging the amoebae adhering to the bottom of the flask.

With a sterile pipette, 1 drop of the amoeba-*Legionella* suspension was placed onto various solid media. The drop was placed in the upper quadrant of the plate, and when dry, the bottom portion of the drop was streaked over the remainder of the plate with a sterile inoculating loop. The media used for plating included BCYE without antibiotics, Trypticase soy agar, BCYE without cysteine or antibiotics, and a variety of other media designed to enhance the detection of variant populations. Controls for each experiment included amoebae that had not been infected with *Legionella* or *Pseudomonas* species, 712 medium alone, and *Legionella* or *Pseudomonas* cells in 712 medium without amoebae. The plating of all controls was the same as that of the amoeba-*Legionella* suspension.

Once plated and streaked, all media containing BCYE were incubated at 37°C for 1 to 2 weeks and then transferred to room temperature. The remaining solid media were incubated at room temperature. The cultures were observed for a period of at least 6 months.

As expected, the bacterial inoculum was the predominating bacteria recovered from the infected amoebae. In each of eight experiments with *L. pneumophila* as the inoculum, a small subpopulation of colonies not indicative of legionellae also appeared on the streak lines of the test agar plates

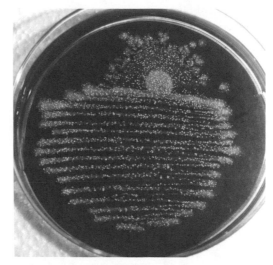

FIG. 1. *A. royreba* infected with *L. pneumophila* streaked on BCYE medium, showing *Legionella* outgrowth and bacteria other than legionellae. Note starburst effect of amoebic outgrowth from point of inoculation.

(Fig. 1). This occurred when either clinically or environmentally derived *Legionella* isolates were used. In addition to BCYE, these bacteria could grow on media that did not support the growth of legionellae. While initially reactive with *Legionella* antibody, these bacteria lost their reactivity on subsequent subculture. These isolates ranged in pigmentation from white to pink and in morphology from gram-negative rods to gram-positive cocci. In 13 separate experiments (Tables 1 and 2) involving five different *Acanthamoeba* species, bacteria other than legionellae were isolated after *Legionella* infection. Conversely, in two tests, *Hartmannella vermiformis* inoculated with legionellae did not yield bacteria other than legionellae. Similarly, in four experiments in which *H. vermiformis* was inoculated with *Pseudomonas* species, only the inoculum was reisolated from the amoebae. However, as with legionellae, acanthamoebae yielded bacteria other than the *Pseudomonas* inoculum in 11 of 15 tests (Tables 1 and 2). Microscopic examination of the *Acanthamoeba royreba* cultures by acridine orange, Giemsa, and Gimenez staining did not reveal the presence of endosymbionts. Conversely, these stains readily detected intracellular bacteria in *Legionella*-infected *Naegleria* species (10) and endosymbionts in *Acanthamoeba* species (5) and *Amoeba proteus* (6).

Various possible scenarios may explain these different observations. (i) Since nonculturable endosymbionts have been seen in acanthamoebae, infection of acanthamoebae by one bacterial spe-

TABLE 1. Growth of newly derived bacterial colonies resulting from coculture of bacteria
with *Acanthamoeba* sp.[a] and *H. vermiformis*

Bacterial inoculum	Growth in coculture with[b]:					
	A. castellanii	*A. lenticulata*	*A. polyphaga*	*A. royreba*	*A. astronyxis*	*H. vermiformis*
Legionellae[c]						
Clinical	+	+	+	+	NT	−
Amoeba derived	+	+	+	+	NT	−
Pseudomonads						
Environmental	NT	NT	NT	+	NT	−
Amoeba derived	+	+	+	+	+	−

[a] With the exception of *A. royreba*, which was originally isolated in our laboratory, all *Acanthamoeba* species were obtained from ATCC.

[b] +, presence of newly derived bacterial colonies; −, no bacterial growth other than from the initial inoculum was detected; NT, not tested.

[c] *L. pneumophila* serogroup 1.

TABLE 2. Summary of experiments showing frequency in which newly derived bacterial colonies arose after
bacterial infection of *Acanthamoeba* sp. and *H. vermiformis*[a]

Bacterial inoculum	No. of experiments showing newly derived bacteria/total no. of experiments after infection of:					
	A. castellanii	*A. lenticulata*	*A. polyphaga*	*A. royreba*	*A. astronyxis*	*H. vermiformis*
Legionella sp.	2/2	3/3	2/2	6/6	NT	0/2
Other gram-negative bacteria	1/3	1/1	2/3	5/5	2/3	0/4

[a] See Table 1 footnotes.

cies may rescue these nonviable bacterial endosymbionts from the amoebae. (ii) Genetic recombination of the bacterial genome from the inoculum with genetic information from bacterial and virus-like particles seen in acanthamoebae by electron microscopy (5, 8, 9) may result in bacteria that were not originally present. (iii) A combination of genetic information with bacterial DNA of the inoculum may result in the formation of newly constituted bacteria. (iv) Although it is unlikely because of exhaustive tests to reveal contaminants, a nonculturable bacterial contaminant may exist in conjunction with the bacterial inoculum and might subsequently be rescued by the amoebae.

Cloning experiments are under way in attempts to derive *A. royreba* cultures which, when inoculated with a known bacterial population, will consistently result in the appearance of the same newly derived bacteria. After such cloned systems are developed, genetic probes prepared against the newly derived bacteria and reacted with amoebic DNA should indicate which of the previously mentioned scenarios are operative.

Whatever the mechanisms, the results to date indicate that some protozoan populations such as acanthamoebae may provide a mechanism for rapid genetic rescue or recombination, resulting in newly derived microbes with as yet unknown pathogenic potential.

We thank Barry Fields of the Centers for Disease Control for supplying *Hartmannella vermiformis*.

REFERENCES

1. **Anand, C., A. Skinner, A. Malic, and J. Kurtz.** 1984. Intracellular replication of *Legionella pneumophila* in *Acanthamoeba palestinensis*, p. 330–332. *In* C. Thornsberry, A. Balows, J. C. Feeley, and W. Jakubowski (ed.), *Legionella: Proceedings of the 2nd International Symposium.* American Society for Microbiology, Washington, D.C.
2. **Fenchel, T.** 1987. *Ecology of Protozoa: The Biology of Free-Living Phagotrophic Protists.* Springer-Verlag, New York.
3. **Fields, B. S., G. N. Saden, J. M. Barbaree, W. W. Morrill, R. M. Wadowsky, E. H. White, and J. C. Feeley.** 1989. Intracellular multiplication of *Legionella pneumophila* in amoebae isolated from hospital hot water tanks. *Curr. Microbiol.* **18:**131–137.
4. **Fields, B. S., E. B. Shotts, Jr., J. C. Feeley, G. W. Gorman, and W. T. Martin.** 1984. Proliferation of *Legionella pneumophila* as an intracellular parasite of the ciliated protozoan *Tetrahymena pyriformis*, p. 327–328. *In* C. Thornsberry, A. Balows, J. C. Feeley, and W. Jakubowski (ed.), *Legionella: Proceedings of the 2nd International Symposium.* American Society for Microbiology, Washington, D.C.
5. **Hall, J., and H. Volez.** 1985. Bacterial endosymbionts of *Acanthamoeba* sp. *J. Parasitol.* **71:**89–95.
6. **Jeon, K. W.** 1987. Change of cellular "pathogens" into required cell components. *Ann. N.Y. Acad. Sci.* **503:**359–371.
7. **Rowbotham, T. J.** 1980. Preliminary report on the pathogenicity of *Legionella pneumophila* for freshwater and soil amoebae. *J. Clin. Pathol.* **33:**1179–1183.

8. **Schuster, F. L., and T. H. Dunnebacke.** 1974. Growth at 37°C of the EGs strain of the amoebo-flagellate *Naegleria gruberi* containing virus-like particles. I. Nuclear changes. *J. Invertebr. Pathol.* **23:**172–181.

9. **Schuster, F. L., and T. H. Dunnebacke.** 1974. Growth at 37°C of the EGs strain of the amoebo-flagellate *Naegleria gruberi* containing virus-like particles. II. Cytoplasmic changes. *J. Invertebr. Pathol.* **23:**182–189.

10. **Tyndall, R. L., and E. L. Domingue.** 1982. Cocultivation of *Legionella pneumophila* and free-living amoebae. *Appl. Environ. Microbiol.* **44:**954–959.

11. **Tyndall, R. L., C. S. Dudney, D. S. Katz, K. S. Ironside, and R. A. Jernigan.** 1987. Identification of bioaerosols and certain particulate emissions into enclosed environments from home humidifiers, vaporizer, and other appliances found in homes. CPSC phases I, II, and III final reports. Consumer Products Safety Commission, Washington, D.C.

12. **Tyndall, R. L., K. S. Ironside, C. D. Little, D. S. Katz, and J. R. Kennedy.** 1991. Free-living amoebae used to isolate consortia capable of degrading trichloroethylene. *Appl. Biochem. Biotechnol.* **28/29:**917–925.

Multiplication of Virulent and Avirulent Strains of *Legionella pneumophila* in Cultures of *Hartmannella vermiformis*

R. M. WADOWSKY, A. FLEISHER, N. J. KAPP, M. EL-MOUFTI, J. N. DOWLING, R. M. AGOSTINI, AND R. B. YEE

University of Pittsburgh, Pittsburgh, Pennsylvania 15261, and Children's Hospital of Pittsburgh, Pittsburgh, Pennsylvania 15213

Hartmannella vermiformis may amplify virulent legionellae in potable water systems of hospitals, hotels, and homes. Plumbing systems are frequently colonized by *H. vermiformis*, *Legionella pneumophila*, and various heterotrophic bacteria, including *Pseudomonas paucimobilis*. Since *H. vermiformis* multiplies in tap water containing killed *P. paucimobilis*, suspensions of these microorganisms are useful for studying the multiplication of legionellae in the presence of multiplying *H. vermiformis*, a condition which likely exists in potable water systems. Only certain strains of legionellae multiply in tap water cocultures (6). Rowbotham (4) has described similar strain-specific interactions between legionellae and free-living amoebae on agar plates. These strain-specific interactions suggest that legionellae require certain virulence factors to infect free-living amoebae. To address this hypothesis, we compare the multiplication of virulent and avirulent strains of *L. pneumophila* in axenic cultures of *H. vermiformis*.

Virulence of strains. A strain of *L. pneumophila* Philadelphia-1 that was grown in embryonated eggs and four isolates (E-52, E-62, E-66, and E-67) of *L. pneumophila* serogroup 1 from the plumbing systems of hospitals were tested for virulence. All of these strains produced plaques on mouse L929 cell culture monolayers and were considered virulent (2). Avirulent strains (E-100, E-101, E-107, and E-108) were derived from these strains by cultivation on supplemented Mueller-Hinton agar (1). The derivative strains did not form plaques.

Multiplication studies. Cultures of *H. vermiformis* (strain 50256; American Type Culture Collection) were incubated in 10 ml of PYNFH medium (no. 1034; American Type Culture Collection) in 25-cm² tissue culture flasks at 37°C.

Cocultures were prepared by replacing the medium from 3-day cultures of *H. vermiformis* (approximately $10^{6.4}$ amoebae per flask) with a suspension of washed legionellae in PYNFH medium (10^7 CFU per flask). Control flasks contained only *L. pneumophila*. Following a 1-h adsorption period, cocultures and controls were washed three times with PYNFH medium. At various times, cocultures and controls were harvested by scraping the flasks with a cell scraper. For measurement of *L. pneumophila* concentrations, culture harvests were sonicated at 40 W for 10 s and then inoculated onto buffered charcoal-yeast extract agar.

The *L. pneumophila* strains multiplied differently in coculture with *H. vermiformis*. The virulent strain of *L. pneumophila* Philadelphia-1 multiplied, whereas the avirulent strain did not. The mean growth yield ($\pm$ standard deviation) at day 7 of incubation obtained from three separate experiments for the virulent strain was 3.3 (± 0.5) log CFU/ml. Each of the parent environmental strains of *L. pneumophila* and the avirulent derivative strains multiplied in the cocultures (Table 1). The growth yields were higher for the parent strains than for the avirulent strains at both day 4

TABLE 1. Multiplication of virulent and avirulent strains of *L. pneumophila* in cultures of *H. vermiformis*

Strain set (virulent/avirulent)	*L. pneumophila* growth yield (log CFU/ml) at indicated time of incubation and with indicated strain type			
	Day 4		Day 7	
	Virulent	Avirulent	Virulent	Avirulent
E-52/E-100	4.2	0.8	4.4	3.5
E-62/E-107	4.8	0.9	5.4	2.0
E-66/E-108	4.0	0.9	4.4	2.1
E-67/E-101	3.8	0.5	5.0	3.2

and day 7. None of the strains multiplied in the amoeba-free control cultures.

Electron microscopy studies. Electron microscopy studies were performed to compare infection of *H. vermiformis* by virulent and avirulent *L. pneumophila*. Our laboratory's standard environmental strain (E-28) of *L. pneumophila* sero-

group 1, which forms plaques in mouse L929 cell culture monolayers, served as the virulent strain. Strain E-100 was used as the avirulent strain. The concentration of the virulent strain increased in the coculture by 4.1 log CFU/ml within 3 days of incubation. In contrast, the avirulent strain multiplied after a lag period of about 7 days. It in-

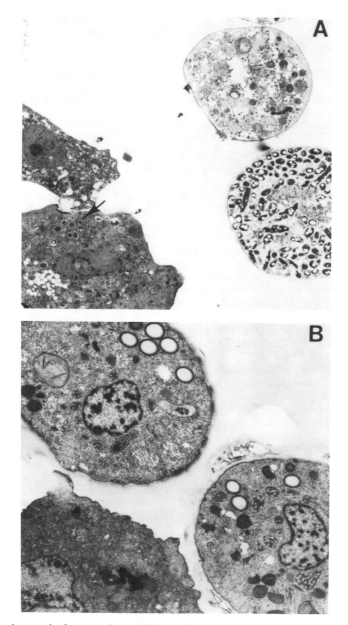

FIG. 1. Electron micrographs from cocultures initiated with virulent or avirulent *L. pneumophila*. (A) Three-day coculture with virulent *L. pneumophila* (strain E-28) (×4,200). An uninfected trophozoite (upper left), a lightly infected trophozoite (lower left; arrow), an uninfected and degenerative rounded form (upper right), and a heavily infected, rounded form with a possible thickened coating (lower right) can be seen. The legionellae in the latter form are extremely electron dense and highly vacuolated. (B) Ten-day coculture with avirulent *L. pneumophila* (strain E-100) (×8,600). An uninfected trophozoite (lower left), an uninfected, early cyst (upper left), and an uninfected cyst (lower right) can be seen.

creased in concentration by 2.1 to 4.3 log CFU/ml between days 10 and 14. Electron micrographs clearly showed a progression of infection in *H. vermiformis* by the virulent strain, whereas infected amoebae were not seen in preparations (over 200 amoebae examined) from the coculture containing the avirulent strain (Fig. 1).

Both virulent and avirulent strains of *L. pneumophila* multiply in coculture with *H. vermiformis* in PYNFH medium. The rate of multiplication is higher for virulent strains than for avirulent strains. Virulent *L. pneumophila* can infect and multiply within *H. vermiformis*. Electron microscopic evidence that avirulent strains infect and multiply within *H. vermiformis* was not obtained; however, sampling error must be considered in electron microscopy studies. The results from the growth studies and electron microscopic observations raise the possibilities that avirulent strains can multiply extracellularly and that extracellular multiplication in addition to intracellular multiplication can occur with virulent strains. Interestingly, none of the avirulent strains of *L. pneumophila* multiplied when incubated in PYNFH medium in the absence of *H. vermiformis*. PYNFH medium contains yeast extract, which probably provides the carbon and energy sources necessary for growth of *L. pneumophila*. We suspect that some component in PYNFH medium is inhibitory to *L. pneumophila*. *H. vermiformis* may neutralize the inhibitory component, thereby facilitating extracellular growth in the medium. Half-strength PYNFH medium is recommended to reduce extracellular growth of *L. pneumophila* in *H. vermiformis* cultures (3). Our results are in general agreement with those of Zraik et al. (6), who reported that environmental isolates of *L. pneumophila* multiply within *Acanthamoeba castellanii* Neff and lose this ability after serial transfer on supplemented Mueller-Hinton agar.

H. vermiformis is susceptible to infection with virulent, environmental strains of *L. pneumophila* and may amplify virulent legionellae in potable water systems.

This work was supported by the U.S. Environmental Protection Agency under cooperative agreements CR 812761 (sponsored by the Center for Environmental Epidemiology of the Graduate School of Public Health of the University of Pittsburgh) and CR 817091-01-0.

REFERENCES

1. **Catrenich, C. E., and W. Johnson.** 1988. Virulence conversion of *Legionella pneumophila*: a one-way phenomenon. *Infect. Immun.* **56:**3121–3125.
2. **Fernandez, R. C., S. H. S. Lee, D. Haldane, R. Sumarah, and K. R. Rozee.** 1989. Plaque assay for virulent *Legionella pneumophila*. *J. Clin. Microbiol.* **27:**1961–1964.
3. **Fields, B. S.** Personal communication.
4. **Rowbotham, T. J.** 1986. Current views on the relationships between amoebae, legionellae and man. *Isr. J. Med. Sci.* **22:**678–689.
5. **Wadowsky, R. M., T. M. Wilson, N. J. Kapp, A. J. West, J. M. Kuchta, S. J. States, J. N. Dowling, and R. B. Yee.** 1991. Multiplication of *Legionella* spp. in tap water containing *Hartmannella vermiformis*. *Appl. Environ. Microbiol.* **57:**1950–1955.

Temperature and the Survival and Multiplication of *Legionella pneumophila* Associated with *Hartmannella vermiformis*

S. J. STATES, J. A. PODORSKI, L. F. CONLEY, W. D. YOUNG, R. M. WADOWSKY, J. N. DOWLING, J. M. KUCHTA, J. S. NAVRATIL, AND R. B. YEE

City of Pittsburgh Water Department, Pittsburgh, Pennsylvania 15238; School of Medicine and Graduate School of Public Health, University of Pittsburgh, Pittsburgh, Pennsylvania 15261; and Children's Hospital of Pittsburgh, Pittsburgh, Pennsylvania 15213

A number of studies have demonstrated that legionellae infect amoebae and ciliated protozoa and reproduce intracellularly (3, 4). Some laboratory studies have also shown that legionellae are able to multiply in potable water only when protozoa are present (5). Protozoa are therefore considered to be natural hosts and amplifiers for *Legionella* spp. in the environment. Knowledge concerning the benefits derived by legionellae from the symbiotic relationship could be used to better control legionellae in aquatic environments such as plumbing systems and cooling towers.

Legionellae are somewhat resistant to elevated temperatures. This property allows *Legionella* spp. to grow in aquatic habitats where many other bacteria are unable to compete and has also complicated efforts to control the legionellae by merely increasing temperature. Additionally, heat enrichment facilitates isolation of legionellae from samples containing other microorganisms. Since some protozoa are also resistant to heat (1), it is possible that they account for the documented heat resistance of legionellae.

The free-living amoeba *Hartmannella vermiformis* is a common contaminant of public water supplies and building plumbing systems. In this study, we investigated the extent to which *H. vermiformis* mediates the effect of temperature on closely associated *Legionella pneumophila*. Specifically, we examined the influence of the amoeba on the multiplication of *L. pneumophila*, at both high and low temperatures, and considered the possible protective effect of the protozoan against inactivation of *L. pneumophila* by short-term exposure to elevated temperatures.

The *H. vermiformis* and *L. pneumophila* serogroup 1 strains used in this study were originally isolated from potable plumbing systems. *H. vermiformis* was maintained in PYNFH medium (American Type Culture Collection medium 1034). *L. pneumophila* was maintained as a frozen stock and was transferred to buffered charcoal-yeast agar (BCYE) prior to each experiment.

To examine the influence of hartmannellid amoebae on the multiplication of legionellae at various temperatures, growth experiments involving cultures of *L. pneumophila* and cocultures of *L. pneumophila* and *H. vermiformis* were conducted at temperatures ranging from 10 to 44°C. *L. pneumophila* was grown in the presence of *H. vermiformis* in PYNFH medium. However, because legionellae do not multiply in PYNFH medium in the absence of amoebae, experiments involving *L. pneumophila* alone were carried out by using buffered yeast extract broth (BYEB). The cultures and cocultures were suspended in 10 ml of broth, in 50-ml plastic tissue culture flasks, with an initial *L. pneumophila* density of 1,000 CFU/ml and an *H. vermiformis* density of 50,000 cells/ml. Replicate suspensions were maintained at the test temperatures for 15 days, and individual flasks were removed and cultured for legionellae on BCYE at several-day intervals.

To determine whether hartmannellid amoebae protect legionellae against short-term exposure to heat, inactivation experiments involving cocultures of *L. pneumophila* and *H. vermiformis* were conducted at temperatures of 55 and 60°C. Prior to the experiments, *H. vermiformis* cultures were grown for 3 days in 50-ml plastic tissue culture flasks containing PYNFH medium. The cultures were then inoculated with 10-ml volumes of *L. pneumophila* (5×10^7 CFU/ml) that had been harvested after 3 days of growth on BCYE plates. The cocultures were incubated (37°C) for 2 additional days to encourage ingestion and intracellular multiplication of legionellae within the amoebae and were subsequently incubated for 3 days in the constant-pH encystment medium of Neff et al. (2) to induce formation of amoebic cysts. The cocultures were then transferred to sterile water and filtered through a 1.0-μm-pore-size polycarbonate membrane filter to separate extracellular legionellae from amoebae and from those legionellae that were sequestered within or closely associated with *H. vermiformis*. The retentate was washed twice with sterile water to remove the remaining loosely associated bacteria. Afterwards, 5-ml aliquots of resuspended retentate and 5-ml aliquots of filtrate, containing loosely held extracellular legionellae, were exposed to 55 or 60°C for 5 min in a water bath. The samples were finally cultured on BCYE to measure survival of *L. pneumophila*.

Table 1 summarizes the results of the multiplication experiments. *L. pneumophila*, alone in BYEB, multiplied at temperatures ranging from 15 to 40°C, with optimum growth at 30 to 37°C. These results are comparable to data from published studies which showed that legionellae from hospital plumbing systems grow at 32 to 42°C (7) and that naturally occurring *L. pneumophila* multiplies in tap water at 25 to 37°C (6). The ability of legionellae in this investigation to multiply at temperatures as low as 15°C may be related to the use of nutrient-rich BYEB medium. At temperatures ranging from 10 to 40°C, legionellae grew more poorly in the presence of amoebae in PYNFH medium than when alone in BYEB. This lower growth rate could be due to amoebae feeding on legionellae. However, at 42°C *L. pneumophila* consistently multiplied (in three separate experiments) only when associated with *H. vermiformis*. The amoebae, therefore, provided a limited increase in the temperature range for *L. pneumophila* multiplication. A similar extension of growth range was not observed at low temperatures.

The results of the heat inactivation experiments (55 and 60°C, 5-min exposure) are shown in Table 2. The extent of heat inactivation of *L. pneumophila* organisms that were associated with amoebae does not appear to differ significantly from that of extracellular legionellae. This result suggests that association with *H. vermiformis* does not significantly increase the heat resistance of *L. pneumophila* to short-term exposure to heat. The

TABLE 1. Influence of temperature on multiplication of *L. pneumophila* alone and in coculture with *H. vermiformis*

Temp (°C)	Growth yield (log CFU/ml) of *L. pneumophila* in:	
	BYEB	PYNFH medium with *H. vermiformis*
10	0.10	<0.01
15	2.01	<0.01
20	5.40	<0.01
30	6.02	4.45
37	6.06	4.92
40	5.68	3.50
42	<0.01	2.63
43	<0.01	<0.01
44	<0.01	<0.01

TABLE 2. Inactivation of *L. pneumophila* by short-term exposure to elevated temperatures

Legionellae inactivated	% Kill (log CFU/ml decease) of *L. pneumophila* following 5-min exposure to:	
	55°C	60°C
Extracellular	62.5 (0.55)	99.2 (2.29)
Associated with *H. vermiformis*	59.3 (0.43)	99.8 (2.72)

actual proportion of legionellae sequestered within the amoebae has not been established. Additional electron microscopic work is under way to determine the exact location of the legionellae cells relative to hartmannellid amoebae in this experimental model. However, multiple washings of the filter retentate suggest that after two washings, most of the easily removed extracellular bacteria have already been freed from the retentate. Therefore, the remaining legionellae are either present within or located in close association with the amoebae.

These experiments, then, indicate that the tolerance of legionellae to extreme temperatures is increased by amoebae to only a limited extent. This finding suggests that the observed resistance of legionellae to elevated temperatures is probably due to other factors such as cell wall composition or protection afforded by association with a biofilm. It further suggests that the benefits obtained by legionellae from the observed symbiotic relationship lie in other aspects of the bacteria's ecology.

This work was supported by the U.S. Environmental Protection Agency under cooperative agreements CR 812761 (sponsored by the Center for Environmental Epidemiology at the Graduate School of Public Health of the University of Pittsburgh) and CR 817091-01-0.

REFERENCES

1. **Chang, S. L.** 1978. Resistance of pathogenic *Naegleria* to some common physical and chemical agents. *Appl. Environ. Microbiol.* **35:**368–375.
2. **Neff, R. J., S. A. Ray, W. F. Benton, and M. Wilborn.** 1964. Induction of synchronous encystment (differentiation) in *Acanthamoeba* sp., p. 55–83. *In* D. M. Prescott (ed.), *Methods in Cell Physiology*, vol. 1. Academic Press, London.
3. **Rowbotham, T. J.** 1980. Preliminary report on the pathogenicity of *Legionella pneumophila* for freshwater and soil amoebae. *J. Clin. Pathol.* **33:**1179–1183.
4. **Rowbotham, T. J.** 1983. Isolation of *Legionella pneumophila* from clinical specimens via amoebae and the interaction of those and other isolates with amoebae. *J. Clin. Pathol.* **36:**978–986.
5. **Wadowsky, R. M., L. J. Butler, M. K. Cook, S. M. Verma, M. A. Paul, B. S. Fields, G. Keleti, J. L. Sykora, and R. B. Yee.** 1988. Growth-supporting activity for *Legionella pneumophila* in tap water cultures and implication of hartmannellid amoebae as growth factors. *Appl. Environ. Microbiol.* **54:**2677–2682.
6. **Wadowsky, R. M., R. Wolford, A. M. McNamara, and R. B. Yee.** 1985. Effect of temperature, pH, and oxygen level on the multiplication of naturally occurring *Legionella pneumophila* in potable water. *Appl. Environ. Microbiol.* **49:**1197–1205.
7. **Yee, R. B., and R. M. Wadowsky.** 1982. Multiplication of *Legionella pneumophila* in unsterilized tap water. *Appl. Environ. Microbiol.* **43:**1330–1334.

Temperature-Dependent Replication of Virulent and Avirulent *Legionella pneumophila* Isolates in *Acanthamoeba castellanii*

MANFRED OTT, MICHAEL STEINERT, LARISA BENDER, BIRGIT LUDWIG, P. CHRISTIAN LÜCK, AND JÖRG HACKER

Institut für Genetik and Mikrobiologie, Universität Würzburg, Würzburg D-W-8700, and Medizinische Akademie Dresden, Dresden D-O-8019, Germany

Legionella pneumophila is an intracellular parasite of phagocytosing cells (present as macrophages during the infection) and in the environment of free-living protists. *Acanthamoeba castellanii* was shown to be among the protozoan hosts that support growth of legionellae in water systems (6). The objective of this study was to investigate the interaction of *L. pneumophila* with *A. castellanii* and to correlate the ability of virulent *L. pneumophila* to infect macrophages with survival and replication in *A. castellanii*.

Virulent *L. pneumophila* replicates intracellularly in *A. castellanii*. *A. castellanii* (ATCC 30011) was grown axenically in PYG 712 medium (American Type Culture Collection) at 37°C and infected with *L. pneumophila* Philadelphia-1 at a multiplicity of infection of 10 in 96-well microtiter plates in a final volume of 1 ml. After 2 h of incubation, extracellular legionellae were removed by thoroughly washing the plates and adding PYG 712 medium containing 80 µg of gentamicin per ml for 1 h; extracellular legionellae were effectively killed at this concentration of gentamicin (data not shown). Following gentamicin treatment (time zero), antibiotic-free medium was replaced for further cultivation of the infected *A. castellanii*. After 0 to 3 h and 1 day,

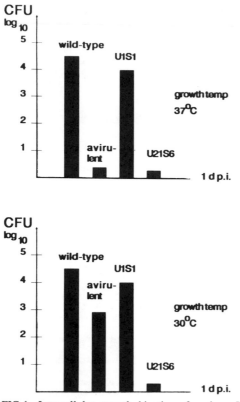

FIG.1. Intracellular growth kinetics of various *L. pneumophila* isolates in *A. castellanii* grown at 37 or 30°C. CFUs were determined after 1 day and are mean values of triplicate determinations.

the multiplication (CFU) of intracellular legionellae was determined by plating the content of each well on buffered charcoal-yeast extract agar in serial dilutions. As depicted in Fig. 1, we found that the virulent variant of the Philadelphia-1 strain multiplied in *A. castellanii*, while an avirulent variant, obtained by passage on supplemented Mueller-Hinton agar (1, 4), was unable to

survive and replicate inside *A. castellanii* at a growth temperature of 37°C. Electron microscopic analysis of thin sections of *A. castellanii* infected by the virulent strain confirmed the intracellular location of legionellae (data not shown).

The growth temperature of *A. castellanii* influences intracellular replication of *L. pneumophila*. We analyzed the effect of the growth temperature of the amoeba on intracellular replication of legionellae. The virulent and avirulent variants of the Philadelphia-1 strain and two environmental isolates, U1S1 and U21S6 (1, 4), obtained from a hot water tank, were analyzed (Table 1; Fig. 1). We found that at 30°C, the avirulent variant of the Philadelphia-1 strain multiplied in coculture with *A. castellanii*. However, the CFUs were not as high as those obtained for the virulent variant. The serogroup 6 environmental isolate (U21S6) was not able to survive and multiply at either temperature. Isolate U1S1 (serogroup 1) behaved similarly to the virulent variant of the Philadelphia-1 strain, as multiplication could be observed at both temperatures.

Intracellular replication of *L. pneumophila* in *A. castellanii* correlates with survivability in macrophage-like (U937) cells and infectivity in the guinea pig model. The *L. pneumophila* variants described above were analyzed for intracellular replication in U937 macrophage-like cells, in an assay similar to that used for *Acanthamoeba* infection, by eliminating extracellular legionellae through use of gentamicin (5). Furthermore, intraperitoneal infection of guinea pigs was attempted to differentiate virulent from avirulent variants in vivo. Table 1 shows that isolates multiplying in *A. castellanii* at 37°C also were able to survive and replicate in macrophage-like cells; in addition, they were infective for guinea pigs (7). The avirulent variant of the Philadelphia-1 strain as well as strain U21S6 did not display infectivity in guinea pigs as they were not able to multiply in U937 cells.

The entry of *L. pneumophila* into *A. castellanii* is independent of microfilament poly-

TABLE 1. Intracellular replication of *L. pneumophila* isolates in *A. castellanii* and U937 macrophage-like cells and virulence in guinea pigs

	Characteristic			
			Multiplication in:	
				A. castellanii	
L. pneumophila isolate	Guinea pig infectivity (intraperitoneal)	U-937 cells	37°C	30°C
Philadelphia-1 variants				
Virulent	+	+	+	+
Avirulent	−	−	−	+
Environmental				
U1S1	+	+	+	+
U21S6	−	−	−	−

merization. Since it had been shown that cytochalasin inhibition of actin microfilament polymerization prevents entry of *L. pneumophila* into macrophages by inhibiting phagocytosis (2), we analyzed the effect of cytochalasin B on the growth kinetics of virulent *L. pneumophila* at 37°C in *A. castellanii* treated with cytochalasin B (4 μg/ml). This treatment did not affect the CFU values obtained after 0 to 3 h and 1 day (see above), which indicates an alternative mode of invasion, independent of microfilament polymerization requiring phagocytosis (data not shown).

The *A. castellanii* model is useful for distinguishing virulent from avirulent variants and enables differentiation between avirulent variants. Our results suggest that *A. castellanii* can be used to distinguish between virulent and avirulent variants of *L. pneumophila,* consistent with a report by Moffat and Tompkins (3). The survivability of avirulent variants in coculture with amoebae at 30°C might be useful for differentiation of avirulent variants, arguing for different "stages" obtained by avirulent variants.

REFERENCES

1. **Bender, L., M. Ott, R. Marre, and J. Hacker.** 1990. Genome analysis of *Legionella* spp. by orthogonal field alternation gel electrophoresis (OFAGE). *FEMS Microbiol. Lett.* **72:**253–258.
2. **Elliot, J. A., and W. C. Winn.** 1986. Treatment of alveolar macrophages with cytochalasin D inhibits uptake and subsequent growth of *Legionella pneumophila. Infect. Immun.* **51:**31–36.
3. **Lück, P. C., et al.** Unpublished data.
4. **Moffat, J. F., and L. S. Tompkins.** 1992. A quantitative model of intracellular growth of *Legionella pneumophila* in *Acanthamoeba castellanii. Infect. Immun.* **60:**296–301.
5. **Ott, M., P. Messner, J. Hessemann, R. Marre, and J. Hacker.** 1991. Temperature dependent expression of flagella in *Legionella. J. Gen. Microbiol.* **137:**1955–1961.
6. **Pearlman, E., A. H. Jiwa, N. C. Engleberg, and B. I. Eisenstein.** 1988. Growth of *Legionella pneumophila* in a human macrophage-like (U937) cell line. *Microb. Pathog.* **5:**87–95.
7. **Rowbotham, T. J.** 1986. Current views on the relationship between amoeba, legionellae and man. *Isr. J. Med. Sci.* **22:**678–689.

Detection of *Legionella* spp. in Environmental Water Samples and Free-Living Amoebae by Using DNA Amplification

B. JAULHAC, C. HARF, M. NOWICKI, AND H. MONTEIL

Institut de Bactériologie de la Faculté de Médecine, Université Louis Pasteur, 3 rue Koeberlé 67000 Strasbourg; Laboratoire d'Hydrobiologie de l'Environment, Université Louis Pasteur, BP 24, 67401 Illkirch; and Centre d'Etudes et de Recherches Bactériologiques, Institut Pasteur de Lyon, Faculté Alexis Carrel, rue Paradin, 69372 Lyon, France

The presence of *Legionella* spp. in environmental water is common, but their recovery by direct growth is time-consuming and not always successful. Since Rowbotham first demonstrated that *Legionella* spp. could infect amoebae (8), several in vitro studies on *Legionella*-amoeba interactions have shown intracellular multiplication of *Legionella* spp. within phagosomes of amoeba trophozoites (6, 11). The occurrence of interactions between *Legionella* spp. and amoeba trophozoites in environmental waters was also demonstrated by immunofluorescence assay (IFA) and inoculation to guinea pigs (3). It remains unknown whether these bacteria are present in the natural environment within amoeba cysts, giving to *Legionella* spp. an opportunity to survive under unfavorable conditions.

To overcome the problems of culturing *Legionella* spp. from biological samples, the polymerase chain reaction (PCR) may serve as a useful tool. Recently, the use of PCR to detect *Legionella* spp. in bronchoalveolar lavage fluid specimens and water samples was reported (2, 5, 9).

The aim of this study was to improve the detection of *Legionella* spp. in river water samples by using PCR. *Legionella* spp. may be present as free-living bacteria or as bacteria harbored in amoeba trophozoites or cysts. Whereas lysis of *Legionella* spp. and trophozoites is achieved by thermal shock or proteinase K treatment, *Acanthamoeba* cysts are extremely resistant to these procedures. Moreover, sediments collected with environmental waters had an inhibitory effect on the detection method. Sample preparation protocols had to be developed in order to overcome these difficulties.

Detection of *Legionella* spp. by PCR in amoeba trophozoites fed in vitro with *Legionella pneumophila*. To assess detection of legionellae in amoeba trophozoites and cysts, *Acanthamoeba griffini* reference strain S7 (kind gift of O. De Jonckheere, Brussels, Belgium) was cultured at 30°C on 2% agar plates previously seeded with *L. pneumophila* serogroup 1 (ATCC 33152) in order to obtain amoebae harboring legionellae. Amoeba trophozoites were harvested from 1-week-old cultures and washed twice in buffered saline solution. Mature amoeba cysts were collected after 1 month of culture and washed twice in buffered saline solution.

DNA was extracted from legionellae and

amoeba trophozoites after centrifugation. Briefly, the pellet obtained was treated with lysis buffer containing 50 μg of proteinase K, 0.5% (vol/vol) Nonidet P-40, and 0.5% (vol/vol) Tween 20 in 500 μl of 10 mM Tris-HCl (pH 8)–50 mM KCl–50 mM MgCl$_2$, allowing lysis of *Legionella* spp. and trophozoites. DNA was then purified by phenol-chloroform-isoamyl alcohol extraction and ethanol precipitation. The air-dried pellet was resuspended in TE buffer (10 mM Tris-HCl [pH 8], 1 mM EDTA), heated for 10 min at 95°C, and submitted to 40 cycles of amplification in a 100-μl volume as previously described (5). The primers used, the conditions of DNA amplification, gel electrophoresis and Southern blot hybridization, and the precautions taken to avoid DNA contaminations were the same as previously reported (5). Detection of DNA from *L. pneumophila* serogroups 1 to 14, *L. micdadei*, and *L. bozemanii* serogroup 1 was possible with a sensitivity of 50 CFU in the samples tested.

By using this lysis procedure, a positive signal was obtained for trophozoites previously fed with *Legionella* spp. As control, no amplification was observed with bacteria usually isolated from environmental water or with *Acanthamoeba* and *Naegleria* trophozoites previously fed with *Escherichia coli*. We were unable to obtain any amoeba cyst lysis either by this procedure or by thermal lysis.

Detection by PCR of legionellae in amoeba cysts previously fed in vitro with *L. pneu-*

mophila. DNA extraction was performed after centrifugation of the microorganisms harvested from 1-month-old cultures. Lysis performed by the procedure described above ensured the removal of intact amoeba cysts from bacterial and trophozoite lysis extracts by differential centrifugation (250 × g for 3 min). The supernatant was subjected to DNA purification and PCR as described above in order to detect free-living legionellae and legionellae within trophozoites. The cyst pellet was resuspended in 0.5 ml of lysis buffer supplemented with approximately 150 mg of glass beads (0.2-mm diameter, Sigma) and shaken vigorously for 5 min as described by Abbaszadegan et al. (1). The samples were then incubated for 2 h at 55°C in order to release *Legionella* DNA from cysts. DNA purification and PCR were then performed as described above for the supernatant.

As expected, a 630-bp DNA fragment was visualized by gel electrophoresis and Southern hybridization only for the samples containing *Acanthamoeba* cysts previously fed in vitro with *L. pneumophila* (Fig. 1). As control, no signal was observed for *Acanthamoeba* cysts previously fed with *E. coli*.

Testing of river water samples. The differential method was then applied to river water samples after separation of the sediments. Several 250-ml aliquots of water with sediments were collected in August 1991 from the Rhine river (France) in a location known to contain *Legionella*

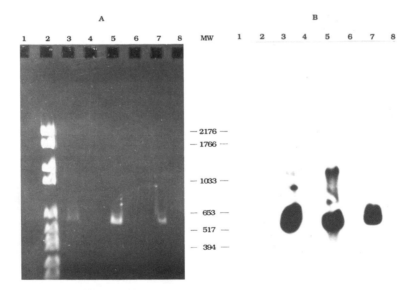

FIG. 1. Agarose gel electrophoresis (A) and Southern blot analysis (B) of amplified DNA (40 cycles) from *Legionella* spp. and from amoebae, using primers Lpm-1 and Lpm-2 and detection probe Lpm-3. Lanes: 1, no DNA; 2, *Bg*lI and *Hin*fI-digested plasmid pBR328 as molecular weight markers (Boehringer Mannheim); 3, 100 pg of *L. pneumophila* serogroup 1 DNA; 4, *Acanthamoeba* trophozoites fed with *E. coli*; 5, *Acanthamoeba* trophozoites fed with *L. pneumophila*; 6, *Acanthamoeba* cysts fed with *E. coli*; 7, *Acanthamoeba* cysts fed with *L. pneumophila*.

spp. (3). The water temperature was 20 to 24°C. Each aliquot was first concentrated by centrifugation (22,000 × g for 1 h at 6°C) to a 5-ml volume.

Because of the inhibitory effect of sediments present in river water samples, a purification step was necessary to remove sediments from microorganisms prior to DNA extraction and PCR. Four methods were compared: (i) differential centrifugation (300 × g for 5 min followed by centrifugation of the supernatant at 5,000 × g for 20 min), (ii) acid-washed polyvinylpolypyrrolidone treatment (4), (iii) sucrose gradient centrifugation (7), and (iv) sodium dodecyl sulfate (SDS) treatment (10). The number of amoeba cysts was then determined by phase-contrast microscopic examination. The greatest number of amoeba cysts was obtained after the SDS treatment.

Among the four separation methods tested, the differential centrifugation and sucrose gradient protocols were unable to detect Legionella spp. in river water samples tested after proteinase K lysis without shaking with glass beads. A weak signal was obtained with the polyvinylpolypyrrolidone method, and the strongest signal was obtained after SDS treatment, indicating the presence of Legionella spp. in the river water samples either as free-living bacteria or as organisms within trophozoites. This result was confirmed by IFA performed on another aliquot of the same river water sample. IFA performed with antiserum pools A, B, and C, obtained from the Centers for Disease Control, was positive with antiserum pool A. Direct culture on defined media of the pellet obtained after the concentration step remained negative for Legionella spp. but showed the presence of Acanthamoeba spp. However, with use of glass bead lysis, no Legionella spp. were detected by DNA amplification from the amoeba cysts in the river water samples tested.

In conclusion, we detected Legionella spp. in river water samples by a PCR assay after a first step separating microorganisms from sediments. This step, performed by the SDS treatment procedure, was important for detecting Legionella spp. by DNA amplification. In addition, we developed a method for lysing amoeba cysts, improving the possibility of detecting Legionella

spp. in the natural environment. Unfortunately, we were unable to show the presence of Legionella spp. in cysts collected during summer, when trophozoites are able to multiply in warm waters and Legionella spp. seem to be more frequent as free-living bacteria or within trophozoites than within cysts.

We thank D. Herb and M. T. Vetter for skillful technical assistance. This work was supported in part by a grant (CRE no. 900316) from INSERM and by GUREN (Université Louis Pasteur).

REFERENCES

1. **Abbaszadegan, M., C. P. Gerba, and J. B. Rose.** 1991. Detection of Giardia cysts with a cDNA probe and applications to water samples. *Appl. Environ. Microbiol.* **57:**927–931.
2. **Bej, A. K., M. H. Mahbubani, and R. M. Atlas.** 1991. Detection of viable Legionella pneumophila in water by polymerase chain reaction and gene probe methods. *Appl. Environ. Microbiol.* **57:**597–600.
3. **Harf, C., and H. Monteil.** 1988. Interactions between free-living amoebae and Legionella in the environment. *Water Sci. Technol.* **20:**235–239.
4. **Holben, W. E., J. K. Jansson, B. K. Chelm, and J. M. Tiedje.** 1988. DNA probe method for the detection of specific microorganisms in the soil bacterial community. *Appl. Environ. Microbiol.* **54:**703–711.
5. **Jaulhac, B., M. Nowicki, N. Bornstein, O. Meunier, G. Prevost, Y. Piemont, J. Fleurette, and H. Monteil.** 1992. Detection of Legionella spp. in bronchoalveolar lavage fluids by DNA amplification. *J. Clin. Microbiol.* **30:**920–924.
6. **Newsome, A. L., L. R. Baker, R. D. Miller, and R. R. Arnold.** 1985. Interactions between Naegleria fowleri and Legionella pneumophila. *Infect. Immun.* **50:**449–452.
7. **Pillai, S. D., K. L. Josephson, R. L. Bailey, C. P. Gerba, and I. L. Pepper.** 1991. Rapid method for processing soil samples for polymerase chain reaction amplification of specific gene sequences. *Appl. Environ. Microbiol.* **57:**2283–2286.
8. **Rowbotham, T. J.** 1980. Preliminary report on the pathogenicity of Legionella pneumophila for freshwater and soil amoebae. *J. Clin. Pathol.* **33:**1179–1183.
9. **Starnbach, M. N., S. Falkow, and L. C. Tompkins.** 1989. Species-specific detection of Legionella pneumophila in water by DNA amplification and hybridization. *J. Clin. Microbiol.* **23:**1257–1261.
10. **Steffan, R. J., and R. M. Atlas.** 1988. DNA amplification to enhance detection of genetically engineered bacteria in environmental samples. *Appl. Environ. Microbiol.* **54:**2185–2191.
11. **Tyndall, R. L., and E. L. Domingue.** 1982. Cocultivation of Legionella pneumophila and free-living amoebae. *Appl. Environ. Microbiol.* **44:**954–959.

Kinetic Studies of *Legionella* Interactions with Protozoa

N. S. PANIKOV, A. E. MERKUROV, AND I. S. TARTAKOVSKII

Institute of Microbiology, Russian Academy of Sciences, and Gamaleya Research Institute of Epidemiology and Microbiology, Russian Academy of Medical Sciences, Moscow, Russia

The interactions of legionellae with soil and water protozoa were shown to be one of the most important factors in the maintenance of pathogens in the natural environment (5–7). These interactions are investigated primarily in a purely qualitative way, e.g., by means of microscopic observation of infected protozoan cells (1). However, many aspects of studies of legionellae must be carried out quantitatively, particularly for analyzing *Legionella* population dynamics and for selecting the optimal strategies for pest control and testing of different epidemiological scenarios.

In this report, we discuss the applicability of the kinetic approach, i.e., the combination of dynamic experiments with mechanistic mathematical modeling, for studies of *Legionella*-protozoa interactions. Mathematical modeling provides a precise and unambiguous representation of proposed mechanisms involved in biological processes. Hence, it helps to differentiate true and false concepts by comparison of the observed dynamic pattern with the calculated pattern.

General kinetic features of interactions of protozoa with bacteria. Protozoa-bacteria interactions are described by different kinds of prey-predator models (2, 4), i.e.,

dynamics of bacteria   (1)
$$dx/dt = ux - a_x x - W(x) y/Y_y$$
dynamics of protozoa
$$dy/dt = w(x)y - a_y y$$

where x is the bacterial population, y is the protozoan population. Y_y is the yield constant for protozoan growth on bacterial cells, a_x and a_y are decay constants for bacteria and protozoa, respectively, and u and $W(x)$ are specific growth rates of bacteria and protozoa, respectively. Such experimental data are obtained primarily for such microbial preys as *Escherichia coli*, *Enterobacter aerogenes*, and *Pseudomonas fluorescens* and for such predators as *Dictyostelium discoideum*, *Paramecium* sp., and *Tetrahymena pyriformis*. In our extensive studies of *Pseudomonas-Tetrahymena* coculture (3), we have found the following kinetic features of protozoan feeding on bacteria.

(i) The dependence of grazing rate $W(x)$ on bacterial population density x could be approximated by the equation

$$W(x) = W_{max} \cdot (x - x^*)/[K_x + (x - x^*) \quad (2)$$
$$+ (x - x^*)^2/K_{xx}]$$

where W_{max} is the maximal specific growth rate, K_x is the saturation constant, and K_{xx} is the substrate inhibition constant. The mechanism of predator inhibition by high bacterial density is not clear but probably is determined by the negative effects of some bacterial metabolites. It was very important that protozoa never consume all of the bacteria in the coculture. When the bacterial concentration fell to some threshold level x^*, then the chance of collision between prey and predator became extremely small, residual bacterial preys being unavailable for further grazing.

(ii) The rate of grazing is dependent on the physiological state of the bacteria. Metabolically active, rapidly growing bacteria were more susceptible to protozoan consumption than were old, starving cells. This finding was explained by modification of the bacterial cell composition during starvation (decrease of RNA and protein content, formation of a polysacharide capsule, etc.).

(iii) The protozoan population survived for a long time in coculture with *T. pyriformis* under starvation conditions (when $x < x^*$). The protozoan cell number remained constant despite the decrease of total biomass as a result of the ability of protozoa to adaptively decrease their maintenance requirements and turnover (decay) rate. To describe this phenomenon, parameter a_y in model 1 was explained as follows. Starvation initially promotes a_y to increase (acceleration of cell turnover and synthesis of new starvation cell components), and then after constant time period t^*, parameter a_y decreases to zero, providing the transition of protozoan cells to a quasi-resting state. Recovery from the dormant state occurs within 1 to 2 h after enrichment of the medium with new bacterial cells.

Specific features of interactions of legionellae with protozoa. The principal peculiarity of the behavior of legionellae in coculture with protozoa is its dependence on the incubation temperature. Under low and moderate temperature conditions (up to 25 to 30°C), bacteria are still consumed by protozoa. At higher temperatures (35 to 37°C), the prey-predator interactions are transformed to a parasite-host type; i.e., bacteria become intracellular parasites of protozoa and replicate within protozoan cells. The results of typical dynamic experiments at 35 to 37°C are shown in Fig. 1. Legionellae in the control trial (without protozoa) were not able to grow and died out at a constant specific death rate. In the presence of protozoa, the dynamic curve of legionellae had a rather complicated shape. For the first day of incubation, the number of CFU decreased at a higher rate than in the control; then the bacterial population increased by several orders of magnitude, reaching the maximum level on day 5. At the same time, the protozoan population decreased from 10^4 cells per ml to 1 to 5 cells per ml.

To describe mathematically the observed dynamics, we used several consecutive approximations. First, we considered the simplest case of parasite-host interactions,

dynamics of bacteria $dx/dt = ux - a_x x$ (3)
dynamics of protozoa $dy/dt = - u \cdot x/Y_x - a y_y$

where u is the specific growth rate of legionellae on protozoa and Y_x is the growth yield expressed as the number of bacterial cells (CFU) released into the medium from one protozoan cell.

However, this simplest simulation deviated significantly from the observed dynamics. Therefore,

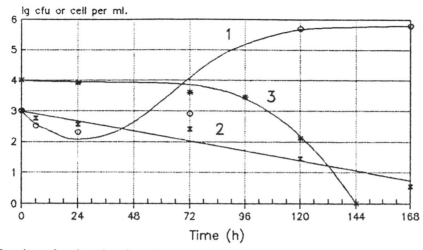

FIG. 1. Experimental study and mathematical simulation of the interaction of legionellae with protozoa (8). *L. pneumophila* Philadelphia-1 was grown at 35°C in coculture with *T. pyriformis* on 3% brain-heart extract. 1, the *Legionella* population in the presence of protozoa (the number of CFU upon plating on charcoal-yeast agar); 2, the same population in control flasks (without protozoa); 3, the number of *T. pyriformis* cells (direct microscopic count). The curves are calculated according to model 6.

we refined the model by taking into account (i) the heterogeneity of the bacterial population, which as a first approximation is represented by virulent (x') and avirulent (x'') forms (virulent bacteria can damage protozoa, whereas avirulent forms cannot multiply inside the host); (ii) the possibility that avirulent legionellae cells are consumed by protozoa according to equation

$$dx''/dt = - a_x x'' - Q_x y x''/(K_x + x'') \quad (4)$$

where Q_x and K_x are maximal uptake rate and saturation constant, respectively, for bacterial grazing by protozoa; and (iii) the dependence of u on y of the Monod type,

$$u(y) = u_m y/(K_y + y) \quad (5)$$

where u_m is the maximal specific growth rate of bacteria and K_y is the saturation constant (population of protozoa in the medium that provides a growth rate of $0.5 u_m$). Finally, we obtained the following modification of model 3:

total bacteria $dx/dt = dx'/dt + dx''/dt \quad (6)$

virulent bacteria $dx'/dt = u(y)x' - a_x x' =$

$\qquad\qquad\qquad u_m y/(K_y + y) - a_x x'$

avirulent bacteria $dx''/dt = - ax'' -$

$\qquad\qquad\qquad Q_x y x''/(K_x + x'')$

protozoa $dy/dt = - ux'/Y_x - a_y y$

The results of simulations are presented in Fig. 1. We can see that model 6 is able to describe all specific features of *Legionellae-Tetrahymena* interactions; for example, it generates the shape of

dynamic curves, including the decline of legionellae during the first day of the experiment, and describes the negative correlation between bacteria and protozoa populations.

After verification of the model, we can discuss its biological interpretation. At this time, we should stress the importance of temperature as the main controlling factor. Temperature has a threshold effect on the type of bacteria-protozoa interaction; i.e., after a transition from 30 to 35°C, it changes from a prey-predator to a parasite-host type. Second, the kinetic analysis revealed the significance of population heterogeneity of interacting species. Only a small proportion of the total bacterial population appeared to be virulent (about 1 cell per 1,000). Their growth rate in protozoan cells was rather high: $u = 2.37\ d^{-1}$, which corresponds to a generation time of 7.0 h. The remaining cells in the original *Legionellae* population were avirulent and lysed by *T. pyriformis* as they were at a low incubation temperature.

Similar behavior was observed in coculture of *T. pyriformis* with another soil-inhabiting pathogen, *Listeria monocytogenes*. At high incubation temperatures (35 to 37°C), *Listeria* cells were able to grow within protozoan cells but less intensively than legionellae (generation time of 14.4 h).

REFERENCES

1. **Anand, C., A. Skinner, and J. Kurtz.** 1983. Interaction of *Legionella pneumophila* and a free-living amoeba (*Acanthamoeba palestinensis*). *J. Hyg.* (Cambridge) **91:**167–178.
2. **Graham, J. M., and R. P. Canale.** 1982 Experimental and modeling studies of a four-trophic level predator-prey system. *Microb. Ecol.* **8:**217–232.

3. **Panikov, N. S.** 1991. *Microbial Growth Kinetics: General Principles and Ecological Applications.* Nauka, Moscow. (In Russian.)
4. **Pirt, S. J.** 1975. *Principles of Microbe and Cell Cultivation,* p. 205–208. Blackwell Scientific Publications, Oxford.
5. **Rowbotham, T. J.** 1980. Preliminary report on the pathogenicity of *Legionella pneumophila* for freshwater and soil amoebae. *J. Clin. Pathol.* **33:**1179–1183.
6. **Rowbotham, T. J.** 1980. Pontiac fever explained? *Lancet*

ii:969.
7. **Tartakovskii, I. S., V. J. Litveen, and S. V. Prozorovsky.** 1988. Ecological aspects of legionnaires' disease. *Zh. Mikrobial. Epidemiol. Immunobiol.* **8:**122–125. (In Russian.)
8. **Tartakovskii, I. S., N. S. Panikov, A. E. Merkurov, and S. V. Prozorovsky.** 1991. Mathematical model of *Legionella pneumophila* growth in the presence of *Tetrahymena pyriformis. Zh. Mikrobiol. Epidemiol. Immunobiol.* **9:**7–9. (In Russian.)

Relationships among Different Serogroups of Legionellae within the Ciliated Protozoan *Tetrahymena pyriformis*

K. NAHAPETIAN, O. CHALLEMEL, S. DUBROU, C. TRAM, AND F. SQUINAZI

Laboratoire d'Hygiène de la Ville de Paris (Prof. B. Festy), 11 rue George Eastman, 75013 Paris, and Institut Pasteur, Unité de Bactériologie Moléculaire et Médicale, 75015, Paris, France

Legionella pneumophila is a facultative intracellular pathogen that is especially fastidious in its growth requirements in the laboratory. It is also a ubiquitous member of the aquatic environment and survives quite well in habitats that would seem inhospitable to such finicky bacteria. In the dark (e.g., in the plumbing systems of hospitals or hotels), the organism grows to surprisingly high levels and can survive for a long period of time. *L. pneumophila* is a freshwater inhabitant (in very low concentration) whose presence is not always associated with legionellosis, whereas a higher concentration of this bacterium is an important factor in the pathogenesis of *Legionella* infection. Several studies have reported that free-living amoebae and the ciliated protozoan *Tetrahymena*

pyriformis can support the multiplication of *L. pneumophila* (4). Combined aquatic environmental factors such as temperature, stagnation, sediment formation, and the presence of biodegradable substances and bacterial flora provide favorable circumstances for interactions between legionellae and protozoa and thus augment the survival potential of the bacteria, which in turn leads to greatly increased *Legionella* populations.

A total of 24 strains of legionellae were studied: 20 strains of *L. pneumophila* serogroups 1 to 10, including 4 strains of patient isolates and 16 strains of hospital environmental isolates; 4 strains of the family *Legionellaceae* (other than *L. pneumophila*), including 1 strain of *L. micdadei* (Centers for Disease Control reference strain ATCC

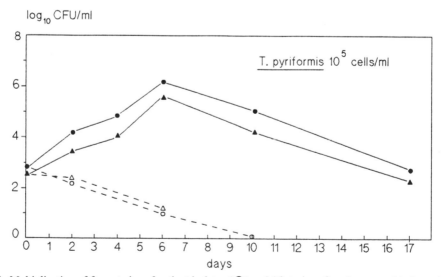

FIG. 1. Multiplication of four strains of patient isolates (●) and 16 strains of environmental isolates (▲) of *L. pneumophila* incubated with *T. pyriformis.* Results for control samples free of *T. pyriformis* (○, △) are also shown.

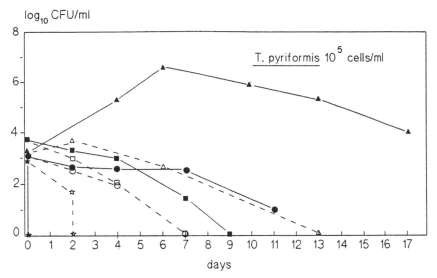

FIG. 2. Coculture of *L. micdadei* (▲), *L. anisa* (■), *L. parisiensis* (●), and *L. rubrilucens* (★) with *T. pyriformis*. Results for control samples free of *T. pyriformis* (△, □, ○, ☆) are also shown.

33128) and 3 strains of environmental origin (*L. anisa, L. parisiensis,* and *L. rubrilucens*).

The clinical isolates used in this study were recultured once or twice on buffered charcoal-yeast extract agar supplemented with α-ketoglutarate after isolation and then cocultured with *T. pyriformis*. All of the remaining strains had been frozen in glycerol-containing brain heart infusion broth (5%) at −74°C for periods ranging from several months to 9 years. *T. pyriformis* cultures were obtained from the Centers for Disease Control stock strain grown in dilute Elliot's medium and maintained at 25°C.

Tissue culture flasks (25 cm²) containing 3.5 ml of Elliot's medium and 3.5 ml of sterile tap water were inoculated with 1 ml of *T. pyriformis* from 48- to 72-h cultures. After 4 days of incubation at 25°C, the numbers of *T. pyriformis* were adjusted to 10^5 cells per ml. The flasks were then inoculated with 1 ml of sterile tap water containing 10^5 *Legionella* cells per ml plus 1 ml of heated *Escherichia coli* as described by Fields et al. (2). The same study was carried out with attenuated *L. pneumophila* clinical isolates of serogroups 1 and 6.

Virulent strains were cultured on charcoal-yeast extract agar and Mueller-Hinton agar (BBL Microbiology Systems) supplemented with 0.025% ferric citrate and 0.025% cysteine (SMH agar). Attenuated strains, obtained after passaging virulent cultures 5 times on charcoal-yeast extract agar and 25 times on SMH agar (1), were cocultured with *T. pyriformis*.

Six male Hartley guinea pigs weighing 250 to 299 g were obtained from local suppliers.

All strains of *L. pneumophila* serogroups 1 to 10 and *L. micdadei* multiplied in cocultures with *T. pyriformis*. The increased numbers of legionellae cocultured with *T. pyriformis* are shown in Fig. 1 and 2; intracellular multiplication is shown in Fig. 3.

In contrast, *L. anisa, L. parisiensis,* and *L. rubrilucens* failed to multiply (Fig. 2). Attenuated strains of *L. pneumophila* serogroups 1 and 6 also failed to multiply, whereas the number of virulent strains of the same isolates increased >2 log_{10} (Fig. 4).

No signs of infection were evident in either of two guinea pigs inoculated with 1 ml of an attenuated strain (10^9 cells per ml), whereas both guinea pigs inoculated with a virulent strain died within 3 days. Numerous *L. pneumophila* serogroup 1 cells were isolated from a spleen suspension (Fig. 5).

The ability to generate an avirulent culture of *L. pneumophila* from a virulent parent culture by successive passages on SMH agar has been well established. *Legionella* growth in protozoa as an important factor of multiplication in the aquatic environment gives us special insight into the pathogenesis of *Legionella* infection. This study demonstrates another variable in the *Legionella*-protozoa interaction, the *Legionella* strain used (3, 5). We have shown that environmental isolates differ in the virulence, and our results suggest a correlation of virulence with the effect of legionellae on the ciliated protozoan *T. pyriformis*.

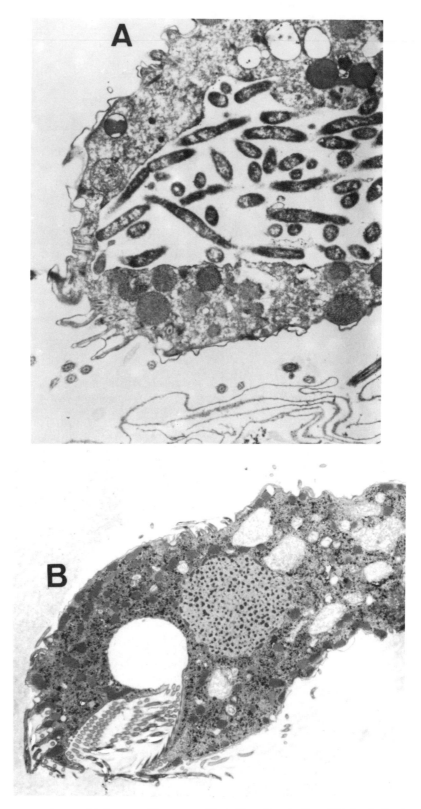

FIG. 3. (A) Intracellular multiplication of *L. pneumophila* in *T. pyriformis* after a 30-h incubation (magnification, ×9,500); (B) control sample free of *L. pneumophila*.

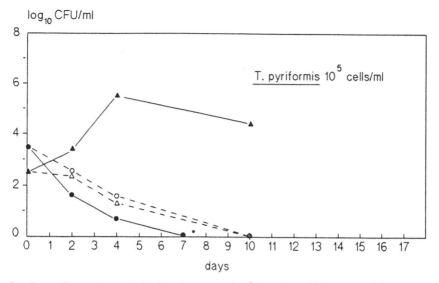

FIG. 4. Coculture of nonattenuated (▲) and attenuated (●) strains of *L. pneumophila* patient isolates of serogroups 1 and 6 with *T. pyriformis*. Results for control samples free of *T. pyriformis* (△, ○) are also shown.

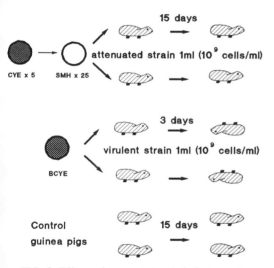

FIG. 5. Effects of attenuated and virulent nonattenuated serogroup 1 strains (both patient isolates) on guinea pigs. CYE, charcoal-yeast extract medium; BCYE, buffered charcoal-yeast extract medium.

Some strains of legionellae and avirulent strains of *L. pneumophila* serogroups 1 and 6 (attenuated strains) could not replicate in protozoa. The obser-vation of intracellular multiplication of legionellae within *T. pyriformis* can be used as a criterion for determining the virulence of certain isolates of *Le-gionella* spp.

We thank P. Gounon for preparation of the electron micro-graphs and Y. Le Moullec for preparation of the figures.

REFERENCES

1. **Catrenich, E. C., and W. Johnson.** 1988. Virulence con-version of *Legionella pneumophila*: a one-way phenome-non. *Infect Immun.* **56:**3121–3125.
2. **Fields, B. S., J. M. Barbaree, E. B. Shotts, Jr., J. C. Feeley, W. E. Morill, G. N. Sanden, and M. J. Dykstra.** 1986. Comparison of guinea pig and protozoan models for determining virulence of *Legionella* species. *Infect. Immun.* **53:**553–559.
3. **Fields, B. S., G. N. Sanden, J. M. Barbaree, W. E. Morill, R. M. Wadowsky, E. H. White, and J.C. Feeley.** 1989. Intracellular multiplication of *Legionella pneu-mophila* in amoebae isolated from hospital hot water tanks. *Curr. Microbiol.* **18:**131–137.
4. **Nahapetian, K., O. Challemel, D. Beurtin, S. Dubrou, P. Gounon, and F. Squinazi.** 1991. The intracellular multi-plication of *Legionella pneumophila* in protozoa from hospi-tal plumbing systems. *Res. Microbiol.* **142:**677–685.
5. **Spriggs, D. R.** 1987. *Legionella,* microbiology, ecology and inconspicuous consumption. *J. Infect. Dis.* **155:**1086–1087.

IV. DETECTION AND CHARACTERIZATION OF LEGIONELLAE

Detection of *Legionella* by Molecular Methods

LUCY S. TOMPKINS AND JEFFREY S. LOUTIT

Division of Infectious Diseases, Department of Medicine, and Department of Microbiology and Immunology, Stanford University Medical Center, Stanford, California 94305

DNA PROBE DEVELOPMENT

Shortly after the discovery of *Legionella* species by investigators from the Centers for Disease Control (CDC), many clinical laboratories began to search for legionellae in clinical specimens, with variable success. Although culture remains the "gold standard" against which other methods are compared, only a modest number of clinical laboratories, usually those in major teaching hospitals, have continued to routinely culture respiratory tract specimens on *Legionella* medium (buffered charcoal-yeast extract [BCYE]), and virtually none attempt to detect legionellae in water samples. Regarding rapid detection methods, Edelstein et al. found that the direct fluorescence antibody (DFA) screen on sputum was reasonably sensitive (2); however, this has not been the experience of other laboratories, including our own. Undoubtedly, the sensitivity of such a subjective test depends on the ability and experience of the microscopist; given that in most clinical laboratories many different technologists may be called upon to perform this test, it is not surprising that sensitivity and specificity have not approached the levels reported by others. For example, in the Stanford University Medical Center (SUMC) clinical microbiology laboratory, we found that the sensitivity of DFA in comparison with culture was only 30%, and the specificity was also dismally low.

Nucleic acid hybridization methods to detect microbial targets in clinical materials offer sensitivity and specificity levels many orders of magnitude greater than those obtainable by conventional techniques. Grimont et al. (6) were among the first to report a DNA hybridization method for detecting *Legionella pneumophila*. Using random endonuclease digestion fragment probes selected to be depleted of cross-hybridizing sequences and a dot blot format, they reported a calculated sensitivity of 10^4 to 10^5 CFU. Although this method was not applied to clinical specimens directly, they showed the potential application of the probe to confirm identification of plate-grown colonies isolated from a clinical specimen. Specificity of the probe was determined by density of the autoradiograph; the probe cross-hybridized with other *Legionella* species and with non-*Legionella* bacteria, making the specificity relative.

Subsequently, scientists at Gen-Probe developed a commercial system to detect legionellae in clinical specimens, using a cDNA probe complementary to specific regions of *Legionella* 16S rRNA and a liquid solution hybridization format. This test had several advantages, including increased sensitivity due to the intrinsic amplification of target RNA molecules (each bacterial cell contains approximately 10^5 16S rRNA molecules) and increased rate of reaction provided by solution hybridization conditions. The sensitivity of this method when tested against purified DNA was extrapolated to be 10^3 CFU (4). Using the first-generation Gen-Probe kit, Edelstein et al. reported results on 342 clinical specimens that had been frozen after testing by DFA and culture (3). Of these, 112 had been culture and/or DFA positive, showing the high prevalence of infection in this population. The sensitivity of the hybridization kit was 56 to 74%, depending on whether 17 specimens were eliminated as being uninterpretable; specificity was 100%. Pfaller subsequently used the Gen-Probe kit to examine 202 respiratory tract specimens from a lower-prevalence population (13). Sensitivity and specificity (67 and 100%, respectively) were quite similar to the results of Edelstein et al. These investigators also showed that the DNA probe assay detected 7 of 11 culture-positive specimens, while the DFA test detected only 4 of 11. False-negative results were obtained when the specimen contained very low numbers of CFU. Among the advantages of this method were that results could be obtained more quickly than with culture, allowing the clinician more specific information about the patient in a timely fashion. It should be noted that the method was not devised to detect legionellae in water samples, for which a more sensitive method was thought to be necessary.

LEGIONELLOSIS AT SUMC

Beginning in 1983, we began to document cases of nosocomial legionellosis occurring at SUMC. Since then, more than 75 cases have been detected, many of which had atypical, unusual features. Although we were unable to determine the reservoir or the major mode of transmission during the first 7 years of this endemic infection, recent epidemiological studies have elucidated the probable mode of transmission, and molecular and microbiological studies on potable water samples have definitively identified the relevant reservoir. Subsequently, we have applied these molecular methods to detect *Legionella* species in water samples collected from two other outbreaks and compared them with the standard means of identifying legionellae in water.

Using molecular fingerprinting methods, we were able to show that SUMC patients were infected by a single clone of *L. pneumophila* serogroup 1 and a single strain of *L. dumoffii* (17). In six cases, both species were detected in clinical samples. These data confirmed the results of epidemiological analyses showing that the infections were nosocomial. Although the SUMC *L. pneumophila* strain restriction endonuclease analysis and alloenzyme type were unique among California isolates, this alloenzyme type was shared by isolates collected in other geographic areas (17). The SUMC *L. dumoffii* strain is unique among the collection at CDC. Using culture methods, we were also able to isolate *L. pneumophila* isolates having the same genotypic pattern as disclosed by restriction endonuclease and alloenzyme type analyses (17) from many potable water sources at SUMC. In this regard, the outbreak at SUMC was typical of a continuing-source, nosocomial endemic infection. However, from the outset it was clear that the SUMC outbreak of *L. pneumophila* and *L. dumoffii* infections had unusual features.

First, the overwhelming majority of patients had undergone cardiothoracic surgery requiring the use of cardiac bypass equipment. The reasons for surgery included heart and/or lung transplant, coronary artery bypass graft surgery, prosthetic valve surgery, and aortic aneurysm. Of note is that virtually all patients required mediastinal or pleural chest tubes (often both) to drain fluid during the initial postoperative period. Second, many of the patients developed extrapulmonary infections, including prosthetic valve endocarditis (16), sternal wound infections (9), and pleuritis, pericarditis, or mediastinitis (10). True extrapulmonary *Legionella* infections have been infrequently documented (reviewed in reference 10), and there were no previous reports of prosthetic valve endocarditis or sternal postoperative wound infections as of 1989. Third, although a significant number of patients were immunocompromised by virtue of

having heart or heart/lung transplantation, many were not immunocompromised and had no known risk factors. Fourth, *L. dumoffii* infections at SUMC were nearly as frequent as *L. pneumophila* infections, even though infection by this species has rarely been documented in other hospitals. In addition, previous studies suggested that the SUMC *L. dumoffii* strain was essentially nonpathogenic when administered via intraperitoneal injection into guinea pigs (5).

Another interesting feature of the SUMC patients was the indolent nature of the infections. A case control analysis of prosthetic valve endocarditis suggested that infection was acquired in the perioperative period even though the clinical manifestations were subtle (16). Taken together, these data strongly suggested that nosocomial acquisition was associated with cardiothoracic surgery and that transmission may have occurred through direct contact with a contaminated reservoir as opposed to the more usual aerosol route. However, we were unable to identify any potential reservoir in the operating rooms per se, and there was nothing in the liquid solutions used in surgery, the cardiac bypass equipment, or the surgical procedure itself that could reasonably account for intraoperative exposure.

Early in 1984, we began a routine program to culture water sources obtained from many locations throughout SUMC, including samples from the cooling towers, the hot water tanks, and faucets in patient care areas. In collaboration with investigators at CDC, we collected multiple samples over a 7-year interval. At CDC, 1 liter of water was concentrated by centrifugation and plated onto selective and nonselective BCYE agar; at SUMC, we plated 0.5 ml of unconcentrated water directly onto selective agar containing dyes, glycine, vancomycin, and polymyxin B. In most instances, sources that contained cultivatable *L. pneumophila* by the CDC concentration method were also positive at SUMC, although the colony counts were 3 log units greater by the CDC method by virtue of concentration of a larger volume of water. Of interest was our finding that for the majority of positive water samples, the number of CFU by either method was surprisingly low, ranging from 1 to 50/ml; a few sources had a significantly greater number of cultivatable legionellae, and overgrowth by *Pseudomonas aeruginosa* was not unusual. This finding was expected, since the concentration of chlorine in the SUMC potable water was negligible.

The results of the culture surveillance demonstrated that the SUMC strain of *L. pneumophila* could be found in the main hot water tanks supplying the clinical care units and in the faucet water of several hospital rooms; although the cooling towers contained other *Legionella* species, neither the SUMC *L. pneumophila* or *L. dumoffii* strain was isolated from them. At no time during the interval from 1984 through 1989 were we or CDC investigators able to isolate *L. dumoffii*, even during periods when clinical cases of *L. dumoffii* had occurred (9).

It has been suggested that some outbreaks of Legionnaires disease occurred in institutions in which no cultivatable legionellae could be detected (7), but coccoid forms could be demonstrated by epifluorescence and fluorescence microscopy. These findings have given rise to the hypothesis that legionellae may exist in some environmental reservoirs as noncultivatable, viable bacteria which might proliferate in culture given optimal conditions. Others have suggested that amoeba species in water support the growth of legionellae and thereby serve as a sort of intermediate host to sequester legionellae and render them nonculturable; amoebae could also provide a mechanism to amplify extracellular bacteria. Since the SUMC water contained minimal concentrations of chlorine, it is not surprising that we were able to identify acanthamoebae in a few potable water samples (unpublished results).

DEVELOPMENT OF PCR TO DETECT LEGIONELLAE AT SUMC

On the basis of these ideas and results, we hypothesized that the SUMC potable water was the major reservoir of both *L. pneumophila* and *L. dumoffii* and that a molecular method which could detect noncultivatable forms of *Legionella* species might be useful in documenting this hypothesis and also might aid in our epidemiological investigations to pinpoint the mode(s) of transmission. To this end, we began a series of experiments to develop *L. pneumophila* and *L. dumoffii*-specific oligonucleotide primers and DNA probes for polymerase chain reaction (PCR) amplification of *Legionella* target sequences in potable water samples. To detect *L. pneumophila*, we identified a chromosomal DNA sequence of *L. pneumophila* that was unique to strains of this species (14). The approach was to hybridize whole cell genomic DNA extracted from a variety of *Legionella* species to *L. pneumophila* restriction endonuclease fragments arrayed in a gel. We then selected an 800-bp fragment of *L. pneumophila* DNA which reacted only with *L. pneumophila* genomic DNA; after being cloned and sequenced, this fragment served as the template for oligonucleotide primers and probe. Parenthetically, we subsequently showed that the metalloprotease gene (*pro*) is highly conserved among only *L. pneumophila* strains and could also serve as a species-specific probe and primer template. Following 35 rounds of amplification at high stringency, the sensitivity of PCR amplification for *L. pneumophila* DNA and viable bacteria in mock-infected potable water

samples was on the order of 35 bacteria, and the primers did not amplify DNA of any other bacterial species.

More recently we have developed a second set of primers and probes to detect *L. dumoffii*, using a similar strategy to select a species-specific sequence (8). Sensitivity on mock-infected water ranged from 1 to 500 bacteria per sample under conditions of high stringency, and the specificity was 100% following PCR amplification of other *Legionella* species and water bacteria.

Atlas and colleagues have also utilized PCR to detect legionellae in mock-contaminated water samples, using *L. pneumophila*-specific primers and probes containing the *mip* gene and the gene encoding 5S rRNA as templates for oligonucleotide and probe synthesis (1, 11). Purified DNA extracted from all *Legionella* species and 15 serogroups of *L. pneumophila* was amplified with the 5S rRNA oligonucleotides. Probe hybridization was tested on Southern blots and dot blots. None of five other bacterial species was detected. Use of oligonucleotides complementary to the ends of a 650-bp sequence originally reported by Engleberg et al. (3a) provided specific amplification of *L. pneumophila* only. The sensitivity was determined by testing serial dilutions of purified *L. pneumophila* DNA analyzed by dot blot hybridization. Amplification of 10 fg of genomic DNA was detected by the *mip* probe (calculated to be equivalent to 1 ag of target DNA), whereas the 5S rDNA probes detected 1 fg of purified DNA. Bej et al. reported incorporation of these probes into a muliplex PCR amplification system to detect legionellae, and immobilized capture probes were used to detect amplified DNA (1). This study suggested that by using PCR amplification with biotin labeling and immobilized capture probe hybridization, as few as one to two bacterial cells could be detected theoretically. It should be noted that these studies were performed on mock-contaminated water samples but have not been repeated on environmental samples.

APPLICATION OF PCR TO POTABLE WATER SAMPLES

We have recently concluded a series of experiments to test the utility of species-specific primers and probes to detect legionellae in water samples collected from outbreak-associated environments. These experiments provided us with the first opportunity to examine the basis for our inability to detect *L. dumoffii* in water at SUMC during a prolonged period during which many cases of nosocomial infection occurred. At the outset, we posed three hypothetical possibilities to account for our inability to culture *L. dumoffii*: (i) we had not sampled the relevant reservoir, (ii) *L. dumoffii* was present in a viable but noncultivatable state throughout the outbreak, and (iii) the concentration of *L. dumoffii* varied episodically and had been too low to detect by culture.

Water samples collected over the period from 1984 through 1991 were stored at 4°C until we tested them; in some cases, samples were 5 years old at the time of PCR amplification. For PCR analysis, we sampled 1 ml from each potable water sample. Tubes containing the water were centrifuged at high speed for 1 h, and the supernatant was discarded. The residual pellet was resuspended in 100 μl of PCR buffer, and a 10-μl aliquot was transferred into PCR amplification tubes. Negative controls were run to check for carryover contamination. Following 35 rounds of amplification under high stringency, using each set of primers independently, the amplification products were electrophoresed and probed with species-specific primers and probes in a Southern hybridization format on nitrocellulose. Results were scored as positive or negative and compared with CFU results obtained at the time of sample collection; in some cases, we had CFU results obtained at CDC and at SUMC, whereas other samples were tested only at SUMC by direct plating.

Of 41 water samples tested for *L. pneumophila*, 8 were PCR positive, compared with 10 that were culture positive. PCR was negative in five samples that were culture positive (sensitivity of 50%); however, three samples were PCR positive and culture negative. Specificity was quite high. It is likely that these "false-positive" results were actually true positives, reflecting the greater sensitivity of PCR. Specificity of the probes and primers was reflected by the finding that some of the water samples contained *P. aeruginosa* which did not cross-hybridize with the primers and was not amplified. Six of the SUMC 41 water samples contained *L. dumoffii* by culture; all 6 were PCR positive, giving a sensitivity of 100% and a specificity of 100%. Of interest was the finding that PCR did not disclose additional positive samples. These results suggest, but do not prove, that PCR detected legionellae in culture-negative samples merely because the concentration of viable bacteria was beyond the limits of detection by plating. The PCR-negative, culture-positive SUMC samples had very small numbers of viable bacteria, between 1 and 10 per 1,000 ml, as determined by concentration-culture at CDC. Since we initially sampled 1 ml for the PCR test, we would not have been able to detect bacteria in these samples. It is important to recognize that if the calculated number of detectable bacteria is one, PCR amplification and culture could lead to either a positive or negative result, and at this level it would be difficult to compare methods. It should be noted that we did not control for possible inhibitory substances present in the potable water, and some of

the PCR-negative, culture-positive results could have been due to this fact. Experiments are currently under way to use an internal target and primers to determine whether the samples inhibited the activity of the *Taq* polymerase, and we will repeat PCR testing with a larger volume of water that will be concentrated by centrifugation.

The probable basis for our inability to detect *L. dumoffii* from water samples collected from 1983 through 1989 by either culture or PCR was the recent discovery that *L. dumoffii* may be persistent in the pipes carrying water to only a few rooms in the postoperative intensive-care unit (ICU). This discovery was made when two patients developed *L. dumoffii* infection in 1989; both patients had undergone cardiovascular surgery during the same 48-h period and were located in adjacent rooms in the ICU. Water obtained from these rooms and another adjacent ICU room was culture and PCR positive for *L. dumoffii* on the day of sampling; however, we were not able to detect *L. dumoffii* by culture or PCR subsequently. As we later realized, none of these rooms had been sampled before, although other ICU rooms were routinely sampled on many occasions.

The potable water system was chlorinated in 1989, and no further cases occurred for 24 months. However, three clinical infections were documented in 1991. In one instance, the patient had been bathed postoperatively in a rarely used ICU room located at the end of the water distribution system; the concentration of chlorine in the hot water supplying this room was far below the desired concentration of 2 ppm. These results suggest that legionellae might have persisted in certain plumbing fixtures or lines, and during unpredictable periods, the concentration could have suddenly reached levels at which infection can occur and which can be detected. We speculate that in the peripherally located ICU rooms, the chlorine concentration was negligible and legionellae that had persisted in these pipes reached a high concentration as a result of relative stasis. Thus, the first few liters of water collected when the faucets were first turned probably contained a much higher concentration of bacteria than did water obtained later in the day. In addition, the acanthamoebae in the potable water could have certainly served as the silent reservoir under environmental conditions, such as high heat, that are not suitable for intracellular replication. Later, during intervals when the chlorine concentration fell or the temperature was lowered, legionellae could have replicated in these hosts. Following replication, legionellae are able to break out of the amoebae, causing a high concentration of extracellular bacteria. This hypothesis is supported by other studies performed by Jennifer Moffat, a graduate student in the laboratory, who has developed an intracellular growth model for *Acanth-*

amoeba castellanii (12).

We have also examined water samples collected during two other outbreaks, including potable water samples linked to community-acquired Legionnaires disease in Pittsburgh, Pa. (15), and potable water samples from the Packard Children's Hospital in Stanford, Calif. To summarize, PCR sensitivity for the Pittsburgh samples was 60%, and specificity was 100%. As in the case of the SUMC samples, PCR amplification testing was falsely negative when the sample contained fewer than 10 bacteria per ml. Combining the results from all water samples, we observed a sensitivity of 57% for PCR compared with culture; specificity was 93%, and the positive and negative predictive values were each 80%. These preliminary findings provide sufficient evidence that when optimized, PCR methods are applicable to potable water samples, providing that the effect of inhibitory substances in the water samples can be controlled.

OTHER MOLECULAR METHODS TO AMPLIFY BACTERIAL TARGETS

Another hybridization-based amplification system that holds promise for incorporating a higher level of specificity, called ligase chain reaction (LCR), has recently been developed. Both PCR and LCR amplification methods utilize oligonucleotides that hybridize to the target, priming the reaction for subsequent amplification. In contrast to PCR, LCR oligonucleotides are designed to completely cover the target, such that one set of oligonucleotides hybridizes with the left half of the target while another set hybridizes with the right half. The ligase enzyme then seals the nick between the two halves, thereby creating a full-length complementary sequence. Amplification of the target sequences via the polymerase enzyme subsequently occurs by the usual mechanism. The key to LCR's utility is that the ligase enzyme will not seal gaps between oligonucleotides that are not abutting perfectly, such that even though the mismatched oligonucleotides may hybridize to the target, they will not be held together to permit subsequent priming for amplification. The advantage of LCR is that very minor mutations, including single base substitutions or deletions, can be detected by using oligonucleotides that are complementary to the mutation.

SHOULD PCR BE USED TO MONITOR WATER QUALITY?

Theoretically, PCR should be able to amplify the number of targets 10^6-fold; consequently, 1 to 10 bacteria per liter should be detectable by this method as compared with culture, in which the plating efficiency is probably not 100%. Therefore, it will probably be important to collect and test larger sample volumes in order to compare the true sensitivities of both methods. We suggest that the most important measure of the applicability of PCR for detection is examination of water samples taken from outbreaks of clinical and subclinical infection to ascertain the relevant concentrations of bacteria that are linked to increased infection rates. The concentration of bacteria sufficient to cause infection may depend on the route of infection. Thus, most of the available data suggest that when Legionnaires disease develops, *Legionella* concentrations in aerosols are relatively high and can be detected readily by culture of the water reservoir. On the other hand, our experience at SUMC with extrapulmonary infections, such as mediastinitis and sternal wound infections, suggests that relatively low concentrations of bacteria can lead to infection in the presence of fresh surgical wounds and indwelling drainage catheters. In such situations when topical application of contaminated potable water has occurred (9), even a "nonvirulent" species like *L. dumoffii* can gain a foothold and cause localized tissue infection, with subsequent spread to contiguous structures. Therefore, standards of acceptable concentrations of bacteria might differ according to the route of transmission and other clinical factors.

A possible application of LCR technology would be the use of oligonucleotides that can differentiate between two species or strains of *Legionella*. For example, the difference between so-called virulent *L. pneumophila* serogroup 1 and avirulent strains may be based on a minor molecular change that could be differentiated by specific oligonucleotides. One could employ LCR to amplify only virulent *L. pneumophila* targets. This methodology should be especially applicable to specifically monitor water quality for potentially virulent strains, since discovery of nonpathogenic *Legionella* species may have no clinical significance.

Currently, recommendations to routinely test potable water and environmental water supplies for legionellae have not been made unless results of prior epidemiological and clinical studies suggest that a particular source is incriminated in an outbreak. However, assessment of the case rate in the usual situation in which clinical infections occur endemically and are unpredictable is difficult and requires resources beyond the capability of most infection control programs. Furthermore, most hospital clinical laboratories, including those in some teaching hospitals, still do not consistently include *Legionella* cultures or other specific detection methods in their routine procedures, and few laboratories routinely examine clinical specimens obtained from extrapulmonary sources. We suggest that it now makes good sense to monitor the potable water system in certain hospitals in a systematic and prospective manner with PCR or LCR (or both), especially in large medical centers that have a substantial number of high-risk patients who could be expected to be susceptible to legionellosis. From our experience, prospective molecular screening of potential reservoirs of legionellosis is feasible, and it is far more cost-effective to prevent infection than to identify and treat clinical infections after they have occurred. Therefore, we are suggesting that prevention, rather than detection, of nosocomial legionellosis should be a goal, just as we currently deal with the prevention of aspergillosis in hospitals. The objective is to prevent infection among high-risk patients by reducing or eliminating exposure by providing a safe environment for the duration of the period of increased susceptibility to infection. Molecular methods offer us the opportunity to determine the efficacy of systems currently under development that could more cost-effectively decontaminate hospital potable water and could provide a rational basis upon which we can predict the desired level of safety in the environment.

REFERENCES

1. **Bej, A. K., M. H. Mahbubani, R. Miller, J. L. DiCesare, L. Haff, and R. M. Atlas.** 1990. Multiplex PCR amplification and immobilized capture probes for detection of bacterial pathogens and indicators in water. *Mol. Cell. Probes* **4**:353–365.

2. **Edelstein P. H., K. B. Beer, J. D. Sturge, A. J. Watson, and L. C. Goldstein.** 1985. Clinical utility of a monoclonal direct fluorescent agent specific for *Legionella pneumophila*: comparative study with other reagents. *J. Clin. Microbiol.* **22**:419–421.

3. **Edelstein, P. H., R. N. Bryan, R. K. Enns, D. E. Kohne, and D. L. Kaclaw.** 1987. Retrospective study of Gen-Probe Rapid Diagnosis System for detection of legionellae in frozen clinical respiratory tract samples. *J. Clin. Microbiol.* **25**:1022–1026.

3a. **Engleberg, N. C., C. Carter, D. R. Weber, N. P. Cianciotto, and B. I. Eisenstein.** 1989. DNA sequence of *mip*, a *Legionella pneumophila* gene associated with macrophage infectivity. *Infect. Immun.* **57**:1263–1270.

4. **Enns, R. K.** 1988. DNA probes: an overview and comparison with current methods. *Lab. Med.* **19**:295–300.

5. **Fields, B. S., J. M. Barbaree, E. M. Shotts, Jr., J. C. Feeley, W. E. Morrill, G. N. Sanden, and M. J. Dykstra.** 1986. Comparison of guinea pig and protozoan models for determining virulence of *Legionella* species. *Infect. Immun.* **53**: 553–559.

6. **Grimont, A. D., F. Grimont, N. Desplaces, and P. Tchen.** 1985. DNA probe specific for *Legionella pneumophila. J. Clin. Microbiol.* **21**:431–437.

7. **Hussong, D., R. R. Colwell, M. O'Brien, E. Weiss, A. D. Pearson, R. M. Weiner, and W. D. Burge.** 1987. Viable *Legionella pneumophila* not detectable by culture on agar media. *Bio/Technology* **5**:947–950.

8. **Loutit, J. S., and L. S. Tompkins.** 1990. Detection of *Legionella dumoffii* in water by DNA amplification and hybridization, abstr. 1033, p. 258. *Program Abstr. 30th Intersci. Conf. Antimicrob. Agents Chemother.*

9. **Lowry, P. W., R. J. Blankenship, W. Gridley, N. J. Troup, and L. S. Tompkins.** 1991. A cluster of *Legionella* sternal-wound infections due to postoperative topical exposure to contaminated tap water. *N. Engl. J. Med.* **324**:109–112.

10. **Lowry, P. W., and L. S. Tompkins.** Extrapulmonary nosocomial Legionellosis: a clinical entity not to be overlooked. *Am. J. Infect. Control,* in press.

11. **Mahbubani, M. H., A. K. Bej, R. Miller, L. Haff, J. DiCesare, and R. M. Atlas.** 1990. Detection of *Legionella* with polymerase chain reaction and gene probe methods. *Mol. Cell. Probes* **4**:175–187.

12. **Moffat, J. F., and L. S. Tompkins.** 1992. A quantitative model of intracellular growth of *Legionella pneumophila* in *Acanthamoeba castellani. Infect. Immun.* **60**:296–301.

13. **Pfaller, M. A.** 1988. Laboratory diagnosis of infections due to *Legionella* species: practical application of DNA probes in the clinical microbiology laboratory. *Lab. Med.* **19**:301–304.

14. **Starnbach, M. N., S. Falkow, and L. S. Tompkins.** 1989. Species-specific detection of *Legionella pneumophila* in water by DNA amplification and hybridization. *J. Clin. Microbiol.* **27**:1257–1261.

15. **Stout, J. E., V. L. Yu, P. Muraca, J. Joly, N. Troup, and L. S. Tompkins.** 1992. Potable water as a cause of sporadic cases of community-acquired Legionnaire's disease. *N. Engl. J. Med.* **326**:151–155.

16. **Tompkins, L. S., B. Roessler, S. C. Redd, L. E. Markowitz, and M. L. Cohen.** 1988. *Legionella* prosthetic valve endocarditis. *N. Engl. J. Med.* **318**:530–535.

17. **Tompkins, L. S., N. J. Troup, T. Woods, W. F. Bibb, and R. M. McKinney.** 1987. Molecular epidemiology of *Legionella* species by restriction endonuclease and alloenzyme analysis. *J. Clin. Microbiol.* **25**:1875–1880.

Selecting a Subtyping Technique for Use in Investigations of Legionellosis Epidemics

JAMES M. BARBAREE

Botany and Microbiology Department, Auburn University, Auburn University, Alabama 36849

The identification of *Legionella* isolates continues to become more complex as additional species and serogroups are recognized. Currently, there are over 29 *Legionella* species (2, 19). Also, it has been shown that there are over 40 subtypes of *Legionella pneumophila* (22). This diversity of types and subtypes (strain differences within a species) and the ubiquitous occurrence of legionellae in water or moist environments make it difficult to identify epidemic strains. Furthermore, it is not uncommon to isolate different legionellae from a single plate of primary isolation medium. Thus, the recognition of an epidemic strain (one the same as clinical isolates from cases in an outbreak) can be a difficult task. Conclusions from other epidemiologic data are weakened unless the data show that the strains isolated from the source for dissemination are the same as isolates from confirmed cases. Subtyping procedures are used to show that the strains are the same or different.

Subtyping procedures used with legionellae include serologic techniques, plasmid analyses, electrophoretic alloenzyme typing (ET), restriction fragment length polymorphism analysis, RNA or DNA probing of DNA digests, and other methods such as pulsed-field gel electrophoresis of DNA digests. The purpose of this report is to review these methods and their application to legionellosis epidemics. The data will show that they are complementary.

SEROLOGIC PROCEDURES

Serologic procedures to subtype legionellae include the use of polyvalent antibodies and monoclonal antibodies (MAbs). Techniques used to date include direct and indirect fluorescent antibody, slide agglutination, and dot enzyme-linked immunosorbent assay procedures (3, 5, 28).

POLYVALENT ANTISERA

A variety of strain differences of *L. pneumophila* serogroup 1 (Lp1) have been demonstrated by using polyvalent antisera. Using rabbit antisera absorbed with different formalin-killed antigens, Thomason and Bibb (24) showed 17 antigenic subtypes among 176 Lp1 strains. The five Lp1 strains used to make the antisera were Knoxville-1, OLDA, Albuquerque-1, Bellingham-1, and San Francisco-9.

This method of subtyping was used in a retrospective study of four epidemics caused by Lp1 (24). The epidemic strains exhibited four different patterns of reactivity (Table 1). No environmental cultures were obtained in the Philadelphia and Burlington outbreaks, but Lp1 case isolates were obtained, and all of them showed one distinct reactivity pattern within each outbreak. Corresponding environmental and clinical strains were found in the Los Angeles outbreak collection. Only one antigenic type was found in sentinel guinea pig lung tissue saved from the 1968 Pontiac fever outbreak in Pontiac, Mich.

MAbs

Several MAb panels have been developed for subtyping Lp1. Joly et al. (9) proposed the use of an international panel of seven MAbs from three laboratories. The sources for these antibodies were R. M. McKinney (United States), I. D. Watkins (United Kingdom), and J. R. Joly (Canada). Use of the panel makes it possible to classify Lp1 into at least 12 subtypes (Table 2).

The selection of the seven MAbs for the panel was done to make a standard MAb panel for Lp1. However, other panels have been used. Among these are panels developed in Columbus, Ohio (United States) (17), and Oxford (United Kingdom) (27) (Table 3). There are advantages for subtyping with each one. For example, the Oxford panel subdivides Lp1 strains in the international Oxford 4032E subgroup into seven subtypes. Conversely, the international panel separates strains in the OLDA-2c subgroup in the Oxford panel into four subtypes. The five MAbs in the Columbus panel allow the subdivision of the Philadelphia-1 subgroup into four subtypes. However, the international panel subdivides the Columbus A-1 subgroup into five subtypes. Obviously, use

TABLE 1. Use of polyvalent antisera to show antigenic subtypes in four
legionellosis outbreaks caused by Lp1

| Outbreak | Antigenic profiles[a] | |
	Environmental samples	Patient samples
Los Angeles, Calif.	2, 5, 6[b]	2, 5, 6
	3, 4, 5	
Philadelphia, Pa.		2, 4, 5
Pontiac, Mich.	2, 3, 4, 5[c]	
Burlington, Vt.		3, 4, 5

[a]Reactivity to the indicated antigens.
[b]Reactivity of antigens 1 to 6 present cumulatively on Knoxville-1, OLDA, Albuquerque-1, Bellingham-1, and San Francisco-9 strains.
[c]Reactivity of Lp1 from sentinel guinea pig tissue.

of MAbs from different sources increases the discriminatory power of subtyping because the panels are complementary. Since only MAbs 1, 2, and 3 are currently available commercially in the United States, some laboratories have only limited ability to use MAb subtyping.

In an outbreak investigated by the Centers for Disease Control, MAb reactivity with the international panel was used in the absence of cultures to subtype the epidemic strain (11). Thirty-two cases were confirmed serologically in this outbreak. A misting device in a grocery store was implicated epidemiologically; it yielded cultures of Lp1 with a Philadelphia-1 reactivity pattern (reactivity with MAbs 1, 2, 5, and 6) in the panel. Since there were no clinical isolates, the epidemic Lp1 strain was subtyped directly in the lung tissues of two deceased patients. The Lp1 cells in the lung tissue exhibited the same pattern (1-2-5-6 reactivity pattern) as did the misting device strain.

PLASMID ANALYSES

Plasmid analyses have been used to subtype legionellae, but the results show this procedure to be of limited use. Plasmidless strains are not uncom-

TABLE 2. International panel of MAbs for Lp1

Subgroup	MAb reactivity pattern[a]
Philadelphia-1	1-2-5-6
Allentown-1	1-2-5
Benidorm 030E	1-2-5-7
Knoxville-1	1-2-3-(6)
France 5811	1-2
OLDA	1-6-7
Oxford 4032E	1-6
Heysham-1	1-3-6-7
Camperdown-1	1
Bellingham-1	1-4-7
Other	1-3-6
Other	Nonreactive

[a]MAbs: 1, MAb 1; 2, MAb 2; 3, MAb 3; 4, W32; 5, 33G2; 6, 32A12; 7, 144C2.
Numbers represent positive reactivity with the designated MAb. (6), variable results with MAb 6. Data are from reference 9.

mon. In fact, Brown et al. reported that the clinical strains in a cluster of cases were plasmidless and the environmental strains contained plasmids (4). One to four plasmids have been reported in individual strains. The sizes of these plasmids vary from very small (1.9 MDa) to very large (135 MDa) (1, 8, 10, 23).

Nolte et al. (14) examined Lpl isolates in an outbreak and reported that the clinical and hot water tank strains were the same (i.e., each had 21- and 49-MDa plasmids), whereas, Lp1 from the cooling tower was different. Stout et al. (23) studied 159 isolates from seven institutions and found matching clinical and environmental strains when plasmid-containing strains were present. Brown et al. (4) used a combination of plasmid and peptide analyses to match epidemic strains.

ELECTROPHORETIC ALLOENZYME TYPING

Application of the ET procedure by Selander et al. (22) increased the ability to subdivide epidemic strains of legionellae. Use of a regimen of 22 enzyme tests to show the allelic variation or similarities of strains enables the separation of *L. pneumophila* into over 40 subtypes. Tobin et al. (25) reported the subdivision of the Philadelphia 1 MAb subgroup into five ET subtypes. In one hospital, Tompkins et al. (26) found clinical and environmental strains that were the same by ET. The ET procedure is very labor-intensive, which makes the technique less desirable in many laboratories.

RIBOTYPING

Grimont et al. (6, 7) reported the use of ribotyping to subtype various species of legionellae. In this technique, the DNA is extracted, nicked with an endonuclease, and probed with labeled 16S and 23S rRNAs from *Escherichia coli*. This procedure has been used at the Centers for Disease Control to subtype Lp1 and Lp3 strains in several U.S. outbreaks.

TABLE 3. Comparison of MAb panels for subtyping Lp1

Strain	No. of strains	Reactivity in international panel subgroups[a]
Oxford panel subgroups		
Pontiac-1a	11	Benidorm (9), Knoxville (2)
Pontiac-2a/c/e	4	Philadelphia (4)
Pontiac-4e	1	Philadelphia (1)
OLDA-1	9	OLDA (8), Oxford 4032E (1)
OLDA-1b	6	OLDA (5), Oxford 4032E (1)
OLDA-2a	39	OLDA (27), Oxford 4032E (4), Heysham (7), nonreactive (1)
OLDA-2b	16	OLDA (9), Oxford 4032E (1), Heysham (6)
OLDA-2c	11	OLDA (1), Oxford 4032E (1), Heysham (8), nonreactive (1)
OLDA-3a	3	Oxford 4032E (1), Heysham (2)
OLDA-3c	4	Oxford 4032E (2), Camperdown (2)
Columbus panel subgroups		
A-1	53	Philadelphia (9), Benidorm (4), Knoxville (1), France (1), Allentown (38)
A-2	15	Philadelphia (15)
A-3	4	Philadelphia (4)
A-4	2	Philadelphia (2)
C	29	OLDA (3), Oxford 4032E (26)

[a]Numbers in parentheses are numbers of strains per subgroup. Data are from references 9, 17, 23, and 27.

Studies by Mao et al. (13) at the Centers for Disease Control with 45 strains of Lp1 showed endonuclease *Cla*I to be the most effective of 12 endonucleases in fragmenting the DNA of Lp1 before probing with labeled rRNA. The Lp1 strains were separated into nine subgroups with this technique. Each international MAb subgroup contained one to three ribotypes.

In one legionellosis outbreak investigated by the Centers for Disease Control (12), the epidemic strains from patients matched isolates from the potable water system at two lodges where the patients stayed. Other Lp1 strains from two control lodges and an industrial plant visited by the patients were compared by MAb reactivity, ribotyping, and ET. Results comparing the use of three different endonucleases before probing with rRNA showed that the clinical and environmental isolates from the two suspect lodges were identical and that the others were different. Further comparison of the epidemic strains with a Benidorm type strain (1-2-5-7 reactivity pattern) from Los Angeles showed that the Los Angeles strain was the same by MAb reactivity and ET but different by ribotyping.

The ribotyping procedure was used by Pang et al. (16) to compare Lp3 strains in two epidemics. *Hind*III, *Eco*RV, and *Cla*I digests each yielded matching environmental and clinical subtypes. Further examination of other strains of Lp3 showed as many as 19 different restriction fragment length polymorphism patterns and a maximum of eight ribotypes with *Cla*I digests and five ribotypes each with *Hind*III and *Eco*RV. However, the visualization of bands after treatment with an endonuclease was more subjective than ribotyping.

OTHER MOLECULAR METHODS

Results reported by Saunders et al. (20, 21) show that the use of the biotinylated probes NS20 and NS21 after digestion with *Nci*I could be more effective than standard ribotyping. Examination of a large number of strains with this technique showed that at least 39 distinct patterns could be seen with Lp1 strains. Seven to ten bands were generated. Eight clinical isolates from the Stafford outbreak were indistinguishable, and one of six environmental isolates from the outbreak at the British Broadcasting Corporation had a pattern identical to that of the clinical strains. The use of the pentanucleotide site-specific *Nci*I endonuclease was superior by Simpson's discrimination indices to use of *Cla*I, a hexanucleotide site-specific enzyme. It is interesting to note that eight phenotypically distinct strains from a single environmental source were indistinguishable. The authors propose that variants from a single genomic type might account for this occurrence.

Other subtyping techniques such as pulsed field electrophoresis of DNA (15) and outer membrane analyses (23) should also be mentioned as candidates for subtyping.

SUMMARY

All of the techniques discussed in this report are useful and complementary. MAb reactivity remains a useful screening procedure. However, the use of DNA or RNA probes to hybridize with DNA nicked by an endonuclease such as *Nci*I is a very discriminating procedure. Recent advances with the use of *Sfi*I to restrict DNA that is separated by pulsed-field gel electrophoresis has enabled effective use of this tool to separate *Legionella* strains (15).

Obviously, the application of DNA separation techniques to subtyping is most productive. As we improve our capabilities with the polymerase chain reaction technology, perhaps we can subtype as we detect. Ultimately, recognition of specific portions of amplified DNA should allow us to subtype legionellae directly from clinical or environmental samples.

REFERENCES

1. Aye, T., K. Wachsmuth, J. C. Feeley, R. J. Gibson, and S. R. Johnson. 1981. Plasmid profiles of *Legionella* species. *Curr. Microbiol.* **6**:389–394.
2. Barbaree, J. M. 1991. Legionnaires' disease: factors affecting the transmission of *Legionella* species form aerosol-emitting equipment to people. *ASHRAE J.* **33**:38–42.
3. Barbaree, J. M., and W. Martin. 1988. Rapid dot blot procedure for identification of *Legionella*, abstr. C-52, p. 340. *Abstr. 88th Annu. Meet. Am. Soc. Microbiol. 1988.*
4. Brown, A., M. Lema, C. A. Ciesielski, and M. J. Blaser. 1985. Combined plasmid and peptide analysis of clinical and environmental *Legionella pneumophila* strains associated with a small cluster of Legionnaires' disease cases. *Infection* **13**:163–166.
5. Cherry, W. B., B. Pittman, P. P. Harris, G. A. Herbert, B. M. Thomason, L. Thacker, and R. E. Weaver. 1978. Detection of Legionnaires' disease bacteria by direct immunofluorescent staining. *J. Clin. Microbiol.* **8**:329–338.
6. Grimont, F., M. Lefevre, E. Ageron, and P. A. D. Grimont. 1989. rRNA gene restriction patterns of *Legionella* species: a molecular identification system. *Res. Microbiol.* **140**:615–626.
7. Grimont, F., M. Lefevre, and P. Grimont. 1987. Taxonomic des *Legionella*, p. 3–8. *In* J. Fleurette, N. Bornstein, D. Marmet, and M. Surgot (ed.), *Colloque Legionella.* Faculté de Médecine, Alexis Carrel, Lyon, France.
8. Johnson, S. R., and W. O. Shallo. 1982. Plasmids of serogroup-1 strains of *Legionella pneumophila. Curr. Microbiol.* **7**:143–146.
9. Joly, J. R., R. M. McKinney, J. O. Tobin, W. F. Bibb, I. D. Watkins, and D. Ramsay. 1986. Development of a standardized subgrouping scheme for *Legionella pneumophila* serogroup 1 using monoclonal antibodies. *J. Clin. Microbiol.* **23**:768–771.
10. Maher, W. E., J. F. Plouffe, and M. F. Para. 1983. Plasmid profiles of clinical and environmental isolates of *Legionella pneumophila* serogroup 1. *J. Clin. Microbiol.* **18**:1422–1423.
11. Mahoney, F. J., C. W. Hoge, T. A. Farley, J. M. Barbaree, R. F. Breiman, R. F. Benson, and L. M. McFarland. 1992. Communitywide outbreak of Legionnaires' disease associated with a grocery store mist machine. *J. Infect. Dis.* **165**:736–739.
12. Mamolen, M., R. Breiman, J. Barbaree, K. Stone, J. Spika, D. Dennis, and R. Vogt. 1989. Legionnaires' dis-

ease outbreak due to identical strains at 2 lodges, abstr. C-376, p. 456. *Abstr. 89th Annu. Meet. Am. Soc. Microbiol. 1989.*
13. Mao, S., J. M. Barbaree, Y. Wang, L. M. Graves, B. Swaminathan, M. Mamolen, and R. F. Breiman. 1989. Ribotypes of *Legionella pneumophila* serogroup 1, abstr. D-183, p. 113. *Abstr. 89th Annu. Meet. Am. Soc. Microbiol. 1989.*
14. Nolte, F. S., C. A. Conlin, A. J. M. Roisin, and S. R. Redmond. 1984. Plasmids as epidemiological markers in nosocomial Legionnaires' disease. *J. Infect. Dis.* **149**:251–256.
15. Ott, M., L. Bender, R. Marre, and J. Hacker. 1991. Pulsed field electrophoresis of genomic restriction fragments for the detection of nosocomial *Legionella pneumophila* in hospital water supplies. *J. Clin. Microbiol.* **29**:813–815.
16. Pang, Y., J. Barbaree, B. Swaminathan, W. Morrill, G. Sanden, T. Mastro, and P. Houck. 1990. Molecular epidemiology of *Legionella pneumophila* serogroup 3 using restriction fragment length polymorphism and ribotyping, abstr. D-44, p. 87. *Abstr. 90th Annu. Meet. Am. Soc. Microbiol. 1990.*
17. Para, M. F., and J. F. Plouffe. 1983. Production of monoclonal antibodies to *Legionella pneumophila* serogroups 1 and 6. *J. Clin. Microbiol.* **18**:895–900.
18. Plouffe, J. F., M. F. Para, W. E. Maher, B. Hackman, and W. L. Webster. 1983. Subtypes of *Legionella pneumophila* serogroup 1 associated with different attack rates. *Lancet* **ii**:649–650.
19. Rogers, F. G., and A. W. Pasculle. 1991. *Legionella*, p. 442–453. *In* A. Balows, W. J. Hausler, Jr., K. L. Herrmann, H. D. Isenberg, and H. J. Shadomy (ed.), *Manual of Clinical Microbiology*, 5th ed. American Society for Microbiology, Washington, D. C.
20. Saunders, N. A., T. G. Harrison, A. Haththotuwa, N. Kachwalla, and A. G. Taylor. 1990. A method for typing strains of *Legionella pneumophila* serogroup 1 by analysis of restriction fragment length polymorphisms. *J. Med. Microbiol.* **31**:45–55.
21. Saunders, N. A., T. G. Harrison, A. Haththotuwa, and A. G. Taylor. 1991. A comparison of probes for restriction fragment length polymorphism (RFLP) typing of *Legionella pneumophila* serogroup 1 strain. *J. Med. Microbiol.* **35**:152–158.
22. Selander, R. K., R. M. McKinney, T. S. Whittam, W. F. Bibb, D. J. Brenner, F. S. Nolte, and P. E. Pattison. 1985. Genetic structure of populations of *Legionella pneumophila. J. Bacteriol.* **163**:1021–1037.
23. Stout, J. E., J. Joly, M. Para, J. Plouffe, C. Ciesielski, M. J. Blaser, and V. L. Yu. 1988. Comparison of molecular methods for subtyping patients and epidemiologically linked environmental isolates of *Legionella pneumophila. J. Infect. Dis.* **157**:486–495.
24. Thomason, B. M., and W. F. Bibb. 1984. Use of absorbed antisera for demonstration of antigenic variation among strains of *Legionella pneumophila* serogroup 1. *J. Clin. Microbiol.* **19**:794–797.
25. Tobin, J. O., I. D. Watkins, S. Woodhead, and R. G. Mitchell. 1986. Epidemiological studies using monoclonal antibodies to *Legionella pneumophila* serogroup 1. *Isr. J. Med. Sci.* **22**:711–714.
26. Tompkins, L. S., N. J. Troup, T. Woods, W. Bibb, and R. M. McKinney. 1987. Molecular epidemiology of *Legionella* species by restriction endonuclease and alloenzyme analysis. *J. Clin. Microbiol.* **25**:1875–1880.
27. Watkins, I. D., J. O. Tobin, P. J. Dennis, W. Brown, R. Newnham, and J. B. Kurtz. *Legionella pneumophila* serogroup 1 subgrouping by monoclonal antibodies—an epidemiological tool. *J. Hyg.* **95**:211–216.
28. Wilkinson, H. W., and B. J. Fikes. 1980. Slide agglutination test for serogrouping *Legionella pneumophila* and atypical *Legionella*-like organisms. *J. Clin. Microbiol.* **11**:99–101.

Detection and Molecular Serogrouping of *Legionella pneumophila* by Polymerase Chain Reaction Amplification and Restriction Enzyme Analysis

ASIM K. BEJ, MEENA H. MAHBUBANI, AND RONALD M. ATLAS

Department of Biology, University of Alabama at Birmingham, UAB Station, Birmingham, Alabama 35294–1170, and Department of Biology, University of Louisville, Belknap Campus, Louisville, Kentucky 40292

Background and objectives. Gram-negative bacteria of *Legionella* spp. are natural inhabitants of water bodies (5) and infect humans via contaminated aerosols. Most outbreaks of legionellosis have been determined to have been community acquired (4). Of all *Legionella* spp., *Legionella pneumophila* has been found to be the common cause of pulmonary infections in patients. Reingold et al. (11) reported that 80 to 85% of *Legionella* infections are caused by various serogroups of *L. pneumophila*. Furthermore, their study showed that approximately 70 to 75% of the *L. pneumophila* infections are caused by serogroups 1 and 6. In a separate study, Tram et al. (15) reported that in the United States 61% and in France 89% of clinical isolates belong to serogroup 1 and that 6% of clinical isolates belong to serogroup 3. Epidemiological study of a pathogen provides valuable information about the source of an outbreak of a disease. With this information, further spread of the disease can be prevented by eradicating the causative pathogen from the source. Subtyping of a pathogen, which is an essential component of an epidemiological study, has been reported for *L. pneumophila* by serogrouping (7), plasmid analysis (6), peptide profiling (9), immunochemical methods that use absorbed antisera and monoclonal antibodies (6), alloenzyme analysis (13), and restriction endonuclease analysis of whole cell DNA (14). Restriction endonuclease analysis of total genomic DNA has the advantage of discriminating among *L. pneumophila* strains lacking plasmids (14, 16). However, electrophoretic patterns of the total genomic DNA digests are often difficult to interpret. To overcome this problem, Tram et al. (15) have described an alternative approach that uses radiolabeled probe fingerprint analysis following restriction endonuclease digestion of the total genomic DNA of *L. pneumophila*. Application of the polymerase chain reaction (PCR) method (12) allows a unique DNA segment characteristic of a target microbial pathogen to be amplified to 10^6 copies (1, 3). All 14 serogroups of *L. pneumophila* have been identified by PCR amplification of a portion of the macrophage infectivity potentiator (*mip*) gene (10). However, application

of the PCR method for differentiating various serogroups of *L. pneumophila* has not been reported. In this study, we used PCR amplification followed by restriction endonuclease analysis of a portion of the amplified *mip* gene as a potential tool for identifying (and possibly subtyping) various *L. pneumophila* serogroups.

Approach. The *L. pneumophila* strains used in this study are described in Table 1. Total genomic DNAs from all strains of *L. pneumophila* were purified as described elsewhere (2). Purified genomic DNA from each strain was subjected to PCR amplification using two 21-mer primers, *Lmip*L920 (5'-GCTACAGACAAGGATAAGTTG-3') and *Lmip* R1548 (5'-GTTTTGTATGACTTTAATTCA-3') (10). PCR amplification conditions were as follows. After initial denaturation of the template DNA at 94°C for 3 min, 25 cycles of PCR amplification of the target *mip* gene were performed; each cycle consisted of denaturation of the template DNA at 94°C for 1 min, primer annealing to the template DNA at 55°C for 1 min, and primer extension at 72°C for 2 min. In each PCR cycle, 0.5 μM each primer, 200 μM each deoxynucleoside triphosphate, 2.5 U of AmpliTaq DNA polymerase (Perkin-Elmer Cetus), and a 1× PCR reaction buffer containing 50 mM Tris-Cl (pH 8.9), 50 mM

TABLE 1. *L. pneumophila* strains used in this study

Strain	Serogroup	Source
Knoxville-1	1	CDC[a]
Togus-1	2	CDC
Bloomington-2	3	CDC
Los Angeles-1	4	ATCC 33156
Dallas-1E	5	ATCC 33216
Chicago-2	6	CDC
Chicago-8	7	ATCC 33823
Concord-3	8	ATCC 35096
IN-23-G1-Cs	9	ATCC 35289
Leiden	10	ATCC 43283
797-PA-H	11	ATCC 43130
570-PA-H	12	ATCC 43290
82A3105	13	ATCC 43736
1169-MN-H	14	ATCC 43703

[a]CDC, Centers for Disease Control.

173

KCl, and 2.5 mM MgCl$_2$ were used. An aliquot of the PCR-amplified DNA was directly used for restriction endonuclease treatment according to the procedure described by the manufacturer. The nucleotide sequence of the *L. pneumophila mip* gene reported by Engleberg et al. (8) was analyzed for the presence of possible restriction enzyme sites within the amplified region of the gene by using the program PC-Gene.

Polymorphism of the PCR-amplified *mip* gene. The PCR-amplified DNAs from all 14 serogroups of *L. pneumophila* were analyzed by gel electrophoresis and showed slight variations in size. *L. pneumophila* serogroups 1 to 3 and 6 to 8 showed the expected amplified DNA bands of 0.65 kb, whereas larger DNA bands were observed for serogroups 5, 9, 10, 12, and 14, and slightly smaller amplified DNA bands were found for serogroups 4, 11, and 13. This result suggests that although the *mip* gene has been reported to be conserved in *L. pneumophila* (10), it is polymorphic. This information can be useful for epidemiological investigations.

Restriction endonuclease analysis of PCR-amplified *mip* DNA. *L. pneumophila* serogroup 1, which is found to be prevalent during outbreaks of legionellosis, showed a unique restriction pattern when treated with *Alu*I. Also, digestion with *Hae*III differentiated serogroup 11 from the other serogroups, and single digestion with *Fok*I, *Rsa*I, *Mae*II, *Hpa*II, *Hae*III, and *Alu*I differentiated serogroup 5 from the other serogroups. Treatment with *Scr*FI separated serogroup 8 from the other serogroups, and Serogroup 6 could be distinguished by treatment with *Hpa*II. Serogroup 5 showed maximum diversity with most of the restriction endonucleases.

Utility of this study. Variations in sizes of the amplified *mip* gene of all 14 serogroups of *L. pneumophila* tested in this study indicated the presence of polymorphism within the gene. This approach can be adopted for subtyping various isolates of *L. pneumophila*. However, the differences in sizes of the amplified DNA within various serogroups of *L. pneumophila* are so small that it may be difficult to interpret the result. This study showed that treatment with various restriction enzymes following PCR amplification may provide more definitive information about various serogroups of *L. pneumophila*. In addition, several serogroups can be differentiated upon treatment with specific restriction enzymes. The information from this study needs to be tested for consistency and reproducibility on various isolates of a specific serogroup before the method is used as a tool for epidemiological study during an outbreak of *Legionella*-caused pneumonia. However, subtyping of *L. pneumophila* by using PCR ampli-

fication of the *mip* gene followed by restriction enzyme treatment has the potential to provide valuable epidemiological information in such an event.

REFERENCES

1. **Atlas, R. M., and A. K. Bej.** 1990. Detecting bacterial pathogens in environmental water samples by using PCR and gene probes, p. 399–406. *In* M. Innis, D. Gelfand, D. Sninsky, and T. White (ed.), *PCR Protocols: a Guide to Methods and Applications.* Academic Press, New York.
2. **Ausubel, F. M., R. Brent, R. E. Kingston, D. D. Moore, J. A. Smith, J. G. Sideman, and K. Struhl** (ed.). 1987. *Current Protocols in Molecular Biology.* John Wiley & Sons, Inc., New York.
3. **Bej, A. K., and M. H. Mahbubani.** 1992. Application of the polymerase chain reaction in environmental microbiology. *PCR Methods Appl.* **1:**151–159.
4. **Best, M., V. L. Yu, J. Stout, A. Goetz, R. R. Muder, and F. Tayler.** 1983. Epidemiologic assessment of methods of transmission of legionellosis. *Zentralbl. Bakteriol. Mikrobiol. Hyg. 1 Abt. Orig.* A **255:**52–57.
5. **Broome, C. V.** 1983. Epidemiologic assessment of methods of transmission of legionellosis. *Zentralbl. Bakteriol. Mikrobiol. Hyg. 1 Abt. Orig.* A **255:**52–57.
6. **Brown, A., R. M. Vickers, E. M. Elder, M. Lema, and G. M. Garrity.** 1982. Plasmid and surface antigen markers of endemic and epidemic *Legionella pneumophila* strains. *J. Clin. Microbiol.* **16:**230–235.
7. **Conlan, J. W., and L. W. Ashworth.** 1986. The relationship between the serogroup antigen and lipopolysaccharide of *Legionella pneumophila.* *J. Hyg.* **96:**39–48.
8. **Engleberg, N. C., C. Carter, D. R. Weber, N. P. Cianciotto, and B. I. Eisenstein.** 1989. DNA sequence of *mip*, a *Legionella pneumophila* gene associated with macrophage infectivity. *Infect. Immun.* **57:**1263–1270.
9. **Lema, M., and A. Brown.** 1983. Electrophoretic characterization of soluble protein extracts of *Legionella pneumophila* and other members of the family *Legionellaceae.* *J. Clin. Microbiol.* **17:**1132–1140.
10. **Mahbubani, M. H., A. K. Bej, R. Miller, L. Haff, J. DiCesare, and R. M. Atlas.** 1990. Detection of *Legionella* with polymerase chain reaction and gene probe methods. *Mol. Cell. Probes* **4:**175–187.
11. **Reingold, A. R., B. M. Thomason, B. J. Brake, L. Thacker, H. W. Wilkinson, and J. N. Kuritsky.** 1984. Legionella pneumonia in the United States: the distribution of serogroups and species causing human illness. *J. Infect. Dis.* **148:**819.
12. **Saiki, R. K., S. Scharf, F. Faloona, K. B. Mullis, G. T. Horn, H. A. Erlich, and N. Arnheim.** 1985. Enzymatic amplification of β-globin genomic sequences and restriction site analysis for diagnosis of sickle cell anemia. *Science* **230:**1350–1353.
13. **Selander, R. K., R. M. McKinney, T. S. Whittman, W. F. Bibb, D. J. Brenner, F. S. Nolte, and P. E. Pattison.** 1985. Genetic structure of populations of *Legionella pneumophila.* *J. Bacteriol.* **163:**1021–1037.
14. **Tompkins, L. S., N. J. Troup, T. Woods, W. F. Bibb, and R. M. McKinney.** 1987. Molecular epidemiology of *Legionella* species by restriction endonuclease and alloenzyme analysis. *J. Clin. Microbiol.* **25:**1875–1880.
15. **Tram C., M. Simonet, M. Nicholas, C. Offredo, F. Grimont, M. Lefevre, E. Ageron, A. Debure, and P. A. D. Grimont.** 1990. Molecular typing of nosocomial isolates of *Legionella pneumophila* serogroup 3. *J. Clin. Microbiol.* **28:**242–245.
16. **van Ketel, R. J., J. ter Schegget, and H. C. Zanen.** 1984. Molecular epidemiology of *Legionella pneumophila* serogroup 1. *J. Clin. Microbiol.* **20:**362–364.

Comparison of Culture and Polymerase Chain Reaction To Detect Legionellae in Environmental Samples

W. T. MARTIN, B. S. FIELDS, AND L. C. HUTWAGONER

National Center for Infectious Diseases, Centers for Disease Control, Atlanta, Georgia 30333

Water samples were collected as part of an epidemiological investigation of nosocomial legionellosis. Aliquots (2 to 100 ml) of 99 samples (5 to 1,000 ml) were frozen at −70°C for subsequent testing by the polymerase chain reaction (PCR). The samples were cultured for legionellae by using Centers for Disease Control isolation procedures. Selective and nonselective α-ketoglutarate-supplemented buffered charcoal-yeast extract agar was used to isolate legionellae. Water samples were (i) plated directly, (ii) filter concentrated and plated, (iii) acid treated and plated, or (iv) subjected to a combination of these procedures, depending on the number of indigenous bacteria in the water sample (1).

Developmental *Legionella* PCR kits and protocols supplied by Perkin-Elmer Cetus Corp. (now Roche Molecular Systems; Perkin-Elmer is the exclusive vendor) were the EnvironAmp Sample Preparation Kit, the EnvironAmp PCR Amplification Kit, and the EnvironAmp PCR Detection Kit. Briefly, samples were filter concentrated, and cells were lysed on the filters. An aliquot of each lysed sample was added to the PCR reaction mix containing the primers that specify which DNA sequences to amplify. The PCR reaction tubes were placed in a Perkin-Elmer Cetus Thermal Cycler and amplified for 30 cycles. Selected samples were retested at 35 cycles. The PCR products were confirmed by hybridization to immobilized biotinylated probes specific for the PCR-amplified DNA sequences of *Legionella pneumophila*, *Legionella* species, and an internal positive control. Ninety-nine water samples were tested by PCR, and the results were compared with the culture results for each sample (Table 1). Of 99 samples, 48 were culture positive for legionellae. Twenty-five samples inhibited the PCR, as indicated by the absence of any reaction, including the internal positive control, at 30 and 35 cycles. Thirteen of these 25 PCR-inhibited samples were culture positive. Another 13 samples were negative by PCR (positive only on the internal positive control), and all 13 were culture negative. Twenty-nine samples were positive for *L. pneumophila* by PCR, and 23 of these samples were also culture positive. An additional 32 samples were positive for *Legionella* species other than *L. pneumophila* by PCR, and 12 of these samples were culture positive. When the 13 PCR-negative, culture-negative samples were retested at 35 cycles, 1 sample remained negative, 1 became positive for *L. pneumophila*, and 11 became positive for other legionellae, some of which may have been

TABLE 1. Detection of legionellae by culture and PCR

PCR	Culture		
	Positive	Negative	Total
Inhibited	13	12	25
Negative	0	13	13
L. pneumophila positive	23[a]	6	29
Legionella species positive[b]	12[c]	20	32
Total	48[d]	51	99

[a] Twenty-one *L. pneumophila* isolates plus two *Legionella* spp. other than *L. pneumophila*.
[b] *L. pneumophila* is excluded.
[c] Eight *L. pneumophila* isolates plus four *Legionella* spp. other than *L. pneumophila*.
[d] One culture-negative, PCR *L. pneumophila*-positive sample was recultured and grew *L. pneumophila*. This isolate was added to the culture-positive tally.

nonspecific reactions. For those samples which did not inhibit amplification, PCR detected *L. pneumophila* in 29 samples, 6 more than were detected by culture. *Legionella* species other than *L. pneumophila* were found in 32 samples, 12 of which were culture positive. Overall, excluding inhibited samples, the number of positive samples detected by PCR was significantly greater than the number positive by culture (61 versus 35; McNemar's test for matched pairs; P < 0.005). Some *Legionella* species are known to grow more slowly and to be more fastidious than *L. pneumophila*, which could account for some of the greater sensitivity of PCR. The culture results were not categorized by species because *L. pneumophila* in low numbers can combine with low numbers of other legionellae to give a positive PCR reaction to *Legionella* species. Excepting inhibited samples, the PCR results for *L. pneumophila* appear to be sensitive and specific. Either the detection of non-*L. pneumophila* species is more sensitive by PCR than by culture or some nonspecific reactions occurred. This question is especially apparent when one considers that after 35 cycles, 12 of 13 culture-negative, PCR negative (30 cycles) samples became PCR positive. The inhibition of PCR by some water samples is being investigated, as is the possibility of nonspecificity with some of the non-*L. pneumophila* primers. A new formulation of the PCR reaction mix and a new thermocycler program are now under evaluation.

REFERENCE

1. **Gorman, G. W., J. M. Barbaree, and J. C. Feeley.** 1983. *Procedures for the Recovery of Legionella from Water.* Centers for Disease Control, Atlanta.

Evaluation of a DNA Amplification Procedure for Detection of *Legionella pneumophila* and *Legionella dumoffii* in Water

J. S. LOUTIT AND L. S. TOMPKINS

Division of Infectious Disease, Department of Medicine, and Department of Microbiology and Immunology, Stanford University, Stanford, California 94305

Legionella pneumophila and *Legionella dumoffii* have been significant causes of morbidity and mortality in patients undergoing cardiothoracic surgery at Stanford University Medical Center (SUMC) since 1980. Despite extensive epidemiologic investigations from 1980 through 1989, no link between culture-positive potable water for *L. pneumophila* and infected patients could be made. In addition, no water samples were culture positive for *L. dumoffii* until 1989. At that time, tap water culture positive for *L. dumoffii* from three rooms in the intensive-care unit was epidemiologically linked to three patients with sternal wound infections (3). It is unclear why this is the only time that we were able to culture *L. dumoffii* from an epidemiologic source even though a significant number of patients were infected with *L. dumoffii*. It had been previously suggested that the bacteria may be in a "non-cultivatable" or "nonviable" form (1); this hypothesis suggested that culture of water samples may be too insensitive to be used in epidemiologic investigations, which might explain the previous inability to grow *L. dumoffii*.

Amplification of target DNA sequences of *L. pneumophila* and *L. dumoffii* before probing with specific chromosomal DNA fragments should overcome these difficulties and allow detection of these forms. Our group has developed and reported a polymerase chain reaction (PCR) amplification/DNA dot blot or Southern hybridization detection method for both *L. pneumophila* (8) and *L. dumoffii* (2). This detection method using PCR primers from random fragments of chromosomal DNA from these two organisms is both sensitive and species specific.

Other authors have described the use of PCR amplification for the detection of legionellae in water. PCR primers derived from the 5S rRNA gene will detect all *Legionella* species, while primers from a portion of the coding region of the macrophage infectivity potentiator protein can be used to detect all serogroups of *L. pneumophila* (4). While these methods are very sensitive and species specific, there have been no published trials of their use in epidemiologic investigations.

We describe the use of this PCR amplification/Southern hybridization method for the detection of *L. pneumophila* and *L. dumoffii* in water samples collected from 1980 through 1989 at SUMC and samples collected during a recent epidemiologic investigation in Pittsburgh, Pa., of community-acquired Legionnaires disease.

Water samples were collected in sterile plastic containers and stored at 4°C. Water collected in Pittsburgh was analyzed within 4 months of collection, while those collected at SUMC were stored for 2 to 8 years before analysis. Primer and probe sequences used for *L. pneumophila* and *L. dumoffii* have previously been reported (2, 8). These samples were then subjected to the following methods. Water samples (1 ml) were centrifuged at 12,000 rpm for 20 min and then resuspended in 100 μl of digestion buffer (6, 9) containing 100 mM Tris-HCl, 1 mM EDTA (pH 8.5), 2% Laureth-12 (PPG/Mazer Chemicals, Gurnee, Ill.), and 400 μg of proteinase K per ml. Following incubation at 55°C for 2 h and then at 95°C for 10 min, 10 μl of this mixture was added to each PCR tube. Amplification mixture was added so that each tube contained the following: 50 mM KCl, 10 mM Tris-chloride (pH 8.3), 1.5 mM MgCl$_2$, 200 μM each deoxynucleoside triphosphate, 0.2 μM each deoxyoligonucleotide (LEG 1:LEG 2 or LDBKS-1:LDBKS-3), and 1.25 U of AmpliTaq DNA polymerase (Perkin-Elmer Cetus, Norwalk, Conn.). Sterile distilled water was added so that the final sample volume was 50 μl in each tube, and then the contents were overlaid with 40 μl of filter-sterilized mineral oil. Amplification was carried out in a programmable thermal controller (MJ Research, Inc., Watertown, Mass.) for 35 cycles, with each cycle consisting of 1 min at 94°C, 1 min at 55°C, and 2 min at 74°C.

The amplified DNA was electrophoresed through 1.0% agarose gels, denatured (0.4 N NaOH, 0.6 M NaCl), renatured (0.5 M Tris HCl [pH 7.5], 1.5 M NaCl), and transferred to Hybond-N (Amersham, Arlington Heights, Ill.) transfer membranes by the method of Southern (7). The membranes were incubated in prehybridization buffer of 6× NaCl/EDTA/Tris (1× NaCl/EDTA/Tris is 0.15 M NaCl, 1 mM EDTA, and 0.03 M Tris-HCl [pH 8.0]), 0.5% Nonidet P-40, and denatured salmon sperm DNA (100 μg/ml) for 3 h at 65°C. The probe (LEG 3 or LDBKS-4) was end labeled with [γ-^{32}P] dATP by using polynucleotide kinase (5). Hybridization was done at 42°C for 16 to 18 h in 6× NaCl/EDTA/Tris-0.5% Nonidet P-40–250 μg of yeast tRNA per ml–50 ng of the probe per ml. Following hybridization, the nylon membranes were washed three times in 50 ml of 6× SSC (1× SSC is 0.15 M

NaCl plus 0.015 M sodium citrate) for 5 min at 42°C, allowed to dry, and exposed to Kodak XAR-5 film (Eastman Kodak, Rochester, N.Y.).

Forty-one water samples from SUMC collected over the 7-year period were analyzed for the presence of *L. pneumophila* (Table 1, comparison A). In the five samples that were culture positive and PCR negative, the bacterial counts were all less than 3 CFU/ml. Three samples were culture negative and PCR positive. In these samples, the hybridization signal after probing with LEG 3 was weak, indicating the low number of organisms present.

These same 41 water samples from SUMC were analyzed for the presence of *L. dumoffii* (Table 1, comparison A). No culture-negative, PCR-positive or culture-positive, PCR-negative samples were detected.

In addition, 15 samples collected in Pittsburgh as part of an epidemiologic investigation of community-acquired Legionnaires disease were tested for *L. pneumophila*. The results of culture and PCR analysis are shown in Table 1, comparison B. No culture-negative, PCR-positive samples were observed.

The overall results of these amplification systems for *L. pneumophila* and *L. dumoffii* as compared with culture for the two sets of samples are summarized in Table 1, comparison C. The results for *L. dumoffii* showed very high sensitivity and specificity, but no water samples with colony counts of less than 30/ml were analyzed. The results for *L. pneumophila* showed a decreased sensitivity but high specificity and good predictive values for this method of detection.

The overall sensitivity of this method as compared with culture for detection of *L. pneumophila* in water samples collected during these two epidemiologic studies was 53% (Table 1, comparison C), with minimal improvement detected when water samples were tested promptly after collection. The lack of agreement between the culture and PCR results occurred most commonly when colony counts were less than 10/ml. This relatively low sensitivity may reflect the small volume (1 ml) of water that was tested, sampling variability, DNA degradation, or the presence of inhibitors in the samples.

The detection method for *L. dumoffii* was highly sensitive and specific, with no culture-positive PCR-negative results being observed. The water samples that were culture positive and PCR positive had colony counts of >30/ml. It is likely that a decrease in sensitivity and specificity, such as seen with *L. pneumophila*, would be observed if water samples with lower colony counts were tested.

Overall, the PCR amplification/Southern hybridization detection method that we used for *L. pneumophila* and *L. dumoffii* did not appear to be

TABLE 1. Comparisons of PCR and culture results

Comparison[a]	Organism	No. of strains					Sensitivity (%)	Specificity (%)	Predictive value	
		Culture +, PCR+	Culture −s, PCR+	Culture+, PCR−	Culture+, PCR−	Culture −, PCR−			Positive	Negative
A	*L. pneumophila* (n = 41)	5	3		5	28	50	90	0.62	0.85
	L. dumoffii (n = 41)	6	0		0	35	100	100	1	1
B	*L. pneumophila* (n = 15)	3	0		2	10	60	100	1	0.83
C	*L. pneumophila* (n = 56)	8	3		7	38	53	93	0.73	0.84
	L. dumoffii (n = 41)	6	0		0	35	100	100	1	1

[a] A, PCR amplification detection system for *L. pneumophila* and *L. dumoffii* versus culture on water samples collected during epidemiologic investigations at SUMC; B, PCR amplification detection system for *L. pneumophila* versus culture on water samples collected during an epidemiologic investigation in Pittsburgh; C, overall combined results for a PCR amplification detection system for *L. pneumophila* and *L. dumoffii* versus culture on water samples collected during epidemiologic investigations at SUMC (A) and Pittsburgh (B).

more sensitive than established culture techniques, and no significant new reservoirs for these organisms were detected.

The PCR amplification method of detection for *L. dumoffii* was highly sensitive and species specific; however, further testing of larger volumes of water samples containing fewer organisms is necessary.

These studies were supported in part by NIH grant AI30618 and a Technology Transfer Award from Stanford University Hospital, both to L.S.T.

REFERENCES

1. **Hussong, D., R. R. Colwell, M. O'Brien, E. Weiss, A. D. Pearson, R. M. Weiner, and W. D. Burge.** 1987. Viable *Legionella pneumophila* not detectable by culture on agar media. *Bio/Technology* **5**:947–950.
2. **Loutit, J. S., and L. S. Tompkins.** 1990. Detection of *Legionella dumoffii* in water by DNA amplification and hybridization, abstr. 1033, p. 258. *Program Abstr. 30th Intersci. Conf. Antimicrob. Agents Chemother.*
3. **Lowry, P. W., R. J. Blankenship, W. Gridley, N. J. Troup, and L. S. Tompkins.** 1991. A cluster of legionella sternal wound infections due to postoperative topical exposure to contaminated tap water. *N. Engl. J. Med.* **324**:109–113.
4. **Mahbubani, M. H., A. K. Bej, R. Miller, L. Haff, J. DiCesare, and R. M. Atlas.** 1990. Detection of *Legionella* with the polymerase chain reaction and gene probe methods. *Mol. Cell. Probes* **4**:175–187.
5. **Sambrook, J., E. F. Fritsch, and T. Maniatis.** 1989. *Molecular Cloning: a Laboratory Manual.* Cold Spring Harbor Laboratory, Cold Spring Harbor, N.Y.
6. **Shibata, D. K., N. Arnheim, and W. J. Martin.** 1988. Detection of human papilloma virus in paraffin-embedded tissue using the polymerase chain reaction. *J. Exp. Med.* **167**:225–230.
7. **Southern, E. M.** 1975. Detection of specific sequences among DNA fragments separated by gel electrophoresis. *J. Mol. Biol.* **98**:503–517.
8. **Starnbach, M. N., S. Falkow, and L. S. Tompkins.** 1989. Species-specific detection of *Legionella pneumophila* in water by DNA amplification and hybridization. *J. Clin. Microbiol.* **27**:1257–1261.
9. **Wright, D., and M. Manos.** 1990. Sample preparation from paraffin-embedded tissues, p. 153–158. *In* M. Innis, D. Gelfand, J. Sninsky, and T. White (ed.), *PCR Protocols: a Guide to Methods and Applications.* Academic Press, Inc., San Diego, Calif.

Rapid Detection of Legionellae in Clinical and Environmental Samples by Polymerase Chain Reaction

M. NOWICKI, N. BORNSTEIN, B. JAULHAC, Y. PIEMONT, H. MONTEIL, AND J. FLEURETTE

Centre d'Etudes et de Recherches Bactériologiques, Institut Pasteur de Lyon, and Laboratoire National de la Santé, Centre National de Référence des Légionelloses, Faculté de Médecine Alexis Carrel, rue Guillaume Paradin, 69372 Lyon, and Institut de Bactériologie de la Faculté de Médecine, Université Louis Pasteur, 3 rue Koeberlé, 67000 Strasbourg, France

Among members of the family *Legionellaceae*, *Legionella pneumophila* is the main etiological agent of legionellosis. This gram-negative bacterium, a natural inhabitant of environmental water, may infect people via contaminated aerosols from natural reservoirs, water distribution systems, and air conditioning systems. The aerosols may also be induced by hospital equipment such as showers, humidifiers, or respiratory equipment (5). Detection of legionellae in clinical and environmental samples is currently based on the direct fluorescent antibody assay (DFA), which lacks sensitivity, and on time-consuming methods. DNA amplification, recently reported for water samples artificially contaminated with legionellae (1, 6), may represent an interesting tool for detection of the organisms in various types of samples.

The aim of this study was to develop a polymerase chain reaction (PCR) technique based on the amplification of a portion of the *mip* gene (3) for the detection of legionellae in clinical and environmental samples and compare the results with those obtained by DFA and culture techniques.

The sensitivity and specificity of DNA amplification were previously evaluated (4) from *Legionella* reference strains and from non-*Legionella* bacterial species frequently isolated from environmental waters and the respiratory tract.

Bronchoalveolar lavage (BAL) fluids obtained from 96 patients were tested. Among these samples, 36 were culture positive for *legionellae* and 60 were negative.

Fifty-three water samples from different sources (tap, shower, pond, and spring water) were tested. Legionellae were isolated from 23 samples, and 30 were culture negative. The majority of water samples were contaminated with non-*Legionella* bacteria.

For sample preparation, a 2-ml aliquot of each BAL fluid was mixed with an equal volume of phosphate-buffered saline and centrifuged for 15 min at $3,500 \times g$. This wash step was repeated twice. Water samples (1 liter) were first concentrated to a 10-ml volume by centrifugation and/or filtration (2). The concentrated samples were then centrifuged for 10 min at $3,500 \times g$. The pellets obtained from BAL or water samples were subjected to a previously described cell lysis protocol (4).

Two primers bracketing a 630-bp-long fragment

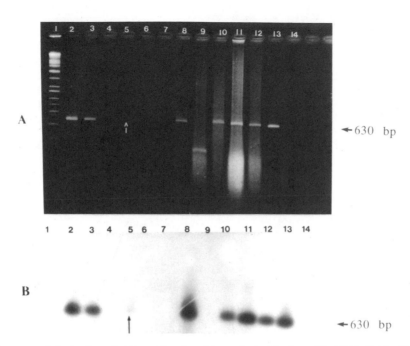

FIG. 1. Agarose gel electrophoresis (A) and Southern blot analysis (B) of amplified BAL fluids. Molecular size markers: lane 1, Raoul Appligene; lane 2, preamplified products. PCR controls: lane 3, 10 ng of DNA from *L. pneumophila* serogroup 1; lane 4, MilliQ water (Millipore). In the other lanes, the numbers (CFU per milliliter) of *L. pneumophila* serogroup 1 in BAL fluids were as follows: lane 5, 90; lane 6, 10; lane 7, 10; lane 8, 2×10^2; lane 10, 2×10^2; lane 11, 5×10^2; lane 12, 10^3; lane 13, 9×10^2; and lane 14, 0. Lane 9, 10 CFU of *L. jordanis* per ml.

from the *mip* gene sequence were chosen as described elsewhere (4) and synthesized. Primer 1 (Lmp-1) (5'-GGTGACTGCGGCTGTTATGG-3') was located between nucleotides 853 and 872 following the initiation codon, and primer 2 (Lpm-2) (5'-GGCCAATAGGTCCGCCAACG-3') was located at nucleotides 1465 to 1484 complementary to the coding strand. A detection probe (Lpm-3) (5'-CAGCAATGGCTGCAAC-CATGCCAC-3') located at nucleotides 888 to 912 from the coding strand was also synthesized and 5' labeled with $[\gamma\text{-}^{32}\text{P}]\text{ATP}$ (>3,000 Ci/mmol; Amersham International, Amersham, United Kingdom).

The samples (20 µl) were amplified within a 100-µl PCR reaction mixture. Then 40 cycles of amplification were performed in a DNA thermal cycler (PHC2 Techne) as follows: 2 min for denaturation at 92°C, 2 min for annealing at 62°C, and 2 min for primer extension at 74°C. After the last amplification cycle, the temperature was kept at 74°C for 5 min for a final extension step. To avoid contamination of samples, sample preparation, PCR amplification, and electrophoresis were performed in three different rooms. Each PCR run included a negative control consisting of the reaction mixture without any DNA. Electrophoresis and Southern blot hybridization were performed

as previously described (4).

The primers and probe used permitted the detection of *L. pneumophila* serogroups 1 to 14, *L. micdadei*, and *L. bozemanii* serogroup 1. The DNA from other *Legionella* species was not amplified (Figure 1). None of the DNAs obtained from the other bacterial species tested was amplified. The lowest level of detection was reproducibly estimated to be 50 CFU when Southern blot hybridization was used (4).

After DNA amplification, 100% of BAL fluids with *Legionella* concentrations of between 40 and 3×10^3 CFU/ml were found to be PCR positive (Table 1). Moreover, 50% of BAL fluids containing 10 or 20 CFU were also PCR positive. The lowest detection level for the DFA assay was determined to be 10^2 CFU.

Among the 60 BAL fluids that were culture negative, 7 were positive after DNA amplification. The clinical records of these seven patients showed that four of them had serologically diagnosed clinical legionellosis. For the three patients with suspected legionellosis, no serological diagnosis was made, but all other etiologies were excluded.

For 18 of 23 water samples containing legionellae (Table 2) as detected by culture, a positive signal was visualized at 630 bp. The

TABLE 1.   Detection of *Legionella* spp. in culture-positive BAL fluids by DNA amplification

No. of samples	DFA	No. of legionellae in BAL fluids (CFU/ml)	Strain isolated	Result after amplification	
				Gel electrophoresis	Southern blot hybridization
6	+	$1 \times 10^3 - 3 \times 10^3$	*L. pneumophila* serogroup 1	+	+
6	+	$4 \times 10^2 - 9 \times 10^2$	*L. pneumophila* serogroup 1	+	+
2	+	10^2	*L. pneumophila* serogroup 1	+	+
3	−	90	*L. pneumophila* serogroup 1	−	+
1	−	40	*L. pneumophila* serogroup 1	−	+
1	−	20	*L. pneumophila* serogroup 1	−	+
4	−	10	*L. pneumophila* serogroup 1	−	+
1	−	20	*L. pneumophila* serogroup 1	−	−
5	−	10	*L. pneumophila* serogroup 1	−	−
1	+	4×10^3	*L. pneumophila* serogroup 3	+	+
1	−	40	*L. pneumophila* serogroup 3	−	+
1	+	2×10^3	*L. pneumophila* serogroup 5	+	+
1	+	10^3	*L. pneumophila* serogroup 6	+	+
1	+	2×10^2	*L. bozemanii* serogroup 1	+	+
1	+	80	*L. micdadei*	+	+
1	−	10	*L. jordanis*	−	−

TABLE 2.   Detection of *Legionella* spp. by DNA amplification in culture-positive samples collected from environmental waters

No. of samples	Origin[a]	No. of legionellae in concentrate (CFU)	Results after amplification	
			Gel electrophoresis	Southern blot hybridization
3	SSW	$1 \times 10^4 - 2.3 \times 10^4$	+	+
7	SSW	$1 \times 10^3 - 6 \times 10^3$	+	+
6	WDS	$1 \times 10^2 - 5.8 \times 10^2$	+	+
1	SSW	60	−	+
1	SSW	58	−	+
1	WDS	3.6×10^{2b}	−	−
1	SSW	1.3×10^{2c}	−	−
1	SSW	3×10^{2d}	−	−
1	WDS	48	−	−
1	WDS	8	−	−

[a]SSW, spa spring water; WDS, water distribution system.
[b]*L. pneumophila* (20%), *L. oakridgensis*, and *L. dumoffii*.
[c]*L. pneumophila* (50%) and *L. oakridgensis*.
[d]*L. pneumophila* (50%) and *L. dumoffii*.

negativity of the test for 5 of the 23 culture-positive samples is probably due to a low concentration of *L. pneumophila*. Two of these samples contained a single *Legionella* species. *L. pneumophila*, at low concentrations (8 and 48 CFU). The three negative samples contained a mix of two *Legionella* species, but the predominant species isolated (*L. dumoffii* or *L. oakridgensis*) could not be amplified by the primers used; the associated *L. pneumophila* species was not detected. The 30 water samples without legionellae in culture were all negative by DNA amplification even when they were contaminated with other bacterial species.

All samples gave similar results when the tests were repeated. The DNA amplification technique described here, using primers and a detection probe from the *mip* gene sequence, enables detection of the *Legionella* species most frequently implicated in respiratory tract infections. The detection level achieved in water samples was about 100 CFU/liter, lower than the theoretical infectivity level for humans (10^3 CFU/liter), which makes this method potentially useful for epidemiological surveys. In conclusion, the genomic amplification method described here appears to be a promising tool for the rapid detection of legionellae in clinical and environmental samples.

REFERENCES

1. **Bej, A. K., M. H. Mahbubani, and R. M. Atlas.** 1991. Detection of viable *Legionella pneumophila* in water by polymerase chain reaction and gene probe methods. *Appl. Environ. Microbiol.* **57:**597–600.

2. **Bornstein, N., C. Vieilly, D. Marmet, M. Surgot, and J. Fleurette.** 1985. Isolation of *Legionella anisa* from a hospital hot water system. *Eur. J. Clin. Microbiol.* **4**:327–330.
3. **Engleberg, N. C., C. Carter, D. R. Weber, W. P. Cianciotto, and B. I. Edelstein.** 1989. DNA sequence of *mip*, a *Legionella pneumophila* gene associated with macrophage infectivity. *Infect. Immun.* **57**:1263–1270.
4. **Jaulhac, B., M. Nowicki, N. Bornstein, O. Meunier, G. Prévost, Y. Piemont, J. Fleurette, and H. Monteil.** 1992. Detection of *Legionella* spp. in bronchoalveolar lavage fluids by DNA amplification. *J. Clin. Microbiol.* **30**:920–924.
5. **Mastro, T. D., B. S. Fields, R. F. Breiman, J. Campbell, B. D. Plikaytis, and J. S. Spika.** 1991. Nosocomial Legionnaires' disease and use of medication nebulizers. *J. Infect. Dis.* **163**:667–671.
6. **Starnbach, M. N., S. Falkow, and L. S. Tompkins.** 1989. Species-specific detection of *Legionella pneumophila* in water by DNA amplification and hybridization. *J. Clin. Microbiol.* **27**:1257–1261.

Polymerase Chain Reaction, Gene Probe, and Direct Fluorescent Antibody Staining of *Legionella pneumophila* Serogroup 1 in Drinking Water and Environmental Samples

C. PASZKO-KOLVA, H. YAMAMOTO, M. SHAHAMAT, AND R. R. COLWELL

Advanced Technology Laboratories, Alta Loma, California 91701; Department of Microbiology, University of Maryland, College Park, Maryland 20742; and Gifu University School of Medicine, Tsukasa-Machi 40, Gifu, Japan

Classical methods for the detection of *Legionella* species involved guinea pig inoculation or direct culture of the organisms on laboratory media (3, 6). Subsequently, direct detection methods employed commercially available fluorescent antibody conjugates (4, 9). More recently, the polymerase chain reaction (PCR) and nucleic acid probe detection methods have been introduced (2, 11). Several techniques based on these methods have been either newly developed or adapted from earlier methods for environmental monitoring. These newer developments, which include monoclonal antibodies directed against heat shock proteins, PCR directed against mRNAs, and gene probes (2, 11, 12), have been able to detect either unique epitopes on the cell surface or nucleic acid sequences through amplification and hybridization. Current research (2, 12) has established that these new techniques are able to detect "healthy" cells (i.e., cells in active culture). However, little is known concerning the ability of immunological and nucleic acid techniques to detect injured, starved, or nonculturable cells (10). Before new methodologies can be implemented in routine monitoring of the environment, extensive laboratory and field evaluations are required, and the results derived therefrom must be carefully analyzed. The objective of our study was to evaluate the efficacy of culture, immunological, and nucleic acid techniques in the detection of *Legionella* species after long-term storage (for 1.5 to 3 years) of the *Legionella* cells under oligotrophic conditions.

An environmental isolate of *Legionella pneumophila* serogroup 1, designated strain 082 and characterized by previously described biochemical, serological, and nucleic acid techniques (9),

was used in this study. Microcosms were used as the test system to examine long-term survival of the cells in both drinking and creek water. Cells grown in α-ketoglutarate-supplemented buffered charcoal-yeast extract (BCYEα) broth were harvested by centrifugation and washed to reduce carryover of nutrients into the microcosms. After washing, cells were inoculated at initial concentrations of 10^7 and 10^4/ml in acid-washed glass bottles containing 900 ml of autoclaved and filtered drinking or creek water. One set of microcosms (initial cell concentration of 10^4/ml) was incubated at ambient temperature (23°C) without agitation. The second set (initial cell concentration of 10^7/ml) was incubated at 15°C on a shaker (100 rpm). Microcosms containing strain 082 were routinely monitored for 535 days. Samples were aseptically removed from the microcosms, cultured on BCYEα, and simultaneously enumerated by acridine orange direct counts (AODC) (7) and direct fluorescent antibody (DFA) staining (4).

In addition, a 10-ml subsample was removed from each microcosm, concentrated by centrifugation, and prepared for DNA amplification. The primer pair (LP-A [5'-GTC ATG AGG CTC GCT G-3'] and LP-B [5'-CTG GCT TCT TCC AGC TTC A 3']) described by Starnbach et al. (11) was used to amplify a species-specific DNA sequence (800 bp) of *L. pneumophila*. Amplified DNA was detected by using gel electrophoresis, biotin-labeled probes (8), and ethidium bromide staining, with visualization using a UV transilluminator.

Figure 1 illustrates the survival of *L. pneumophila* serogroup 1 initial concentration of 10^7 cells/per ml) in sterile creek and drinking water microcosms, as measured by CFU per milliliter and fluorescence microscopy (AODC). *Le-*

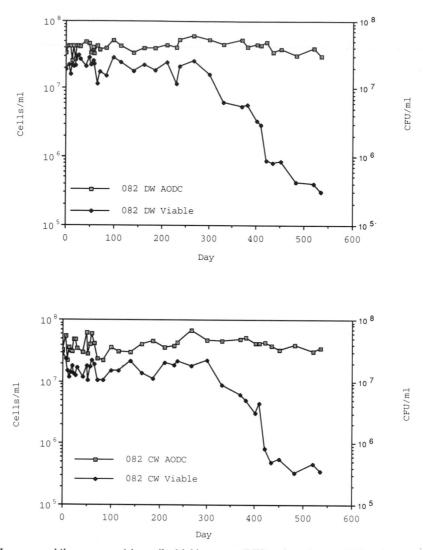

FIG. 1. *L. pneumophila* serogroup 1 in sterile drinking water (DW) and creek water (CW) microcosms incubated at 15°C for 535 days. Colony counts of cells (CFU per milliliter) and direct counts (AODC) are shown.

gionella cells in the microcosms during 1.5 to 3 years in both waters revealed strong DFA staining reactions throughout the study period. Viable counts of both microcosms declined by 2 logs to 10^5 cells per ml. Even after 1.5 years in the microcosm, the *Legionella* cells remained culturable. The *Legionella* cells (initial concentration of 10^7 cells per ml) were readily detected by PCR and gene probe techniques, as was expected (Fig. 2, lanes 2 and 3). The drinking water microcosm containing an initial *Legionella* concentration of 10^4 cells per ml became nonculturable (9, 10) after 51 days (data not shown). However, the microcosm was held for 1.5 years, after which the cells were subjected to DFA staining and to PCR and gene probe analyses. *Legionella* cells were detected by DFA staining at concentrations of 10^3

cells per ml. Probe results from the non-culturable *Legionella* microcosm were negative, and amplified products were not detected by agarose gel electrophoresis (lane 4), even after double PCR (lane 5). It is believed that the chromosomal DNA of many of the *Legionella* cells which were nonculturable after incubation for 51 days in the drinking water microcosms underwent subsequent degradation.

DFA staining as presently done does not provide information on viability. PCR and gene probes, employing suitable primers to detect mRNAs or genes involved in vital cell processes, may be more useful in this regard (2). However, the sensitivity of PCR has to be established as being greater than that of DFA staining for analyzing environmental samples. Inhibitors of the PCR

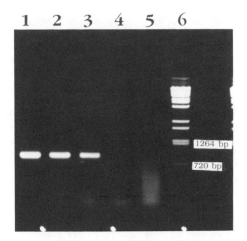

1264 bp

720 bp

FIG. 2. Ethidium bromide-stained agarose gel electrophoresis of PCR amplification products, using 35 cycles of PCR. Lanes: 1, *L. pneumophila* GIFU 9134 (10^5 cells per ml); 2, *L. pneumophila* 082 CW (10^5 cells per ml); 3, *L. pneumophila* 082 DW (10^5 cells per ml); 4, nonculturable *L. pneumophila* 082 TW; 5, additional PCR of the sample in lane 4; 6, λ DNA digested with *Bst*PI.

must be identified and removed before the results are conclusive. It is suggested that for detection of legionellae in environmental samples, PCR and gene probes be used in conjunction with DFA staining. Together, these techniques provide a total count of *Legionella* cells and an estimate of cell integrity, i.e., retention of at least a significant portion of the genome. It is concluded that *Legionella* cells whose chromosomal DNA may have undergone partial lysis or damage after long-term storage in water remain intact and detectable by DFA staining. Further research is required to determine the effects of environmental and chemical parameters, including temperature, pH, predation, ozone, and chlorine, on the ability of PCR and gene probes to detect their specific nucleic acid targets. When the latter have been suitably developed for environmental samples, the combination of PCR and gene probes with DFA staining will provide a powerful method for detection of *Legionella* species and other pathogens in the environment.

REFERENCES

1. **Anand, C. M., A. R. Skinner, A. Malic, and J. B. Kurtz.** 1983. Interaction of *Legionella pneumophila* and a free-living amoeba (*Acanthamoeba palestinensis*). *J. Hyg.* **91:**167–178.
2. **Bej, A. K., M. H. Mahbubani, and R. M. Atlas.** 1991. Detection of viable *Legionella pneumophila* in water by polymerase chain reaction and gene probe methods. *Appl. Environ. Microbiol.* **57:**597–600.
3. **Benson, R. F., W. L. Thacker, R. P. Waters, P. A. Quinlivan, W. R. Mayberry, D. J. Brenner, and H. W. Wilkinson.** 1989. *Legionella quinlivanii* sp. nov. isolated from water. *Curr. Microbiol.* **18:**195–197.
4. **Cherry, W. B., P. P. Pittman, G. A. Harris, B. M. Herbert, L. Thomason, W. L. Thacker, and R. E. Weaver.** 1978. Detection of Legionnaires' disease bacteria by direct immunofluorescent staining. *J. Clin. Microbiol.* **8:**329–338.
5. **Ezaki, T., S. Dejsirilert, H. Yamamoto, N. Takeuchi, S. Liu, and E. Yabuuchi.** 1988. Simple and rapid genetic identification of *Legionella* species with aphotobiotin-labeled DNA. *J. Gen. Appl. Microbiol.* **34:**191–199.
6. **Fliermans, C. B., W. B. Cherry, L. H. Orrison, and L. Thacker.** 1979. Isolation of *Legionella pneumophila* from nonepidemic related aquatic habitats. *Appl. Environ. Microbiol.* **37:**1239–1242.
7. **Hobbie, J. E., R. J. Daley, and S. Jasper.** 1977. Use of Nuclepore filters for counting bacteria by fluorescence microscopy. *Appl. Environ. Microbiol.* **33:**1225–1228.
8. **Lo, Y.-M., W. Z. Mehal, and K. A. Fleming.** 1988. Rapid production of vector-free biotinylated probes using the polymerase chain reaction. *Nucleic Acids Res.* **16:**8719.
9. **Paszko-Kolva, C., H. Yamamoto, M. Shahamat, T. K. Sawyer, G. Morris, and R. R. Colwell.** 1991. Isolation of amoebae and *Pseudomonas* and *Legionella* spp. from eyewash stations. *Appl. Environ. Microbiol.* **57:**163–167.
10. **Rozak, D. B., and R. R. Colwell.** 1987. Survival strategies of bacteria in the natural environment. *Microbiol. Rev.* **52:**365–379.
11. **Starnbach, M. N., S. Falkow, and L. S. Tompkins.** 1989. Species-specific detection of *Legionella pneumophila* in water by DNA amplification and hybridization. *J. Clin. Microbiol.* **27:**1257–1261.
12. **Steinmetz, I., C. Rheinheimer, I. Hubner, and D. Bitter-Suermann.** 1991. Genus-specific epitope on the 60-kilodalton *Legionella* heat shock protein recognized by a monoclonal antibody. *J. Clin. Microbiol.* **29:**346–354.
13. **Wright, J. B., I. Ruseska, M. A. Athar, S. Cobert, and J. W. Costerton.** 1989. *Legionella pneumophila* grows adherent to surfaces in vitro and in situ. *Infect. Control Hosp. Epidemiol.* **10:**408–415.

Comparison of Methods for Subtyping *Legionella pneumophila*

MARC J. STRUELENS, NICOLE MAES, ARIANE DEPLANO, NICOLE BORNSTEIN, AND FRANCINE GRIMONT

Microbiology Laboratory, Hôpital Erasme, University of Brussels, Brussels 1070, Belgium; Centre National de Référence des Légionelloses, Faculté de Médecine Alexis Carrel, 69372 Lyon Cedex 2, France; and Unité des Entérobactéries, Unité INSERM 199, Institut Pasteur, F-75724 Paris Cedex 15, France

Because *Legionella pneumophila* serogroup 1 is the *Legionella* species most frequently isolated from infected patients and the environment, epidemiologic studies on the sources of sporadic and epidemic Legionnaires disease require subtyping of clinical and environmental isolates (2–4, 6, 9).

Monoclonal antibodies (MAbs) have been commonly used to screen phenotypic differences between *L. pneumophila* strains, and several methods of DNA fingerprinting have been applied for further discrimination (2, 3, 6, 8–10). In contrast to the majority of investigations, in which matching of phenotypes and genotypes confirmed the source of infections (2, 3, 6, 9, 10), we observed a discrepancy between MAb types isolated from patients and the epidemiologically linked water source during a nosocomial outbreak in a university hospital (7). These findings prompted us to further characterize these outbreak-related and control *L. pneumophila* isolates by means of four discriminating molecular methods.

Clinical isolates of *L. pneumophila* (serogroups 1 and 6) from 20 patients with nosocomial infections were compared with *L. pneumophila* (serogroup 1) isolates from the hospital hot water system. Eighteen control isolates of *L. pneumophila* (serogroups 1 and 6) included epidemiologically unrelated isolates from Belgian patients with sporadic infection, environmental isolates from other Belgian hospitals, and type strains. MAb typing was performed with the Oxford panel (8) and repeated in two other laboratories with the Oxford and the standardized panels (3). Restriction endonuclease analysis was performed with *Eco*RI and *Hind*III (2), and Southern hybridization was carried out with the randomly cloned chromosomal DNA probe λL2 from an *L. pneumophila* (serogroup 3) strain (9). Multilocus enzyme electrophoresis of 19 enzymes was performed as previously described (5). Pulsed-field gel electrophoresis of macrorestriction fragments of genomic DNA digested with *Not*I, *Nhe*I, and *Sma*I was performed in 1% agarose in Tris-borate-EDTA buffer (200 V), using a CHEF-DR II apparatus (Bio-Rad Laboratories, Nazareth, Belgium) (4). For *Not*I digests, pulses were increased from 60 to 90 s for 24 h and maintained at 90 s for 3 h; for *Nhe*I and *Sma*I fragments, pulses were increased from 0.5 to 2 s for 12 h then ramped from 4 to 8 s for 12 h.

MAb typing indicated that the Pontiac/Benidorm subtype accounted for 18 of 22 isolates from patients with nosocomial *L. pneumophila* serogroup 1 infection. In contrast, this subtype was not found in 42 water isolates of this serogroup recovered during the outbreak, and it was present in only 6 of 105 isolates recovered during the 4-year surveillance of the disinfected hot water system ($P < 0.0001$, Fisher exact test). The remaining clinical isolates as well as the majority of water isolates belonged to the Bellingham subtype. By multilocus enzyme electrophoresis, restriction endonuclease analysis, and Southern hybridization, all nosocomial isolates from Erasme Hospital belonged to one of two clones of *L. pneumophila* serogroup 1 and serogroup 6, re-

spectively, and all hospital water isolates belonged to the first clone (Table 1).

By pulsed-field electrophoresis of macrorestriction fragments, outbreak-associated isolates of *L. pneumophila* serogroup 1 were confirmed to be clonally related. Identical restriction patterns were obtained in all isolates with *Nhe*I and *Sma*I (29 and 28 fragments, respectively), whereas a minor variation between two restriction profiles of 5 and 6 fragments (patterns Ia and Ib, respectively) was observed with the rare cutter *Not*I. Interestingly, these genotypic variants correlated with the MAb subtype (Table 1).

By the combined genotypic techniques, the epidemic clone was distinct from control stains of *L. pneumophila* serogroup 1 ($P < 0.001$, Fisher exact test). The highest discriminatory power was obtained with pulsed-field gel electrophoresis of macrorestriction fragments, followed by restriction endonuclease analysis, multilocus electrophoresis, Southern blot analysis, and MAb typing. In addition to its high discriminatory ability, macrorestriction analysis provided well-resolved, easily compared patterns, thereby allowing determination of interstrain relatedness. This technique, therefore, appears very promising for the epidemiologic and phylogenetic study of *Legionella* and other bacterial species.

In contrast to most previous investigations of outbreaks of legionellosis (2, 6, 8), MAb typing in this study showed discordant results between clinical isolates and isolates from the epidemiologically linked source of infection. In one study, two of seven hospital outbreaks were associated with predominance of Pontiac, or MAb 2-positive, strains in patients, while Bellingham strains predominated in the environmental source (6), as was observed in our setting. From a practical point of view, our early results with MAb typing could have led us to the incorrect conclusion that the water system was not the source of the majority of nosocomial infections. The combination of four genotypic methods, on the other hand, proved highly discriminating: each control strain showed a distinct DNA type, whereas all nosocomial patient isolates of *L. pneumophila* serogroup 1 matched the water isolates as belonging to a single clone. Successful epidemic control by means of water disinfection confirmed the accuracy of genotypic results (7).

What are the possible explanations for this discrepancy between phenotypic and genotypic results? The first hypothesis to consider is that of sampling bias. Assuming that two *Legionella* strains colonized the water system and infected hospitalized patients, our difficulty in identifying the predominant epidemic MAb type in the water reservoir may have been due to the sampling of sites not representative of the actual sources or to preferential isolation of one subtype by environ-

TABLE 1. Phenotypic and genotypic characteristics of *L. pneumophila* isolates from Erasme Hospital and epidemiologically unrelated sources

Category	Source	Serogroup	MAb		MEE[a]	REA[b]	SB[c]	MREA[d]
			Oxford panel	Standardized panel				
Erasme Hospital	Patients ($n = 5$)	1	Pontiac	Benidorm	1	A	a	Ia
	Patient ($n = 1$)	1	Pontiac	Philadelphia	1	A	a	Ib
	Patients ($n = 4$)	1	Bellingham	Bellingham	1	A	a	Ib
	Water ($n = 2$)	1	Pontiac	Benidorm	1	A	a	Ia
	Water ($n = 6$)	1	Bellingham	Bellingham	1	A	a	Ib
	Patients ($n = 2$)	6			9, —	M_1, M_2	f	—
Unrelated sources	Patient; CA[e]	1	Pontiac	Benidorm	8	C	d	II
	Patient; CA	1	OLDA	Oxford	6	I	—	III
	Patient; CA	1	OLDA		—	H	a	IV
	Patient; CA	1	Pontiac		—	K	e	V
	Patient; CA	1	Pontiac		—	K	e	V
	Hospital A; water	1	Bellingham	Bellingham	7	E	b	VI
	Hospital B; patient	1	Pontiac		5	F	c	VII
	Hospital C; patient	1	Pontiac		1	G	a	VIII
	Factory A; water	1	Pontiac		1	A	a	IX
	NCTC[f]; Philadelphia-1	1	Pontiac	Philadelphia	3	B	c	X
	NCTC; Bellingham-1	1	Bellingham	Bellingham	2	D	b	XI
	NCTC; OLDA	1	OLDA	OLDA	4	A	a	Ic
	Erasme Hospital; patient, CA	6			—	N	c	—
	Nursing home; water ($n = 3$)	6			—	O_1, O_2	c, —	—
	NCTC; Chicago-2	6			—	P	c	—
	Factory B; water ($n = 2$)	6			—	Q	—	—

[a]MEE, multilocus enzyme electrophoresis.

[b]REA, restriction enzyme analysis of total DNA with *Eco*RI and *Hind*III. Letters indicate major restriction profiles, and numbers indicate variants distinguished by one restriction fragment difference.

[c]sb, Southern blot hybridization of *Hind*III-restricted DNA with a λ L2 probe.

[d]MREA, macrorestriction analysis of genomic DNA with *Not*I, *Sma*I, and *Nhe*I. Roman numerals denote major restriction profiles, and letters indicate variants distinguished by one restriction fragment difference.

[e]CA, community acquired.

[f]NCTC, National Collection of Type Cultures.

mental versus clinical culture techniques. This hypothesis is not supported by the methods used for sampling environmental sites, which included several hundred specimens from outlets located in the rooms where acquisition of legionellae was documented. In addition, water and clinical specimens were processed by similar isolation techniques (acid decontamination, selective and nonselective buffered charcoal-yeast extract medium incubated for 10 days at 37°C). A second explanation is that a higher attack rate may have been associated with the MAb 2/Pontiac strain, which is considered to be more virulent. This would explain the inverse proportion of Pontiac/Bellingham subtypes in isolates from patients versus the environmental reservoir. No significant difference in 50% lethal dose for guinea pigs infected by the aerosol route could be found among four representative isolates of both subtypes (10), although this model may not have been sensitive enough to detect differential strain survival in aerosol. Finally, a third possibility to consider is that of phenotypic instability in the environment or during patient infection, a possibility also suggested in a detailed environmental investigation by Harrison et al. (1). Like these authors, we were able to correlate some variations in MAb reactivity with a minor genomic polymorphism within a clonally related group of isolates from an environmental reservoir. It appears unlikely that two strains would have converged to such highly related genotypes; a more likely explanation is that a minor genomic rearrangement occurred in a parent strain. Although we were unable to document in vitro variation in either MAb type or genotype after five subcultures on buffered charcoal-yeast extract medium, Rogers et al. (this volume) have reported in vitro loss of MAb 2 reactivity at a frequency of 10^{-3}. These observations raise questions about the reliability of MAb typing for the epidemiologic study of *L. pneumophila* serogroup 1. We suggest that DNA fingerprinting, by a technique such as pulsed-field gel electrophoresis, may provide a more accurate typing tool.

REFERENCES

1. **Harrison, T. G., N. A. Saunders, A. Haththotuwa, G. Hallas, R. J. Birtles, and A. G. Taylor.** 1990. Phenotypic variation amongst genotypically homogeneous *Legionella pneumophila* serogroup 1 isolates: implications for the investigation of outbreaks of Legionnaires' disease. *Epidemiol. Infect.* **104:**171–180.
2. **Janet, E., M. S. Stout, V. L. Yu, P. Muraca, J. Joly, N. Troup, and L. S. Tompkins.** 1992. Potable water as a cause of sporadic cases of community-acquired Legionnaires' disease. *N. Engl. J. Med.* **3:**151–155.
3. **Joly, J. R., R. M. McKinney, J. O. Tobin, W. F. Bibb, I. D. Watkins, and D. Ramsay.** 1986. Development of a standardized subgrouping scheme for *Legionella pneumophila* serogroup 1 using monoclonal antibodies. *J. Clin. Microbiol.* **23:**768–771.
4. **Ott, M., L. Bender, R. Marre, and J. Hacker.** 1991. Pulsed-field electrophoresis of genomic restriction fragments for the detection of nosocomial *Legionella pneumophila* in hospital water supplies. *J. Clin. Microbiol.* **29:**813–815.
5. **Selander, R. K., R. M. McKinney, T. S. Whittam, W. F. Bibb, D. J. Brenner, F. S. Nolte, and P. E. Pattison.** 1985. Genetic structure of populations of *Legionella pneumophila*. *J. Bacteriol.* **163:**1021–1037.
6. **Stout, J. E., J. Joly, M. Para, J. Plouffe, C. Ciesielski, M. J. Blaser, and V. L. Yu.** 1988. Comparison of molecular methods for subtyping patients and epidemiologically linked environmental isolates of *Legionella pneumophila*. *J. Infect. Dis.* **157:**486–495.
7. **Struelens, M. J., N. Maes, F. Rost, A. Deplano, F. Jacobs, C. Liesnard, N. Bornstein, F. Grimont, S. Lauwers, M. P. McIntyre, and E. Serruys.** 1992. Genotypic and phenotypic methods for the investigation of a nosocomial *Legionella pneumophila* outbreak and efficacy of control measures. *J. Infect. Dis.* **166:**22–30.
8. **Tobin, J. O. H., I. D. Watkins, S. Woodhead, and R. G. Mitchell.** 1986. Epidemiological studies using monoclonal antibodies to *Legionella pneumophila* serogroup 1. *Isr. J. Med. Sci.* **22:**711–714.
9. **Tram, C., M. Simonet, M. H. Nicolas, C. Offredo, F. Grimont, M. Lefevre, E. Ageron, A. Debure, and P. A. D. Grimont.** 1990. Molecular typing of nosocomial isolates of *Legionella pneumophila* serogroup 3. *J. Clin. Microbiol.* **28:**242–245.
10. **Tully, M.** Unpublished data.

Molecular Epidemiology of Outbreak-Associated Serogroup 1 Isolates of *Legionella pneumophila*

W. EHRET, G. ANDING, I. TARTAKOVSKII, AND G. RUCKDESCHEL

Max v. Pettenkofer Institute for Medical Microbiology, University of Munich, Munich, Germany, and Gamaleya Institute of Epidemiology and Microbiology, Academy of Medical Sciences, Moscow, Russia

Legionellosis is a disease that has been reported worldwide. Though the incidence of disease seems to be highly variable among countries, the relative frequency of Legionnaires disease in western and central Europe is probably similar to that of North America. A study performed in the United States in 1990 found *Legionella* species to be the third most frequently isolated etiologic agent (6.7%) in 359 patients with community-acquired pneumonia; in a similar study in Germany, 5.9% of 476 pneumonia patients were diagnosed as suffering from *Legionella* pneumonia (10, 13).

To better understand the epidemiology of Legionnaires disease and to develop appropriate eradication measures, we must be able to identify the water sources involved. In most cases, airborne transmission of bacteria from cooling towers or from potable water systems has been implicated in the spread of disease.

Although more than 30 different *Legionella* species, most of them pathogenic for humans, are currently known, the vast majority of infections are caused by *Legionella pneumophila*. Fourteen serogroups of this species have been identified thus far (2), but most human infections, including the majority of reported outbreaks, are caused by serogroup 1.

L. pneumophila serogroup 1 is not homogeneous, however. Some attempts have been made to develop subgrouping schemes based on monoclonal antibody (MAb) typing. The most widely accepted scheme is that of Joly et al., which resulted in 10 MAb-defined subtypes of serogroup 1 (12). Tobin et al. have reported a subtyping scheme consisting of the three major subgroups, OLDA, Bellingham, and Pontiac (14). The latter subgroup is probably identical with the 1a subgroup of the typing scheme of Joly et al.

Like a number of other authors, we have found a MAb that is able to discriminate between clinical and environmental strains of *L. pneumophila* serogroup 1 (8). In subsequent studies, we found that our MAb B-1 was of the same specificity as the MAb of Tobin et al. for the Pontiac subtype.

Several reports have described molecular tools for the epidemiological characterization of *Legionella* strains. These techniques have used soluble protein patterns (11), DNA restriction endonuclease profiles (15), multilocus enzyme analysis (16), or orthogonal-field-alternation gel electrophoresis (1).

In this study, we compared three methods: protein analysis by sodium dodecyl sulfate-polyacrylamide electrophoresis (SDS-PAGE), restriction enzyme cleavage of genomic bacterial DNA followed by conventional agarose gel electrophoresis (REA), and analysis of the patterns of DNA fragments separated by pulsed-field gel electrophoresis (PFGE). Using these methods, we analyzed strains from a nosocomial outbreak of Legionnaires disease in Bayreuth, Germany, in 1990 with isolates from 11 cases, 3 of them with fatal outcome. A second outbreak from which strains were obtained occurred in a rubber-manufacturing plant in the Russian town of Armavir in 1987.

Clinical and environmental isolates were cultured on α-ketoglutarate-supplemented buffered charcoal-yeast extract (BCYE-α) agar as recommended by Edelstein et al. (6). Bacteria from water samples were concentrated by filtering 500 ml through 0.45-μm-pore-size polycarbonate filters;

the filtrate was suspended in sterile water and inoculated on BCYE-α agar.

The organisms were identified with our own fluorescein-labeled rabbit antisera to the serogroup prototype strains according to the method of Cherry et al. (4). In addition, the ubiquinone content was determined and used to classify the isolates as *L. pneumophila* as described previously (7). Our own MAbs were used to identify the isolates as described elsewhere (8).

The method of membrane protein isolation from *L. pneumophila* strains followed by SDS-PAGE was described in 1985 (9). The technique used for extraction and digestion of bacterial DNA was similar to van Ketel's procedure (15); *Hind*III- and *Eco*RI-cleaved DNA was separated in a 0.7% agarose gel at 1.6 V/cm for 17 h in Tris-borate buffer (pH 8.3). For PFGE, bacterial DNA preparations were cleaved with *Sma*I and *Nae*I in thinly sliced blocks and then electrophoresed through a 1% agarose gel in TBE buffer (44.5 mM Tris-boric acid, 1 mM EDTA [pH 8.3]) at 10°C by using a contour-clamped homogeneous electric field. The conditions for electrophoresis were 200 V for 18 h with pulse times of 1 s. Thereafter, the gels were stained with ethidium bromide and photographed.

While a comparison of the membrane proteins

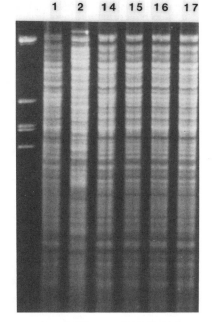

FIG. 1. Cleavage patterns of *Eco*RI-digested genomic DNA of *L. pneumophila* Philadelphia-1 (lane 1) and Knoxville-1 (lane 2) and of strains from different sources from the Armavir outbreak: Armavir-3a (lane 14), Armavir-6a (lane 15), Armavir-7a (lane 16), and Armavir-19a (lane 17).

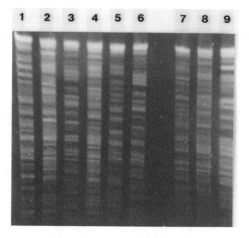

FIG. 2. Comparison of epidemiologically unrelated strains of *L. pneumophila* serogroup 1 by PFGE following *Sma*I cleavage of genomic DNA. Lanes: 1, Philadelphia-1; 2, Knoxville-1; 3, Bellingham-1; 4, OLDA; 5, Stockholm-1; 6, Munich-U-1; 7, Vienna-1; 8, Munich-1; 9, Zurich-1.

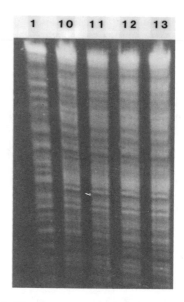

FIG. 3. Cleavage patterns produced by *Sma*I cleavage of genomic DNA separated by PFGE. Lane 1, strain Philadelphia-1; lanes 10 to 13, isolates So 13 (potable water), So 23 (patient lung), So 26 (potable water), and So 27 (potable water), respectively, from the Bayreuth outbreak.

of 11 different epidemiologically unrelated *L. pneumophila* serogroup 1 strains obtained from different parts of the world showed significantly different patterns, the strains from the Bayreuth outbreak were homogeneous in this respect. The strain isolated from a patient's lung exhibited the same membrane protein pattern as did those isolated from different points of the potable water system of this hospital.

Comparison of REA patterns gave the same result. Different DNA fingerprints were observable with epidemiologically unrelated isolates, while the strains from the Bayreuth outbreak (patient and water isolates) were homogeneous by this technique.

The usefulness of the REA technique was also demonstrated by analysis of the strains from the Armavir outbreak (Fig. 1). A homogeneous DNA fragment pattern indicated the clonal identity of the outbreak strain.

Comparison of the *Sma*I-cleaved DNA fragments by PFGE using epidemiologically unrelated *L. pneumophila* serogroup 1 strains resulted in very distinct patterns (Fig. 2). The same result was obtained by using *Nae*I cleavage instead of *Sma*I cleavage of the bacterial DNA. In contrast to these results, the strains from the Bayreuth outbreak showed identical DNA fingerprints with the two enzymes (Fig. 3).

It was interesting that all of our outbreak-associated *L. pneumophila* serogroup 1 strains were attributable to the Pontiac subtype by MAb analysis. This result supports the earlier assumption that the Pontiac subtype may represent a more virulent subgroup (3, 5, 8) or a more predominant environ-

mental strain. Because of this homogeneity, MAb analysis may in certain cases be not discriminatory enough for the study of outbreak strains.

For identification of the clonal identity of an outbreak strain, the various molecular biological techniques proved to be more efficient than MAb analysis. The discriminatory power of SDS-PAGE of bacterial proteins was similar to that of restriction enzyme cleavage of genomic DNA. Clearly superior to both of these techniques was PFGE of genomic bacterial DNA cleaved by *Sma*I or *Nae*I. Although the latter method is somewhat more laborious, it allows clear-cut identification of a specific bacterial clone from an aquatic habitat that may be responsible for cases of Legionnaires disease.

REFERENCES

1. **Bender, L., M. Ott, R. Marre, and J. Hacker.** 1990. Genome analysis of *Legionella* ssp. by orthogonal field alternation gel electrophoresis (OFAGE). *FEMS Microbiol. Lett.* **60:**253–257.
2. **Benson, R. F., W. L. Thacker, H. W. Wilkinson, R. J. Fallon, and D. J. Brenner.** 1988. *Legionella pneumophila* serogroup 14 isolated from patients with fatal pneumonia. *J. Clin. Microbiol.* **26:**382.
3. **Bollin, G. E., J. F. Plouffe, M. F. Para, and R. B. Prior.** 1985. Difference in virulence of environmental isolates of *Legionella pneumophila. J. Clin. Microbiol.* **21:**674–677.
4. **Cherry, W. B., and R. M. McKinney.** 1978. Detection in clinical specimens by direct immunofluorescence, p. 130–145. *In* G. L. Jones and G. A. Hebert (ed.), *Legionnaires'—the Disease, the Bacterium and Methodology.* Centers for Disease Control, Atlanta.

5. Dournon, E., N. Desplaces, P. Rajagopalan, W. F. Bibb and R. M. McKinney. 1986. Recognition of virulent *L. pneumophila* serogroup 1 strains with monoclonal antibodies. *Isr. J. Med. Sci.* **22**:756.

6. Edelstein, P. H., J. B. Snitzer, and S. M. Finegold. 1982. Isolation of *Legionella pneumophila* from hospital potable water specimens: comparison of direct plating with guinea pig inoculation. *J. Clin. Microbiol.* **15**:1092–1096.

7. Ehret, W., K. Jacob, and G. Ruckdeschel. 1987. Identification of clinical and environmental isolates of *Legionella pneumophila* by analysis of outer-membrane proteins, ubiquinones and fatty acids. *Zentralbl. Bakteriol. Hyg. A* **266**:261–275.

8. Ehret, W., B. U. von Specht, and G. Ruckdeschel. 1986. Discrimination between clinical and environmental strains of *Legionella pneumophila* by a monoclonal antibody. *Isr. J. Med. Sci.* **22**:715–723.

9. Ehret, W., and G. Ruckdeschel. 1985. Membrane proteins of *Legionellaceae*. I. Membrane proteins of different strains and serogroups of *Legionella pneumophila*. *Zentralbl. Bakteriol. Hyg. A* **259**:433–445.

10. Fang, G. D., M. Fine, J. Orloff, D. Arisumu, V. L. Yu, W. Kapoor, J. T. Grayston, S. P. Wang, R. Kohler, and R. R. Muder. 1990. New and emerging etiologies for community-acquired pneumonia with implications for therapy. A prospective multicenter study of 359 cases. *Med. Baltimore* **69**:307–316.

11. Ferguson, D. A., Jr., and W. R. Mayberry. 1987. Differentiation of *Legionella* species by soluble protein patterns in polyacrylamide slab gels. *Microbios* **52**:105–114.

12. Joly, J. R., R. M. McKinney, J. O. Tobin, W. F. Bibb, I. D. Watkins, and D. Ramsay. 1986. Development of a standardized subgrouping scheme for *Legionella pneumophila* serogroup 1 using monoclonal antibodies. *J. Clin. Microbiol.* **23**:768–771.

13. Ruf, B., D. Schürmann, I. Horbach, F. J. Fehrenbach, and H. D. Pohle. 1989. The incidence of *Legionella* pneumonia: a 1-year prospective study in a large community hospital. *Lung* **167**:11–22.

14. Tobin, J. O., I. D. Watkins, S. Woodhead, and R. G. Mitchell. 1986. Epidemiological studies using monoclonal antibodies to *Legionella pneumophila* serogroup 1. *Isr. J. Med. Sci.* **22**:711–714.

15. van Ketel, R. J. 1988. Similar DNA restriction endonuclease profiles in strains of *Legionella pneumophila* from different serogroups. *J. Clin. Microbiol.* **26**:1838–1841.

16. Woods, T. C., R. M. McKinney, B. D. Plikaytis, A. G. Steigerwalt, W. F. Bibb, and D. J. Brenner. 1988. Multilocus enzyme analysis of *Legionella dumoffii*. *J. Clin. Microbiol.* **26**:799–803.

Investigation of Nosocomial Legionellosis Using Restriction Enzyme Analysis by Pulsed-Field Gel Electrophoresis

DIANNA J. SCHOONMAKER AND STAN F. KONDRACKI

Wadsworth Center for Laboratories and Research and Bureau of Communicable Disease Control, New York State Department of Health, Box 509, Albany, New York 12201-0509

Epidemiologic investigation of legionellosis is complicated by the ubiquity of legionellae in aquatic habitats. Discriminatory subtyping systems are needed in the investigation of legionellosis to identify common source cases and to identify and control *Legionella pneumophila* in aquatic habitats that serve as sources of exposure for susceptible individuals. Although several techniques, such as monoclonal antibody subtyping (6), plasmid analysis (8), and restriction enzyme analysis (11), have been used in epidemiologic investigations, many of the current subtyping systems cannot readily differentiate between organisms of the same serogroup. Because genetic polymorphism among various bacterial species has been successfully detected by using pulsed-field gel electrophoresis (PFGE) to separate large chromosomal restriction endonuclease fragments (1, 2, 7, 9), a study was initiated to determine whether this technique could be applied to differentiate *L. pneumophila* strains obtained during investigations of outbreaks.

The bacteria used in this study included 52 *L. pneumophila* serogroup 1 and serogroup 6 strains isolated from patient and environmental sources from five nosocomial outbreaks and six control strains (*L. pneumophila* serogroup 1: Knoxville-1, Philadelphia-1, LB376-89, LB394-89, and LB311-89; *L. pneumophila* serogroup 6: Chicago-2) (Table 1). Samples from the respiratory tracts of patients, with and without acid washing (3), were plated on α-ketoglutarate-supplemented buffered charcoal-yeast extract agar (BCYEα) and on BCYEα with added antibiotics, either BCYEα with cefamandole, polymyxin B, and anisomycin (BMPAα) (4) or BCYEα with cephalothin, colistin, vancomycin, and cycloheximide (3). Environmental samples were acid washed, concentrated, or diluted, as needed, and plated on BCYEα, BMPAα, and modified Wadowsky-Yee medium (4, 5). Multiple colonies selected from the same source are designated by a numeral following the specimen number (e.g., LB299-1).

Genomic DNA was prepared by a modification of the procedure of Smith and Cantor (10), using cells that had been grown for 48 h at 37°C on BCYEα slants. To prevent the breakage of DNA that occurs during preparation in solution, bacteria were embedded in agarose prior to lysis. The agarose matrix keeps large DNA molecules intact during detergent and protease treatment, washing, and digestion. *Sfi*I was used for restriction endonuclease digestion. The large chromosomal fragments were separated on a clamped homogeneous electric field apparatus (CHEF-DR II; Bio-Rad Laboratories, Richmond, Calif.) at 200 V with the initial pulse time of 7 s increased linearly to 74 s

TABLE 1. Restriction enzyme analysis using PFGE of *L. pneumophila* serogroup 1 and serogroup 6 isolates

Type of isolate	Serogroup	Patient isolates		Environmental isolates	
		No.	PFGE pattern	No.	PFGE pattern
Outbreak					
1	1	8	5	3	5
2	6	1	12	8	12, 12a, 15, 15a
3	1	3	1	3	1
4	6	2	10	2	10
5	1	3	1		
	6	3	6, 7	16	6, 7, 9, 13, 14
Non-outbreak	1	4	3, 4, 11, 16	1	2
	6	1	8		

over 24 h. Gels were then stained with ethidium bromide, destained in water, and photographed.

In this study, a confirmed case of Legionnaires disease was defined as one in which a patient had fever and radiographic evidence of pneumonia and from whom *L. pneumophila* was isolated from respiratory secretions. To be classified as a nosocomial case, a patient had to have been hospitalized for between 2 and 10 days before the onset of symptoms or to have been readmitted within 10 days of previous discharge.

Investigation of the five nosocomial outbreaks was conducted jointly by personnel from the state and local health departments and the respective hospital infection control unit. All five outbreaks occurred in acute-care hospitals located in upstate New York between June 1989 and January 1992. Epidemiologic follow-up included case/chart review, environmental assessment to identify potential sources, and collection of clinical specimens and environmental water samples. Potable water was implicated as the source in all five outbreaks from the epidemiologic data and by identification of the same serogroup in both clinical and environmental (water) specimens. Cooling towers, humidifiers, air handling systems, or other potential sources were not associated with any of the outbreaks. Two of the outbreaks involved *L. pneumophila* serogroup 1, two involved *L. pneumophila* serogroup 6, and one involved both of these serogroups (Table 1).

Restriction enzyme analysis using PFGE detected 16 banding patterns in the outbreak and control isolates tested (Table 1). Patterns present in patient isolates were identical to patterns found in isolates from the potable water supply of the outbreak hospital in all five instances. With one exception, the PFGE patterns within each outbreak were distinct from patterns present in the other outbreaks and in controls. (*L. pneumophila* serogroup 1 isolates from outbreak 3 and outbreak 5 both had PFGE pattern 1.)

Figures 1 to 4 show the patterns seen by restriction enzyme analysis using PFGE in the nosocomial outbreak and control isolates. Outbreak 1 involved 13 cases that occurred between January and June 1990 in a 220-bed community hospital. Epidemiologic investigation indicated that the cases were confined to the patient care areas of the main building. Environmental sampling in June 1990 resulted in isolation of *L. pneumophila* serogroup 1 from the hot water supply of the main building, with 9 of 13 sites positive. Water samples were negative for the west wing patient care areas, which were also free of legionellosis cases. Central air conditioning cooling towers were not in use when the first cases occurred, and the rooms in the main area of the hospital had individual room air conditioners. The pattern seen in *L. pneumophila* serogroup 1 isolates from patients with nosocomial legionellosis in outbreak 1 (Fig. 1, lanes 2 to 4 and 6 to 10) was identical to the pattern seen in isolates from the main building hot water tank (lane 11) and from hot water in patient room sinks of the main building (lanes 12 and 13). The restriction pattern by PFGE in combination with the results of the epidemiologic investigation suggested that the water system was the source of the *Legionella* infections. The restriction pattern of an isolate (LB376) from a patient who was admitted to the outbreak hospital with legionellosis acquired during vacation to an adjacent state was very similar to the pattern seen in the outbreak isolates, with only minor but reproducible differences (lane 5). The pattern from the nonoutbreak isolate (LB376) had one broad band at approximately 260 kb instead of two bands seen in the outbreak isolates, an additional band at 165 kb, and no band at 97 kb. In most instances, the pattern differences between strains were easily distinguishable.

Figure 2 shows the restriction patterns obtained by PFGE in *L. pneumophila* serogroup 6 isolates from outbreak 2 (lanes 2 to 8) and *L. pneumophila* serogroup 1 isolates from outbreak 3 (lanes 9 to 15). Outbreak 2 involved eight cases in a large teaching hospital. Multiple patterns were seen in the *L. pneumophila* serogroup 6 isolates from out-

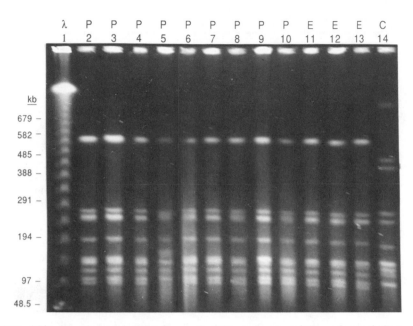

FIG. 1. PFGE of *Sfi*I-cleaved genomic DNA from patient (P), environmental (E), and control (C) *L. pneumophila* serogroup 1 isolates from outbreak 1. Lanes: 2, LB131; 3, LB134; 4, LB246; 5, LB376; 6, LB409; 7, LB506; 8, LB80; 9, LB82; 10, LB90; 11, LB339; 12, LB345; 13, LB351; 14, Knoxville-1. Lambda concatemers (lane 1) were used as molecular size standards (48.5 kb).

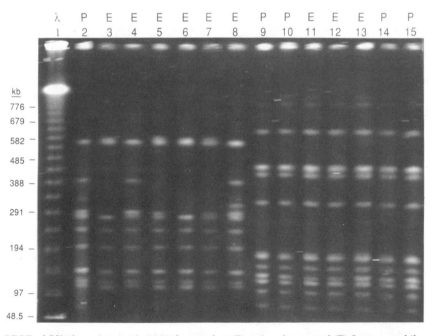

FIG. 2. PFGE of *Sfi*I-cleaved genomic DNA from patient (P) and environmental (E) *L. pneumophila* serogroup 6 (lanes 2 to 8, outbreak 2) and *L. pneumophila* serogroup 1 (lanes 9 to 15, outbreak 3) isolates. Lanes: 2, LB637; 3, LB198; 4, LB199; 5, LB203; 6, LB204; 7, LB238; 8, LB241; 9, LB295; 10, LB293; 11, LB323; 12, LB324; 13, LB327; 14, LB337-1; 15, LB337-2. Lambda concatemers (lane 1) were used as molecular size standards (48.5 kb).

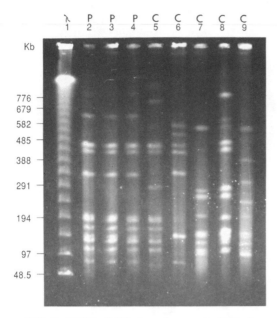

FIG. 3. PFGE of *Sfi*I-cleaved genomic DNA from patient (P) and control (C) *L. pneumophila* serogroup 1 isolates from outbreak 5. Lanes: 2, LB309; 3, LB310; 4, LB469; 5, LB311; 6, LB394; 7, LB246; 8, Knoxville-1; 9, Philadelphia-1. Lambda concatemers (lane 1) were used as molecular size standards (48.5 kb).

break 2. However, identical PFGE patterns were seen in patient (lane 2) and hot water tank 1 (lane 4) isolates. An isolate from a patient room sink showed a very similar pattern (lane 8). Environmental isolates from hot water tank 2 (lane 5) and isolates from room sinks (lanes 3, 6, and 7) had similar patterns. A minor difference was detected between the PFGE pattern of isolates from two room sinks (lanes 3 and 6), which had a single band at approximately 290 kb, and that of isolates from hot water tank 2 and a room sink (lanes 5 and 7), which had a double band at this location. However, the significance of minor differences between strains is not clear at this time, and the possibility that changes in band patterns can occur over time in a dynamic population must also be considered. The PFGE patterns of isolates from this outbreak are very similar, especially when compared with those of epidemiologically unrelated isolates, suggesting that the outbreak isolates are closely related to one another.

Outbreak 3 isolates from patients (Fig. 2, lanes 9, 10, 14, and 15), two hot water tanks (lanes 12 and 13), and the patient shower (lane 11) had identical restriction patterns as detected by PFGE. During the epidemiologic investigation of this outbreak, which occurred in June 1991 at a 420-bed community hospital, it was determined that the cooling towers that serve the air conditioning system had an excellent maintenance program, with biocide treatment every week. Attempts to isolate *Legionella* sp. from the cooling towers were unsuccessful. The fact that the patient and environmental isolates had identical PFGE restriction patterns, together with data from the epidemiologic investigation, indicate that the water supply was the probable source of the *L. pneumophila* infections.

Outbreak 4 involved only two legionellosis cases, both in elderly patients who had been on ventilators in the intensive-care unit of a 550-bed community hospital during March 1990. *L. pneumophila* serogroup 6 was isolated from patients, from the hot water return, and at numerous peripheral sites of the constant-heat, continuous-loop design hot water system in use at this hospital. The PFGE restriction pattern seen in the two patient isolates was identical to the pattern seen in an isolate from the hot water return and in an isolate from the sink in the room occupied by one of the patients. Samples from the roof modules that serviced the air conditioning system (which was not in service at the time of the outbreak) and collection points in the water distribution system upstream from the hot water return were negative for *Legionella* sp. An example of the PFGE pattern of these isolates is shown in Fig. 4, lane 12 (LB104, a hot water return isolate).

Outbreak 5 involved six cases of legionellosis, three caused by *L. pneumophila* serogroup 1 and three caused by *L. pneumophila* serogroup 6. These occurred in the renal transplant unit of a tertiary-care facility. The three *L. pneumophila* serogroup 1 isolates from patients with nosocomial legionellosis had identical PFGE restriction endonuclease patterns (Fig. 3, lanes 2 to 4), suggesting a common source of exposure, even though *L. pneumophila* serogroup 1 was not found in the hospital environment (9a). By contrast, five PFGE patterns were seen in the *L. pneumophila* serogroup 6 isolates from the outbreak. One pattern seen in the *L. pneumophila* serogroup 6 isolate from one patient (Fig. 4, lane 6) was the same as that of the environmental isolates from the hot water tank (lane 8), a patient room sink (lane 7), a second patient room sink (data not shown), and the ultrasound room sink (data not shown). The potable water was therefore felt to be the source of the patient's infection. A second restriction pattern was seen in the *L. pneumophila* serogroup 6 isolates from two other legionellosis cases (Fig. 2, lanes 2 and 3) and in an isolate from the patient shower (Fig. 4, lane 4). Both patients reported using the patient shower, which was therefore felt to be the source of exposure for these patients. A third restriction pattern, not seen in isolates from legionellosis cases, was seen in an *L. pneumophila* serogroup 6 isolate from the hot water tank (Fig. 4, lane 5). *L. pneumophila* serogroup 6

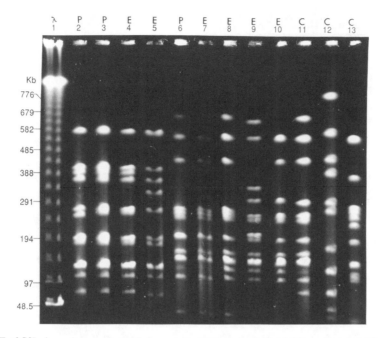

FIG. 4. PFGE of *Sfi*I-cleaved genomic DNA from patient (P), environmental (E), and control (C) *L. pneumophila* serogroup 6 isolates from outbreak 5. Lanes: 2, LB308; 3, LB412; 4, LB286-3; 5, LB299-2; 6, LB312; 7, LB292; 8, LB299-1; 9, LB303; 10, LB329-5; 11, Chicago-2; 12, LB104; 13, LB635. Lambda concatemers (lane 1) were used as molecular size standards (48.5 kb).

was also isolated from two cooling towers. Epidemiologic investigation suggested that these towers were not a likely source of the patients' infections because of their distant, upwind location from the renal transplant unit and the use of individual room air conditioners in patients' rooms rather than opening of room windows. Analysis by PFGE showed that the *L. pneumophila* serogroup 6 isolates from the two towers (Fig. 4, lanes 9 and 10) had PFGE patterns different from those seen in the isolates from the patients and from the water supply. These results suggest that the cooling towers were not the source of the patients' infections or the source of the contamination of the water system. Restriction enzyme analysis using PFGE on isolates from this outbreak indicate that this technique detects sufficient heterogeneity to differentiate strains associated with disease from those in the hospital environment that are not the cause of legionellosis cases.

In summary, restriction enzyme analysis using PFGE detected 16 patterns among 58 *L. pneumophila* isolates from five nosocomial outbreaks and unrelated sources. The identity of the patterns seen in patient and water supply isolates from each outbreak, in combination with epidemiologic data, indicated that the water supply was the source of the strains associated with legionellosis cases in all five instances. Restriction enzyme

analysis using PFGE appears to be a highly discriminatory tool that, when combined with epidemiologic investigation, provides useful information for the detection of common-source cases and the identification of sources of exposure.

REFERENCES

1. **Allardet-Servent, A., N. Bouziges, M.-J. Carles-Nurit, G. Bourg, A. Gouby, and M. Ramuz.** 1989. Use of low-frequency-cleavage restriction endonucleases for DNA analysis in epidemiological investigations of nosocomial bacterial infections. *J. Clin. Microbiol.* **27:**2057–2061.

2. **Anderson, D. J., J. S. Kuhns, M. L. Vasil, D. N. Gerding, and E. N. Janoff.** 1991. DNA fingerprinting by pulsed-field gel electrophoresis and ribotyping to distinguish *Pseudomonas cepacia* isolates from a nosocomial outbreak. *J. Clin. Microbiol.* **29:**648–649.

3. **Bopp, C. A., J. W. Sumner, G. K. Morris, and J. G. Wells.** 1981. Isolation of *Legionella* spp. from environmental water samples by low-pH treatment and use of a selective medium. *J. Clin. Microbiol.* **13:**714–719.

4. **Edelstein, P. H.** 1981. Improved semiselective media for isolation of *Legionella pneumophila* from contaminated clinical and environmental specimens. *J. Clin. Microbiol.* **14:**298–303.

5. **Edelstein, P. H.** 1982. Comparative study of selective media for isolation of *Legionella pneumophila* from potable water. *J. Clin. Microbiol.* **16:**697–699.

6. **Joly, J. R., R. M. McKinney, J. O. Tobin, W. F. Bibb, I. D. Watkins, and D. Ramsay.** 1986. Development of a standardized subgrouping scheme for *Legionella pneumophila* serogroup 1 using monoclonal antibodies. *J. Clin. Microbiol.* **23:**768–771.

7. **Murray, B. E., K. V. Singh, J. D. Heath, B. R.**

Sharma, and G. M. Weinstock. 1990. Comparison of genomic DNAs of different enterococcal isolates using restriction endonucleases with infrequent recognition sites. *J. Clin. Microbiol.* **28:**2059–2063.

8. Nolte, F. S., C. A. Conlin, A. J. M. Roisin, and S. R. Redmond. 1984. Plasmids as epidemiological markers in nosocomial Legionnaires' disease. *J. Infect. Dis.* **149:**251–256.

9. Ott, M., L. Bender, R. Marre, and J. Hacker. 1991. Pulsed-field electrophoresis of genomic restriction fragments for the detection of nosocomial *Legionella pneu*-mophila in hospital water supplies. *J. Clin. Microbiol.* **29:**813–815.

9a. Schoonmaker, D. J., T. Heimberger, and G. Birkhead. 1992. *J. Clin. Microbiol.* **30:**1491–1498.

10. Smith, C. L., and C. R. Cantor. 1987. Purification, specific fragmentation, and separation of large DNA molecules. *Methods Enzymol.* **155:**449–467.

11. Tompkins, L. S., N. J. Troup, T. Woods, W. Bibb, and R. M. McKinney. 1987. Molecular epidemiology of *Legionella* species by restriction endonuclease and alloenzyme analysis. *J. Clin. Microbiol.* **25:**1875–1880.

Complementary Identification of *Legionella* Species by Electrophoretic Characterization of Soluble Protein Extracts

N. BORNSTEIN, M. H. DUMAINE, F. FOREY, AND J. FLEURETTE

Centre National de Référence des Légionelloses, Laboratoire National de la Santé, and Laboratoire de Bactériologie, Faculté de Médecine Alexis Carrel, rue Guillaume Paradin, 69372 Lyon, France

Different species and serogroups of the genus *Legionella* continue to be described, and they remain difficult to identify. Despite the availability of several methods, such as cultural, biochemical, and antigenic studies, as well as fatty acid and ubiquinone analysis, complete identification to the species level cannot always be achieved.

Electrophoresis of soluble protein extracts has been used as a complementary test to identify many bacteria (6–8). Until now, this method has been applied to very few *Legionella* species and mainly for epidemiological purposes, particularly when *Legionella pneumophila* serogroup 1 is involved (2, 4, 7). In this study, we have tried to assess the utility of sodium dodecyl sulfate (SDS)-polyacrylamide gel electrophoresis protein pattern analysis as a complementary method of *Legionella* identification just before the last step of hybridization, which involves specialized laboratories.

We have studied the following 61 reference strains, representative of 57 *Legionella* species and serogroups: *L. pneumophila* serogroup 1 (Philadelphia-1 [ATCC33152]), *L. pneumophila* serogroup 2 (Togus-1 [ATCC 33154]), *L. pneumophila* serogroup 3 (Bloomington-2 [ATCC 33155]), *L. pneumophila* serogroup 4 (Los Angeles-1 [ATCC 33156] and Portland-1), *L. pneumophila* serogroup 5 (Cambridge-2 and Dallas-1E [ATCC 33216]), *L. pneumophila* serogroup 6 (Chicago-2 [ATCC 33215]), *L. pneumophila* serogroup 7 (ATCC 33823), *L. pneumophila* serogroup 8 (ATCC 35096), *L. pneumophila* serogroup 9 (ATCC 35289), *L. pneumophila* serogroup 10 (ATCC 43283), *L. pneumophila* serogroup 11 (ATCC 43130), *L. pneumophila* serogroup 12 (ATCC 43290), *L. pneumophila* serogroup 13 (ATCC 43736), *L. pneumophila* serogroup 14 (ATCC-43703), *L. pneumophila* Lansing-3 (ATCC 35251), *L. adelaidensis* (ATCC 49625), *L. anisa* (ATCC 35292, CH47-C1, and CH47-C3), *L. birminghamensis* (ATCC 43702), *L. bozemanii* serogroup 1 (ATCC 33217), *L. bozemanii* serogroup 2 (ATCC 35545), *L. brunensis* (ATCC 43878), *L. cherrii* (ATCC 35252), *L. cincinnatiensis* (ATCC 43753), *L. dumoffii* (ATCC 33279), *L. erythra* (ATCC 35303), *L. fairfieldensis* (ATCC 49588), *L. feeleii* serogroup 1 (ATCC 35072), *L. feeleii* serogroup 2 (ATCC 35849), "*L. geestiana*," *L. gormanii* (ATCC 33297), *L. gratiana* (ATCC 49413), *L. hackeliae* serogroup 1 (ATCC 35250), *L. hackeliae* serogroup 2 (ATCC 35999), *L. israelensis* (ATCC 43119), *L. jamestowniensis* (ATCC 35298), *L. jordanis* (ATCC 33623), "*L. londiniensis*" serogroup 1, "*L. londiniensis*" serogroup 2, *L. longbeachae* serogroup 1 (ATCC 33462). *L. longbeachae* serogroup 2 (ATCC 33484), *L. maceachernii* (ATCC 35300), *L. micdadei* (ATCC 33218), *L. moravica* (ATCC 43877), "*L. nautarum*," *L. oakridgensis* (ATCC 33761), *L. parisiensis* (ATCC 35299), "*L. quateirensis*," *L. quinlivanii* (ATCC 43830), *L. rubrilucens* (ATCC 35304), *L. sainthelensi* serogroup 1 (ATCC 35248), *L. sainthelensi* serogroup 2 (ATCC 49322), *L. santicrucis* (ATCC 35301), *L. spiritensis* (ATCC 35249), *L. steigerwaltii* (ATCC 35302), *L. tucsonensis* (ATCC 49180), *L. wadsworthii* (ATCC 33877), and "*L. worsleiensis*."

Seventy-two laboratory isolates of clinical and environmental origin were also tested. Among these strains, 56 were clearly identified by using the classical identification protocol: characterization of cultural and biochemical properties, antigenic study by direct immunofluorescence assay using specific immune sera, and cell wall fatty acid and ubiquinone analysis by gas-liquid chromatography and high-performance liquid chromatography, respectively (1). The remaining 16 strains were unclassified. All strains were plated on buffered charcoal-yeast extract agar for 72 h at

TABLE 1. Average similarity percentages (DC) of protein profiles for *Legionella* strains isolated and identified by classical techniques

| Species | No. of strains studied | % Similarity in comparison with: | |
		Isolates and reference strain	Isolates
L. anisa	6	82–95	87–98
L. birminghamensis	6	81–87	85–100
L. bozemanii serogroup 1	11	80–95	80–97
L. dumoffii	6	89–90	92–100
L. erythra	3	88–90	83–90
L. feeleii	1	83	
L. gormanii	6	85–92	85–100
L. hackeliae	1	86	
L. jordanis	1	98	
L. londiniensis	3	82–95	86–97
L. longbeachae	2	82–100	92
L. oakridgensis	3	85–97	84–98
L. rubrilucens	6	84–91	81–94
L. sainthelensi	1	88	
Total	56	80–100	80–100

$35°C$ without CO_2.

Soluble proteins were extracted by a modification of the method of Lema and Brown (7). Twenty-six microliters of a solution containing SDS (20%, wt/vol), EDTA (3.8%, wt/vol), bromophenol blue (0.01%, wt/vol), β-mercaptoethanol (5%, wt/vol), and glycerol (5%, wt/vol) was added to 74 μl of *Legionella* suspension. Samples were boiled for 15 min and centrifuged (15,000 rpm). To enable accurate comparison of the different protein patterns, a constant concentration (3 mg/ml) of lysostaphin (Sigma) was added to each suspension.

Electrophoresis was performed in a 12.5% (wt/vol) polyacrylamide gel (PhastGel homogeneous 12.5) in a Phast system (Pharmacia, Uppsala, Sweden) at 250 V and 10 mA. Two PhastGel-SDS buffer strips were used for each gel. Samples were applied to gels with PhastGel applicators (12 wells, 0.3 μl per well). Whole-cell protein bands were silver stained (Merck) as recommended by Pharmacia.

To perform gel analysis, protein profiles obtained for each strain studied were represented in schematic form, and the average similarity percentage between any two *Legionella* protein electrophoretic patterns was assessed by using the Dice coefficient (DC) (3): (number of matching bands × 2)/(total number of bands in both isolates). Each comparison between strains was established by using extracts run on the same gel.

The similarity percentages between reference *Legionella* strains representative of different species varied from 17 to 69%. Conversely, for refer-

ence strains belonging to the same species and to the same or a different serogroup, DC values ranged from 84 to 95% (not shown).

The results were similar for the well-identified laboratory isolates; in comparisons with the same species, reference strains, or other isolates, DC values varied from 80 to 100% (Table 1). However, this method did not differentiate among serogroups of the same *Legionella* species. For the 14 serogroups of *L. pneumophila* and *L. pneumophila* Lansing-3 tested, DC values were between 70 and 96%. The lowest DC values (70% $\leq DC < 80$%) were obtained for *L. pneumophila* serogroup 4 (Los Angeles and Portland strains) compared with serogroups 10 to 14. For all other serogroups of *L. pneumophila*, the values were above 80%.

By protein pattern analysis, 6 of the 16 isolates not included in a given *Legionella* species could be identified as *L. anisa*, *L. spiritensis*, *L. micdadei*, or *L. oakridgensis*, with DC values from 83 to 98% (Table 2); 5 other strains were found to be *Legionella* sp., as confirmed by analysis of rRNA gene restriction patterns (5). The latter five strains are still under investigation.

In conclusion, our results are in accordance with previous studies showing the value of this test for taxonomic or epidemiologic purposes. Its application here to a large number of strains representative of all *Legionella* species currently described allowed us to determine a similarity percentage of 80% for two *Legionella* strains belonging to the same species. Electrophoretic characterization of soluble proteins was confirmed as

TABLE 2. Process for identification of 16 laboratory isolates

Isolate(s)	Autofluorescence[a]	Direct immunofluorescence[b]	Fatty acid analysis		Ubiquinone analysis		DC		Final identification
			Fatty acid	Possible identification	Ubiquinone	Possible identification	Possible identification	% Similarity	
1	BW	*L. gratiana, L. anisa* *L. bozemanii*	C_{15}–C_{16}	*L. anisa*	Q9–Q12	*L. anisa* *L. bozemanii*	*L. anisa* *L. bozemanii*	93–95 63–65	*L. anisa*
2	BW	*L. anisa,* *L. bozemanii,* *L. tucsonensis,* *L. longbeachae* *L. gratiana,* *L. parisiensis* *L. micdadei*	C_{15}–C_{16}	*L. anisa* *L. tucsonensis* *L. parisiensis*	Q9–Q12	*L. anisa* *L. parisiensis* *L. longbeachae* *L. bozemanii*	*L. anisa* *L. parisiensis* *L. bozemanii*	92–98 62 64	*L. anisa*
3	BW	*L. tucsonensis,* *L. gratiana* *L. bozemanii,* *L. longbeachae,* *L. anisa* *L. micdadei*	C_{15}–C_{16}	*L. anisa* *L. tucsonensis*	Q9–Q12	*L. anisa* *L. bozemanii* *L. longbeachae*	*L. anisa* *L. tucsonensis* *L. bozemanii* *L. longbeachae*	92–93 34 42–45 51	*L. anisa*
4	–	*L. erythra* *L. spiritensis* *L. santicrucis*	C_{16}	*L. erythra* *L. spiritensis* *L. santicrucis*	Q13	*L. spiritensis*	*L. spiritensis*	84	*L. spiritensis*
5	–	*L. micdadei,* *L. maceachernii* *L. bozemanii* *L. nautarum*	C_{15}	*L. micdadei*	Q13	*L. micdadei*	*L. micdadei*	83	*L. micdadei*

No.	Fluorescence[a]	Species	C	Species	Q	Species	%	Species
6	—	L. sainthelensi, L. hackeliae, L. oakridgensis	C$_{16}$	L. oakridgensis	Q10	L. oakridgensis, L. sainthelensi, L. hackeliae, L. spiritensis	86, 47, 50, 50	L. oakridgensis
7, 8	—	L. spiritensis (L. santicrucis)	C$_{16}$	L. spiritensis, L. santicrucis	Q12	L. spiritensis	50	Legionella sp.[c]
9	—	L. anisa	C$_{16}$	L. anisa	Q12	L. anisa, L. pneumophila, L. birminghamensis, L. israelensis	52–57, 52, 64, 37	Legionella sp.
10, 11	—	—	C$_{16}$	—	Q12			Legionella sp.
12	BW	L. bozemanii, L. gratiana, L. anisa, L. jordanis	C$_{15}$	L. bozemanii, L. jordanis	Q12	L. bozemanii, L. jordanis, L. gratiana, L. anisa	57–67, 46, 52, 52–62	—[d]
13	—	L. londiniensis	C$_{17}$	L. londiniensis	Q11	L. londiniensis	60–63	—
14	—	L. londiniensis	C$_{16}$		Q10	L. londiniensis	51–54	—
15	—	L. hackeliae, L. longbeachae, L. oakridgensis, L. sainthelensi, L. longbeachae	C$_{16}$	L. longbeachae, L. oakridgensis	Q12	L. longbeachae, L. oakridgensis, L. hackeliae	53–56, 49, 54	—
16	BW	L. bozemanii, L. anisa, L. gratiana, L. tucsonensis, L. longbeachae	C$_{15}$–C$_{16}$	L. anisa, L. tucsonensis	Q9–Q12	L. anisa, L. tucsonensis, L. bozemanii, L. longbeachae	37–45, 47, 51, 61	—

[a]BW, blue-white fluorescence; —, no fluorescence.
[b]Intensity of reaction indicated as follows: ++++, bold italics; +++, italics; ++, underline; +, broken underline; +f, parentheses.
[c]Confirmed by analysis of rRNA gene restriction patterns.
[d]—, strains are still being studied.

being a useful tool for *Legionella* identification in the laboratory.

We thank F. Grimont (Unité des Entérobactéries, Institut Pasteur, Paris, France) for helpful collaboration in performing rRNA gene restriction patterns of strains.

REFERENCES

1. **Bornstein, N., D. Marmet, M. Surgot, M. Nowicki, H. Meugnier, J. Fleurette, E. Ageron, F. Grimont, P. A. D. Grimont, W. L. Thacker, R. F. Benson, and D. J. Brenner.** 1989. *Legionella gratiana* sp. nov. isolated from French spa water. *Res. Microbiol.* **140:**541–542.
2. **Brown, A., M. Lema, C. A. Ciesielski, and M. J. Blaser.** 1985. Combined plasmid and peptide analysis of clinical and environmental *L. pneumophila* strains associated with a small cluster of Legionnaires' disease cases. *Infection* **13:**163–165.
3. **Dice, L. R.** 1945. Measures of the amount of ecological association between species. *Ecology* **26:**297–302.
4. **Ehret, W., and G. Ruckdeschel.** 1985. Membrane proteins of Legionellaceae. I. Membrane proteins of different strains and serogroups of *Legionella pneumophila*. *Zentralbl. Bakteriol. Hyg. A* **259:**433–445.
5. **Grimont, F., M. Lefèvre, E. Ageron, and P. A. D. Grimont.** 1989. rRNA gene restriction patterns of Legionella species: a molecular identification system. *Res. Microbiol.* **140:**615–626.
6. **Kersters, K., and J. De Ley.** 1975. Identification and grouping of bacteria by numerical analysis of electrophoretic protein patterns. *J. Gen. Microbiol.* **87:**333–342.
7. **Lema M., and A. Brown.** 1983. Electrophoretic characterization of soluble protein extracts of *Legionella pneumophila* and other members of the family *Legionellaceae*. *J. Clin. Microbiol.* **17:**1132–1140.
8. **Thomson Carter, F. M., and T. H. Pennington.** 1989. Characterization of methicillin-resistant isolates of *Staphylococcus aureus* by analysis of whole-cell and exported proteins. *J. Med. Microbiol.* **28:**25–32.

Comparison of Different Detection Methods for Isolation of *Legionella pneumophila* from Water Supplies of Alpine Hotel Resorts

F. TIEFENBRUNNER, A. ARNOLD, E. TARABOI, U. CERNECK, AND K. EMDE

Institute of Hygiene, Faculty of Medicine, University of Innsbruck, Fritz Pregl Strasse 3, A-6010 Innsbruck, Tirol, Austria, and Department of Civil Engineering, University of Alberta, Edmonton, Alberta T6G 2E1, Canada

With the increase in public health and regulatory concerns about waterborne legionellae, there is a need for improved detection methods. Reliable, easy to use procedures and media are required to selectively isolate legionellae from environmental water samples. It has been recognized that no single medium will be optimal for all environmental samples containing *Legionellaceae* (1–4). These samples often contain large numbers of contaminating heterotrophs. Despite advances in medium formulation and pretreatment techniques, recovery of legionellae from these samples can still be quite low, difficult, and time-consuming.

From 1989 to 1990, 35 hotels in the province of Tyrol, Austria, were surveyed to determine types of microorganisms, including *Legionella* species, able to colonize the hot/mixed (i.e., warm) and cold water distribution systems. The objectives of this research were to compare and evaluate the different methods for the isolation of *Legionella pneumophila* from environmental water samples and to evaluate the influence of water temperature on the isolation and relative colonization of plumbing system components by *L. pneumophila*.

In the first phase of the study, 35 hotels in Tyrol were surveyed to determine the microbial composition of the various components of the water distribution system. Water samples were plated for total heterotrophic bacteria, *Legionella* species,

Pseudomonas species, and total coliforms. Methods used for Legionella species included "classical" *Legionella* membrane filtration (0.45-μm-pore-size cellulose-nitrate filter, 100-ml sample volume) (1, 4) (method A); classical *Legionella* membrane filtration but with substitution of a 0.45-μm-pore-size polycarbonate filter and sonication (300 ml of sample filtered, 0.3 ml plated) (method B), and classical *Legionella* membrane filtration with a 0.45-μm-pore-size polycarbonate filter, sonication, and acid pretreatment (300 ml of sample filtered, 0.3 ml plated) (method C).

All *Legionella*-positive hotels were resampled and treated by a number of different methods. These methods were compared and evaluated. Hot and mixed water systems were sampled on separate occasions from cold water systems. Additional inhibitors were used in buffered charcoal-yeast extract *Legionella* medium (3 g of glycine, 50T polymycin, 80 mg of anisomycin, 1 mg of vancomycin). Bromthymol blue and bromcresol purple were also added. Filtration methods, in addition to those already described, included classical *Legionella* membrane filtration (0.45-μm-pore-size polycarbonate filters, sonication, and acid pretreatment, 100 ml of sample filtered, 0.1 ml plated) (method D); centrifugation and concentration of the original water sample, resuspension of the pellet, and plating directly on *Legionella*

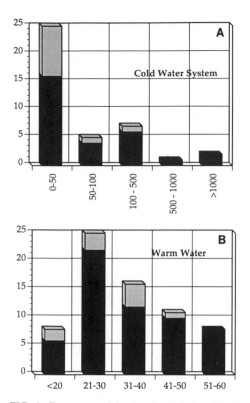

FIG. 1. Frequency of *Legionella* isolation (A) from cold water samples as a function of the total count, and (B) as a function of warm water temperature (°C). Solid area, *Legionella*-negative samples; shaded area, *Legionella*-positive samples.

medium (method E); sonication for 15 min of 0.3 ml of the suspension described in method E and then plating on *Legionella* medium (method F); and sonication for 15 min of 0.3 ml of the suspension described in method E and then acid treatment prior to plating onto *Legionella* medium.

The cold water systems of 31% of the hotels surveyed were found to be positive for *L. pneumophila*. The hot and/or mixed water systems of 26% of the hotels surveyed were positive for *L. pneumophila*. Of these, approximately 33% had *Legionella* counts ranging from 100 to 500 CFU/100 ml. The balance of positive hotels had *Legionella* counts ranging from 1 to 100 CFU/100 ml. Although legionellae may enter the building from municipally supplied water, the building plumbing system was found to be the major site for growth and further dissemination of legionellae. The plumbing system configuration, water use patterns, and degree of corrosion appear to combine to favor the survival and growth of legionellae in oligotrophic environments. In both water systems, first-flush samples had much higher levels of legionellae than did samples taken after 5 or 10 min of flushing. This finding indicates that the amount of biofilm accumulation on

the inner pipe surface and at the fixture itself is significant to the levels of legionellae isolated. The cold water system appears to be as important as the hot/mixed water system for amplification of legionellae. Addition of cold water to hot at the shower (mixed system) yielded significantly higher total heterotroph counts as well as higher *Legionella* counts. The results of cold water sampling suggest that *L. pneumophila* can proliferate in water temperatures ranging from < 8 to 20°C as well as at the temperatures found in the hot/mixed water system. Figure 1 shows correlations between levels of legionellae isolated in this study and water temperature.

Results of this study showed that method D was the best method for isolation of *L. pneumophila* from cold water samples. Methods A and B were comparable in isolation of legionellae from cold water systems. Method A was able to isolate a broader spectrum of heterotrophs than did methods B or C. This was a deterrent to its use because of the potentially high contaminant levels. Addition of a sonication step in method B substantially reduced levels of competing pseudomonads, yeasts, and gram-positive and gram-negative rods. Addition of an acid pretreatment in method C almost entirely eliminated these contaminants. Methods E, F, and G did not prove to be advantageous for isolation of legionellae from cold water systems. This finding may be in part a function of the relatively small sample size used for the study. Method E appeared to be the most successful for isolation of legionellae from hot and mixed water systems. Figure 2 illustrates average counts of *L. pneumophila* obtained for each of the isolation methods evaluated. Sonication and/or acid pretreatment had relatively little effect on levels of gram-positive and gram-negative cocci, legionellae, and sporeformers.

The majority of *L. pneumophila* isolates from cold water systems belonged to serogroups 1 and 8. In the hot/mixed water system, the predominant serotype isolated was serogroup 8 (Concord); it

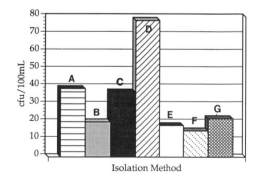

FIG. 2. Average *L. pneumophila* counts in relation to isolation method. Bars labeled according to method.

was isolated in 40% of positive hotels. Comparison and evaluation of results from both water systems suggest that use of a single *Legionella* isolation medium and/or technique is not suitable for all types of water systems. Cold water system samples tend to have higher levels of contaminating bacteria, which can interfere with the success of *Legionella* isolation. In hot and/or mixed (>40°C) water systems, the sample water temperature has an inhibitory effect that reduces the level of contamination. There also appeared to be differences in serogroups of *L. pneumophila* isolated in the systems studied. Further research is required to determine whether this is a phenomenon peculiar to the hotels sampled or a function of water temperature. To maximize isolation of *Legionella* species from environmental water samples, consideration needs to be given to the water temperature of the distribution system being sampled along with selection of an appropriate pre-treatment method(s) and media.

REFERENCES

1. **American Public Health Association, American Water Works Association, and Water Pollution Control Federation.** 1989. *Standard Methods for the Examination of Water and Wastewater,* 17th ed. American Public Health Association, Washington, D.C.
2. **Dennis, P. J., C. L. R. Bartlett, and A. E. Wright.** 1983. A comparison of isolation methods for *Legionellaceae*, p. 294–296. *Proc. 2nd Int. Symp. Legionella.* American Society for Microbiology, Washington, D.C.
3. **Edelstein, P. H.** 1981. Improved semiselective medium for isolation of *Legionella pneumophila* from contaminated clinical and environmental specimens. *J. Clin. Microbiol.* **14:**298–303.
4. **Jones, G. L., and G. A. Hebert.** 1979. *Legionnaires—the Disease, the Bacterium and Methodology.* Centers for Disease Control, Atlanta.
5. **Morris, G. K., C. M. Patton, J. C. Feeley, S. E. Johnson, G. Gorman, W. T. Martin, P. Skaliy, G. F. Mallison, B. D. Politi, and D. C. Mackel.** 1979. Isolation of the Legionnaires' disease bacterium from environmental samples. *Ann. Intern. Med.* **90:**664–666.

Recovery of *Legionella* spp. from Water Samples by Four Different Methods

HANNELE R. JOUSIMIES-SOMER, SIRKKU WAARALA, AND MARJA-LIISA VÄISÄNEN

Legionella Reference Unit, National Public Health Institute, Mannerheimintie 166, SF-00300 Helsinki, Finland

In water samples, the concentrations of *Legionella* spp. are often lower than those of heterotrophic bacteria. Therefore, concentration of the sample as well as pretreatment and plating on selective media are used to enrich the legionellae and to reduce the number of accompanying bacteria. The aim of this study was to test the ability of four different methods to recover *Legionella* spp. from water samples.

Processing of Water Samples. One-liter water samples positive for *Legionella* spp. from 16 community taps and five industrial process water basins were processed in the following way. A 0.1-ml volume of the native sample was inoculated on a modified Wadowsky-Yee medium (MWY) agar plate (2) (method N). The 1-liter sample was concentrated by filtration through a 0.2-μm-pore-size nylon membrane (N66 Posidyne; Pall Trinity Micro Corp., Cortland, N.Y.), which was cut in small strips; the strips were suspended in 5 ml of the original water and vigorously shaken strokewise with glass beads for 30 s by a Vortex mixer (method C). Then 0.1 ml of the concentrate was plated on MWY and CCVC (selective medium with cephalotin, cycloheximide, vancomycin, and polymyxin E) (2) plates. Another 0.1 ml of the concentrate was acid washed by adding 0.9 ml of HCl-KCl solution (pH 2.2) to the tube. The mixture was vortexed and allowed to stand at room temperature for 4 min (1) (method A). Then 0.1 ml of the acid-washed sample was plated on MWY and BCYEα [buffered charcoal-yeast extract medium with *N*-(2-acetamido)-2-aminoethanesulfonic acid (ACES) buffer and α-ketoglutarate] agar media (2). Finally, 0.5 ml of the concentrate was heated at 50°C for 30 min (1) (method H), and 0.1 ml of the heat-treated concentrate was inoculated on BCYEα and MWY agar media.

All media were incubated at 36°C in a humid chamber in air for up to 10 days. The heterotrophic counts of native samples were determined on plate count agar after 10 to 14 days of incubation at room temperature.

Recovery of legionellae. Of the 21 samples tested, the number positive for *Legionella* spp. by the four methods were as follows: N, 7; C, 14; A, 12; and H, 20. The positive results obtained by each method alone and in combination are given in Table 1.

All samples yielded *Legionella pneumophila.* The tap water isolates were of serogroup 1, and the industrial isolates were of serogroups 6 (three samples) and 4 (two samples).

The concentrations of *Legionella* spp. in the samples ranged from 50 to 2×10^6 CFU/liter. The theoretical detection thresholds for methods N, C, A, and H were, respectively, 10^4, 50, 500,

TABLE 1. Number of samples positive for *Legionella* spp. by various methods

Method	Plating medium(a)	No. of samples positive/21 tested	
N	MWY	7	(N only, 0)
C	MWY, CCVC	14	(C only, 1)
A	MWY, BCYEα	12	(A only, 0)
H	MWY, BCYEα	20	(H only, 3)
C + H		3	
A + H		3	
N + C + H		2	
N + A + H		1	
C + A + H		4	
N + C + A + H		4	

TABLE 2. *Legionella* counts in relation to heterotrophic counts of 21 water samples

Heterotrophic count (CFU/liter)	No. of samples	*Legionella* counts (CFU/liter)
$< 10^6$	5	50, 4×10^3, 2×10^4, 2×10^4, 2×10^6
$\geq 10^6 < 10^7$	8	200, 200, 200, 560, 3×10^3, 10^4, 10^4, 6×10^4
$\geq 10^7 < 10^8$	4	50, 50^a, 250, 2.5×10^3
$\geq 10^8 < 10^9$	1	50^a
$\geq 10^9$	3	50^a, 2.4×10^{3a}, 10^{5a}

[a]Industrial water sample.

and 50 CFU/liter. The corresponding counts for the heterotrophic bacteria in the same samples ranged from 5×10^5 to 10^9 CFU/liter. The quantitative recovery of *Legionella* spp. in relation to the heterotrophic counts is presented in Table 2. There was a tendency for higher *Legionella* concentrations from samples with lower heterotrophic counts.

The numbers of colonies recovered on MWY agar and on BCYEα agar after acid wash or heat treatment were relatively concordant. However, the MWY plates were easier to interpret because accompanying flora was seldom interfering.

Conclusions. Heat treatment was the most effective single method to detect *L. pneumophila*

serogroups 1, 4, and 6 from the water samples, followed by concentration alone and acid wash. Plating of native water yielded the lowest number of positive results. Heat treatment combined with plating on MWY agar most effectively allowed isolation of *Legionella* spp. by suppressing the contaminating flora. There was a tendency for better recovery and higher *Legionella* counts from samples with lower counts of heterotrophic bacteria.

REFERENCES

1. **Dennis, P. J.** 1988. Isolation of legionellae from environmental specimens, p. 31–44. *In* T. G. Harrison and A. G. Taylor (ed.), *A Laboratory Manual for Legionella*. J. Wiley & Sons, Chichester, England.
2. **Edelstein, P. H.** 1985. *Legionnaires' Disease Laboratory Manual*. National Technical Information Service, Springfield, Va.

Lack of Dormancy in *Legionella pneumophila*?

A. A. WEST, J. ROGERS, J. V. LEE, AND C. W. KEEVIL

Public Health Laboratory Service Centre for Applied Microbiology and Research, Porton Down, Salisbury, Wiltshire SP4 0JG United Kingdom

Legionella pneumophila, the principal agent of Legionnaires disease, although found in aquatic environments over a wide range of temperatures, is most frequently isolated from warm waters (3, 7, 13). The microorganism is not thermophilic, but it exhibits a tolerance to higher temperatures which gives it an ecological advantage ideally suited to man-made water systems (6). Epidemiological studies of outbreaks have provided good evidence that domestic hot water and cooling waters in large buildings are the prime source of infection (2).

Dormancy prevents a number of bacteria from dying when sufficient substrate is not available for growth (9). For example, waterborne pathogens such as *Vibrio cholerae* and members of the family *Pseudomonadaceae* become dormant in

low-nutrient environments, entering a viable but nonculturable state (1). These nutrient-limited microorganisms can undergo a number of morphological and physiological changes (1). Perhaps associated with this phenomenon, *L. pneumophila* and several other *Legionella* species respond to sharp rises in temperature with a coordinated increase in the rate of synthesis of a set of proteins similar to those observed in other microorganisms tested (8, 10, 12).

Previously, Colbourne and Dennis (4) concluded that *L. pneumophila* was made culture positive after heat shock treatment. In this study, we investigated the relationship between dormancy and heat shock in *L. pneumophila* serogroup 1.

L. pneumophila serogroup 1 subtype Pontiac, as determined by the monoclonal antibody typing system of Watkins et al. (14), was used in this study. Pontiac is the subgroup most commonly associated with disease, although it does not appear to be as common in the environment as are the other two subgroups (14).

The domestic softened cold water used in the experiment was sterilized by the method of Colbourne et al. (5). The water was inoculated with *L. pneumophila* serogroup 1 subgroup Pontiac (10^3 ml^{-1}) and incubated at 23°C. The numbers of culturable legionellae were monitored by plating onto buffered charcoal-yeast extract (BCYE) agar (11), which was then incubated for up to 7 days. The numbers of *Legionella* colonies were then counted, and the numbers of culturable legionellae were plotted against day of incubation in the water. Because legionellae grow slowly on laboratory media, their enumeration by culture (viable count) is a lengthy process. The viable count method of detecting CFU is complicated by the fact that BCYE agar is very rich in nutrients in comparison with the levels found in natural water. Because bacteria may die as a result of nutrient shock, plate counts may not give a true picture of the viability of the microorganisms in the original water sample; the observed viable counts may be considerably lower than the actual viabilities. For these reasons, in addition to plate counts, ATP in the microorganisms and the waters was measured by using luciferin-luciferase reagents (Lumac, Schaesberg, The Netherlands). Numbers of legionellae were also counted by using the indirect immunofluorescence assay. Samples (5 µl) were dried onto a Multispot microscope slide, fixed in acetone, and then coated with 5 µl of a polyclonal or monoclonal antibody. The samples were incubated for 1 h in a moist atmosphere at 37°C, washed with three changes of phosphate-buffered saline and one change of water, and dried. The samples were coated with 5 µl of anti-rabbit or anti-mouse (for the polyclonal or monoclonal antibody, respectively) immunoglobulin G-fluorescein isothyiocyanate conjugate and incubated for 30 min in a moist atmosphere at 37°C. The samples were again washed as before, dried, and viewed with a fluorescence microscope at 336 nm.

Heat shock experiments were carried out by incubating legionellae in domestic tap water until they became nonculturable (i.e., until it was no longer possible to detect colonies on BCYE agar plates). The samples were heat shocked by incubation at 45°C for 10 min and then either plated directly onto BCYE agar or incubated at 23°C for 3 days and plated onto BCYE agar (Fig. 1). Planktonic-phase or copper, glass, or plastic biofilms from a continuous mixed culture containing legionellae were also heat shocked, and the numbers of culturable legionellae were compared with those from non-heat-shocked cultures, using the heat shock/non-heat shock ratio (Fig. 2).

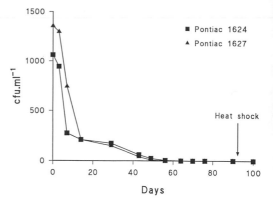

FIG. 1. Loss of culturability of *L. pneumophila*.

Incubation of legionellae in sterile water caused a gradual decrease in the numbers of culturable legionellae; after 60 days, no culturable legionellae could be detected on BCYE agar (Fig. 1). However, high numbers of legionellae similar to those of the initial inoculum could still be detected by the indirect immunofluorescence assay after the 60-day period (results not shown), indicating that the *Legionella* cells were still intact in the water although not culturable. Moreover, viable ATP detection (results not shown) indicated that although some of the legionellae had become nonculturable, they might still be viable, i.e., in a dormant (9) state or susceptible to nutrient shock on BCYE recovery agar.

Heat shock failed to revive the legionellae. Heat shock of culturable legionellae resulted in a decrease in culturable microorganisms (Fig. 1). No difference was observed between cultures plated out immediately after heat shock and those incubated for 72 h and then plated out. The ratios of heat-shocked to non-heat-shocked legionellae from the mixed-culture heat shock experiment (Fig. 2) indicated that the numbers of culturable

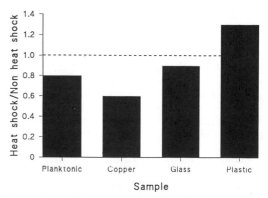

FIG. 2. Ratio of recovery of heat shocked to non-heat-shocked legionellae.

legionellae from heat-shocked planktonic-phase mixed cultures were lower than those of non-heat-shocked controls.

Decreases were also found in culturable legionellae from mixed biofilm cultures of glass and copper surfaces. The ratio was lower for the copper surfaces than for the glass surfaces, probably indicating an inhibitory effect of the copper surface itself. Legionellae from mixed biofilms on plastic surfaces increased in culturability when heat shocked. These biofilms were considerably thicker than those of the copper and glass surfaces; therefore, heat shock of these films may act as a method of breaking up the biofilm clumps and releasing more colonies of legionellae that then become culturable. Therefore, contrary to the results of Colbourne and Dennis (4), we found that heat shock of legionellae had a detrimental effect on the culturability of the microorganisms (i.e., dormancy could not be confirmed by using classical heat shock techniques).

REFERENCES

1. **Baker, R. M., F. L. Singleton, and M. A. Hood.** 1983. Effects of nutrient deprivation on *Vibrio cholerae. Appl. Environ. Microbiol.* **46**:930–940.
2. **Bartlett, L. R., A. D. Macrae, and J. T. Macfarlane.** 1986. *Legionella Infections.* Edward Arnold, London.
3. **Best, M., J. Stout, R. R. Muder, V. L. Yu, A. Goetz, and F. Taylor.** 1983. Legionellaceae in the hospital water supply. *Lancet* ii:307–310.
4. **Colbourne, J. S., and P. J. Dennis.** 1989. The ecology and survival of *Legionella pneumophila. J. IWEM* **3**:345–350.
5. **Colbourne, J. S., R. M. Trew, and P. J. Dennis.** 1988. Treatment of water for aquatic bacterial growth studies. *J. Appl. Bacteriol.* **65**:1–7.
6. **Dennis, P. J., D. Green, and B. P. C. Jones.** 1984. A note on temperature tolerance of Legionella. *J. Appl. Bacteriol.* **56**:349–350.
7. **Fliermans, C. B., W. B. Cherry, L. H. Orrison, S. J. Smith, D. L. Tison, and D. H. Pope.** 1985. Ecological distribution of *Legionella pneumophila. Appl. Environ. Microbiol.* **41**:9–16.
8. **Hoffman, P. S., L. Houston, and C. A. Butler.** 1990. *Legionella pneumophila htpAB* heat shock operon: nucleotide sequence and expression of the 60-kilodalton antigen in *L. pneumophila*-infected HeLa cells. *Infect. Immun.* **58**:3380–3387.
9. **Kjelleberg, S., M. Hermansson, and P. Mardén.** 1987. The transient phase between growth and nongrowth of heterotrophic bacteria, with emphasis on the marine environment. *Annu. Rev. Microbiol.* **41**:25–49.
10. **Lema, M. W., A. Brown, and G. C. C. Chen.** 1986. Altered rate of synthesis of specific peptides in the legionellae in response to growth temperature. *Curr. Microbiol.* **12**:699–701.
11. **Pasculle, A. W., J. C. Feeley, R. J. Gibson, L. G. Cordes, R. L. Myerowitz, C. M. Patton, G. W. Gorman, C. L. Carmack, J. W. Ezzell, and J. N. Dowling.** 1980. Pittsburgh pneumonia agent: direct isolation from human lung tissue. *J. Infect. Dis.* **141**:727–732.
12. **Schlesinger, M. J., G. Aliperti, and P. M. Kelley.** 1982. The response of cells to heat shock. *Trends Biochem. Sci.* **7**:222–225.
13. **Stout, J., V. L. Yu, R. M. Vickers, J. Zuraleff, M. Best, A. Brown, R. B. Yee, and R. Wadowsky.** 1982. Ubiquitousness of *Legionella pneumophila* in the water supply of hospital with endemic Legionnaires' disease. *N. Engl. J. Med.* **306**:466–468.
14. **Watkins, I. D., J. O. Tobin, P. J. Dennis, W. Brown, R. Newnham, and J. B. Kurtz.** 1985. *Legionella pneumophila* serogroup 1 subgrouping by monoclonal antibodies—an epidemiological tool. *J. Hyg.* **95**:211–216.

Inhibitory Effect of Heterotrophic Bacteria on the Cultivation of *Legionella dumoffii*

CHRISTINE PASZKO-KOLVA, PATRICK A. HACKER, MIC H. STEWART, AND ROY L. WOLFE

Metropolitan Water District of Southern California, Water Quality Division, La Verne, California 91750

The presence of legionellae in potable water supplies and natural reservoirs such as lakes, rivers, and ponds has been well established (2, 3, 6, 9). It has long been postulated that the source of *Legionella* contamination in potable water systems may be the municipal water supply, which could seed plumbing systems of homes, hospitals, and institutions. However, a recent study conducted by States et al. (7) failed to recover *Legionella* species in municipal drinking water systems, despite the use of several isolation techniques. Investigators believed that *Legionella* cells may have been injured or inactivated by the presence of a chlorine residual maintained throughout the distribution system.

The Metropolitan Water District of Southern California conducted a *Legionella* survey of its distribution system, employing direct fluorescent antibody (DFA) staining and culture. Twenty-liter water samples were collected from source waters, finished waters, and backwash waters of conventional treatment plants that use flocculation, sedimentation, and filtration followed by postdisinfection (chloramination). The finished water has a chloramine residual of 1.5 mg/liter at a chlorine-to-ammonia weight ratio of 5:1.

The samples were concentrated on polysulfone filters, which were then placed into sterile bottles containing 250 ml of the same water and shaken vigorously (at 300 rpm) for 1 h. Acridine orange staining was performed on the unconcentrated sample. The concentrated sample was subjected to DFA staining with two polyvalent conjugates: (i) *Legionella pneumophila* serogroups 1 to 6 and (ii)

TABLE 1. Results of water samples analyzed by DFA staining

		% Positive		
Water	Total no. of samples	L. pneumophila serogroups 1–6[a]	Poly[b]	L. pneumophila serogroups 1–6 + Poly
Source	44	48	41	34
Effluent	19	16	0	0
Backwash	10	50	50	30
Total	73	40	32	25

[a]Polyvalent antisera to L. pneumophila serogroups 1 to 6.
[b]Poly, polyvalent antisera to L. bozemanii, L. micdadei, L. dumoffii, L. jordanis, L. longbeachae serogroups 1 and 2 and L. gormanii.

L. bozemanii, L. micdadei, L. dumoffii, L. jordanis, L. gormanii, and L. longbeachae serogroups 1 and 2 (Scimedx).

Concentrated samples were spread plated in duplicate onto buffered charcoal-yeast extract agar amended with α-ketoglutarate (BCYEα), both alone and supplemented with glycine, vancomycin, polymyxin B, and cycloheximide. In addition, the samples were plated on Legionella transparent medium (1). Heat and acid treatments and sequential culturing were applied when deemed appropriate (6). The samples were incubated at 37°C in 2.5% CO_2 in a humid environment for 2 to 3 days.

Although Legionella species were detected by DFA staining in source, effluent, and backwash waters (Table 1), all culture results were negative. Some 40% of all samples were positive for the presence of L. pneumophila serogroups 1 to 6, whereas 25% of the samples were positive against both polyvalent conjugates used. Three of 19 effluent waters analyzed were positive for L. pneumophila serogroups 1 to 6, but at low concentrations (1 to 16 cells per ml). The highest concentrations of legionellae were found in source and backwash samples at 10^2 and 10^3 cells per ml, respectively. Table 2 provides mean general water quality data and Legionella monitoring results for the source, effluent, and backwash samples examined. It is apparent that Legionella populations make up a very small percentage (0.0012%) of the total count. Since high concentrations of hetero-

trophic bacteria were found, either competition or inhibition of Legionella may have been occurring.

To determine whether inhibition of legionellae by heterotrophic bacteria was occurring, L. dumoffii was selected because of its ability to fluoresce blue-white under long-wave UV light, making it an ideal model with which to study inhibition. Concentrated samples of the various waters were spiked (at previously determined dilutions) with an environmental isolate of L. dumoffii (ATCC 33279) along with filtered-water controls. The samples were examined after 48, 72, and 96 h under long-wave UV light. Colonies appearing to inhibit L. dumoffii growth (visualized as zones of no fluorescence) were isolated and transferred to R2A agar for identification with the use of API Rapid NFT strips (Analytab Products, Inc.). Although inhibition was concurrently observed on Legionella transparent medium, many isolates had a tendency to swarm on this medium; therefore, its use is not recommended for spread plating of environmental samples.

In contrast to other studies (8, 9), which found pigmented colonies responsible for supplying L. pneumophila growth-supporting factors, only nonpigmented colonies inhibitory to L. dumoffii were isolated in this study. Nonpigmented inhibitory colonies were identified as members of the genera Pseudomonas, Aeromonas, and Flavobacterium. Isolates identified to the species level included Aeromonas hydrophila, Aeromonas salmonicida, Flavobacterium meningosepticum,

TABLE 2. Mean values for water quality parameters

	Mean Value						
						DFA (cells/ml)[b]	
Water	pH	Turbidity	Temp (°C)	Acridine orange direct count (cells/ml)	Heterotrophic plate count (CFU/ml)[a]	L. pneumophila serogroups 1–6	Poly
Source	8.01	1.02	19.8	1.85×10^6	8.25×10^4	12	13
Effluent	7.85	0.33	19.4	5.78×10^4	4.8	12	0
Backwash	7.58	16.81	18.6	6.38×10^6	1.88×10^5	17	29

[a]Enumerated by membrane filtration and plating onto R2A medium for 7 days at 28°C.
[b]The conjugates used are described in Table 1, footnotes a and b.

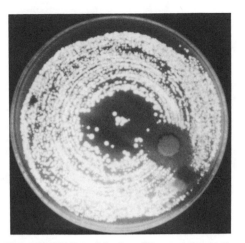

FIG. 1. Inhibition of *L. dumoffii* growth by a colony of *Pseudomonas* sp. on BCYEα, viewed under longwave UV light.

and *Pseudomonas aeruginosa*. Strains that inhibited the growth of *L. dumoffii* were isolated from source, backwash, and effluent waters. These microoganisms, like *Streptomyces* species, are believed to secrete extracellular (bactericidal) products into the surrounding media, and *L. dumoffii* appears to be particularly susceptible to these products.

The growth of *L. dumoffii* colonies was inhibited to various degrees. As shown in Fig. 1, some colonies produced inhibition zones similar to those produced in a Kirby-Bauer antibiotic assay. Zones of inhibition ranged in size from 2 to 6 mm on a lawn of *L. dumoffii* (containing 10^8 cells per ml). Another group of heterotrophic microorganisms inhibited the growth of *L. dumoffii* cells directly under them, as evidenced by lack of fluorescence and growth when the cells were transferred. Noninhibitory heterotrophic isolates were identified by *L. dumoffii* cells fluorescing beneath them.

Many studies have concentrated on growth-supporting factors for *Legionella* species associated with potable water supplies (8, 9); however, few studies have focused on biological inhibition. Growth-supporting factors include interrelationships with certain protozoa, algae, biofilms, and other microorganisms (8, 9). These interrelationships are of particular importance in the amplification and dissemination of *Legionella* species and associated disease. Environmental control through predation and interaction with inhibitory microorganisms may limit the outbreaks associated with natural waters (3, 5). An equally important aspect of *Legionella* epidemiology is laboratory isolation from environmental samples, which has been difficult at best. Numerous reasons have been given for the poor recovery efficiency on laboratory media, including the stress of heat and acid pretreatments, the susceptibility of certain species to antibiotics, overgrowth by naturally occurring microorganisms, the presence of viable but nonculturable cells, and nutrient shock (4, 6). The results of this study suggest that certain indigenous waterborne bacteria can dramatically inhibit the growth of *L. dumoffii* on laboratory media.

REFERENCES

1. **Armon, R., and P. Payment.** 1990. A transparent medium for isolation of *Legionella pneumophila* from environmental water sources. *J. Microbiol. Methods* **11**:65–71.
2. **Fliermans, C. B., W. B. Cherry, L. H. Orrison, S. J. Smith, D. L. Tison, and D. H. Pope.** 1981. Ecological distribution of *Legionella pneumophila*. *Appl. Environ. Microbiol.* **41**:9–16.
3. **Fliermans, C. B., W. B. Cherry, L. H. Orrison, and L. Thacker.** 1979. Isolation of *Legionella pneumophila* from nonepidemic related aquatic habitats. *Appl. Environ. Microbiol.* **37**:1239–1242.
4. **Hussong, D., R. R. Colwell, M. O'Brien, A. D. Weiss, A. D. Pearson, R. M. Weiner, and W. D. Burge.** 1987. Viable *Legionella pneumophila* not detectable by culture on agar media. *Bio/Technology* **5**:947–950.
5. **Paszko-Kolva, C., M. Shahamat, H. Yamamoto, T. K. Sawyer, J. Vives-Rego, and R. R. Colwell.** 1991. Survival of *Legionella pneumophila* in the aquatic environment. *Microb. Ecol.* **22**:75–83.
6. **Shahamat, M., C. Paszko-Kolva, J. Keiser, and R. R. Colwell.** 1991. Sequential culturing method improves recovery of *Legionella* spp. from contaminated environmental samples. *Zentralbl. Bakteriol. Hyg.* **275**:312–319.
7. **States, S. J., L. F. Conley, J. M. Kuchta, B. M. Oleck, M. J. Lipovich, R. S. Wolford, R. M. Wadowsky, A. M. McNamara, J. L. Sykora, G. Keleti, and R. B. Yee.** 1987. Survival and multiplication of *Legionella pneumophila* in municipal drinking water systems. *Appl. Environ. Microbiol.* **53**:970–986.
8. **Wadowsky, R. M., and R. B. Yee.** 1983. Satellite growth of *Legionella pneumophila* with an environmental isolate of *Flavobacterium breve*. *Appl. Environ. Microbiol.* **46**:1447–1449.
9. **Wadowsky, R. M., and R. B. Yee.** 1985. Effect of nonlegionellae bacteria on the multiplication of *Legionella pneumophila* in potable water. *Appl. Environ. Microbiol.* **49**:1206–1210.

Enzymatic Activities of *Legionella* spp. Characterized Using API Enzyme Research Kits

M. MANAFI, R. SOMMER, AND G. WEWALKA

Hygiene Institute, University of Vienna, Kinderspitalgasse 15, A-1095 Vienna, Austria

The identification of *Legionella* spp., in particular *Legionella pneumophila*, has been accomplished by methods such as radioimmunoassay, enzyme-linked immunosorbent assay, latex agglutination test, fluorescent antibody assay, use of nucleic acid probes, and polymerase chain reaction. The biochemical characterization of this species is complicated because of the unique metabolism of these bacteria, characterized by the ability to use amino acids as the major sources of energy and carbon (5). The organisms do not utilize carbohydrates other than starch.

Several authors have used chromogenic enzyme substrates to investigate the enzymatic activities of *Legionella* spp. (1–4, 6–8). The aim of this study was to establish an extensive enzymatic characterization of *Legionella* spp., in particular different serogroups of *L. pneumophila* strains, using chromogenic enzyme research kits.

Four strains of *L. pneumophila* designated Philadelphia-1 (serogroup 1), Togus-1 (serogroup 2), Bloomington-2 (serogroup 3), and Chicago-2 (serogroup 6), as well as one strain each of *L. dumoffii* (NY-23), *L. gormanii* (LS-13), *L. jordanis* (BL-540), *L. feeleii* (ATCC 35072), *L. micdadei* (Tatlock), *L. bozemanii* (ATCC 35545), *L. sainthelensi* (ATCC 35248), *L. oakridgensis* (Oak Ridge 10), and *L. longbeachae* (Longbeach-4), were studied. All strains were plated on buffered charcoal-yeast extract agar and incubated for 48 h at 37°C in an atmosphere of 5% CO_2 in air. Dense cell suspensions were prepared in 5 ml of 10 m sterile phosphate buffer (pH 7.5) and adjusted to a turbidity approximating that of a McFarland no. 5 standard.

The commercially available API ZYM and experimental API galleries of esterases and aminopeptidases (API Systems SA, Montalieu-Vercieu, France) were used. A total of 84 enzymes were tested: 63 arylpeptidases, 10 esterases, alkaline phosphatase, acid phosphatase, 8 glycosidases, and phosphoamidase.

The test strips were placed in moistened plastic incubation trays, and 100 μl of the cell suspensions was added to each cupule of the strips. All of the galleries were incubated for 6 h at 37°C. After incubation, 1 drop each of reagent A (Tris, 25 g/100 ml; hydrochloric acid [37%], 11 ml; lauryl sulfate, 10 g) and reagent B (0.35% fast blue BB salt in 2-methoxyethanol) were added to each cupule, which were then exposed to a 1,000-W light source for 5 min to destroy excess reagent B. The

color was allowed to develop for 5 to 15 min. Enzymatic activities by API ZYM were graded according to the intensity of color with the API ZYM color reaction chart (0, negative; 1, very weak positive; 2 and 3, positive; 4 and 5, strong positive). Strip tests show positive reactions in appearance of violet color for esterases and orange color for aminopeptidases.

The results obtained with the API enzyme kits were reproducible and gave clear reactions.

Enzymes apparently absent in all *Legionella* strains tested were lipases of myristate, palmitate, and stearate; α-galactosidase; β-galactosidase; β-glucuronidase; α-glucosidase; β-glucosidase; *N*-acetyl-β-glucosaminidase; α-mannosidase; and α-fucosidase. Enzymes apparently present in all *Legionella* strains tested were arylamidases of valine, L-phenylalanine, L-lysine, L-histidine, L-arginine, L-alanine, methionine, L-glutamine, L-ornithine, L-proline, L-serine, L-threonine, L-tryptophan, β-alanine, glycylglycine, glycylphenylalanine, glycylproline, leucylglycine, L-seryltyrosine, L-alanyl-L-arginine, glycyl-L-alanine, glycyl-L-arginine, glycyl-L-tryptophan, L-histidyl-L-serine, L-leucyl-L-alanine, L-lysyl-L-alanine, L-lysyl-L-lysine, L-phenylalanyl-L-arginine, L-phenylalanyl-L-proline, L-seryl-L-methionine, L-histidyl-L-phenylalanine, L-alanyl-L-phenylalanyl-L-proline, L-phenylalanyl-L-prolyl-L-alanine, L-valyl-L-tyrosyl-L-serine, L-lysyl-L-serine-4-methoxy, L-alanyl-L-phenylalanyl-L-prolyl-L-alanine, and L-leucyl-L-leucyl-L-valyl-L-tyronyl-L-serine; esterases of butyrate, valerate, caproate, caprylate, nananoate, and caprate; alkaline phosphatase; acid phosphatase; and phosphoamidase.

The variable enzymatic activities assayed are presented in Table 1. The similarities among the strains tested are illustrated in a dendrogram derived by single-linkage cluster analysis (Fig. 1). As shown in Table 1, strains of *Legionella* species are heterogenic in their enzyme profiles.

In our study, we found a distinct homogeneity within *L. pneumophila* strains, which was in accordance with results of other studies (1, 4). However, three differences within this species could be found. *L. pneumophila* serogroup 6 did not show L-prolyl-L-arginine arylamidase activity, in contrast to serogroups 1, 2, and 3. On the other hand, serogroup 6 possesses *N*-CBZ-arginine-4-methoxy arylamidase and serogroup 2 possesses *N*-benzoylleucine arylamidase, which could not

TABLE 1. Variable enzymatic activities of *Legionella* spp. as tested by the API enzyme system

Enzyme test	A	B	C	D	E	F	G	H	I	J	K	L	M
Leucine arylamidase	×	×	×	×	×	+	×	×	×	−	×	×	×
Cystine arylamidase	+	+	+	+	· +	−	+	+	+	×	+	+	+
Trypsin	−	−	−	−	−	−	−	−	−	×	−	−	−
Chymotrypsin	−	−	−	−	−	+	−	−	−	+	−	−	−
L-Tyrosine arylamidase	+	+	+	+	−	+	+	−	+	−	+	+	−
L-Pyrrolidone arylamidase	+	+	+	+	−	−	+	−	+	−	+	+	−
L-Hydroxyproline arylamidase	+	+	+	+	+	+	+	+	+	+	−	+	+
Glycine arylamidase	×	×	+	+	+	+	×	+	−	+	+	+	+
L-Aspartate arylamidase	×	×	×	×	×	×	×	+	−	+	×	−	+
α-L-Glutamate arylamidase	+	+	+	×	×	+	+	+	+	×	×	×	+
L-Isoleucine arylamidase	+	+	+	+	×	+	×	+	+	+	−	+	−
γ-Glutamyltransferase	+	×	+	+	×	+	+	+	+	+	+	−	+
N-Benzoylleucine arylamidase	−	+	−	−	+	−	−	+	−	+	+	+	−
S-Benzylcysteine arylamidase	+	+	×	×	+	+	×	+	×	−	+	+	+
L-Arginyl-L-arginine arylamidase	+	+	+	×	+	×	−	×	+	×	+	+	+
α-L-Aspartyl-L-alanine arylamidase	×	×	+	×	+	×	−	×	+	×	+	+	+
α-L-Aspartyl-L-arginine arylamidase	×	×	+	+	+	+	−	+	−	×	×	+	+
α-L-Glutamyl-α-L-glutamic arylamidase	×	×	+	+	−	+	−	+	+	+	+	×	+
α-L-Glutamyl-L-histidine arylamidase	×	×	+	+	−	+	−	+	+	+	+	×	+
L-Prolyl-L-arginine arylamidase	+	+	+	−	+	+	+	+	+	+	×	+	+
N-CBZ-arginine-4-methoxy arylamidase	−	−	−	+	−	−	−	−	−	+	−	−	−
N-CBZ-glycylglycyl-L-arginine arylamidase	+	+	+	+	−	+	×	−	−	+	−	×	−
L-Histidyl-L-leucyl-L-histidine arylamidase	+	+	+	+	×	+	+	+	+	×	×	×	−
N-Benzyl-L-alanine-4-methoxy arylamidase	−	−	−	−	−	+	−	−	−	−	−	−	−
N-CBZ-arginyl-4-methoxy arylamidase	−	−	−	−	−	−	+	−	−	+	−	−	−
N-Acetylglycyl-L-lysine arylamidase	+	+	×	+	−	+	×	−	−	+	−	−	−
Laurate lipase	−	−	−	−	+	+	+	+	+	+	×	−	−

[a]A, *L. pneumophila* serogroup 1; B, *L. pneumophila* serogroup 2; C, *L. pneumophila* serogroup 3; D, *L. pneumophila* serogroup 6; E, *L. dumoffii*; F, *L. gormanii*; G, *L. jordanis*; H, *L. feeleii*; I, *L. micdadei*; J, *L. bozemanii*; K, *L. sainthelensi*; L, *L. oakridgensis*; M, *L. longbeachae*. Reactions are indicated as follows: −, negative or very weak positive; +, positive; ×, strong positive.

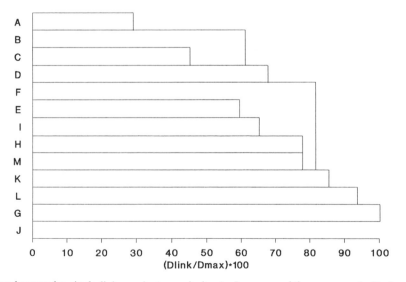

FIG. 1. Dendrogram by single-linkage cluster analysis. A, *L. pneumophila* serogroup 1; B, *L. pneumophila* serogroup 2; C, *L. pneumophila* serogroup 3; D, *L. pneumophila* serogroup 6; E, *L. dumoffii*; F, *L. gormanii*; G, *L. jordanis*; H, *L. feeleii*; I, *L. micdadei*; J, *L. bozemanii*; K, *L. sainthelensi*; L, *L. oakridgensis*; M, *L. longbeachae*.

be detected in other serogroups.

In agreement with other researchers (7, 8), we found in all strains tested strong activities of phosphoamidase and of acid and alkaline phosphatases (pH range from 5.4 to 8.5) but no activities of glycosidases and lipases of myristate, palmitate, and stearate. Laurate lipase was absent only in strains of *L. pneumophila*, *L. oakridgensis*, and *L. longbeachae*.

Müller (7) reported that *L. pneumophila* has a wide range of aminopeptidase activities with the exceptions of L-proline and L-hydroxyproline arylamidases. Contrary to his finding, only weakly positive activities of these two enzymes were detectable in our study.

The absence of trypsin in all strains except *L. bozemanii* is in agreement with other reports (7, 8).

We found detectable chymotrypsin activities in *L. bozemanii* and *L. gormanii* and a very weak reaction by *L. pneumophila* serogroup 2, *L. dumoffii*, and *L. micdadei*. In contrast, Berdal et al. (4) found strong chymotrypsin-like activity with use of chromogenic succinyl-methoxy-carbonylpropionyl-arginylprolyl-tyrosine-*p*-nitroanilide. It appears that the detection of chymotrypsin activity depends on use of an appropriate chromogenic substrate; this question should be further investigated.

In conclusion, the enzymatic activities of *L. pneumophila* showed great similarities. Thus, these strains can be clearly distinguished from strains of other *Legionella* species, in particular by their arylpeptidase activities.

REFERENCES

1. **Berdal, B. P., O. Hushovd, O. Olsvik, O. R. Odegard, and T. Bergan.** 1982. Demonstration of extracellular proteolytic enzymes from *Legionella* species strains by using synthetic chromogenic peptide substrates. *Acta Pathol. Microbiol. Immunol. Scand. Sect. B* **90:**119–123.
2. **Berdal, B. P., B. Kjell, O. Olsvik, and T. Omland.** 1983. Patterns of extracellular proline-specific endopeptidases in *Legionella* and *Flavobacterium* spp. demonstrated by use of chromogenic peptides. *J. Clin. Microbiol.* **17:**970–974.
3. **Berdal, B. P., and O. Olsvik.** 1983. *Legionella* extracellular protease activity on chromogenic peptides: a simplified procedure for biochemical enzyme identification. *Acta Pathol. Microbiol. Immunol. Scand. Sect. B* **91:**89–91.
4. **Berdal, B. P., O. Olsvik, S. Myhre, and T. Omland.** 1982. Demonstration of extracellular chymotrypsin-like activity from various *Legionella* species. *J. Clin. Microbiol.* **16:**452–457.
5. **George, J. R., L. Pine, M. W. Reeves, and W. K. Harrel.** 1980. Amino acid requirements of *Legionella pneumophila*. *J. Clin Microbiol.* **11:**286–291.
6. **McIntyre, M., F. D. Quinn, P. I. Fields, and B. P. Berdal.** 1990. Rapid identification of *Legionella pneumophila* zinc metalloprotease using chromogenic detection. *APMIS* **99:**316–320.
7. **Müller, M.** 1981. Enzymatic profile of *Legionella pneumophila*. *J. Clin. Microbiol.* **13:**423–426.
8. **Nolte, F. S., G. E. Hollick, and R. G. Robertson.** 1982. Enzymatic activities of *Legionella pneumophila* and *Legionella*-like organisms. *J. Clin. Microbiol.* **15:**175–177.

V. PREVENTION AND CONTROL OF LEGIONELLOSIS

Monitoring for the Presence of *Legionella:* Where, When, and How?

JEAN R. JOLY

Groupe de Recherche en Épidémiologie de l'Université Laval, Hôpital du Saint-Sacrement, 1050 Chemin Sainte-Foy, Quebec G1S 4L8, and Département de Microbiologie, Faculté de Médecine, Université Laval, Quebec G1K 7P4, Canada

Monitoring for the presence of a pathogen in the environment was initially implemented for the determination of potable water quality with bacterial counts. In the United States, the Public Health Service Drinking Water Standards were first adopted in 1914 (32). Since 1968, public beaches have also been monitored for the presence of specific bacterial species used as markers for fecal contamination (10). The supply of adequate potable water and the monitoring of both potable and recreational waters for the presence of fecal contamination has been one of the major achievements of public health programs. In recent years, it was found that other pathogens are also present in potable water supplies and that some of them may be responsible for severe and even life-threatening infections. Atypical mycobacteria and legionellae are among these bacteria (1, 14, 25, 42, 43, 47). Since our previous success with the control of enteric pathogens was partly due to an adequate monitoring system, it is tempting to introduce similar strategies for these previously unrecognized pathogens.

It is, however, important to remember that not all of our monitoring efforts were as successful as those for enteric pathogens in potable water. In the early 1960s, it was considered appropriate practice to monitor the presence of air or surface bacteria in the hospital environment, a practice that has largely been abandoned in the 1970s and 1980s (3, 19). The latter monitoring practices were occasionally introducing a false sense of security and relaxation in the application of more appropriate prevention measures.

Whereas there is a scientific basis for the monitoring of enteric pathogens in potable water or public beaches, a similar demonstration for air or surface culture of samples from the hospital environment was never achieved. It is the purpose of this article to review the evidence for and against the implementation of a monitoring policy for legionellae. Obviously, our knowledge of the importance of the different environments favoring the transmission of legionellosis is imperfect, and it is impossible to generalize monitoring strategies from one ecological niche that harbors legionellae to another. In the following few pages, I will review the different environments that have been associated with Legionnaires disease and the evidence that may suggest a public health benefit in monitoring for the presence of these bacteria. In the last section, I will briefly review the methods that are used to identify members of the family *Legionellaceae* in both natural and man-made environments.

NATURAL ENVIRONMENT

The ubiquity of legionellae in lakes and rivers throughout the world is well known. Fliermans et al. have shown that nearly 100% of lakes and rivers in the southeastern United States are contaminated (21, 22). Similar figures have been reported in Puerto Rico, and 50% of lake and river samples in Canada were also found to contain *Legionellaceae* (29, 38). The concentration of legionellae in these waters is usually low (21). Because of this, and despite the extensive aerosolization that may take place in, for instance, natural waterfalls, no known case of legionellosis related to this type of exposure has ever been reported. Without cases, monitoring of the natural environment would be not only useless but also extremely expensive.

The sole exception to this rule may be the contamination of hot spring spas, if these may be considered natural environments. Bornstein et al. reported the occurrence of Legionnaires disease in five patients and therapists at a French hot spring spa (8). Despite the presence of fairly large concentrations of *Legionellaceae* (10^3 to 10^5 CFU/liter), it was impossible to implement a hyperchlorination program since this would have altered the medicinal qualities of the water, a modification that is forbidden by French law. Obviously, heating water to 60°C was not an alternative. The only acceptable solution was the implementation of drastic housekeeping procedures when the levels of legionellae were considered unsafe.

Following this outbreak, monitoring for the presence of *Legionellaceae* was implemented in all French hot spring spas, a policy that required the licensing of laboratories and implementation of a proficiency testing program for these laboratories. When unsafe levels of legionellae were found in a spa, a thorough cleansing of the facility was required. Unsafe levels of legionellae are, however, extremely difficult to determine, since the human infective dose is unknown and probably largely dependent on the immune status of the host and the possibilities of aerosolization in that facility. Because of this, implementation of stringent housekeeping procedures in all of these spas and case surveillance should be sufficient. Such a policy would, however, need to be validated before implementation.

MAN-MADE ENVIRONMENTS

Hospitals. Hospitals as well as other large buildings are frequently contaminated by *Legionellaceae* (1, 5a, 6, 14, 39, 42–45, 47). In the United Kingdom, United States, and Canada, 75, 60, and 75% of sampled institutions were contaminated by these bacteria (1, 5a, 46). These high proportions are most probably minimum figures, since they are based on limited sampling for a restricted time in each institution. Indeed, it has been our experience that the level of contamination within an institution will be highly variable without any specific intervention (1). In a hospital where quarterly monitoring of the same 10 sites was routinely performed, more than 60 samples had to be analyzed before a single one was found to be positive; then, within a month, 80% of these sites were contaminated by legionellae. Not a single factor could be identified in that hospital to explain the sudden surge in the proportion of positive samples. It is thus quite probable that most hospital potable water supplies will eventually be found to be contaminated by these bacteria. Finally, contamination of the hospital environment is related to the location of the institution, the age of the building, the size of the largest hot water reservoir, and the temperature of the hot water, all factors (except the last) that are largely beyond our control (1, 26).

The irregular contamination pattern makes it difficult to determine the frequency of monitoring and the number of sites within an institution that should be sampled (4). The literature is extremely poor when it comes to the methodology of site selection within an institution (random sampling throughout the hospital, only in areas where high risk patients are hospitalized, etc.) and the monitoring schedule (every year, month, week, after repair on the plumbing system, etc.). Finally, if monitoring is decided upon, the procedure that

should be used not only to culture the bacteria but also to address the elusive issue of viable but nonculturable organisms is also a highly debatable issue. An answer to most if not all of these questions would certainly be useful before a rational monitoring program is instituted.

The presence of legionellae in the hospital environment has frequently been associated with the presence of nosocomial legionellosis (6, 27, 35, 37, 42–44). Moreover, in some institutions where no known cases of legionellosis had been identified in the previous months or years, the implementation of routine surveillance of nosocomial pneumonia disclosed major problems if adequate laboratory support for the detection of legionellae was also provided (35). In some of these instances, Legionnaires disease accounted for over 14% of all cases of nosocomial pneumonia (35). Yet in other institutions, although legionellae were routinely recovered from the potable water supply, no known cases were found despite adequate surveillance (14, 45, 47). The factors that could account for these discrepant results are largely unknown. Certain serogroups and subtypes of *Legionella pneumophila* are known to be more virulent than others, or at least to be more frequently associated with outbreaks of legionellosis (41). Could this be the only significant difference between institutions with and without cases? This is improbable, since numerous hospitals colonized with "avirulent strains" had nosocomial infections caused by *L. pneumophila*. Different studies have demonstrated that some plumbing devices (e.g., aerators) and designs (e.g., presence of dead ends) were more frequently contaminated by legionellae (12) or that certain plumbing material provided the appropriate nutrients for the growth of *L. pneumophila* (13).

Despite these observations, we still do not know whether the presence of legionellae in the water distribution system of a hospital will necessarily lead to the occurrence of nosocomial legionellosis. This is a crucial question, as it relates directly to the issue of monitoring. At this meeting, Michel Alary and I presented preliminary results on this issue (Joly and Alary, this volume). Ten hospitals known to have a potable water supply contaminated by *L. pneumophila* serogroup 1 were matched with a similar number of institutions from whose water supply these bacteria could not be recovered. In each institution, active surveillance of all cases of nosocomial pneumonia was established for 9 months. One institution in the contaminated group dropped out of the study, whereas one that was initially thought to be noncontaminated was later found to harbor legionellae. In 4 of the 10 contaminated institutions, nosocomial legionellosis was identified. Of the nine uncontaminated hospitals, none had nosocomial infections caused by legionellae ($P =$ 0.056, Fisher's exact test). If confirmed, these results would suggest that a significant number (>40%) of hospitals with a potable water supply contaminated by *L. pneumophila* serogroup 1 would have cases of nosocomial legionellosis within a few months. Whether all of these institutions would have cases is still unknown, and longer follow-up periods would be necessary to demonstrate this possibility.

Because of the latter result, because of the ubiquity of legionellae in the hospital environment, because of the large fluctuations in the number of culture-positive outlets in a single institution, and because Legionnaires disease is frequently overlooked as a nosocomial infection, even in institutions where *L. pneumophila* accounted for more than 30% of all nosocomial pneumonia, I would suggest that all hospital potable water systems should be considered contaminated and that appropriate preventive measures should be taken regardless of the results of environmental cultures. With such a policy, since all institutions would be considered contaminated, monitoring would be useless. Environmental cultures should be done only during recognized outbreaks when one is examining known and potential new environmental sources of legionellae.

Although the costs of these measures could be substantial and a formal cost analysis study should be done, it is quite probable that the reduction in time of hospitalization, loss of productivity, and potential liabilities would offset the costs. Whether hyperchlorination, increased water temperature, or any other engineering measure should be adopted should be dictated by the local situation. A careful analysis of the presence of known risk factors and their elimination should be an essential part of any preventive program for legionellosis. Since aerators are known to increase the contamination of the outlets by legionellae, could faucets without these devices be used in all hospitals? Could dead ends be eliminated?

Alternatives to this primary prevention strategy should be examined. The possibility that ingestion of contaminated water can lead to legionellosis in high-risk subjects has recently been suggested. In a study done at the Victoria General Hospital in Halifax, it was found that patients with nasogastric tubes were at high risk of acquiring legionellosis (34). Irrigation of these tubes was usually done with tap water. Following this observation, sterile water was used for irrigation, with a concomitant decrease in the number of cases of nosocomial legionellosis. Despite this measure, cases of Legionnaires disease still occurred in hospitalized patients. Further study of these patients revealed that all were highly immunosuppressed. Once these high-risk individuals were given sterile water as drinking water, no further nosocomial

infections caused by *L. pneumophila* were found. The annual cost of such a policy was approximately $12,000, a figure comparable to the cost of hyperchlorination or heating the hot water supply to 60°C. Unfortunately, the major problem with such a simple policy is compliance. Convincing these high-risk individuals of the potential benefits of this solution is often a very difficult task.

Cooling towers. Cooling towers are also frequently contaminated by *Legionellaceae* (15, 23, 31). Miller and Kenepp (this volume) have shown that 36% of the cooling towers sampled in the Washington, D.C., area contained *Legionellaceae*. In some instances, the number of *L. pneumophila* found in these cooling towers was extremely high (up to 2×10^7/liter). Cooling towers not only provide an excellent amplifier for *Legionellae*, but also are efficient disseminators of these bacteria.

Cooling towers have been associated with numerous outbreaks (15, 23, 31). The best evidence for this causal relationship was established in the Burlington, Vt., outbreak, when a direct relationship between the distance from the cooling tower and the attack rate was demonstrated (9, 31). When a subject worked between 0 and 200 m from the implicated cooling tower, the attack rate was 67.3/10,000. For individuals working between 200 and 700 m from the tower, the attack rate was reduced to 4.3/10,000. In addition, the bacteria that were isolated from the cooling tower were identical to those found in the tracheobronchial secretions of patients with Legionnaires disease (30). A further line of evidence for the association between cooling towers and legionellosis comes from an epidemiological study done in Glasgow (6a). In a case control study of subjects with sporadic community-acquired Legionnaires disease, the attack rate for the infection was related to the distance of the subject house to the nearest cooling tower. There are thus good indications that both epidemic and sporadic community-acquired Legionnaires diseases can be acquired from contaminated cooling towers.

Legionellaceae are relatively difficult to isolate from grossly contaminated environments and are fastidious in their growth requirements, a situation somewhat similar to that of certain known enteric pathogens. Because of this, should we look for a surrogate marker for their presence, just as fecal coliforms are markers of fecal contamination in potable water? Again, evidence presented at this meeting does not support this possibility. Indeed, in the study presented by Miller and Kenepp (this volume), *L. pneumophila* levels could not be related to the presence of any heterotrophic bacteria or to use of biocide.

Given the known relationship between cooling towers with outbreaks of legionellosis and their possible association with sporadic cases, should we adopt a monitoring policy for these apparatuses? Given the aforementioned difficulties, should not all cooling towers be considered contaminated? Good housekeeping practices for these mechanical devices (including adequate maintenance and routine use of appropriate biocides) should be implemented. New designs aimed at reducing the amount of drift as proposed by the Australians should be encouraged. Monitoring for the presence of legionellae and the reported absence of these bacteria during routine monitoring should not be considered a substitute for good maintenance of these towers. Indeed, in two of the most deadly and publicized outbreaks to occur in the United Kingdom (the British Broadcasting Corporation and Staffordshire outbreaks), both cooling towers implicated as sources of *L. pneumophila* were routinely monitored for the presence of these bacteria. Monitoring can have perverse effects, providing a false sense of security when negative results are obtained and, as a consequence, fostering a disregard of appropriate preventive measures.

Hotels. Whether hotel potable water supplies should be monitored for the presence of legionellae is another difficult question. Obviously, hotels have been implicated in some outbreaks (5). Given the relatively small (but certainly grossly underestimated) number of outbreaks that have been related to this type of exposure, continuous monitoring of all of these institutions is probably not warranted. However, I would suggest that international monitoring of cases using the case definition provided by the World Health Organization is warranted (49). The British experience in establishing relationships between sporadic legionellosis and prior hotel exposure has been extremely fruitful. Indeed, by simply linking cases to previous hotel exposure and by cross-tabulating these exposures with other cases in which such exposure had occurred, British epidemiologists showed that numerous point source outbreaks related to hotels could be identified and that preventive measures could be implemented. This extremely simple and inexpensive measure should be applied on a more global scale, and international reporting should be encouraged. The European Working Group on Legionella has been instrumental in developing such an approach in Europe, and similar protocols should be implemented worldwide. Routine surveillance of cases appears to be the best possible approach in this specific instance.

Workplace. The workplace has undoubtedly been related to outbreaks of legionellosis. The *L. feeleii* outbreak in an engine assembly plant in North America and the British Broadcasting Corporation outbreak are good examples (28, 36). Does the occurrence of these few reported incidents warrant routine monitoring of all industries

and companies? Data to support such a policy are simply nonexistent.

In the presence of a single case of legionellosis that might be related to workplace exposure, should a full investigation be launched? Although labor unions will demand such an inquiry the probability that a single case will be related to this type of exposure appears to be so low as to preclude such measures on a routine basis. However, the finding of a second case in the same environment should be enough to warrant a full investigation, including environmental cultures. Once the cause has been identified and proper measures have been implemented, there is little evidence in the scientific literature to suggest that continuous monitoring of that environment would provide any additional safety measure. The authorities responsible for maintenance of the source of these few cases should be held accountable for its proper maintenance.

Domestic environment. Until recently, the domestic environment was not thought to be an important source of legionellosis. A recent report demonstrated that a substantial but small proportion of sporadic cases was related to this type of exposure (40). Given the diversity of domestic environments, the number of exposed individuals might range from a single family for a private house to a few hundred or possibly thousands in large multiapartment buildings. Should we monitor for the presence of legionellae in these residences without a previously reported case? Obviously not. Once a case is identified, should we launch a full-scale environmental investigation? During a research project, such a measure is probably justified, but establishing this measure as a routine public health strategy would possibly divert significant resources to a problem that may not be important enough to warrant the procedure. Obviously, additional studies in this area are needed.

MONITORING TECHNIQUES

The recovery of *Legionellaceae* from the environment was initially achieved through animal inoculation. Initial studies on the environmental distribution of these bacteria were also realized through animal inoculation and immunofluorescence techniques (11, 21, 22). With the introduction of more efficient and semiselective culture media and the identification of enrichment procedures, animal inoculation became obsolete (16–18, 20). Numerous laboratories now isolate legionellae from the environment by using semiselective media (48) and an acid enrichment procedure (7).

The role of direct or indirect immunofluorescence technique in the identification of legionellae in the environment is still highly debated. Whereas some will cite the high specificity and sensitivity of this technique (22), others have found it to be nonspecific and nonsensitive (2, 24). Whether this disagreement is related to the issue of viable but nonculturable bacteria is still unresolved. The demonstration that a specific environment is related to cases of Legionnaires disease still requires the isolation of legionellae from that source. Although important, this prerequisite does not by itself imply that the culture-positive environment is the source of legionellosis. This determination must be made through an adequate epidemiological study.

In the last few years, the polymerase chain reaction has been introduced for the detection of legionellae in the environment (33). Up to now, most studies have been restricted to seeded samples or non-outbreak-related water samples, and the sensitivity and specificity of the technique appear to be high. Whether this will hold true for samples that originate directly from potential sources of legionellosis remains to be seen. Nonetheless, the polymerase chain reaction appears to be a promising tool for detection of legionellae in the environment.

CONCLUSION

Monitoring for the presence of legionellae in the hospital environment and in most if not all other environments is based largely on the intuitive feeling that knowledge of the presence of these bacteria in a given habitat will somehow increase our ability to prevent or recognize Legionnaires disease, a postulate that still needs to be proven. Given that numerous laboratories are still unable to isolate legionellae, monitoring would require an intense training effort as well as the introduction of a good proficiency testing program. In an era of limited resources and hard choices, the efforts devoted to these activities would necessarily have to be eliminated from other important prevention activities.

Before any of these prevention activities can be given priority, it will be important to define the attributable risk related to different types of exposure. We know that between 60 and 80% of all reported cases are sporadic. The sources of these infections are still largely unknown, although 40% of the cases in one study could be attributed to a given source. Further studies along this line are needed to better identify the sources of each of these cases. Only then will we be able to adequately address the issue of primary prevention.

REFERENCES

1. **Alary, M., and J. R. Joly.** 1992. Factors contributing to the contamination of hospital water distribution systems by Legionellae. *J. Infect. Dis.* **165:**565–569.
2. **Alary, M., and J. R. Joly.** 1992. Comparison of culture methods and an immunofluorescence assay for the detection of *Legionella pneumophila* in domestic hot water devices. *Curr. Microbiol.* **25:**19–23.
3. **American Hospital Association Committee on Infections within Hospitals.** 1974. Statement on microbiologic sampling in the hospital. *Hospitals* **48:**125–6.
4. **Barbaree, J. M., G. W. Gorman, W. T. Martin, B. S. Fields, and W. E. Morril.** 1987. Protocol for sampling environmental sites for legionellae. *Appl. Environ. Microbiol.* **53:**1454–1458.
5. **Bartlett, C. L. R., and L. F. Bibby.** 1983. Epidemic legionellosis in England and Wales 1979–1982. *Zentralbl. Bakteriol. Mikrobiol. Hyg. Abt. 1 Orig. Reihe A* **255:**64–70.
5a. **Bartlett, C. L. R., J. B. Kurtz, J. G. P. Hutchinson, G. P. Turner, and A. E. Wright.** 1983. Legionella in hospital and hotel water supplies. *Lancet* **ii:**1315.
6. **Best, M., V. L. Yu, J. Stout, A. Goetz, R. R. Muder, and F. Taylor.** 1983. *Legionellaceae* in the hospital water supply. Epidemiological link with disease and evaluation of a method for control of nosocomial Legionnaires' disease and Pittsburgh pneumonia. *Lancet* **ii:**307–310.
6a. **Bhopal, R. S., R. J. Fallon, E. C. Buist, R. J. Black, and J. D. Urquhart.** 1991. Proximity of the home to a cooling tower and risk of non-outbreak Legionnaires' disease. *Br. Med. J.* **302:**378–383.
7. **Bopp, C. A., J. W. Sumner, G. K. Morris, and J. G. Wells.** 1981. Isolation of *Legionella* spp. from environmental water samples by low-pH treatment and use of a selective medium. *J. Clin. Microbiol.* **13:**714–719.
8. **Bornstein, N., D. Marmet, M. Surgot, M. Nowicki, A. Arslan, J. Esteve, and J. Fleurette.** 1989. Exposure to *Legionellaceae* at a hot spring spa: a prospective clinical and serological study. *Epidemiol. Infect.* **102:**31–36.
9. **Broome, C. V., S. A. Goings, S. B. Thacker, R. L. Gogt, H. N. Beaty, and D. W. Fraser.** 1979. The Vermont epidemic of Legionnaires' disease. *Ann. Intern. Med.* **90:**573–577.
10. **Cabelli, V. J., A. P. Dufour, L. J. McCabe, and M. A. Leven.** 1982. Swimming associated gastroenteritis and water quality. *Am. J. Epidemiol.* **115:**606–616.
11. **Cherry, W. B., B. B. Pittman, P. P. Harris, G. A. Hebert, B. M. Thomason, L. Thacker, and R. E. Weaver.** 1978. Detection of Legionnaires disease bacteria by direct immunofluorescent staining. *J. Clin. Microbiol.* **8:**329–338.
12. **Ciesielski, C. A., M. J. Blaser, and W. L. Wang.** 1984. Role of stagnation and obstruction of water flow in isolation of *Legionella pneumophila* from hospital plumbing. *Appl. Environ. Microbiol.* **48:**984–987.
13. **Colbourne, J. S., D. J. Pratt, M. G. Smith, S. P. Fisher-Hoch, and D. Harper.** 1984. Water fittings as sources of Legionella pneumophila in a hospital plumbing system. *Lancet* **i:**210–213.
14. **Dennis, P. J., J. A. Taylor, R. B. Fitzgeorge, C. L. R. Bartlett, and G. I. Barrow.** 1982. *Legionella pneumophila* in water plumbing systems. *Lancet* **i:**949–951.
15. **Dondero, T. J., Jr., R. C. Rendtorff, G. F. Mallison, R. M. Weeks, J. S. Levy, E. W. Wong, and W. Schaffner.** 1980. An outbreak of Legionnaires' disease associated with a contaminated air cooling tower. *N. Engl. J. Med.* **302:**365–370.
16. **Edelstein, P. H.** 1981. Improved semi-selective medium for isolation of *Legionella pneumophila* from contaminated clinical and environmental specimens. *J. Clin. Microbiol.* **14:**298–303.
17. **Edelstein, P. H.** 1982. Comparative study of selective media for isolation of *Legionella pneumophila* from potable water. *J. Clin. Microbiol.* **16:**697–699.
18. **Edelstein, P. H., J. B. Snitzer, and S. M. Finegold.** 1982. Isolation of *Legionella pneumophila* from hospital potable water specimens: comparison of direct plating with guinea pig inoculation. *J. Clin. Microbiol.* **15:**1092–1096.

19. **Eickhoff, T. C.** 1970. Microbiologic sampling. *Hospitals* **44:**86–87.

20. **Fitzgeorge, R. B., and P. J. Dennis.** 1983. Isolation of *Legionella pneumophila* from water supplies: comparison of methods based on the guinea-pig and culture media. *J. Hyg.* (Cambridge) **91:**179–187.

21. **Fliermans, C. B., W. B. Cherry, L. H. Orrison, S. J. Smith, D. L. Tison, and D. H. Pope.** 1981. Ecological distribution of *Legionella pneumophila. Appl. Environ. Microbiol.* **41:**9–16.

22. **Fliermans, C. B., W. B. Cherry, L. H. Orrison, and L. Thacker.** 1979. Isolation of *Legionella pneumophila* from non-epidemic-related aquatic habitats. *Appl. Environ. Microbiol.* **37:**1239–1242.

23. **Garbe, P. L., B. J. Davis, J. S. Weisfeld, L. Karkowitz, P. Miner, F. Garrity, J. M. Barbaree, and A. R. Reingold.** 1985. Nosocomial Legionnaires' disease. Epidemiologic demonstration of cooling towers as source. *JAMA* **254:**521–524.

24. **Glupczynski, Y., M. Labbe, and E. Yourassowsky.** 1988. Cross-reactivity of environmental bacteria with fluorescent antibody conjugates for *Legionella pneumophila. Eur. J. Clin. Microbiol.* **3:**215.

25. **Goslee, S., and E. Wolinsky,** 1976. Water as a source of potentially pathogenic mycobacteria. *Am. Rev. Respir. Dis.* **113:**287–292.

26. **Groothuis, D. G., H. R. Veenendaal, and H. L. Dijkstra.** 1985. Influence of temperature on the number of *Legionella pneumophila* in hot water systems. *J. Appl. Bacteriol.* **59:**529–536.

27. **Helms, C. M., R. M. Massanari, R. Zeitler, S. Streed, M. J. Gilchrist, N. Hall, W. J. Hausler, Jr., J. Sywassink, W. Johnson, L. Wintermeyer, and J. Hierholzer, Jr.** 1983. Legionnaires' disease associated with a hospital water system: a cluster of 24 nosocomial cases. *Ann. Intern. Med.* **99:**172–178.

28. **Herwaldt, L. A., G. W. Gorman, T. McGrath, S. Toma, B. Brake, A. W. Hightower, J. Jones, A. R. Reingold, P. A. Boxer, P. W. Tang, C. W. Moss, H. Wilkinson, D. J. Brenner, A. G. Steigerwalt, and C. V. Broome.** 1984. A new Legionella species. *Legionella feeleii* species nova, causes Pontiac fever in an automobile plant. *Ann. Intern. Med.* **100:**333–338.

29. **Joly, J. R., M. Boissinot, J. Duchaine, M. Duval, J. Rafrafi, D. Ramsay, and R. Letarte.** 1984. Ecological distribution of *Legionellaceae* in the Quebec city area. *Can. J. Microbiol.* **30:**63–67.

30. **Joly, J. R., and W. C. Winn.** 1984. Correlation of subtypes of *Legionella pneumophila* defined by monoclonal antibodies with epidemiological classification of cases and environmental sources. *J. Infect. Dis.* **150:**667–671.

31. **Klaucke, D. N., R. L. Vogt, D. LaRue, L. E. Witherell, L. A. Orciari, K. C. Spitalny, R. Pelletier, W. B. Cherry, and L. F. Novick.** 1984. Legionnaires' disease: the epidemiology of two outbreaks in Burlington, Vermont, 1980. *Am. J. Epidemiol.* **119:**382–391.

32. **Last, J. M., and R. B. Wallace (ed.)** 1992. *Maxcy-Rosenau-Last Public Health and Preventive Medicine,* 13th ed. Appleton Century Crofts, Norwalk, Conn.

33. **Mahbubani, M. H., A. K. Bej, R. Miller, L. Haff, J. DiCesare, and R. M. Atlas.** 1990. Detection of Legionella with polymerase chain reaction and gene probe methods. *Mol. Cell. Probes* **4:**175–187.

34. **Marrie, T. J., D. Haldane, K. MacDonald, K. Clarke, C. Fanning, S. Le Fort-Jost, G. Bezanson, and J. Joly.** 1991. Control of endemic nosocomial Legionnaires' disease by using sterile potable water for high risk patients.

35. **Muder, R. R., V. L. Yu, J. K. McClure, F. J. Kroboth, S. D. Kominos, and R. M. Lumish.** 1983. Nosocomial Legionnaires' disease uncovered in a prospective pneumonia study: implications for underdiagnosis. *JAMA* **249:**3184–3192.

36. **Muraca, P. W., J. E. Stout, V. L. Yu, and Y. C. Yee.** 1988. Legionnaires' disease in the work environment: implications for environmental health. *Am. Ind. Hyg. Assoc. J.* **49:**584–590.

37. **Neill, M. A., G. W. Gorman, C. Gibert, A. Roussel, A. W. Hightower, R. M. McKinney, and C. V. Broome.** 1985. Nosocomial legionellosis, Paris, France. Evidence of transmission by potable water. *Am. J. Med.* **78:**581–588.

38. **Ortiz-Roque, C. M., and T. C. Hazen.** 1987. Abundance and distribution of *Legionellaceae* in Puerto Rican waters. *Appl. Environ. Microbiol.* **53:**2231–2236.

39. **States, S. J., L. F. Conley, J. M. Kuchta, B. M. Oleck, M. J. Lipovich, R. S. Wolford, R. M. Wadowsky, A. M. McNamara, J. L. Sykora, G. Keleti, and R. B. Yee.** 1987. Survival and multiplication of *Legionella pneumophila* in municipal drinking water systems. *Appl. Environ. Microbiol.* **53:**979–986.

40. **Stout, J., J. R. Joly, J. Plouffee, M. Para, C. Ciesielski, M. J. Blaser, and V. L. Yu.** 1988. Comparison of molecular methods for subtyping patients' and epidemiologically linked environmental isolates of Legionella pneumophila. *J. Infect. Dis.* **157:**486–495.

41. **Stout, J. E., V. L. Yu, P. Muraca, J. Joly, N. Troup, and L. S. Tompkins.** 1992. Potable water as a cause of sporadic cases of community-acquired Legionnaires' disease. *N. Engl. J. Med.* **326:**151–155.

42. **Stout, J. E., V. L. Yu, R. M. Vickers, and J. Shonnard.** 1982. Potable water supply as the hospital reservoir for Pittsburgh pneumonia agent. *Lancet* **i:**471–472.

43. **Stout, J. E., V. L. Yu, R. M. Vickers, J. Zuravleff, M. Best, A. Brown, R. B. Yee, and R. Wadowsky.** 1982. Ubiquitousness of *Legionella pneumophila* in water supply of a hospital with endemic Legionnaires' disease. *N. Engl. J. Med.* **306:**466–468.

44. **Tobin, J. O., M. S. Dunnil, M. French, P. J. Morris, J. Beare, S. Fisher-Hock, R. G. Mitchell, and M. F. Muers.** 1980. Legionnaires' disease in a transplant unit: isolation of the causative agent from shower baths. *Lancet* **ii:**118–121.

45. **Tobin, J. O., R. A. Swann, and C. L. R. Bartlett.** 1981. Isolation of *Legionella pneumophila* from water systems: methods and preliminary results. *Br. Med. J.* **282:**515–517.

46. **Vickers, R. M., V. L. Yu, S. S. Hanna, P. Muraca, W. Diven, N. Carmen, and F. B. Taylor.** 1987. Determinants of *Legionella pneumophila* contamination of water distribution systems: 15-hospital prospective study. *Infect. Control* **8:**357–363.

47. **Wadowsky, R. M., R. B. Yee, L. Mezmar, E. J. Wing, and J. N. Dowling.** 1982. Hot water systems as sources of *Legionella pneumophila* in hospital and nonhospital plumbing fixtures. *Appl. Environ. Microbiol.* **43:**1104–1110.

48. **Wadowsky, R. M., and R. B. Yee.** 1981. Glycine-containing selective medium for isolation of *Legionella pneumophila* from environmental samples. *Appl. Environ. Microbiol.* **42:**768–772.

49. **World Health Organization.** 1990. Epidemiology, prevention and control of legionellosis: memorandum from a WHO meeting. *Bull. W.H.O.* **68:**155–164.

Epidemiol. Infect. **107:**591–605.

Legionella in Cooling Towers: Practical Research, Design, Treatment, and Control Guidelines

CLIVE R. BROADBENT

Federal Department of Administrative Services, Phillip, ACT 2606, Australia

Cooling towers and similar heat rejection devices provide cooling water for a wide variety of applications. These applications include refrigeration plant, water-cooled air compressors, and other industrial processes in which heat is generated. A prime function of cooling towers is to save water that would otherwise be run to waste.

Microorganisms may enter cooling water systems via the water supply, via the air intake, or during tower installation. The constant fall of water through the tower serves to act as an air scrubber. Airborne particulate matter in some urban districts may be in the order of 1.5 g/1,000 m³. Therefore, for a typical tower rejecting 700 kW and handling an airflow of 19,000 liters/s, some 100 kg of solid matter could be drawn into the tower every 1,000 h of operation. Some 200 kg may enter the system as solids in the water supply itself (typically 100 mg of suspended solids per liter in the mains water and 0.5 liters of water consumption per s), for a total of 300 kg. The elevated water temperature, the moisture, the increased oxygen tension at air-water surfaces, and the addition of nutrients present ideal conditions for microbial growth, which is assisted by the large surface area of the basin, fill, pipework, and heat exchanger. Algae, protozoa, fungi, and bacteria, including *Legionella* species, are commonly able to colonize these systems. Cooling towers have been linked to many outbreaks of Legionnaires disease (3, 4, 23). Of course, contaminated water presents a risk only when dispersed into the air in the form of aerosol that may originate as water droplets.

Dissemination of water droplets from cooling towers can be greatly reduced by efficient drift eliminators fitted to the discharge. Although it is small droplets that are of eventual interest as far as the receiving host is concerned, physically large droplets are also of interest, since they are more likely to contain large numbers of bacteria and may dry down to a smaller size before evaporating completely, leaving droplet nuclei that may contain many viable bacteria of a size that can be inhaled to the depths of the lungs.

Manufacturers have greatly improved the performance of drift eliminators in recent years with the development of components vacuum molded to precise geometric patterns. Water lost as drift may now be orders of magnitude lower than in earlier styles. Such eliminator modules may also be retrofitted to older towers. Care should be taken with any eliminator installation to ensure that there is no opportunity for air to bypass the eliminators and so defeat their purpose.

When the tower fan is idle, reverse airflow can take place under adverse wind conditions (9). If the cooling water is inadvertently circulating at the same time, droplets can become entrained in the air leaving the tower at the basin air (intake) opening. This set of circumstances may have prevailed at the cooling tower that led to the outbreak of Legionnaires' disease at Stafford, England, in April 1985 (8). The outside air intake for the air conditioning plant was, in effect, located immediately adjacent to the tower within a roof enclosure. Further, the colocation of air-handling plants and cooling towers in a common ventilated plant room is not unusual. Existing layouts of this type need to be reviewed, and if reversed airflow through the tower can enter the intake to the air-handling plant, the latter should be relocated to draw air directly from outside.

Many countries have produced guidelines or codes of practice relating to the control of *legionellae* (9, 18). An Australian development has been the production of a regulatory standard called AS 3666—1989, "Air-Handling and Water Systems of Buildings, Microbial Control" (27). This standard aims to improve overall health and hygienic aspects of air and water systems. It puts forward reasonable control measures based on the best engineering and scientific knowledge to date and places much importance on design aspects of systems because many previous design practices made effective maintenance difficult. Requirements include the need for building plans that are submitted to regulatory authorities to include a site survey of the new building and adjacent buildings regarding location of cooling towers, air intakes, and exhaust discharges (the separation distance between cooling towers and air intakes should be the maximum that is reasonably possible); detailed system design, installation, and maintenance features; appropriate safety procedures and protective gear; and, the need for trained personnel to carry out maintenance work at cooling towers because the public (and their own) health is potentially at risk.

The incorporation of this Australian standard into health legislation has important ramifications. For example, old dilapidated cooling towers, of which there are many, must be reassessed in light of the legislation. No longer is the issue one of extending the functional life of a particular tower because now the equipment must be viewed as a potential health hazard and a legal liability if the owner is negligent. There are now stiff penalties for failing to maintain and treat cooling tower systems. To improve maintenance standards, several Australian health agencies have initiated compulsory registration of cooling towers, a trend which is apparent elsewhere, notably in the United Kingdom.

A number of Australian regulatory actions such as tower registration resulted from concerns generated by the outbreak (44 cases) in Wollongong in April 1987. This outbreak occurred in a shopping center and, apart from the immediate suffering, long-term shopping, business, and tourism were seriously affected. Several features of the outbreak (11) were as follows: warm, humid, and cloudy weather conditions prevailed, with light coastal evening breezes; the cooling tower implicated was small (air conditioning capacity of about 70 kW); the tower was about 70 m away from the air intake to the ventilation plant serving the premises at which the outbreak occurred; the tower was operated only intermittently in hot weather; the tower was in a poor state of maintenance; no drift eliminators were fitted to the tower; and the public anxiety aroused by this outbreak was intense.

While the need for equipment hygiene is a well-recognized aspect of conventional wisdom on the subject, most of the practices presently in place to control Legionella colonization in cooling towers are almost entirely empirical (5, 14, 24), and confidence in their efficacy is incomplete (2). Published research to substantiate current practices is scarce. Some management strategies are barely adequate, but others, motivated by fear of industrial unrest or the potential for litigation, seem to be excessively costly. A more analytical basis for management approaches is needed.

Barbaree (2) has highlighted the lack of field research data and has pointed out the difficulties in controllling Legionella populations in equipment, such as cooling towers, given the ubiquitous presence of the bacteria in natural and man-made water systems and the complex manner in which legionellae adapt to their environment. He has stressed the need for further research in order to establish better control measures.

In response to this need, a field research project is in progress in Australia. The project aims to establish the maintenance necessary to control Legionella colonization cost-effectively by introducing better analytical methodologies into current management approaches. Three years of ongoing research have now been completed; results after 2 years were reported in the literature (7).

Objectives of the project are to investigate the relationship between Legionella concentrations and conditions normally experienced, including pH, conductivity, water temperature, and ambient air temperatures; routine cleaning; decontamination (generally by high-dosage chlorination and cleaning); seasonal variations; usage, i.e., operating hours and whether continuous or seasonal; effectiveness of biocides; and, presence of growth niches within cooling tower systems. Possible correlations between these factors and Legionella colonization have been investigated by computer-aided statistical analysis.

The towers selected varied considerably in age, condition, and materials of construction but were all of the packaged, compact type; such types have predominated in disease outbreaks, at least in Australia. Initially, some 45 cooling towers, all in Adelaide, South Australia, were monitored; several were subsequently decommissioned, and the sample size was reduced to 36 at the end of 2 years and to 31 after 3 years. Several towers were decommissioned because of consistently high Legionella counts; they were replaced with dry, air-cooled plant.

After 2 years in the study, it was considered necessary to introduce further data from another site (of different latitude, mains water, etc.) to assist in the confirmation of results at that time. Accordingly, water samples from a control group of 34 cooling towers located in Melbourne, Victoria, were collected, and these towers were included in the research study.

Results to date are based on the analysis of approximately 9,000 samples taken from 65 (nominal) cooling towers over the 3-year period. Analysis was by conventional laboratory culturing techniques (13). Most of the Adelaide towers were fitted with hours-run meters, temperature sensors, and other instrumentation to assist with data gathering.

For the duration of the study, all of the Adelaide cooling towers were on similar cleaning and chemical treatment protocols, including continuous scale and corrosion inhibitors and, generally, weekly slug dosages of biocide to control overall microbial populations. Cleaning was initially quarterly (5).

Although the Legionella concentrations in tower water may not be directly related to infectivity (14), precautionary decontamination of cooling towers was carried out when the level of 1,000 CFU/ml was exceeded. Decontamination involved shutdown followed by a sequence of steps that included use of detergents, high-dosage chlorination, flushing, physical cleaning, and further chlorination in accordance with established procedures (5, 17).

Key results to date are as follows. *Legionella* colonization of cooling towers varied seasonally, as reported elsewhere (17). The *Legionella* species isolated were *Legionella pneumophila* serogroup 1 (70%), *L. anisa* (23%), *L. rubrilucens* (6.9%), and *L. pneumophila* serogroups 2 to 13 (0.1%). *Legionella* counts fell below detectable limits when the pH rose above 10.0, but this is an undesirable operating condition for all but unusual cooling tower applications. As in other studies (19, 22), no relationship was established between *Legionella* counts and conductivity, nor was a correlation with total bacterial counts found. Because of difficulties in sediment sample treatment in the laboratory, bulk water was the most reliable practical indicator of *Legionella* colonization. Only rarely in these trials was a positive report from water or slime samples collected from the fill of cooling towers. This site appears to provide a poor environment for *Legionella* amplification in spite of prior concerns about the surface seemingly presenting a suitable environmental niche for colonization and growth. A plausible explanation is that the intermittent drying out of the fill when water is not circulating prevents significant buildup of biofilm there compared with the basin surfaces, which are continuously wet. Legionellae are very susceptible to drying (20). Discrete cleaning events had no significant effect in reducing established *Legionella* concentrations, although the potential for multiplication may be reduced. Therefore, *Legionella* control methods must include supplementary biocidal treatment. Careful cleaning at regular intervals is necessary for overall tower efficiency and also serves to augment the chemical treatment by removing organic accumulations. Decontamination of cooling towers had only a significant short-term effect on high *Legionella* concentrations, again justifying the need for a field-proven supplementary water treatment program. *Legionella* counts were consistently reduced below detection limits, but the bacteria were detected again, usually within 1 month, and often within days, of decontamination. Finally, system water temperature was the most important predictor of *Legionella* concentrations and was influenced not only by the ambient air temperature but also by the degree of tower usage. Frequently operated towers may be expected to be colonized even at cooler ambient temperatures.

The apparent significance of water temperature on colonization led to an investigation of the concept of a critical basin water temperature above which *Legionella* growth is likely to be stimulated. The results of this investigation are shown in Fig. 1 as pooled data. Data were excluded from this analysis if interventions such as decontaminations or changes of biocide might have caused *Legionella* concentrations to fall.

It was found that there is a critical temperature (approximately 16.5°C) below which *Legionella* concentrations appear not to rise and below which there is a very small standard error in the observations. There is another temperature (approximately 23°C) beyond which *Legionella* multiplication may become explosive but which also produces large standard errors.

The lower limit of 16.5°C for significant *Legionella* detection is somewhat lower than that noted in other studies (12). In an operating cooling tower system, the basin temperature is actually the coolest part of the system, being typically about 5°C lower than the temperature of water leaving the condenser (heat source). Taking this factor into consideration, the lower temperature limit is not inconsistent with previous findings, suggesting that it is the heat exchanger rather than the tower basin that is the primary site of *Legionella* multiplication. Clearly, cooling water systems should be operated at as low a temperature as is practicable given the constraints of refrigeration system characteristics and ambient wet bulb conditions.

The effectiveness of readily available proprietary biocides is also being evaluated as part of the Australian field study. Briefly, the findings are as follows.

Sufficient testing has been completed to conclude that chlorinated phenolic thioether (fentichlor) is effective in these trials against legionellae at the maker's recommended dosage, giving 200 ppm retained in the system for 4 h (as a weekly slug dose). This nonoxidizing biocide has a reasonably broad antimicrobial control spectrum but leaves residual cyclic compounds. It is costly to use compared with other biocides. An antifoaming agent may be needed in some applications.

Bromochlorodimethylhydantoin (BCD) has been found in these trials to be effective for *Legionella* control when used in bimonthly doses with a slow-release cartridge giving an initial 300 ppm. Observed halogen free residual concentrations were up to 0.4 ppm but were usually negligible. BCD is a broad-spectrum oxidizing biocide whose activity depends on bromine and chlorine, which are bound to a relatively unstable organic ring structure. The biocide is of low toxicity and is biodegradable. BCD was found to be successful both in laboratory studies and in field studies carried out by the John Radcliffe Hospital, Oxford,

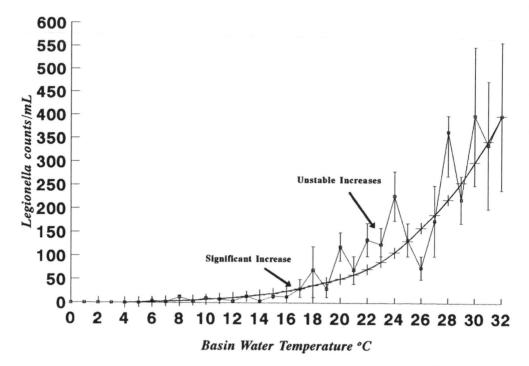

Fig. 1. Mean *Legionella* concentration—basin water temperature relationship ($n = 25$ towers).

England (21), although Fliermans and Harvey (16) found it unsuccessful at a concentration of 2 ppm.

Results for bromonitropropanediol (BNPD) in the Adelaide trials are equivocal, and BNPD cannot be recommended as the biocide of choice. BNPD is a broad-spectrum nonoxidizing biocide that is unlikely to produce any harmful environmental effects. The recommended dosage of 100 ppm has been reported in one study as being effective (15). However, its effectiveness is considerably reduced in water systems having high water hardness, high pH, elevated temperatures, and the presence of oxidizing agents, all of which are commonly found in cooling towers.

Quaternary ammonium compounds were in use in most of the Adelaide towers at the start of the study but permitted the majority of towers to amplify Legionellae, some to concentrations above 1,000 CFU/ml; therefore, these compounds cannot be recommended. Quaternary ammonium compounds are nonoxidizing and are of prime use in algae control. The compound in use in these field trials comprises a mixture of alkyl dimethyl benzyl and alkyl dimethyl ethylbenzyl ammonium chlorides.

The study also included isothiazolinones, which are nonoxidizing biocides. The biocide in common use in the Melbourne-based cooling tower systems is a mixture of methylthiazolinone and methylchlorothiazolinone with additional magne-

sium and copper salts. This biocide permitted many towers to amplify legionellae, some to concentrations above 1,000 CFU/ml, and therefore cannot be recommended. However, in the absence of control towers not on this biocidal regimen (and in the same locality), it has not yet been possible to fully assess effectiveness. This biocide has been reported to be effective in one study (15) but less effective in another (26).

These results point to the importance of appropriate field trials in establishing a suitable biocidal regimen for each unique application (1). The most successful strategy for these towers was the use of chlorinated phenolic thioether (nonoxidizing) rotated with BCD (oxidizing) after an intervention (notably, cleaning). A comprehensive review of the role of biocides in controlling *Legionella* growth is provided by the 1989 "Report of the Expert Advisory Committee on Biocides," U.K. Department of Health.

A further observation from the Australian field study was that high bleed-off (turnover of the water) as a discrete event did not appreciably reduce *Legionella* counts; i.e., retention time of water in the system was not significant (see Bentham et al., this volume) despite the fact that legionellae could not be recovered from concentrated samples of mains water. This finding may have important ramifications for water treatment programs because it highlights the need to address the entire system, including microbial matter that attaches to surfaces but may slough off from time to time. Sessile populations in these niches appear to be the primary sites for multiplication. Strategies that address organisms in the circulating water only, such as nonchemical sidestream techniques, are unlikely to be effective in reducing *Legionella* counts. This finding appears to agree with another Australian study involving a once-through cooling tower system used to cool bore water for a town's supply; legionellae were not detected in the hot bore water but were detected at the cooling tower when the water temperature was brought into the *Legionella* growth range (25).

Christensen et al. (10) recovered legionellae from power station cooling systems employing once-through river water. They observed that *Legionella* organisms recovered in this way were not as infective as for open recirculating cooling tower systems and speculated that such recirculation provided continued thermal stress to legionellae as well as variations in growth conditions.

Finally, it is now well recognized that control of legionellae and other microorganisms plays an important role in the cooling tower life cycle. The factors to be considered would include (24) the following. (i) Planning should consider siting of a tower relative to air intakes and prevailing wind directions (27). (ii) Design criteria should include selection of towers for maintainability, accessibility, cleanability, reliability, and capability (24). Good performance drift eliminators are important for secondary control in the chain of transmission (6). (iii) The commissioning stage is of vital importance. There is often pressure to achieve early completion and handover of facilities. The history of outbreaks such as that at Stafford, England (8), suggests that the health risks increase if building engineering services are not properly commissioned. (iv) Cooling towers should be inspected at, say, monthly intervals (9, 24, 27) for slime and algal growths, deterioration of materials, damage to components (e.g., drift eliminators), blockages, and corrosion effects and for correct operation of fans, motors, and pumps. Weekly inspections are recommended for sensitive sites such as hospitals (5). Good records need to be kept. (v) Maintenance activities should include (5) periodic (generally twice yearly [27]) flushing and physical cleaning of the cooling tower to remove accumulations of sediment and organic matter, attention to the items identified by inspections, and a water treatment program that includes corrosion and scale control and automatic dosing with a biocide to provide a residual effect for the complete system.

Cooling towers are potential amplifiers of legionellae; adequate strategies for hazard control are described in the literature. There is now a need for these strategies to be further refined to reflect better analytical methodology involving limiting water temperature, a cleaning program to suit local conditions, and water treatment compatible with local water characteristics. Such measures are necessary not only for reasons of *Legionella* control but also to reduce energy usage and to improve plant reliability.

REFERENCES

1. **American Society of Heating, Refrigerating and Air-Conditioning Engineers.** 1989. Position paper on Legionellosis. American Society of Heating, Refrigerating and Air-Conditioning Engineers, Atlanta.
2. **Barbaree, J. M.** 1991. Legionnaires' disease: factors affecting the transmission of *Legionella* species from aerosol-emitting equipment to people. *ASHRAE J.* 33(6):38–42.
3. **Bartlett, C. L. R., A. D. Macrae, and J. T. Macfarlane.** 1986. *Legionella Infections.* Edward Arnold, London.
4. **Breiman, R. F., W. Cozen, B. S. Fields, T. D. Mastro, S. J. Carr, J. S. Spika, and L. Mascola.** 1990. Role of air sampling in investigation of an outbreak of Legionnaires' disease associated with exposure to aerosols from an evaporative condenser. *J. Infect. Dis.* 161:1257–1261.
5. **Broadbent, C. R.** 1987. Practical measures to control Legionnaires' disease hazards. *Austral. Refrig. Air Cond. Heat.* 41(7):22–30.
6. **Broadbent, C. R.** 1991. Developments in Australia to control *Legionella*. *ASHRAE Trans.* 97(part 1):258–264.
7. **Broadbent, C. R., L. N. Marwood, and R. H. Bentham.** 1991. *Legionella* in cooling towers: report of a field study in South Australia, p. 55–60. *Trans. Far East Conf. Environ. Qual. Issues.* American Society of Heating, Refrigerating and Air-Conditioning Engineers, Atlanta.
8. **Brundrett, G. W.** 1991. Outbreak of Legionnaires' disease at Stafford District General Hospital. Building services engineering. *Trans. Chart. Inst. Build. Serv. Eng.* 12(2):53–64.
9. **Chartered Institution of Building Services Engineers.** 1991. Minimising the risk of Legionnaires' disease. Technical Memoranda no. 13. The Chartered Institution of Building Services Engineers, London.
10. **Christensen, S. W., R. W. Tyndall, J. A. Solomon, C. B. Fliermans, and S. B. Gough.** 1984. Patterns of *Legionella* spp. infectivity in power plant environments and implications for control, p. 313–315. *In* C. Thornsberry, A. Balows, J. C. Feeley, and W. Jakubowski (ed.), *Legionella: Proceedings of the 2nd International Symposium.* American Society for Microbiology, Washington, D.C.
11. **Christopher, P. J., L. M. Noonan, and R. Chiew.** 1987. Epidemic of Legionnaires' disease in Wollongong. *Med. J. Aust.* 147:127–128.
12. **Colbourne, J. S., and P. J. Dennis.** 1989. The ecology and survival of *Legionella pneumophila*. *J. Inst. Water Environ. Manage.* 3:345–350.
13. **Dennis, P. J.** 1988. Isolation of Legionellae from environmental specimens, p. 31–171. *In* T. G. Harrison and A. G. Taylor (ed.), *A Laboratory Manual for Legionella.* John Wiley & Sons, New York.
14. **Edelstein, P. H.** 1985. Environmental aspects of *Legionella*. *ASM News* 51:460–467.
15. **Elsmore, R.** 1986. Biocidal control of legionellae. *Isr. J. Med. Sci.* 22:647–654.
16. **Fliermans, C. B., and R. S. Harvey.** 1984. Effectiveness of 1-bromo-3-chloro-5, 5-dimethylhydantoin against *Legionella pneumophila* in cooling towers. *Appl. Environ. Microbiol.* 47:1307–1310.
17. **Fliermans, C. B., and J. A. Nygren.** 1987. Maintaining industrial water systems free of *Legionella pneumophila*. *ASHRAE Trans.* 93(part 2):1405–1415.
18. **Health Department, Victoria.** 1989. Guidelines for the control of Legionnaires' disease. *Environmental Health*

Standards. Health Department, Victoria, Australia.

19. **Ikedo, M., and E. Yabuuchi.** 1986. Ecological studies of *Legionella* species. Viable counts of *Legionella pneumophila* in cooling tower water. *Microbiol. Immunol.* **30:**413–423.

20. **Katz, S. M., and J. M. Hammel.** 1987. The effect of drying, heat and pH on the survival of *Legionella pneumophila. Ann. Clin. Lab. Sci.* **17:**150–156.

21. **Kurtz, J. B., and V. Davis.** 1988. Efficacy of bromine biocide in cooling water systems. *Lancet* **i:**304.

22. **Lee, J. V., and A. A. West.** 1991. Survival and growth of *Legionella* species in the environment. *J. Appl. Bacteriol. Suppl.* **70:**121s–129s.

23. **Mitchell, P., A. Chereshsky, A. J. Haskell, and M. A. Brieseman.** 1991. Legionellosis in New Zealand; first recorded outbreak. *N.Z. Med. J.* **104**(915):275–276.

24. **National Health and Medical Research Council.** 1989. Australian guidelines for the control of *Legionella* and Legionnaires' disease. National Health and Medical Research Council, Australian Government Publishing Service, Canberra.

25. **Ng, S., and C. Derbyshire.** 1989. Isolation of *Legionella* from cooling towers supplied by artesian bores. *In Communicable Diseases Intelligence Bulletin 89/16,* 14 August. Federal Department of Health, Housing and Community Services. Canberra, Australia.

26. **Skaliy, P., T. A. Thompson, G. W. Gorman, G. K. Morris, H. V. McEachern, and D. C. Mackel.** 1980. Laboratory studies of disinfectants against *Legionella pneumophila. Appl. Environ. Microbiol.* **40:**697–700.

27. **Standards Australia.** 1989. AS3666, air-handling and water systems of buildings, microbial control. Standards Australia, Sydney.

Potable Water Systems: Insights into Control

P. JULIAN DENNIS

Thames Water Utilities, Environment and Science, Reading RG1 8DB, England

The growth of microorganisms in any water system is governed by temperature (stagnation can lead to warming), pH, redox potential, the type of water treatment, the concentration and persistence of residual disinfectant, the availability of organic and inorganic substrate, and the presence of sediments and corrosion products (6). Growth in water systems forms biofilms or slime layers on the surfaces of pipes and tanks in contact with water.

Biofilms can be regarded as playing a normal role in the life cycle of most microorganisms. They are formed in response to, and for survival in, hostile environments such as those with a low nutrient concentration, e.g., tap water. A diverse population of aquatic microorganisms are able to gain access to and colonize water systems; most are harmless, but a few are able to give rise to opportunistic infections. Of these, *Legionella* is now probably the most notorious.

Legionellae are aquatic organisms that have been isolated from a range of habitats, particularly natural thermal ponds (28) and thermally polluted waters. These bacteria can be regarded as ubiquitous, having also been isolated from streams, rivers, and the shores of lakes (15) and from the ponds located in the blast zone of a volcano (25). They are most commonly isolated from warmer waters (40 to 60°C) (15). *Legionella pneumophila* has been found to be able to derive essential nutrients for growth from amoebae (23), flavobacteria (29), and cyanobacteria (26).

Aquatic microorganisms gain entry to man-made water systems during construction or repair, and under some circumstances, during or after treatment (19). It is inevitable that legionellae are a natural component of the aquatic population of the lakes, streams, and reservoirs from which we draw our water. They will also enter and colonize man-made water systems.

L. pneumophila was first isolated by McDade et al. in 1976 from the lung tissue of American Legionnaires (21). Following attendance at a convention in Philadelphia, the Legionnaires developed pneumonia which in a number of cases was fatal (16). The organism and the disease it produces are however, not new. A bacterium similar to *L. pneumophila* was first isolated in 1947

(20). The first well-documented outbreak of the disease happened in 1957 (22). The epidemiological investigation of the outbreak of *Legionella* pneumonia in Philadelphia concluded that infection was due to inhalation of the bacterium (16). Later epidemiological evidence implicated domestic water systems in large buildings (27) and cooling towers (12) as the source and means of airborne spread.

Aerosols containing legionellae can be produced from faucets and showers (11), cooling towers (12), and humidifiers (32). Relative to other bacteria, *L. pneumophila* survives well in aerosols (17). Many interrelated factors influence the survival of bacteria in aerosols, although those associated with their survival in aerosols from cooling towers may differ from those in the enclosed environment of a shower room. Particle size is particularly important (13, 18), with those of less than 5 μm able to penetrate to the alveoli of the lung. The growth phase of the organism has been shown to affect survival (17), and substances aerosolized with the organism can also improve survival (5).

Large volumes of sludge and slime containing high numbers of legionellae have been responsible for at least one well-documented outbreak of Legionnaires disease (14). In this case, a calorifier that had been out of use for some time was brought into use to satisfy an increase in demand for hot water. Accumulated sludge was discharged throughout the system. Therefore, it is likely that the ability of some strains of legionellae to survive better in aerosols than others (9), as well as the concentration of cells disseminated in aerosols or present in the water in the system, are primary factors in the sequence of events leading to infection. If we consider the susceptibility of those exposed to any aerosol, we can account for the relatively low attack rate of only 5%.

If outbreaks of Legionnaires disease are to be avoided, it is important to focus control methods not just at legionellae, but at the whole microbial community, which supports and protects the legionellae both in the water systems and aerosols. Controlling overall microbial numbers will reduce the numbers of legionellae, reducing the number aerosolized. Thus, the risk to susceptible individuals is minimized.

DOMESTIC WATER PLUMBING SYSTEMS

In the United Kingdom, water for domestic use is derived mainly from the public supply either by direct connection to the rising main or through properly constructed and protected storage cisterns. Water that is stored in tanks (other than those just mentioned) or that is conditioned before heating naturally is not considered potable because it suffers some degree of microbial or chemical deterioration. Private supplies that are not adequately treated suffer similarly. It is the colonization and subsequent growth of legionellae in these non-potable systems in large buildings such as hospitals and hotels that is known to lead to outbreaks of Legionnaires disease. However, it is important to appreciate the fact that legionellae have also been isolated from buildings with no apparent disease (10, 30).

In the United States and the United Kingdom, hot water systems have been found to be the most common source of legionellae (10, 30), with temperatures between 30 and 54 °C favoring growth. Hot water tanks maintained at between 71 and 77 °C were found to be free of the organism (30).

Legionellae are able to extract sufficient nutrients to enable them to grow from other organisms, materials used to construct water systems, and the water. They are able to grow in water that is not sterile, and continue to grow at 42 °C when other organisms in the water fail to do so (31). Natural rubber sealing washers and gaskets have all been found to support the growth of legionellae (7, 24). In one hospital, only replacement of the rubber washers with suitable alternative materials resulted in the eradication of the organism.

MAINTENANCE AND MONITORING

To prevent the accumulation of microbial sludge and slime, a factor known to be associated with outbreaks of Legionnaires disease, domestic water systems should be cleaned regularly. They must be run in such a way that microbial growth is limited or prevented, because it is inappropriate in most circumstances to add biocides or disinfectants to these systems. Hot water should be stored at 60 °C, with a minimum water temperature of 50 °C in the return and at least 50 °C attainable at the faucet within 1 min of running; however, caution must be maintained to avoid scalding. Cold water storage and distribution temperatures should be kept below 20 °C (1–4). Detailed procedures for the management and maintenance of domestic water systems are available (1–4).

To determine whether or not maintenance or the general running of the system has been successful in controlling microbial growth, chemical and microbiological monitoring should be done. This procedure will reveal whether the cleaning has been successful and will provide confidence in running and maintenance procedures. Routine monitoring for *Legionella* is recommended only as part of a structured monitoring regime (8). To be effective, monitoring must be done on a regular basis so that a historical log of the performance of the system can be compiled and a normal baseline established. Recording the monitoring data (and plotting on a graph) will allow deviations from this base line to be easily seen. Corrective or remedial action can be undertaken quickly. The parameters measured and sampling frequency can vary. They depend on the type of system and the way it is used.

Methods to limit or prevent the growth of legionellae are based on the simple understanding of the factors that encourage the survival and growth of the organisms. Avoiding these factors and ensuring that domestic water systems are managed properly will prevent an unnecessary and avoidable disease.

REFERENCES

1. **Anonymous.** 1987. Minimising the risk of Legionnaires' disease. Technical Memorandum (TM13). The Chartered Institution of Building Services Engineers, London.
2. **Anonymous.** 1989. Report of the Expert Advisory Committee on Biocides. H. M. Stationery Office, London.
3. **Anonymous.** 1989. The control of *Legionella* in health care premises. A Code of Practice. H. M. Stationery Office, London.
4. **Anonymous.** 1991. The control of Legionellosis including Legionnaires' disease. Health and Safety booklet HS (G) 70. H. M. Stationery Office, London.
5. **Berendt, R. F.** 1981. Influence of blue-green algae (cyanobacteria) on survival of *Legionella pneumophila* in aerosols. *Infect. Immun.* **32:**690–692.
6. **Colbourne, J. S.** 1986. Materials usage and their effects on the microbiological quality of water supplies, p. 47S–59S. *In* W. R. White and Susan M. Passmore (ed.), *Microbial Aspects of Water Management.* Society for Applied Microbiology Symposium Series, no. 14.
7. **Colbourne, J. S., D. J. Pratt, M. G. Smith, S. P. Fisher-Hoch, and D. Harper.** 1984. Water fittings as sources of *Legionella pneumophila* in a hospital plumbing system. *Lancet* **i:**210–213.
8. **Committee of Enquiry.** 1987. Second report into the outbreak of Legionnaires' Disease in Stafford in April. Comnd 256. H. M. Stationery Office, London.
9. **Dennis, P. J., and J. V. Lee.** 1988. Differences in aerosol survival between pathogenic and non-pathogenic strains of *Legionella pneumophila* serogroup 1. *J. Appl. Bacteriol.* **65:**135–141.
10. **Dennis, P. J., J. A. Taylor, R. B. Fitzgeorge, C. L. R. Bartlett, and G. I. Barrow.** 1982. *Legionella pneumophila* in water plumbing systems. *Lancet* **i:**949–951.
11. **Dennis, P. J. L., A. E. Wright, D. A. Rutter, J. E. Death, and B. P. C. Jones.** 1984. *Legionella pneumophila* in aerosols from shower baths. *J. Hyg.* **93:**349–355.
12. **Dondero, T. J., R. C. Rendtorff, G. F. Mallison, R. M. Weeks, J. S. Levy, E. M. Wong, and W. Schaffner.** 1980. An outbreak of Legionnaires' disease associated with a contaminated air-conditioning cooling tower. *N. Engl. J. Med.* **302:**365–370.

13. **Druett, H. A., D. W. Henderson, L. Packman, and S. Peacock.** 1953. Studies on respiratory infection. 1. The influence of particle size on respiratory infection with anthrax spores. *J. Hyg.* **51:**359–371.

14. **Fisher-Hoch, S. P., M. G. Smith, and J. S. Colbourne.** 1982. *Legionella pneumophila* in a hospital hot water cylinder. *Lancet* **i:**1073.

15. **Fliermans, C. B., W. B. Cherry, L. H. Orrison, S. J. Smith, D. L. Tison, and D. H. Pope.** 1981. Ecological distribution of *Legionella pneumophila*. *Appl. Environ. Microbiol.* **41:**9–16.

16. **Fraser, D. W., T. R. Tsai, W. Orenstein, W. E. Parkin, P. H. J. Beecham, R. G. Sharrar, J. Harris, G. F. Mallison, S. M. Martin, J. E. McDade, C. G. Shepard, P. S. Brachman, and The Field Investigation Team.** 1977. Legionnaires' disease: description of an epidemic of pneumonia. *N. Engl. J. Med.* **297:**1189–1197.

17. **Hambleton, P., M. G. Broster, P. J. Dennis, R. Henstridge, R. Fitzgeorge, and J. W. Conlan.** 1983. Survival of virulent *Legionella pneumophila* in aerosols. *J. Hyg.* **90:**451–460.

18. **Harper, G. J., and J. D. Morton.** 1953. The respiratory retention of aerosols. Experiments with radioactive spores. *J. Hyg.* **51:**372–385.

19. **Hutchinson, M., and J. W. Ridgway.** 1977. Microbiological aspects of drinking water supplies, pp. 179–218. *In* F. A. Skinner and J. M. Shewan (ed.), *Aquatic Microbiology Symposium.* Series no. 6. Academic Press, Ltd., London.

20. **McDade, J. E., D. J. Brenner, and F. M. Bozeman.** 1979. Legionnaires' disease bacterium isolated in 1947. *Ann. Intern. Med.* **90:**659–661.

21. **McDade, J. E., C. C. Shepard, D. W. Fraser, T. R. Tsai, M. A. Redus, W. R. Dowdle, and The Laboratory Investigation Team.** 1977. Legionnaires' disease: isolation of a bacterium and demonstration of its role in respiratory disease. *N. Engl. J. Med.* **297:**1197–1203.

22. **Osterholm, M. T., D. Y. Chin, D. O. Osbourne, H. B. Dull, A. G. Dean, D. W. Fraser, P. S. Hayes, and W. N. Hall.** 1983. A 1957 outbreak of Legionnaires' disease associated with a meat packing plant. *Am. J. Epidemiol.* **117:**60–67.

23. **Rowbotham, T. J.** 1980. Preliminary report on the pathogenicity of *Legionella pneumophila* for freshwater and soil amoebae. *J. Clin. Pathol.* **33:**1179–1183.

24. **Schofield, G. M., and A. E. Wright.** 1984. Survival of *Legionella pneumophila* in a model hot water distribution system. *J. Gen. Microbiol.* **130:**1751–1756.

25. **Tison, D. L., J. A. Baross, and R. J. Seidler.** 1983. *Legionella* in aquatic habitats in the Mount Saint Helens blast zone. *Curr. Microbiol.* **9:**345–348.

26. **Tison, D. L., D. H. Pope, and C. B. Fliermans.** 1980. Utilization of algal extracellular products by *Legionella pneumophila*, abstr. I-40, p. 91. *Abstr. 80th Annu. Meet. Am. Soc. Microbiol. 1980.* American Society for Microbiology, Washington, D.C.

27. **Tobin, J. O., J. Beare, M. S. Dunnill, S. P. Fisher-Hoch, M. French, R. G. Mitchell, P. J. Morris, and M. F. Muers.** 1980. Legionnaires' disease in a transplant unit: isolation of the causative agent from shower baths. *Lancet* **ii:**188–121.

28. **Verissimo, A., G. Marrao, F. Gomes da Silva, and M. S. da Costa.** 1991. Distribution of *Legionella* spp. in hydrothermal areas in continental Portugal and the Island of Sao Miguel, Azores. *Appl. Environ. Microbiol.* **57:**2921–2927.

29. **Wadowsky, R. M., and R. B. Yee.** 1983. Satellite growth of *Legionella pneumophila* with an environmental isolate of *Flavobacterium breve. Appl. Environ. Microbiol.* **46:**1147–1149.

30. **Wadowsky, R. M., R. B. Yee, L. Mezmar, E. J. Wing, and J. N. Dowling.** 1982. Hot water systems as sources of *Legionella pneumophila* in hospital and non-hospital plumbing fixtures. *Appl. Environ. Microbiol.* **43:**1104–1110.

31. **Yee, R. B., and R. M. Wadowsky.** 1982. Multiplication of *Legionella pneumophila* in unsterile tap water. *Appl. Environ. Microbiol.* **43:**1330–1334.

32. **Zuravleff, J. J., V. L. Yu, J. W. Shonnard, J. D. Rihs, and M. Best.** 1983. *Legionella pneumophila* contamination of a hospital humidifier. Demonstration of aerosol transmission and subsequent subclinical infection in exposed guinea-pigs. *Am. Rev. Respir. Dis.* **128:**657–661.

Continuous Hyperchlorination for Control of Nosocomial *Legionella pneumophila* Pneumonia: a Ten-Year Follow-Up of Efficacy, Environmental Effects, and Costs

M. GROSSERODE, R. WENZEL, M. PFALLER, AND C. HELMS

Department of Internal Medicine, University of Iowa College of Medicine, and Epidemiology Program, University of Iowa Hospitals and Clinics, Iowa City, Iowa 52242, and Department of Pathology, Oregon Health Sciences University, Portland, Oregon 97201

The optimum methods of construction and of treatment of potable water systems to prevent and control nosocomial *Legionella* pneumonia are unclear. Treatment modalities studied include ozone (6), UV radiation (8), heat flushing (1, 2, 19), and pulse as well as continuous hyperchlorination (3, 7, 9, 11–14, 16, 17). Reported field experience with some of these methods is sparse, but experience with continuous hyperchlorination is slowly accumulating.

In this report, we summarize findings of 10 years of experience in continuous hyperchlorination following an outbreak of nosocomial *Legionella* pneumonia among immunosuppressed patients in one division (Division C) of the University of Iowa Hospitals and Clinics (11, 12). We evaluate the effects of hyperchlorination on the occurrence of *Legionella* pneumonia and on the isolation of legionellae from the potable water system. We also discuss the effects of hyperchlorination on the integrity of the involved water distribution system and estimate associated costs.

Case definition. The case definition of nosocomial *Legionella pneumophila* pneumonia used throughout this study required onset of illness 48 h or more after admission or within 14 days of discharge, X-ray documentation, and laboratory confirmation (21). The last required at least one of the following: (i) a fourfold or greater rise in titer of indirect immunofluorescent serum antibodies to a titer of ≥ 1:128; (ii) positive direct immunofluorescent antibody testing; (iii) positive DNA probe testing (Gen-Probe, San Diego, Calif.) of respiratory secretions or tissue; and (iv) isolation of *L. pneumophila* from respiratory secretions or tissue.

Case identification. Cases of nosocomial *Legionella* pneumonia were identified by prospective nosocomial infection surveillance and retrospective review of microbiological laboratory results. All units of Division C housing immunosuppressed patients were prospectively surveyed 5 days per week by infection control technicians. The population of immunosuppressed patients surveyed in Division C increased in the 10-year study period. The infection control surveillance system has recently been validated and shown to have a sensitivity of 84% and a specificity of 97% (4).

To identify other cases possibly related to University Hospital, the names of Legionnaires disease patients diagnosed in Iowa over the same time period were checked against University Hospital admission records. No new nosocomial cases were identified by this approach.

Environmental sample collection and specimen processing. Methods of environmental sample collection and specimen processing have remained essentially unchanged during the 10-year study period (11, 12).

The sensitivity of the environmental culturing system was tested in 1991. Two 500-ml hot water samples were inoculated with sufficient *L. pneumophila* serogroup 1 organisms to bring the concentration to approximately 300 or 3,000 CFU/1liter. Laboratory personnel identified both test samples among 12 samples submitted blindly.

Frequency of nosocomial *Legionella* pneumonia. In the 10 years following the outbreak in 1981, only 5 cases of nosocomial *Legionella* pneumonia have been identified among immunosuppressed patients housed in Division C (Table 1). Thus, the high incidence during the outbreak (35/1,000 admissions) has fallen dramatically (< 1/1,000 admissions). In addition, the high frequency of cases of *Legionella* pneumonia among nosocomial pneumonias during the outbreak (16 cases among 21 pneumonias tested) also declined significantly (5 cases among 204 tested) ($P < 0.001$, two-tailed Fisher's exact test).

Surveillance of the potable water system for *Legionella* species. Twelve of 41 samples from Division C in December 1981 yielded isolates of *L. pneumophila* prior to intervention. No *Legionella* species were isolated from over 500 water samples obtained from May 1982, 5 months after initiation of continuous hyperchlorination, through 1991.

Water distribution system integrity and operation. Leaks first appeared in the copper pipes of the water distribution system after hot and cold water chlorine injectors had been in operation in Division C for approximately 2 years (Fig. 1). Pipe samples from hot and cold water systems were sent for analysis. Significant deterioration was noted only in the five pipe samples from the hot water system. Consultants concluded that the chemical composition of the water could have

TABLE 1. Frequency of nosocomial *L. pneumophila* pneumonia among patients on hematology-oncology, bone marrow transplantation, and renal transplantation units of Division C

Period	No. of admissions	No. of nosocomial pneumonia cases (no./1,000 admissions)	No. of pneumonias tested	No. of *L. pneumophila* pneumonia cases (no./1,000 admissions)	Frequency (%) of *L. pneumophila* pneumonia
1981	456	30 (66)	21	16 (35)	76
1982–86	3,947	188 (48)	73	4 (1)	5.5
1987–91	8,081	290 (36)	131	1 (0.1)	0.8

supported a corrosive process because of its softness, alkalinity (pH 9), and high oxygen and CO_2 contents. Chlorination levels were decreased to 3 ppm, but over the next 4 years, the number of leaks increased substantially.

A sodium silicate injector unit was installed in the hot water system in May 1987. It was hypothesized that the silicate would act to coat and protect the interior surface of the piping from further corrosion. The number of leaks decreased markedly after this time, from a rate of approximately 53/ year in 1986 to 10/year in 1990 (Fig. 1). The silicate level in hot water was maintained at 25 to 30 ppm initially but was reduced to 10 to 15 ppm in January 1988 because of the obstructive buildup of calcium carbonate and sodium silicate precipitates in parts of the system.

In August 1990, on the basis of previously negative culturing results and emerging national experience, hyperchlorination was restricted to the hot water distribution system and carried out at levels of approximately 2 ppm.

Costs of hyperchlorination. Direct costs in-

curred and associated with hyperchlorination and silicate injection included (i) $75,800 to install the chlorine injectors, with an annual operating cost of $7,000; (ii) $54,480 to install the silicate injector, with an annual operating cost of $10,814; (iii) $36,250 in repairs; and (iv) $48,000 in consultant fees. Total costs over the 10-year period were estimated at $334,994, or approximately $33,500/ year.

Discussion. Field experience with continuous hyperchlorination of potable water systems for control of nosocomial *Legionella* pneumonia is accumulating slowly. Some institutions have resorted to this approach when previous attempts to control infection with heat flushing and/or pulse chlorination have proved unsuccessful or unsatisfactory (11, 16, 17).

Our past experience indicated that pulse chlorination, elevation of hot water temperatures, and continuous hyperchlorination were effective in controlling an outbreak of nosocomial pneumonia associated with a specific strain of *L. pneumophila* serogroup 1 colonizing a water distribution system

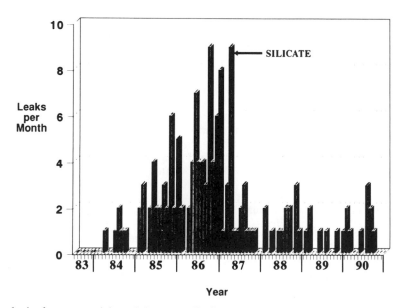

FIG. 1. Leaks in the copper piping of the water distribution system of Division C from July 1983 through December 1990.

at our hospital (12). Follow-up data (11), including those presented here, document that continuous hyperchlorination has not completely eradicated nosocomial *Legionella* pneumonia despite apparent eradication of *Legionella* species from the water distribution system. The rate of nosocomial *Legionella* pneumonia in Division C has been much reduced since the outbreak, but the infection is still detectable. Subtyping of four case isolates of *L. pneumophila* serogroup 1 by monoclonal antibody and plasmid analysis has shown them to differ from the original outbreak strain (11).

The reasons for continuing sporadic nosocomial *Legionella* pneumonia in Division C are potentially many. For example, *Legionella* species may persist at undetectable levels in the water distribution system despite hyperchlorination. If so, the bacteria must be at levels lower than we can detect by our culture system (approximately 300 to 3,000 CFU/liter). Alternatively, secondary reservoirs (i.e., showerheads, aerators, and other end-use hospital faucet fixtures in which water may stand and provide a surface for *L. pneumophila* to colonize) may be few in Division C, and the number of samples done may have been inadequate to detect them. Finally, infections may have been acquired by Division C patients from the potential potable water reservoirs in other parts of the hospital.

Continuous hyperchlorination of the Division C water distribution system has not occurred without substantial costs. Corrosion and pipe leaks in the hot water system are probably related to initially high and erratically controlled chlorine levels (5 to 8 ppm) produced by the injector system. With the addition of silicates, which presumably line and protect the internal surface of the piping, a marked decrease of over 80% in the total number of leaks per year occurred. The silicate system itself initially created some problems as well, in the form of precipitation of sodium silicate and calcium carbonate. Currently, we maintain continuous hyperchlorination of the hot water system alone at levels of about 2 ppm. Silicate levels are maintained at 10 to 15 ppm. To date, total direct attributable costs are estimated at $334,994, or slightly more than one-third of the amount that would be required to replace the copper piping in the water distribution system ($950,000 in 1990).

Many questions about continuous hyperchlorination for the control of nosocomial *Legionella* pneumonia still remain. What are the indications for hyperchlorination? What are the optimum water conditions and chlorine levels necessary to control *Legionella* colonization and minimize damage to water distribution systems? What is the appropriate duration of hyperchlorination?

On the basis of our admittedly limited experience, we would make the following suggestions concerning continuous hyperchlorination for the

control of nosocomial *Legionella* pneumonia.

First, before initiating continuous hyperchlorination, one should verify that the potable water distribution system is the source of the case or case cluster through careful epidemiologic, environmental, and microbiologic studies. Special care should be taken to localize the site of colonization within the water distribution system.

Second, before continuous hyperchlorination is begun, acute systemic treatment of the water distribution system should be attempted, with careful environmental microbiologic follow-up. Heat flushing and pulse chlorination appear to be useful initially, but these strategies may not offer lasting protection and are labor-intensive. One institution estimated costs of heat flushing at over $30,000 in overtime labor alone (17).

Third, before continuous hyperchlorination is initiated, features of the water system predisposing to *Legionella* colonization should be corrected. Sediment and areas of sluggish flow should be eliminated (5, 20). Rubbers containing thiuram do not enhance the growth of *L. pneumophila*, and some have suggested the use of such rubber in water systems (15).

Fourth, continuous hyperchlorination should be considered if cases continue to be identified or if a *Legionella* strain isolated from patients persists in the water distribution system. If *Legionella* isolates are limited to the hot water system, continuous hyperchlorination should be initiated for the hot water system alone. The hot water temperature should be maintained at about 50°C to reduce loss of chlorine due to instability at higher temperatures. Chlorine levels of about 2 ppm in hot water appear to be adequate (17) and to keep trihalomethanes at acceptable levels (11).

Fifth, the hyperchlorinated water distribution system should be prospectively monitored for pipe damage. Assays for levels of copper, lead, and iron and use of Langlier and stability indexes may permit early detection and control of corrosion problems (18). A silicate injector system should be considered early if monitoring indicates new or worsening corrosion.

Sixth, sink and shower outlets in patient rooms and inpatient units should be flushed with hyperchlorinated water prior to patient admission to eliminate potential secondary reservoirs of *Legionella* colonization.

Seventh, to assess the efficacy of the intervention, prospective surveillance for nosocomial *Legionella* pneumonia among high-risk patients should be continued or instituted following initiation of hyperchlorination. Environmental culturing is useful initially to ensure that *Legionella* species are eliminated from previously positive sites. Determining the optimal length for culturing is problematic, since culturing is expensive and probably not useful if subsequent clinical cases cease or occur infrequently.

Eighth, discontinuation of continuous hyperchlorination should be considered after an appropriate period of prospective surveillance has elapsed without cases of nosocomial *Legionella* pneumonia identified and with negative environmental cultures of *Legionella* species. Prospective case surveillance should be continued for a reasonable period after hyperchlorination is interrupted.

The management of epidemics of nosocomial *Legionella* pneumonia has proved to be complex, requiring interdisciplinary cooperation between clinicians, infection control personnel, microbiology laboratory staff, hospital engineers, administrators, and public relations staff (21). The engineering implications, use of personnel, and resource expenditures are substantial (10). Continued careful study of onoging continuous hyperchlorination experiments should result in information leading to better prevention and control measures in the future.

We gratefully acknowledge the help of the following individuals over the course of this study: W. Hierholzer, Jr., R. M. Massanari, W. Johnson, W. Hausler, Jr., L. Wintermeyer, N. Moyer, N. Hall, M. Bale, S. Streed, and D. Rasley. In addition, without the cooperation of administrative and medical staffs at the University of Iowa Hospitals and Clinics, this study would not have been possible.

REFERENCES

1. **Best, M., A. Goetz, and V. L. Yu.** 1984. Heat eradication measures for control of nosocomial Legionnaires' disease. Implementation, education, and cost analysis. *Am. J. Infect. Control* **12:**26–30.
2. **Best, M., V. L. Yu, J. Stout, A. Goetz, R. R. Muder, and F. Taylor.** 1983. *Legionellaceae* in the hospital watersupply. Epidemiological link with disease and evaluation of a method for control of nosocomial legionnaires' disease and Pittsburgh pneumonia. *Lancet* **ii:**307–310.
3. **Bornstein, N., C. Vieilly, M. Nowicki, J. C. Paucod, and J. Fleurette.** 1986. Epidemiological evidence of legionellosis transmission through domestic hot water supply systems and possibilities of control. *Isr. J. Med. Sci.* **22:**655–661.
4. **Broderick, A., M. Mari, M. D. Nettleman, S. A. Streed, and R. P. Wenzel.** 1990. Nosocomial infections: validation of surveillance and computer modeling to identify patients at risk. *Am. J. Epidemiol.* **131:**734–742.
5. **Ciesielski, C. A., M. J. Blaser, and W. L. Wang.** 1984. Role of stagnation and obstruction of water flow in isolation of *Legionella pneumophila* from hospital plumbing. *Appl. Environ. Microbiol.* **48:**984–987.
6. **Edelstein, P. H., R. E. Whittaker, R. L. Kreiling, and C. L. Howell.** 1982. Efficacy of ozone in eradication of *Legionella pneumophila* from hospital plumbing fixtures.

Appl. Environ. Microbiol. **44:**1330–1333.
7. **Ezzeddine, H., C. Van Ossel, M. Delmëe, and G. Wauters.** 1989. *Legionella* spp. in a hospital hot water system: effect of control measures. *J. Hosp. Infect.* **13:**121–131.
8. **Farr, B. M., J. C. Gratz, J. C. Tartaglino, S. I. Getchell-White, and D. H. Gröschell.** 1988. Evaluation of ultraviolet light for disinfection of hospital water contaminated with *Legionella*. *Lancet* **ii:**669–672.
9. **Guiguet, M., J. Pierre, P. Brun, G. Berthelot, S. Gottot, C. Gibert, and A. J. Valleron.** 1987. Epidemiological survey of a major outbreak of nosocomial legionellosis. *Int. J. Epidemiol.* **16:**466–471.
10. **Harper, D.** 1988. Legionnaires' disease outbreaks: the engineering implications. *J. Hosp. Infect.* **11**(Suppl. A):201–208.
11. **Helms, C. M., R. M. Massanari, R. P. Wenzel, M. A. Pfaller, N. P. Moyer, and N. Hall.** 1988. Legionnaires' disease associated with a hospital water system. A five-year progress report on continuous hyperchlorination. *JAMA* **259:**2423–2427.
12. **Helms, C. M., R. M. Massanari, R. Zeitler, S. Streed, M. J. Gilchrist, N. Hall, W. J. Hausler, Jr., J. Sywassink, W. Johnson, L. Wintermeyer, and W. J. Hierholzer, Jr.** 1983. Legionnaires' disease associated with a hospital water system: a cluster of 24 nosocomial cases. *Ann. Intern. Med.* **99:**172–178.
13. **Johnston, J. M., R. H. Latham, F. A. Meier, J. A. Green, R. Boshard, B. R. Mooney, and P. H. Edelstein.** 1987. Nosocomial outbreak of Legionnaires' disease: molecular epidemiology and disease control measures. *Infect. Control* **8:**53–58.
14. **Le Saux, N. M., L. Sekla, J. McLeod, S. Parker, D. Rush, J. R. Jeffery, and R. C. Brunham.** 1989. Epidemic of nosocomial Legionnaires' disease in renal transplant recipients: a case-control and environmental study. *Can. Med. Assoc. J.* **140:**1047–1053.
15. **Niedeveld, C. J., F. M. Pet, and P. L. Meenhorst.** 1986. Effect of rubbers and their constituents on proliferation of *Legionella pneumophila* in naturally contaminated hot water. *Lancet* **ii:**180–184.
16. **Shands, K. N., J. L. Ho, R. D. Meyer, G. W. Gorman, P. H. Edelstein, G. F. Mallison, S. M. Finegold, and D. W. Fraser.** 1985. Potable water as a source of Legionnaires' disease. *JAMA* **253:**1412–1416.
17. **Snyder, M. B., M. Siwicki, J. Wireman, D. Pohlod, M. Grimes, S. Bowman-Riney, and L. D. Saravolatz.** 1990. Reduction in *Legionella pneumophila* through heat flushing followed by continuous supplemental chlorination of hospital hot water. *J. Infect. Dis.* **162:**127–132.
18. **Stone, A., D. Spyridakis, M. Benjamin, J. Ferguson, S. Reiber, and S. Osterhus.** 1987. The effects of short-term changes in water quality on copper and zinc corrosion rates. *J. Am. Water Works Assoc.* **79:**75–82.
19. **Stout, J. E., M. G. Best, and V. L. Yu.** 1986. Susceptibility of members of the family *Legionellaceae* to thermal stress: implications for heat eradication methods in water distribution systems. *Appl. Environ. Microbiol.* **52:**396–399.
20. **Stout, J. E., V. L. Yu, and M. G. Best.** 1985. Ecology of *Legionella pneumophila* within water distribution systems. *Appl. Environ. Microbiol.* **49:**221–228.
21. **Timbury, M. C., J. R. Donaldson, A. C. McCartney, J. H. Winter, and R. J. Fallon.** 1988. How to deal with a hospital outbreak of Legionnaires' disease. *J. Hosp. Infect.* **11**(Suppl. A):189–200.

Legionella Strains in Six Hospital Water Supply Systems

L. FRANZIN, A. SINICCO, P. GIOANNINI, AND M. CASTELLANI PASTORIS

Infectious Diseases Department, University of Turin, Turin 10149, and Istituto Superiore di Sanità, Rome 00161, Italy

Potable water has been frequently reported as the reservoir of legionellae and the source for nosocomial legionellosis. Hospital infections, however, have not been always reported in buildings with contaminated water supplies. On the other hand, clinically unrecognized cases of nosocomial legionellosis have been described in hospitals whose plumbing systems were contaminated by *Legionella pneumophila* (2, 6). The usefulness of *Legionella* surveillance in the hospital environment, even in the absence of recognized legionellosis, has been shown (6, 7, 9).

We carried out an environmental surveillance of the water supplies of six hospitals in Turin (Piedmont, north Italy). The hospitals' plans were inspected to determine the locations and characteristics of the hot and cold potable water supply systems.

A total of 204 samples were examined: cold tap water from the public supply (5 liters), hot and cold tap water from the hospital distribution systems (5 liters), hot and cold tap water from patients' rooms and bathrooms (5 liters), hot water from tanks and instantaneous heaters (5 liters), recycled hot water (5 liters), dialysis water (5 liters), tap water from therapy tanks (5 liters), shower head water (100 ml), air conditioner water (1 liter), and oxygen bubble humidifier water (100 ml).

All samples were concentrated by filtration through cellulose acetate membrane filters (0.2-μm pore size) and resuspended in 10 ml of water. Aliquots (0.1 ml) of the untreated, heat-treated (50°C for 30 min), and acid-washed suspensions (1) were plated onto α-ketoglutarate-supplemented buffered charcoal-yeast extract agar, BMPA (3), and modified Wadowsky-Yee medium MWY (8). The plates were incubated at 37°C in a candle jar for 15 days. The strains of *Legionella* isolated were serologically typed by slide agglutination and by immunofluorescence assay.

Laboratory diagnosis of legionellosis in patients (culture and serodiagnosis by the indirect immunofluorescence assay and by the microagglutination test) was carried out when suspected cases were reported.

No legionellae were isolated from the cold water of the public supply, collected before entry into the hospital distribution systems, and from the hot water collected from the hot water tanks and from the instantaneous heaters. The water temperatures of the heating system were 50 to 55°C, but the distal sites showed variations of between 31 and 50°C.

Legionella strains were isolated from the water supplies of five out of six hospitals. Cultures of the water samples yielded 20 to 8,000 CFU of *Legionella* per liter, while cultures from shower head water yielded 1 to 250 CFU/ml.

L. pneumophila serogroup 3 strains were isolated in hospital 1 (100 to 6,000 CFU/liter) and in hospital 2 (20 to 2,400 CFU/liter). In hospital 1, where the environmental control program was carried out for 6 years, 78% of the hot tap water samples were positive. All of the samples with a temperature of <45°C showed the presence of legionellae. The cultures in 1 of 12 oxygen bubble humidifiers yielded 16 CFU/ml. Despite the repeated isolation of *L. pneumophila* serogroup 3 strains in the water supply, no cases of nosocomial legionellosis have been reported (4).

Strains of *L. pneumophila* serogroup 3 were also isolated in hospital 2, where legionellosis cases have not been described. The cultures from air conditioner water were negative.

In hospital 3, the cultures showed 20 to 8,000 CFU of legionellae per ml, identified as *L. pneumophila* serogroups 2 and 6 (prevalent strains), *L. pneumophila* not serogroups 1 to 10, and *Legionella* spp. (under identification). No cases of *Legionella* pneumonia have been reported by the epidemiological surveillance.

L. pneumophila serogroups 1 and 3, *L. spiritensis*, and other *Legionella* spp. (under identification) were isolated from the water supply of hospital 4 (20 to 8,000 CFU/liter). *L. pneumophila* serogroup 1 and *L. spiritensis* were isolated from the oxygen bubble humidifiers (25 to 200 CFU/ml). Cases of nosocomial legionellosis have been described; they have been associated with the contaminated water supply and with the use of oxygen bubble humidifiers, contaminated by *L. pneumophila* serogroup 1 (5). The environmental surveillance and the serodiagnosis of the patients confirmed the source of infection and the mode of transmission.

L. pneumophila serogroups 1, 6, 8, and not 1–10 and other *Legionella* spp. (under identification) were isolated (20 to 2,000 CFU/liter) in hospital 6. Tap water samples from the therapy tanks were also positive. The occurrence of nosocomial legionellosis in the patients has not been proven, despite the presence of *L. pneumophila* serogroup 1. The risk of *Legionella* infection in long-term patients is under investigation.

Different strains of *L. pneumophila* have been isolated from five of six hospitals of Turin. Repeated isolations confirmed the ubiquitousness of the bacterium.

L. pneumophila serogroups 1, 2, 3, 6, 8, and not 1–10, *L. spiritensis*, and other *Legionella* spp. (under identification) were isolated, but only strains of *L. pneumophila* serogroup 1 have been associated with nosocomial legionellosis in one hospital.

We believe that environmental cultures are useful; the knowledge that legionellae are present in part of the hospital plumbing system should encourage greater attention to hospital-acquired pneumonia and to maintenance.

This work was supported by the Italian National Research Council grant 86.02613.52 and by the Specchio dei Tempi Foundation, La Stampa, Turin, Italy.

REFERENCES

1. **Bopp, C. A., J. W. Summer, G. K. Morris, and J. G. Wells.** 1981. Isolation of *Legionella* spp. from environmental water samples by low-pH treatment and use of a selective medium. *J. Clin. Microbiol.* **13:**714–719.
2. **Brennen, C., R. M. Vickers, V. L. Yu, A. Puntereri, and Y. C. Yee.** 1987. Discovery of occult *Legionella* pneumonia in a long stay hospital: results of prospective serological survey. *Br. Med. J.* **295:**306–307.
3. **Edelstein, P. H.** 1981. Improved semiselective medium for isolation of *Legionella pneumophila* from contaminated clinical and environmental specimens. *J. Clin. Microbiol.* **14:**298–303.
4. **Franzin, L., M. Castellani Pastoris, P. Gioannini, and G. Villani.** 1989. Endemicity of *Legionella pneumophila* serogroup 3 in a hospital water supply. *J. Hosp. Infect.* **13:**281–288.
5. **Franzin, L., P. Cavallo-Perin, M. Borsa, S. Siviero, and P. Gioannini.** 1989. Nosocomial legionellosis associated to oxygen bubble humidifiers, p. 117–119. *Proc. 18th AMCLI Congr.*
6. **Johnson, J. T., V. L. Yu, M. G. Best, R. M. Vickers, A. Goetz, R. Wagner, H. Wicker, and A. Woo.** 1985. Nosocomial legionellosis in surgical patients with head-and-neck cancer: implications for epidemiological reservoir and mode of transmission. *Lancet* **ii:**298–300.
7. **Vickers, R. M., V. L. Yu, S. S. Hanna, P. Muraca, W. Diven, N. Carmen, and F. B. Taylor.** 1987. Determinants of *Legionella pneumophila* contamination of water distribution systems: 15-hospital prospective study. *Infect. Control* **8:**357–363.
8. **Wadowsky, R. M., and R. B. Yee.** 1981. A glycine-containing selective medium for isolation of *Legionella* from environmental specimens. *Appl. Environ. Microbiol.* **42:**768–772.
9. **Yu, V. L., T. R. Beam, R. M. Lumish, R. M. Vickers, J. Fleming, C. McDermott, and J. Romano.** 1987. Routine culturing for *Legionella* in the hospital environment may be a good idea: a three-hospital prospective study. *Am. J. Med. Sci.* **294:**97–99.

Biofilm Formation by *Legionella pneumophila* in a Model Domestic Hot Water System

JOHN W. WIREMAN, ANN SCHMIDT, CELESTE R. SCAVO, AND DAN T. HUTCHINS

Biological Research Solutions, Detroit, Michigan 48201; Wayne State University, Detroit, Michigan 48202; and Dihydro Services, Sterling Heights, Michigan 48310

Survival of aquatic microorganisms in low-nutrient water environments frequently involves attachment to solid surfaces and the formation of biofilms. A mixed population of microorganisms form a biofilm consortium and interact in many ways, including the cometabolic use of nutrients provided from materials in the surface or the water phase.

Two characteristics of *Legionella pneumophila* are particularly puzzling and intriguing: (i) the organism is ubiquitous in aquatic environments and in many ways is typical of bacteria that can survive and grow in very low nutrient environments, but (ii) it is fastidious in the laboratory, and reliable culturing is at best difficult. What is the relationship between these two characteristics, and how can they be reconciled?

The usual (and sometimes adamantly defended) criterion for the presence of legionellae in water is the ability to form colonies on a solid agar surface (3). Is it realistic to require an aquatic bacteria to shift its metabolism from a low-nutrient survival mode in a liquid environment to form colonies on an extremely nutrient rich agar surface (1, 2)? We believe that this is not a realistic expectation and that the phenomenon of viable but nonculturable is the rule with legionellae rather than the rare exception. It would therefore be of great value to develop alternate methods to reliably measure the presence of legionellae in water.

It is difficult to predict, except in a general way, whether the bacterial population will predominately exist in the water phase or as biofilms. It is known that high nutrient concentrations will shift the equilibrium toward colonization of the water phase and that low nutrient concentrations will result in increased biofilm formation. It follows, therefore, that appropriate surfaces submerged in low-nutrient water containing active legionellae should be colonized by a portion of the planktonic population that is at least transiently present in the bulk water phase (4).

The purpose of these studies was to take advantage of this phenomenon to quantitate the activity of legionellae in water by the specific measurement of legionellae in biofilms rather than the criterion of colony formation on an agar surface. These studies therefore test the effect of certain

FIGURE IA

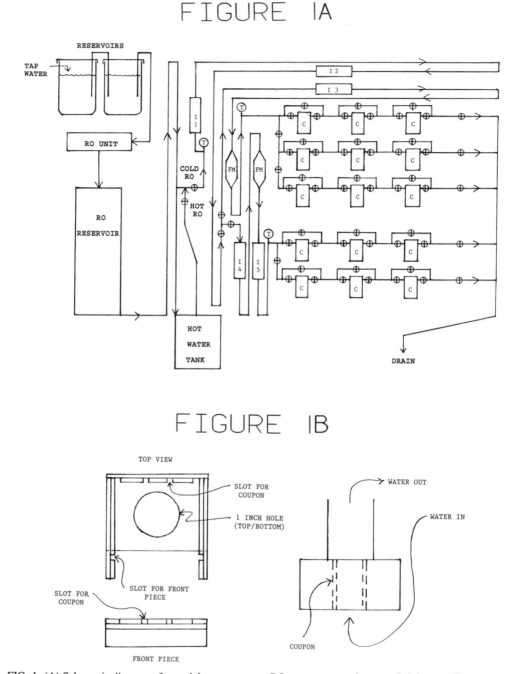

FIGURE IB

FIG. 1. (A) Schematic diagram of a model water system. RO, reverse osmosis water; I, injectors; T, temperature probe; FM, flow meter; C, canisters with coupon holder. (B) Diagram of acrylic coupon holder.

water parameters on the phenomenon of biofilm formation by legionellae in a model water system.

A diagrammatic representation of the model water system is shown in Fig. 1A. The system was designed to simulate point-of-use devices rather than recirculating water; thus, the water flows in one direction and exits to a drain following passage through the system. The source water was reverse osmosis purified and then reconstructed by chemical injection to produce chemically defined water. The temperature of the system was controlled by mixing hot and cold reverse osmosis water, and the flow rate was controlled by flow meters. Calibrated pumps were used to inject chemicals or bacteria at any one of five injector ports. The system is constructed of 0.75-in. (ca. 1.9-cm) chlorinated polyvinyl chloride pipe, with some brass or stainless steel fittings.

Flat coupons of various composition were housed in acrylic boxes that forced the water flow over the coupon surface (Fig. 1B). The coupon boxes were held in canisters (600-ml volume) that remained filled with test water between applications of fresh test water. Each canister contained a bypass pipe that allowed the test coupons to be in line in the water flow or bypassed.

For each experiment, selected water parameters were measured. These parameters included flow rate (gallons [1 gal = 3.785 liters] per minute), temperature (temperature probe), water hardness (EDTA titration), pH, and bacterial concentration (CFU per milliliter on standard methods agar or buffered charcoal yeast-extract).

Biofilms were measured after a specific protocol of exposure to test water. The coupons were rinsed with deionized water two times and then fixed with methanol for 2 min. The fixed, dried surfaces were stained directly with acridine orange on one portion of the surface and fluorescent monoclonal antiserum specific for *L. pneumophila* (Genetic Systems) on another portion of the surface. The stained surfaces were observed by epifluorescence at ×1,000 magnification (oil immersion). The number of fluorescent cells per 25 fields was determined.

These studies were conducted to determine whether quantitative methods could be developed to measure the activity of *L. pneumophila* in a model water system. Activity of legionellae is defined here as the ability or propensity to form stable biofilms, as opposed to the more traditional criterion of the presence of culturable cells in the bulk water phase. Since many studies have shown that *L. pneumophila* participates in biofilm formation at solid-liquid interfaces, it seems feasible to develop a general testing protocol to quantitate legionellae in water by the rate and extent of biofilm formation over a period of time rather than measuring CFU present in a water sample at a single point in time.

Several parameters were measured in this model water system, and several of these could not be determined to be important in their effects on biofilm formation. The noninfluential parameters in this system were, flow rate (1 to 3 gal/min), temperature (37 to 50°C), hardness (50 to 100 ppm), pH (6.0 to 7.0), and frequency of surface contact (1 to 10 times per week). Although these parameters may have effects on biofilm formation by legionellae under other testing protocols or other model system designs, the studies reported here

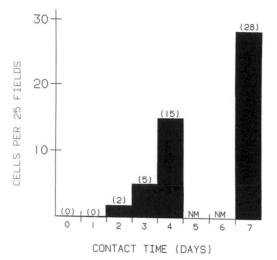

FIG. 2. Rate of attachment of legionellae to gasket rubber coupons (styrene-butadiene). Flow, 2 gal/min; temperature, 46°C; hardness, 80 ppm; pH, 6.1 to 7.0; total flow, 10 gal/day; *Legionella* concentration, 10^4 CFU/ml.

were unable to establish a relationship.

Three parameters were shown to significantly influence biofilm formation by legionellae. The first was time of contact. Although the numbers of *Legionella* cells present on the test surface were not always precisely proportional to the time of contact (days), there was a consistent, direct relationship. An example of such a measurement is shown in Fig. 2.

The second parameter was the concentration of *L. pneumophila*. Fresh suspensions of *L. pneumophila* (serogroup 1, Philadelphia strain) were injected into the water flow via calibrated pumps to achieve various final concentrations. The system was also naturally contaminated with a mixed flora of other heterotrophic bacteria. An example of the effect of the *Legionella* concentration in the water flow is shown in Fig. 3. In this experiment the contact time was 7 days. With different contact times or with different coupon surface types, the extent of attachment of legionellae varies, but there is a consistent increase in the number of attached bacteria as the *Legionella* concentration increases.

The third parameter was the coupon surface type. The attachment of legionellae was, as expected, strongly dependent upon the nature of the coupon surface. The results of a screening of eight different surface types are shown in Fig. 4. The visualization of attached legionellae on various surfaces by monoclonal antiserum was usually straightforward and reproducible, but one surface, natural gum, was difficult to observe because of background fluorescence. Ethylene propylene diene was consistently superior to other surfaces in

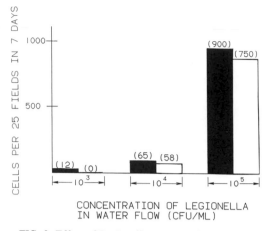

FIG. 3. Effect of *Legionella* concentration on biofilm formation. Flow, 2 gal/min; temperature, 43°C; hardness, 100 ppm; pH, 7.0; total flow, 6 gal/day; contact, five times per 7 days. Solid bars, styrene-butadiene (gasket rubber); open bars, galvanized steel.

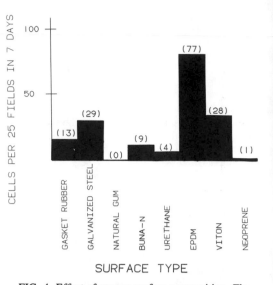

FIG. 4. Effect of coupon surface composition. Flow, = 2 gal/min; temperature, 43°C; hardness, 50 to 70 ppm; pH, 6.5 to 7.2; total flow, 6 gal/day; contact, = two times per 7 days; *Legionella* concentration, 10³ CFU/ml. Materials tested were styrene-butadiene (gasket rubber), galvanized steel, polyisoprene (natural gum), butadiene-acrylonitrile (Buna-N), polyester polyether urethane (urethane), ethylenepropylenediene (EPDM), fluorinated hydrocarbon (Viton), and polycholoprene (neoprene).

the quantitative attachment of legionellae. Although this surface does contain a great deal of visible texture, the detection of attached legionellae was unambiguous.

Even though numerous non-*Legionella* bacteria attached to the various surfaces as measured by acridine staining, legionellae were also visible on the same coupon surface. The ability to stain legionellae even in a thick biofilm is not obscured by the presence of other bacteria.

Legionellae are common in water environments, but they are also fastidious and difficult to culture in the laboratory. Alternate methods for measuring the activity of legionellae, especially in high-risk hospital domestic water, would therefore be valuable.

L. pneumophila, like many other aquatic bacteria that survive and grow under low-nutrient conditions, is a biofilm organism. The studies reported here measured the activity of a laboratory strain of *L. pneumophila* by measuring the rate and extent of biofilm formation on several surfaces.

To develop a quantitative assay for *Legionella* activity, several parameters that could influence biofilm formation were tested. Three parameters that were shown to influence biofilm formation were (i) days of contact, (ii) *Legionella* concentration, and (iii) surface type.

Further studies and field testing will be necessary to determine whether a reliable biofilm detection method can be used to quantitate the activity of legionellae in water, especially the activity of natural strains that have not been subjected to prior culture procedures.

REFERENCES

1. **Buck, J. D.** 1979. The plate count in aquatic microbiology, p. 19–28. *In* J. W. Costerton and R. R. Colwell (ed.), *Native Aquatic Bacteria: Enumeration, Activity, and Ecology.* American Society for Testing and Materials, Philadelphia.
2. **Byrd, J. J., H.-S. Xu, and R. R. Colwell.** 1991. Viable but nonculturable bacteria in drinking water. *Appl. Environ. Microbiol.* **57:**875–878.
3. **Hussong, D., R. R. Colwell, M. O'Brien, E. Weiss, A. D. Pearson, R. M. Weiner, and W. D. Burge.** 1987. Viable *Legionella pneumophila* not detectable by culture on agar media. *Bio/Technology* **5:**947–950.
4. **Wright, J. B., I. Ruseska, M. A. Athar, S. Corbett, and J. W. Costerton.** 1989. *Legionella pneumophila* grows adherent to surfaces in vitro and in situ. *Infect. Control Hosp. Epidemiol.* **10:**408–415.

Occurrence and Distribution of *Legionella pneumophila* in Water Systems of Central European Private Homes

F. TIEFENBRUNNER, A. ARNOLD, M. P. DIERICH, AND K. EMDE

Institute of Hygiene, Faculty of Medicine, University of Innsbruck, Fritz Pregl Strasse 3, A-6010 Innsbruck, Tirol, Austria and Department of Civil Engineering, University of Alberta, Edmonton, Alberta T6G 2E1, Canada

As a result of increased concern about the potential occurrence of *Legionella pneumophila* in potable water supplies (1), homes in central Europe were selected at random and systematically evaluated for factors that might be significant for the contamination and persistence of legionellae within a home plumbing system. Evidence now implicates the components of the home plumbing system as among the single largest factors for widespread proliferation and dissemination of legionellae (7). These health concerns have been expressed in guidelines of both the U.S. Environmental Protection Agency and the European ISO Commission. The new U.S. drinking water regulation has stipulated a maximum contaminate goal level of <1 legionella per 100 ml of drinking water (9). In contrast, the European ISO Commission has proposed a risk threshold of 100 CFU/100 ml of drinking water (7). Both regulatory guidelines apply to water quality as discharged at the faucet or shower head. It has been noted that potable distribution systems are capable of sustaining a diverse population of direct and opportunistic pathogens, including *Legionella* species, with the passing water phase acting as a transmission vector to exposed potential risk groups (2–6). Aerosols created by home plumbing systems may then create significant health risks for exposed, sensitive, or compromised persons.

This research was conducted in two phases. The first phase surveyed 63 homes, chosen at random from a list of a possible 2,000 homes in Germany, the Netherlands, and Austria. Each site was characterized in detail, and duplicate water samples for chemical and microbiological analyses were taken from various sites in the home. One set of samples was analyzed immediately in a mobile, on-site laboratory. The second set was processed at the laboratories of the University of Innsbruck. Microbiological analyses included buffered charcoal-yeast extract agar, *L. pneumophila* selective agar, cetrimide agar, mannitol-salt agar mEndo agar, and total heterotrophic count agar. Presumptive legionellae were subcultured to L-cysteine-free medium and identified by using direct immunofluorescence reaction with a monoclonal (mouse) fluorescein isothiocyanate-labeled antibody specific for *L. pneumophila* serogroups 1 to 8. Serogroup affiliation was confirmed with fluorescein isothiocyanate-labeled anti-*L. pneumophila* immunoglobulin (Fa. Fresenius).

In the second phase, *Legionella*-positive homes had additional sampling ports installed at the water heater and at hot and cold water pipes immediately upstream of the fixture being sampled. These ports did not influence flow through the fixture, nor were the sampling ports influenced by sludge or sediment accumulation in the fixture sampled. Fifteen locations were sampled in each home. Samples were analyzed as described for phase I.

Eight percent of the phase I homes were confirmed positive for *L. pneumophila*. Twenty-one percent of the homes were also found positive for *Escherichia coli*. It was not determined whether *E. coli* was part of the home distribution system biofilm or entered via the municipal water supply. Table 1 lists significant technical factors found at phase I homes. Figure 1 illustrates the occurrence of *L. pneumophila* and other microorganisms isolated at phase I homes. There did not appear to be significant correlation between the types and variety of microorganisms isolated and the occurrence of legionellae. Although there appeared to be some correlation between individual categories of samples with individual sampling locations, it was not possible to establish significant correlations between chemical parameters and incidence of legionellae.

In phase II, it was determined that all *Legionella*-positive homes had copper plumbing, whereas *Legionella*-negative homes had copper, galvanized steel or PE-X piping. Homes with a low daily water consumption tended to have a higher frequency of *Legionella* isolation. Conditions in these homes would favor increased biofilm development, which would be sheared from the internal pipe surface during peak use times (e.g., early morning or evening). These conditions may also favor the attachment and growth of legionellae. Table 2 shows a quanitative analysis of legionellae found at phase II homes. Homes having "sporadic" hot water recirculation systems or no recirculation system tended to be more susceptible to *Legionella* colonization than were homes with a hot water recirculation system.

From the findings of this survey, it was determined that the levels of legionellae tended to be lower in single- and two-family homes (duplexes) than in large, multiresident buildings. This is likely a direct function of the differences in plumbing systems (e.g., length and materials), water use patterns, and the length of time the water is stagnant within the system (7, 8). Residual

TABLE 1. Phase I field site characteristics

Component	Parameter measured	No. found positive or measured value	% of total investigated
Water heater	Instantaneous heaters	13	21
	Water storage heaters	50	79
	Tank capacity (liters; range)	80–250	
	Hot water temp. at storage heater (°C)	42–79	
	Estimated mean water temp. at tank outlet (°C)	57	
Plumbing	Copper	50	79
	Galvanized steel	10	16
	Plastic (PE-X)	3	5
	Avg length of cold water pipe in the home (m)	11.7	
	Avg length of hot water pipe in the home (m)	8.4	
Circulation system	Homes with hot water storage heaters, having:		
	No recirculation plumbing, configuration	24	48
	Recirculation plumbing	26	52
	Pump-driven circulation system	12	46
Fittings	Avg no. of draw-off points/house	12	
	Avg vol withdrawn/ draw-off, point[a] (m³)	17	
	Washbasin fittings		
	Homes with single-lever tap	35	57
	Homes with classic two-lever taps	27	43
	Homes with thermostat	1	1
	Shower and bath fittings		
	Single-lever tap	22	15
	Classic two-lever taps	15	24
	Shower hose	60	92
	Plastic shower hose	44	70
	Metal spiral hose	19	30
	Overhead shower	3	8

[a]Estimated average annual consumption of 200 m³.

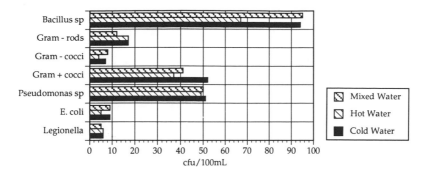

FIG. 1. Microbial composition of phase I homes.

water in the shower head, shower hoses, and spouts of mixed water taps was found to be insignificant relative to the actual amount of stagnant water within the entire plumbing system. Recirculating hot water systems, rather than "fill and draw" systems, were found to minimize the proliferation of legionellae within plumbing materials. Points where the cold water system is subject to warming or the hot water system is cooled by addition of cold water (to prevent scalding) were found to favor *Legionella* growth. This observation is documented in Table 2, which shows that the frequency of *Legionella* isolation

was almost the same at cold, hot, and mixed water sampling locations. Therefore, in a risk evaluation for legionellae, it is important to consider the entire home plumbing system and not only the hot water system.

This project was funded and supported technically by Friedrich Grohe Ltd., Krupp Stahl A.G., Viessmann Ltd., Viega Ltd., and Wilo Ltd.

REFERENCES

1. **Bundesgesundheitsamt Berlin.** 1987. Recommendations of the Federal Ministry of Health on risk minimization for *Legionella* infections. *Bundesgesundheitsblatt* **30:**252–253.

TABLE 2. *Legionella* species found at phase II sampling sites (cfu/100 ml)

	CFU/100 ml at phase II site:				
Sampling point	1	2	3	4	5
Water storage tanks/heaters					
Tank inlet					16
Tank outlet				10	>500
Tank outlet after cooling to <40°C	10			10	139
Base of tank					>500
Recirculation line					14
Washbasins					
Cold water sampling port (upstream from cold water tap)	35			10	
Hot water sampling port (upstream from hot water tap)					>1,000
Cold water tap	10	10			
Hot water tap		50			
Hot water tap after cooling to <40°C			5		>500
Cold water sampling port (upstream from bath/shower fitting)					
Hot water sampling port (upstream from bath/shower fitting)					
Mixed water from shower head				10	10
Shower hose					
Hand spray + shower hose			57		

2. **Colbourne, J. S., and P. J. Dennis.** 1989. The ecology and survival of *Legionella pneumophila*. *J. Inst. Water Environ. Manage.* **3:**345–350.
3. **Emde, K. M. E., D. W. Smith, and R. Facey.** 1992. Initial investigation of microbially influenced corrosion (MIC) in a low temperature water distribution system. *Water Res.* **26:**169–175.
4. **Lee, J. V., and A. A. West.** 1991. Survival and growth of *Legionella* species in the environment. *J. Appl. Bacteriol. Suppl.* **70:**121S–129S.
5. **Lee, T. C., J. E. Stout, and V. L. Yu.** Factors predisposing to *Legionella pneumophila* colonization in residential water systems. *Arch. Environ. Health* **43:**59–62.
6. **Olsen, B. H., and L. A. Nagy.** 1984. Microbiology of potable water. *Adv. Appl. Microbiol.* **30:**73–132.
7. **Tiefenbrunner, F., A. Arnold, E. Taraboi, and U. Czernek.** 1990. Occurrence of *Legionella* in single family homes and hotels. *Proc. 1990 German Assoc. Hyg. Microbiol.* (In German.)
8. **Tiefenbrunner, F., H. Hillbert, E. Braun, and R. Gesslauer.** 1987. Disinfection of water distribution systems in apartment and building complexes. *Forum Staedte Hyg.* **38:**130–135. (In German.)
9. **U.S. Office of the Federal Register.** 1990. *Code of Federal Regulations, Title 40, Protection of Environment.* Government Printing Office, Washington, D.C.

Dynamics of *Legionella pneumophila* in the Potable Water of One Floor of a Hospital

THOMAS J. MARRIE, GREGORY BEZANSON, JONATHAN FOX, ROSEMARY KUEHN, DAVID HALDANE, AND SUSAN BURBRIDGE

Department of Medicine, Victoria General Hospital, Halifax, Nova Scotia B3H 2Y9, and Department of Microbiology, Dalhousie University, Halifax, Nova Scotia B3H 1V8, Canada

Legionella pneumophila serogroup 1 has been present in the potable water of our hospital since 1981, when we first began sampling the water. In a previous study in which we sampled 20 water distribution sites randomly selected throughout the hospital, we found that there was marked intersite variation in the percentage of water samples positive for *L. pneumophila* (range, 25 to 75%) over a 1-year period. However, there was intrasite stability in that the same strain tended to be recovered from the same site. In this study, we examined the dynamics of *L. pneumophila* in the potable water of one floor of our hospital.

The eighth floor of the Victoria General Hospital consists of five wards in two wings. Wards 8A and 8B are in the Centennial Wing, which was built in 1967; wards 8N, 8S, and 8W are in the Victoria Wing, which was built in 1948. All of the wards are interconnected.

The potable water comes from Pockwock Lake, 22 miles away. It is chlorinated at the source. Almost all of the distribution pipes are copper. Some of the risers in the Victoria Wing are brass. The hot water circulates at a temperature of 60°C.

Water was collected from every water outlet on the eighth floor on several occasions from March to August 1991. Water samples were obtained by turning on the hot and cold taps so that the water flowed slowly. The hot and cold water systems were sampled separately once. Two hundred milliliters of water was collected into a sterile bottle containing 0.1 ml of 10% solution sodium thiosulfate. At one site on 8A, water samples were collected once every hour for 23 h.

Water samples (50 ml) were centrifuged at 3,000 rpm for 20 min. The supernatant was removed, leaving approximately 10% of the original volume, in which the sediment was resuspended. A sterile cotton-tipped swab (Salem Manufacturing Co., Salem, Minn.) was then used to inoculate the surface of the following media: 5% sheep blood agar; and buffered charcoal-yeast extract agar (BCYE) containing 0.1% α-ketoglutarate (GIBCO Laboratories, Madison, Wis.) (3). Early in the course of this study, we also used BCYE agar with 0.1% α-ketoglutarate, cefamandole, and polymyxin B as well as BCYE agar with 0.1% α-ketoglutarate, polymyxin B, anisomycin, and vancomycin (GIBCO). These additional plates did not increase our yield over the use of only BCYE agar containing 0.1% α-ketoglutarate. All plates were incubated at 37°C, in a humidified atmosphere containing 5% carbon dioxide, for 7 days and were examined daily. Colonies that morphologically resembled legionellae were cultured onto blood and BCYE agar. Those that failed to grow on blood agar were examined by a direct fluorescent antibody technique (1), using *L. pneumophila* serogroup 1 antisera (Centers for Disease Control, Atlanta, Ga.).

Portions of the growth achieved after 48 h of incubation of the isolates on BCYE agar were suspended in 0.5 ml of TE buffer (0.5 M Tris-HCl [pH 8.0], 0.02 M EDTA). After pelleting and resuspending in 25 μl of TE, plasmid DNA was extracted from the cells by using a modified alkaline sodium dodecyl sulfate procedure (2). The contents of the extracts were determined by electrophoresis in vertical 0.75% agarose gels followed by ethidium bromide staining. The plasmid

TABLE 1. Results of cultures of hot water on 8A and
8B examined in 1991

Date	No. positive for *L. pneumophila*/ no. sampled (% positive)	
	8A	8B
March 1	22/47 (47)	16/23 (70)
March 14	27/39 (69)	13/24 (54)
May 23	21/43 (49)	12/24 (50)

profiles were as follows: 0, no plasmid, II, 20-MDa plasmid; III, 96- and 72-MDa plasmids; IV, 70-MDa plasmid; V, 89-MDa plasmid; VI, 100-MDa plasmid; and VII, 58- and 103-MDa plasmids.

Table 1 shows that when the water sites on wards 8A and 8B were sampled on March 1,

March 14, and May 23, 1991, 54% of the 129 samples obtained on 8A were positive for *L. pneumophila* and 58% of the 71 samples obtained on 8B were positive. Plasmid profile II predominated in both locations, accounting for 84% of the isolates typed from 8A and 96% of those typed from 8B (Table 2).

When 8A and 8B were sampled in July and August 1991, plasmid type II again was predominant (Table 3). However, type VI now accounted for 21% of the isolates on 8B. It is noteworthy that plasmid type III was the predominant type isolated from 8S and 8N water, accounting for 77 and 65% of the isolates typed. The cold water only was rarely positive on 8B (11% of the samples), while on both 8S and 8N, the cold water accounted for most of the isolates (Table 4).

Table 5 shows the results of repeated sampling over one 24-h period of one water site on 8A. All 8 of the samples collected from 2400 to 0700 were

TABLE 2. Results of plasmid typing of *L. pneumophila* isolated in 1991

	8A				8B			
	No. typed	No. (%) type:			No. typed	No. (%) type:		
Date		II	III	VI		II	III	VI
March 1	19	17 (89)	2 (11)	0	7	7 (100)	0	0
March 14	17	12 (74)	4 (24)	1 (5)	5	5 (100)	0	0
May 23	20	18 (90)	4 (10)	0	12	11 (92)	9 (8)	0

TABLE 3. Results of plasmid typing of *L. pneumophila* isolates obtained during July and August 1991

Site	No. plasmid typed	No. (%) with plasmid profile:		
		II	III	VI
8A	5	5 (100)		
8B	38	28 (74)	2 (5)	8 (21)
8S	13	3 (23)	10 (77)	
8N	20	6 (30)	6 (30)	1 (5)

TABLE 4. Results of cultures of hot and cold water on three wards, July and August 1991

Ward	No. of hot-cold pairs sampled	No. (%) hot and cold positive	No. (%) hot positive	No. (%) cold positive	No. (%) hot and cold negative	Range of hot water temp (°C)
8B	28	4 (14)	18 (64)	3 (11)	3 (11)	53–59
8S	18	2 (11)	0	16 (89)	0	47–65
8N	11	0	0	6 (55)	5 (45)	52–65

TABLE 5. Results of repeated sampling of water site
8A, room 100, on June 12 to 13, 1991

Time	*L. pneumophila* isolated	Plasmid profile
0700	Yes	II
0800	No	
0900	No	
1000	No	
1100	Yes	II
1200	Yes	II
1300	Yes	II
1400	No	
1500	Not done	
1600	No	
1700	No	
1800	No	
1900	No	
2000	No	
2100	No	
2200	No	
2300	No	
2400	Yes	VI
0100	Yes	II
0200	Yes	II
0300	Yes	II
0400	Yes	II
0500	Yes	II
0600	Yes	II
Total no. (%)	11/23 (48%)	10/11 (91) type II 1/11 (9) type IV

positive, while only 3 of the 15 collected thereafter were positive ($P < 0.001$).

We conclude the following. (i) There is a marked difference in the ecology of *L. pneumophila* on one floor in our hospital. 8A and 8B water sites are populated predominantly by *L. pneumophila* plasmid type II, while 8N and 8B water sites have predominantly plasmid type III. *L. pneumophila* was isolated mostly from cold water samples on 8S and 8N, while it was isolated chiefly from hot water samples on 8B. (ii) It is likely that the rate of positivity of water samples varies throughout the day.

This study was supported by grant MT-10577 from the Medical Research Council of Canada.

REFERENCES

1. **Cherry, W. B., B. Pittman, P. P. Harris, G. A. Hebert, B. M. Thomason, and R. E. Weaver.** 1981. Detection of Legionnaires' disease bacteria by direct immunofluorescent staining. *J. Clin. Microbiol.* **14:**298–303.
2. **Dillon, J. R., G. S. Bezanson, and K.-H. Yeung.** 1985. Basic techniques, p. 1–126. *In* J. R. Dillon, A. Nasim, and E. Nestman (ed.), *Recombinant DNA Methodology.* J. Wiley & Sons, Inc., Toronto.
3. **Vickers, R. M., J. E. Stout, V. L. Yu, and J. D. Rihs.** 1987. Manual of culture methodology for *Legionella. Semin. Respir. Infect.* **2:**274–279.

Analysis of *Legionella pneumophila* Serogroup 6 Strains Isolated from Dental Units

P. C. LÜCK, L. BENDER, M. OTT, J. H. HELBIG, W. WITZLEB, AND J. HACKER

Institut für Medizinische Mikrobiologie, Medizinische Akademie Dresden, Güntzstrasse 32, D-O-8019 Dresden, and Institut für Genetik, Universität Würzburg, Röntgenstrasse 11, D-W-8700 Würzburg, Germany

Bacteria of the genus *Legionella* are ubiquitous in water environments. They have also been found in dental units (3, 4). We studied the occurrence of *Legionella* species in dental units and the connected water system by which the dental chairs were supplied in the Faculty of Dentistry at the School of Medicine in Dresden. This warm water supply was found to be contaminated with *Legionella pneumophila* serogroup 6 (Lp6) (3).

The aims of this study were to find detectable changes in Lp6 strains isolated from dental units and the connected water system over a 3-year period. For this purpose, we typed Lp6 strains isolated at different times from water samples, using monoclonal antibodies (MAbs) and the *Not*I cleavage pattern of the genomic DNA after pulsed-field gel electrophoresis (PFGE). To estimate the discriminating properties of these subtyping methods, we studied an additional 17 Lp6

strains isolated from 16 different sources in Germany, Czechoslovakia, and Austria. A serogroup-specific MAb and a subgroup-specific MAb were applied in the indirect immunofluorescence (IFA) technique to define subgroups Chicago (reacting with the subgroup-specific MAb) and Dresden (not reacting with the subgroup-specific MAb) (2). Cleaved genomic DNA was separated by PFGE, using a CHEF-DR system (Bio-Rad, Munich, Germany) or a ROTAPHOR apparatus (Biometra, Göttingen, Germany) (2).

Virulence testing was performed on two arbitrarily selected strains from the dental units isolated at the beginning of the study in May 1988 and at the end in February 1990. Virulent (reisolated from the spleen of an intraperitoneally infected guinea pig) and avirulent variants (passaged more than 100 times on buffered charcoal-yeast extract agar) of the Lp6 ATCC type strain Chicago-2 were used for comparison.

To test virulence for guinea pigs, logarithmic dilutions of Lp6 strains in A.bidest were intraperitoneally injected into two animals per dilution. Lp6 strains were reisolated from spleens of the animals that died. Fifty percent lethal doses (LD$_{50}$s) were calculated by the Karber-Spearman method.

Growth kinetics in *Acanthamoeba castellanii* cultures were determined in the following way. Acanthamoebae were precultivated for 48 h and infected with legionellae to give a 1:1 ratio of legionellae to amoebae. Multiplication of legionellae was determined by counting CFU of the amoeba culture supernatant on buffered charcoal-yeast extract agar on days 0 and 7. Growth kinetics were expressed as CFU (day 7)/CFU (day 0).

The prevalence of Lp6 antibodies in various populations with and without exposure to Lp6 from dental units was estimated in the IFA test using heat-killed antigen (6). Reactive sera were retested after absorption with *Escherichia coli*-containing fluid (6). Sera from 37 dentists working at the Dental Faculty of Dresden with Lp6-contaminated dental units, 50 dental assistants from the Dental Faculty, 54 dentists working in other dental clinics of Dresden, 22 dentists working in Görlitz (approximately 80 km away), and 293 healthy persons (no dentists or dental assistants) living in Dresden were tested.

All *Legionella* strains isolated over a 3-year period from dental units and the warm water system were of the same MAb subtype (Dresden) and showed the same *Not*I cleavage pattern in PFGE. Thus, we could find no detectable changes in the *Legionella* population in this water system. The *Not*I cleavage pattern of the Lp6 strains from the Dental Faculty were distinct from those of the other 17 Lp6 strains tested.

For subtyping Lp6 strains, MAb typing is less powerful than long-range genome mapping using PFGE, since only two subtypes were defined by MAbs whereas 13 different genome types were found among 17 strains of different origins with use of the *Not*I pattern.

Two arbitrarily selected Lp6 strains had LD$_{50}$s of 3×10^8 CFU/ml (strain St 37) and 2×10^8 CFU/ml (strain St 221). The growth indices in acanthamoebae were 150 and 175, respectively. For comparison, the LD$_{50}$ of the virulent Chicago-2 variant was $< 10^5$ CFU/ml, and that of the avirulant variant was $> 10^9$. The amoeba growth indices were > 200 and < 1, respectively, for these strains. This finding demonstrates that the two Lp6 strains from dental units had a low virulence for guinea pigs and a medium growth kinetic index value in amoebae.

The prevalence of Lp6 antibodies among dentists working at the Faculty of Dentistry with Lp6-contaminated dental chairs was significantly higher in comparison with findings for dentists from Dresden ($P < 0.05$) and Görlitz and a group of healthy people living in Dresden ($P < 0.01$) (Fig. 1). Dental assistants working at the same faculty have had a not significantly higher preva-

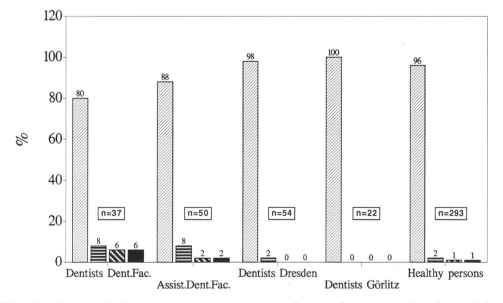

FIG. 1. Prevalence of antibodies against Lp6, among dentists working with *Legionella*-contaminated dental chairs at the Dental Faculty, dentists working in other geographic locations, and healthy persons living in Dresden and not engaged in dentistry-related work. IFA titer: ▨, <64; ▤, 64; ▧, 128; ■, 256.

lence of Lp6 antibodies compared with the dentist groups. In comparison with the group of healthy persons, IFA titers were significantly higher ($P <$ 0.05). Compared with findings for the dentists of the Dental Faculty, the prevalence was lower (not significantly).

It can be concluded from our results that an unchanged Lp6 population induced anti-Lp6 antibodies in dentists working with contaminated dental units. This observation is in agreement with the results of Oppenheim et al. (4) and Reinthaler et al. (5). On the other hand, Oppenheim et al. found no infections among patients treated by these dentists. A possible explanation for this discrepancy is that the virulence of the Legionella strains from the dental units is too low to cause infections following a short time of exposure during dental treatment. The low virulence of our strains supports this observation.

Among the dentists from Dresden, no cases of Legionella pneumonia occurred. Thus, the antibodies are probably due to continuous ingestion of small amounts of legionellae, which led to light (Pontiac fever) or inapparent infections (1) detectable by antibody measurement.

REFERENCES

1. **Bornstein, N., D. Marmet, M. Surgot, M. Novicki, A. Arslan, J. Esteve, and J. Fleurette.** 1989. Exposure to Legionellaceae at a hot spring spa: a prospective clinical and serological study. Epidemiol. Infect. **102**:31–36.

2. **Lück, P. C., L. Bender, M. Ott, J. H. Helbig, and J. Hacker.** 1991. Analysis of Legionella pneumophila serogroup 6 strains isolated from a hospital warm water supply over a three-year period using genomic long range mapping techniques and monoclonal antibodies. Appl. Environ. Microbiol. **57**:3226–3231.

3. **Lück, P. C., S. Seidel, J. H. Helbig, C. Pilz, W. Witzleb, I. Voigt, and T. Henke.** 1990. Anzucht von Legionella pneumophila aus Wasserproben stomatologischer Behandlungseinheiten. Z. Klin. Med. **45**:247–249.

4. **Oppenheim, B. A., A. M. Senfton, N. Gill, J. E. Tyler, M. C. O'Mahony, J. M. Richards, P. J. L. Dennis, and T. G. Harrison.** 1987. Widespread Legionella pneumophila contamination of dental stations in a dental school without apparent human infection. Epidemiol. Infect. **99**:159–166.

5. **Reinthaler, F. F., F. Mascher, and D. Stunzner.** 1988. Serological examinations for antibodies against Legionella species in dental personnel. J. Dent. Res. **67**:942–943.

6. **Wilkinson, H. W., C. E. Farshy, B. J. Fikes, D. D. Cruce, and L. P. Yealy.** Measure of immunoglobulin G-, M-, and A-specific titers against Legionella pneumophila and inhibition of titers against nonspecific, gram-negative bacteria antigens in the indirect immunofluorescence test for legionellosis. J. Clin. Microbiol. **10**:685–689.

Effect of Chlorine on the Survival and Growth of *Legionella pneumophila* and *Hartmannella vermiformis*

JOHN M. KUCHTA, JEANNINE S. NAVRATIL, ROBERT M. WADOWSKY, JOHN N. DOWLING, STANLEY J. STATES, AND ROBERT B. YEE

Department of Water, Pittsburgh, Pennsylvania 15238, Departments of Pathology and Medicine, School of Medicine, and Department of Infectious Diseases and Microbiology, Graduate School of Public Health, University of Pittsburgh, Pittsburgh, Pennsylvania 15261, and Children's Hospital of Pittsburgh, Pittsburgh, Pennsylvania 15213

Legionella pneumophila can exist in potable water systems even though it is exposed to a 0.75 to 1.5 ppm of free chlorine residual for extended times. It can multiply and colonize hot water tanks (1) and other environments ostensibly adverse for bacteria. These anomalies can be resolved at least in part if the bacteria are somehow protected from the environment. Such protection is afforded to legionellae by intracellular growth in certain protozoa, such as *Tetrahymena pyriformis* and *Acanthamoeba castellanii* (3, 6). *Hartmannella* amoebae are common inhabitants in potable water systems (1, 2, 8), and since *Hartmannella vermiformis* promotes intracellular growth of legionellae (1, 2, 8, 9), it is likely that these organisms interact in the natural environment. We have previously shown that *L. pneumophila* isolated from a hot water tank and passaged in tap water is much more resistant to chlorine than are its agar-grown counterparts (5). Besides le-

gionellae, these samples were known to contain amoebae, one of which was isolated and identified as *H. vermiformis* (8, 9), and at least four other bacterial species, including *Pseudomonas paucimobilis* (9). This organism was later used as a food source for *H. vermiformis* in a tap water system developed for additional studies to determine the chlorine resistance of *L. pneumophila* and associated *H. vermiformis* (9). This new system, consisting only of legionellae, amoebae, and dead *P. paucimobilis* for amoebal food in tap water, allowed us to extend our chlorine studies.

In early experiments, tap water-grown legionellae were separated from amoebae by using a 1-μm-pore-size filter and tested for resistance to chlorine. Although chlorine demand was significantly reduced in this new system, it was not eliminated; to achieve the same free chlorine residual between tap water-grown and agar-passaged legionellae, we always added additional chlorine to the tap water-grown sample. Under these conditions, we found that legionellae in the tap water or filtrate samples were very resistant to chlorine, and each was much more resistant than the agar-grown counterparts (7). This finding suggested that possibly some physiological change occurred to legionellae as a result of multiplying inside amoebae, which made them more resistant to chlorine than was the agar-passaged strain. Alternatively, the heat-killed *P. paucimobilis*, through close association with legionellae, may have physically protected them from the effects of chlorine.

To determine the explanation for the enhanced chlorine resistance observed in the tap water culture, a 6-day-old legionella-hartmannella coculture was divided in two, and the samples were treated as follows. One sample was passed through a 1-μm-pore-size filter to separate extracellular legionellae from amoebae (referred to as 1-μm filtrate). The second sample of coculture was not filtered. At the same time, two samples of agar-passaged legionellae were prepared to contain the same number of legionellae as in the tap water-grown cultures. One of these samples was resuspended in tap water, and the other was resuspended in tap water containing 10^9 heat-killed CFU of *P. paucimobilis* per ml to approximate growth conditions in the coculture. All of the samples were washed extensively and resuspended in sterile tap water in demand-free tubes. This washing eliminated any measurable, excess demand in the coculture-grown samples. All four samples were treated with the same amount of chlorine for the same time, neutralized, and plated on buffered charcoal-yeast extract medium. The results strongly suggest that rather than some physiological change occurring in legionellae growing inside amoebae, the extracellular legionellae are more resistant to chlorine purely as a result of physical protection by *P. paucimobilis*. Three of the cultures, i.e., coculture grown, 1-μm filtrate of coculture grown, and most importantly agar grown resuspended in coculture medium containing *P. paucimobilis*, all contained a high percentage (50 to 83%) of surviving legionellae after chlorination. In contrast, only 4% of the legionellae that were agar grown survived the treatment (data not shown). This physical protection afforded to legionellae does not result in a measurable chemical demand to the system, and we termed this phenomenon "micro-demand." Care in experimental design and interpretation of results must be taken if physical protection by organisms, organelles, or cell parts is a possibility.

We next turned our attention to the chlorine resistance of hartmannellae. Since hartmannellae can exist as trophozoites or cysts, depending on environmental conditions, the chlorine resistance of both forms was determined. Also, after each form was chlorinated over a range of concentra-

tions, the amoebae were diluted into fresh medium containing legionellae and heat-killed *P. paucimobilis* to determine whether chlorine-treated amoebal cultures could still support growth of legionellae. It is important to note that in these experiments, legionellae were not present during chlorination. Chlorine concentrations ranged from 0 to 20 ppm, and exposure time was 30 min. As in all experiments, the reaction was stopped with sodium thiosulfate. Two axenic cultures of sterile tap water-grown amoebae were treated: a 1-day-old culture containing at least 95% trophozoites, and a 10-day-old culture containing at least 95% cysts. After treatment, a portion of each neutralized sample was inoculated into fresh tap water medium containing legionellae, and growth of legionellae and amoebae was monitored. The hartmannellid culture containing mostly trophozoites appeared to be slightly more sensitive to chlorine than was the mostly cyst culture (Table 1). At 4 ppm of free chlorine residual, the culture containing mostly cysts supported only about a 2-log growth of legionellae, as opposed to 4-log growth in the mostly cyst cultures not exposed to chlorine (control). Amoebal growth was seen only sporadically in the mostly trophozoite cultures treated with 4 ppm of free chlorine residual; at 5 days after chlorine treatment, a small number of legionellae appeared and grew only 0.5 log by day 7. The growth of legionellae in these cultures could be attributed either to a very small number of trophozoite survivors or to the presence of a few cysts in the culture (Table 1).

Comparison of our results with those of Kilvington and Price (4) indicates that *H. vermiformis* cysts are about 25 times less resistant to chlorine than are *Acanthamoeba polyphaga* cysts. Although cysts of *A. polyphaga* are much more resistant to chlorine than are trophozoite forms, our study did not find an appreciable difference in the chlorine resistance of hartmannellid cultures containing mostly cysts or mostly trophozoites. Our cultures, which contained mostly trophozoites, may have had a sufficient number of cysts to obscure our ability to measure a true difference between cysts and trophozoites of *H. vermiformis*. In a potable water system, the extremely high chlorine resistance of *A. polyphaga* cysts probably does not give this organism an ecological advantage over organisms that are only moderately chlorine resistant, since the concentration of free chlorine in this environment is normally 0.75 to 1.5 ppm. *H. vermiformis* can withstand twice this amount in our tap water system and then support growth of legionellae. Because of its adaptability, *H. vermiformis* is a very common inhabitant of drinking water systems (1, 2, 8).

We next changed the circumstances to determine whether legionellae would grow in tap water

TABLE 1. Effects of free chlorine on *H. vermiformis* cultures and on *H. vermiformis-L. pneumophila* cocultures and subsequent growth of *L. pneumophila* in each

Growth condition in a tap water system	Growth[a] at free chlorine concn (ppm [mg/liter]) of:				
	0	2	4	10	20
H. vermiformis[b]					
Trophozoites	+++	+++	+	−	−
Cysts	++	++	++	−	−
L. pneumophila					
In trophozoite culture	(+++)	(+++)	(+)	(−)	(−)
In cyst culture	(+++)	(+++)	(++)	(+)	(−)
H. vermiformis-L. pneumophila coculture[c]					
H. vermiformis	++	++	++	−	−
L. pneumophila	(+++)	(+++)	(+++)	(−)	(−)

[a]Growth of hartmannellae was determined by hemocytometer counts as described in the text, and the extent of growth was determined after 6 days. +++, >2.0-net-log increase; ++, 1.0 to 2.0-net-log increase; +, <1.0-net-log increase; −, no growth. Calculations were made as the difference between time zero and day 6 averaged from three experiments. ( ), subsequent growth of legionellae.

[b]*L. pneumophila* (10^3 CFU/ml) was added after chlorination of amoebae.

[c]No additional *L. pneumophila* was added after chlorination. Coculture was 2 days old when chlorinated.

cultures if we chlorinated cocultures with different concentrations of chlorine. This experiment differs from previous ones in that a 2-day-old coculture of legionellae and hartmannellae consisting of a mixture of 90% trophozoites and 10% cysts was chlorinated and no additional legionellae were added after chlorination. Chlorination of a coculture, especially at or above 1 ppm of free chlorine residual, should result in a drastic reduction of extracellular legionellae, according to past experiments, while those residing in amoebae would be protected as long as no severe damage to the amoebae occurred. We tested the likelihood that chlorination resulted in the death of mostly extracellular legionellae at chlorine concentrations in the range of 1 to 2 ppm of free chlorine residual. Samples from the coculture and their 1-μm filtrates were chlorinated. The kill rates in the two cases were nearly identical, indicating that mostly extracellular legionellae were killed and that these organisms were reduced to near 0 CFU/ml (data not shown). However, when these cocultures were diluted into fresh medium, as much as 4 logs of legionellae growth occurred. In samples treated with 4.0 ppm of free chlorine residual, however, initial growth was delayed (Table 1). Therefore, a very small number of legionellae surviving chlorination could potentially pass through a water treatment system with the help of amoebae.

Overall, our results indicate that organisms can be physically protected from chlorine disinfection through a phenomenon called micro-demand. Particles, such as dead bacterial cells, in close association with live organisms protect them from chlorine while contributing little if anything to the overall measurable chlorine demand. In addition, it appears that tap water cultures of *H. vermiformis* containing mostly cysts are only nominally more resistant to chlorine disinfection than are cultures containing mostly trophozoites. However, both are capable of existing in potable water supplies with 0.75 to 1.5 ppm of free chlorine residual, which, according to our results, is well below the lethal limit for hartmannellae. At this time, there is no conclusive evidence that legionellae may be sequesterd in *H. vermiformis* cysts. However, trophozoites of this species can contain large numbers of legionellae and protect these intracellular bacteria from the effects of chlorine. The subsequent release of the organisms from trophozoites and infection by them of healthy amoebae may be the preferred mode of colonization of potable water systems by legionellae.

This work was supported by the U.S. Environmental Protection Agency under cooperative agreements CR 812761 (sponsored by the Center for Environmental Epidemiology at the Graduate School of Public Health of the University of Pittsburgh) and CR 817091-01-0.

REFERENCES

1. **Breiman, R. F., B. S. Fields, G. M. Sanden, L. Volmer, A. Meier, and J. Spika.** 1990. Association of shower use with Legionnaire's disease. *JAMA* **263**:2924–2926.
2. **Fields, B. S., G. N. Sanden, J. M. Barbaree, W. E. Morrill, R. M. Wadowsky, E. H. White, and J. C. Feeley.** 1989. Intracellular multiplication of *Legionella pneumophila* in amoebae isolated from hospital hot water tanks. *Curr. Microbiol.* **18**:131–137.
3. **Fields, B. S., E. B. Shotts, Jr., J. C. Feeley, G. W. Gorman, and W. T. Martin.** 1984. Proliferation of *Le-*

gionella pneumophila as an intracellular parasite of the ciliated protozoan *Tetrahymena pyriformis. Appl. Environ.
Microbiol.* **47:**467–471.

4. **Kilvington, S., and J. Price.** 1990. Survival of *Legionella
pneumophila* within cysts of *Acanthamoeba polyphaga* following chlorine exposure. *J. Appl. Bacteriol.* **68:**519–525.

5. **Kuchta, J. M., S. J. States, J. E. McGlaughlin, J. H.
Overmeyer, R. M. Wadowsky, A. M. McNamara, R. S.
Wolford, and Robert B. Yee.** 1985. Enhanced chlorine
resistance of tap water-adapted *Legionella pneumophila* as
compared with agar medium-passaged strains. *Appl. Environ. Microbiol.* **50:**21–26.

6. **Moffat, J. F., and L. S. Tompkins.** 1992. A quantitative
model of intracellular growth of *Legionella pneumophila* in
Acanthamoeba castellanii. Infect. Immun. **60:**292–301.

7. **Navratil, J. S., J. M. Kuchta, R. H. Palmer, S. J. States,
R. M. Wadowsky, and Robert B. Yee.** 1990. *Program
Abstr. Annu. Meet. Am. Soc. Microbiol. 1990,* abstr. Q-82,
p. 302).

8. **Wadowsky, R. M., L. J. Butler, M. K. Cook, S. M
Verma, M. A. Paul, B. S. Fields, G. Keleti, J. L. Sykora, and R. B. Yee.** 1988. Growth-supporting activity for
Legionella pneumophila in tap water cultures and implication of hartmannellid amoebae as growth factors. *Appl. Environ. Microbiol.* **54:**2677–2682.

9. **Wadowsky, R. M., T. M. Wilson, N. J. Kapp, A. J.
West, J. M. Kuchta, S. J. States, J. N. Dowling, and R.
B. Yee.** 1991. Multiplication of *Legionella* spp. in tap water
containing *Hartmannella vermiformis. Appl. Environ. Microbiol.* **57:**1950–1955.

Resistance of a Model Hot Water System to Colonization by *Legionella pneumophila*

D. J. M. HALDANE, G. S. BEZANSON, S. M. BURBRIDGE, R. D. KUEHN, AND T. J. MARRIE

*Department of Microbiology, Victoria General Hospital, Halifax, Nova Scotia B3H 1V8, and Department of Medi-
cine, Dalhousie University, Halifax, Nova Scotia B3H 2Y9, Canada*

Legionella pneumophila is a well-recognized
cause of nosocomial pneumonia. Contaminated
potable water has frequently been implicated as
the source of this microorganism. The potable water supply of our institution has been contaminated
with legionellae for more than 8 years. A model
hot water system was constructed, using the same
materials as in our potable water supply, to determine factors important in the chronic colonization
of these systems. We report our experience in attempting to establish colonization of the model
system.

A model hot water system was constructed with
a loop of copper piping (Fig. 1). Water was heated
in a 12-imperial-gallon (ca. 54.5-liter), 3,000-W
electric water heater. Circulation of water was
constant and maintained by a circulating pump.
The model temperature and pressure were monitored by gauges connected to the loop. One domestic faucet drained directly from the loop, and a
second drained one of two dead-end pipes (dead
end 2). A brass plumbing faucet drained the other
dead end. Inocula were introduced via an injection
pump connected to a closable injection port.
Mains water was used to prime the system initially, the faucet was then closed, and there was a
backflow-preventing valve to protect the mains
supply from contamination. The pressure in the
model was raised during inoculation and sampling
but was otherwise negative relative to the mains
water supply pressure. Each 1 to 2 ml of inoculum
was flushed into the model with approximately
250 ml of filter (0.45-μm-pore-size)-sterilized tap
water, which was also used to replace water
drained from the model during sampling.

The model was inoculated with strain 2579Sm,

a clinical isolate of *L. pneumophila* serogroup 1.
This isolate had previously been well characterized by plasmid analysis, monoclonal antibody
typing, and restriction endonuclease analysis and
was selected for resistance to streptomycin (100
μg/ml). For the final inoculation, *L. pneumophila*
serogroup 1-1109, a similarly characterized strain,
was used. The amoebae used for the final inoculation were limax amoebae isolated from a colonized institution in our area.

L. pneumophila serogroup 1 was grown to con-
fluence on α-ketoglutarate-supplemented buffered
charcoal-yeast extract (BCYEα) medium in 5%
CO_2 at 37°C. A suspension was prepared by
scraping the growth from the medium and suspending it in sterile water. For the initial inoculum, the optical density of the suspension was
adjusted to 0.5 at 620 nm with sterile water, and
then the suspension was diluted to approximately
1.5×10^6 CFU/ml. For heavy inocula, the isolate
was concentrated by centrifugation, the supernatant was discarded, and the pellet was resuspended
in 1 to 2 ml of sterile water. Colony counts were
performed on BCYE-α, using serial 1:10 dilutions. The amoeba was grown on nonnutrient agar
(NNA) plates seeded with killed *Enterobacter
aerogenes* and transferred twice in succession
onto NNA seeded with *L. pneumophila*. After the
growth was harvested by scraping the plate with a
glass rod, a suspension of cysts was prepared in
Page's amoeba saline. Absence of viable coliforms was confirmed by subculture to 5% sheep
blood agar.

The first samples for culture were usually removed within 24 h of inoculation; 100 ml of water
was removed from a dead-end faucet, and 100 ml

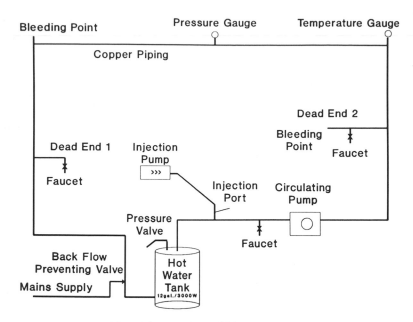

FIG. 1. Diagram of a model hot water system.

was removed from a faucet attached to the circuit. Fifty milliliters of each was used for *Legionella* culture; the sample was centrifuged at 1,200 × *g* for 15 min, and 10 μl of the concentrate was placed on BCYEα agar. The remaining 50 ml was cultured for amoebae by filtration through a 0.45 μm-pore-size filter and placement of the latter on NNA seeded with viable *E. aerogenes*.

After three consecutive negative cultures, the model was disinfected by increasing the water temperature to 70°C for 72 h. Faucets and bleeding points were flushed to ensure heat penetration throughout the system. Before the fifth inoculation, disinfection was not performed. The results are indicated in Table 1.

A model hot water system was constructed to mimic the conditions that exist in a potable water supply. The system was primed with tap water and

disinfected with heat. In this state, the system was, for legionellae, microbiologically virginal. Legionellae introduced to the system in this state were unable to initiate colonization despite large inocula. Inoculations were made at approximately 50°C, to mimic the conditions of a system in use, and at approximately 35°C, to eliminate the effect of temperature stress in reducing the inoculum. As it was not possible to keep the entry port sterile, other organisms, including pseudomonads, were able to colonize the system. This flora was eliminated by using heat in the first inoculations but did not promote colonization when left intact for the fifth inoculation.

There are a number of possible explanations for this failure of colonization. The environment within the model might be hostile, because of metal ion concentrations or lack of dissolved oxy-

TABLE 1. Results of inoculation of the model system with *L. pneumophila* serogroup 1

Inoculum of *L. pneumophila* (CFU)	Water temp (°C)	Concn (CFU/ml) at 24 h postinoculation h[a]
1.5×10^6	50	ND[b]
2×10^6	35	ND
1×10^{11}	50	104
2.4×10^{12}	45	244
2×10^{13}	36	ND
$3 \times 10^8 + 3.5 \times 10^6$ amoebic cysts	35	ND

[a] All cultures were negative at 7 days postinoculation.
[b] ND, not done.

gen or nutrients, or a high pH may have prevented growth. The 50°C temperature may have inhibited colonization, but temperature alone cannot explain our failure to colonize the system, as no growth occurred at 35°C. Legionellae have been shown to tolerate moderate concentrations of metal ions (5) and wide ranges of pH (from 5.5 to 9.2) and to survive in environments with low concentrations of oxygen (6). Although the initial heating (70°C) might remove some of the dissolved gases from the water, the addition of nonheated filter-sterilized water would partially replace them.

The inocula were prepared from isolates that had been grown on agar at 35°C and were suspended in sterile water. It is possible that laboratory adaptation had occurred, but we have been able to inoculate stored isolates to bottles of water that have remained culture positive for extended periods of time. Although the organisms could have become nonculturable, organisms are readily isolated from contaminated potable water systems. The organisms were introduced to the system as planktonic forms. It may be necessary to develop a biofilm to establish colonization, which may require the inoculum to be given over a longer period of time. Although legionellae are able to grow on copper and brass, they colonize these surfaces slowly (2). In our model, there are only small areas of nonmetallic surfaces that could be colonized (i.e., washers on the faucets and gauges). Older systems may favor colonization by the deposition of scale that would cover the less favorable metal surface.

Limitation of nutrients resulting from the exclusion or elimination of other organisms is a possible explanation for the failure of colonization (1, 4, 7). Although photosynthetic organisms are not available in hot water systems, bacteria and protozoa have been demonstrated to support growth of legionellae. The bacterial flora that became established when the model was in use does not reflect the usual flora of our potable water; presumably the flora reflects the mode of entry via the entry port, which has no counterpart in the institutional system. That this flora does not support growth was suggested by the fifth inoculum. Preparations are under way to inoculate the model with the flora colonizing our institution's system.

Other groups have developed model systems. Muraca et al. designed a model and used it to evaluate disinfection methods (3). They inoculated their systems within hours of each experiment. We have attempted to establish chronic colonization of our system to determine the effect of manipulations of the conditions of growth.

Large inocula, given as a single bolus, of *L. pneumophila* serogroup 1 strains did not establish colonization in a model hot water system. Additional, as yet unknown factors are required to establish chronic colonization.

REFERENCES

1. **Hume, R. D., and W. D. Hann.** 1984. Growth relationships of *Legionella pneumophila* with green algae (chlorophyta), p. 323–324. *In* C. Thornsberry, A. Balows, J. C. Feeley, and W. Jakubowski (ed.), *Legionella: Proceedings of the 2nd International Symposium.* American Society for Microbiology, Washington, D.C.
2. **Lee, J. V. and A. W. West.** 1991. Survival and growth of Legionella species in the environment. *J. Appl. Bacteriol. Symp. Suppl.* **70:**1215–1295.
3. **Muraca, P., J. E. Stout, and V. L. Yu.** 1987. Comparative assessment of chlorine, heat, ozone, and UV light for killing *Legionella pneumophila* within a model plumbing system. *Appl. Environ. Microbiol.* **53:**447–453.
4. **Rowbotham, T. J.** 1984. Legionellae and amoebae, p. 325–327. *In* C. Thornsberry, A. Balows, J. C. Feeley, and W. Jakubowski (ed.), *Legionella: Proceedings of the 2nd International Symposium.* American Society for Microbiology, Washington, D.C.
5. **States, S. J., L. F. Conley, M. Ceraso, T. E. Stephenson, R. S. Wolford, R. M. Wadowsky, A. M. McNamara, and R. B. Yee.** 1985. Effects of metals on *Legionella pneumophila* growth in drinking water plumbing systems. *Appl. Environ. Microbiol.* **50:**1149–1154.
6. **Wadowsky, R. M., R. Wolford, A. M. McNamara, and R. B. Yee.** 1985. Effect of temperature, pH, and oxygen level on the multiplication of naturally occurring *Legionella pneumophila* on potable water. *Appl. Environ. Microbiol.* **49:**1197–1205.
7. **Wadowsky, R. M., and R. B. Yee.** 1985. Effect of non-*Legionellaceae* bacteria on the multiplication of *Legionella pneumophila* in potable water. *Appl. Environ. Microbiol.* **49:**1206–1210.

Effects of Water Chemistry and Temperature on the Survival and Growth of *Legionella pneumophila* in Potable Water Systems

JULIE ROGERS, P. J. DENNIS, J. V. LEE, AND C. W. KEEVIL

Pathology Division, Public Health Laboratory Service Centre for Applied Microbiology and Research, Porton Down, Salisbury, Wiltshire SP4 0JG, and Thames Water Utilities, Spencer House Laboratory, Manor Farm, Reading, Berkshire RG2 0JN, United Kingdom

Within low-nutrient environments, *Legionella pneumophila* grows in association with the other organisms that colonize the adjacent surfaces, including flavobacteria (10), cyanobacteria (8), and amoebae (7). The bacteria are able to gain sufficient nutrients by forming a consortium and developing biofilm. The material on which the microorganisms grow, including metal corrosion products (3), may become incorporated into the biofilm. The biofilm may not only serve to allow the growth of bacteria in water systems but may also protect from biocide treatment (2). The objectives of this work were to study the ecology of *L. pneumophila* under conditions that realistically simulated the aquatic environment.

CHEMOSTAT MODEL

A two-stage chemostat model was developed from that previously used (11), using filter-sterilized tap water as the sole growth medium for a mixed population of bacteria, fungi, and protozoa. The inoculum was derived from a calorifier responsible for an outbreak of Legionnaires disease and contained virulent *L. pneumophila*. The water from the calorifier was concentrated by filtration, resuspended, and inoculated into the chemostat. The inoculum contained *Pseudomonas, Alcaligenes, Acinetobacter, Chromobacterium, Aeromonas, Flavobacterium, Methylobacter, Vibrio,* and *Actinomyces* spp. Two vessels were linked in series to simulate the conditions found in a water system. The first vessel, representing, for example, a storage tank, had a dilution rate of $0.05 \, h^{-1}$ and supplied a constant inoculum into the second vessel at a dilution rate of $0.2 \, h^{-1}$. This modeled the distribution system and was used to generate biofilms. Conditions within the chemostats were maintained at 30°C, 20% dissolved oxygen tension, and a fluid velocity of 1 to 2 m/s by using Anglicon microprocessor control units (Process Systems, Newhaven, United Kingdom). Careful selection of only glass, titanium, and silicone materials for the chemostat construction prevented chemical modification of the water chemistry. Biofilm was developed on the surface of 1-cm^2 coupons of sterile materials suspended into the culture. Tiles supporting biofilms were periodically removed from the chemostat and washed in 10 ml of sterile water. Biofilm was removed from the materials with a dental probe and resuspended into 1 ml of sterile water. Vortexing was used to disperse biofilm before serial dilution of the sample. Nonlegionella populations were enumerated in low-nutrient R2A medium (6) to avoid substate shock to oligotrophic species. Buffered charcoal-yeast extract agar (5) and buffered charcoal-yeast extract medium supplemented with glycine, vancomycin, polymyxin, and cycloheximide (1) were used to determine the numbers of *L. pneumophila*. Plates were incubated at 30°C for 7 days prior to counting. The bacteria isolated from the biofilm and planktonic phases were identified by using the Biolog gram-negative identification system and data base (Biolog, Hayward, Calif.). *L. pneumophila* isolates were identified by using an additional data base for legionellae (4).

INFLUENCE OF WATER CHEMISTRY ON GROWTH OF *L. PNEUMOPHILA*

The experimental model was used to culture the inocula described above with different tap waters. A softened river-derived water from a lowland catchment area, a medium-hard river-derived water, and a hard borehole water were compared for the ability to support the growth of *L. pneumophila*. In the case of the medium-hard river-derived water, it was necessary to reduce the dilution rates in order to maintain the *L. pneumophila* in the chemostat culture. The dilution rates were reduced to $0.04 \, h^{-1}$ in the first vessel and $0.16 \, h^{-1}$ in the second vessel. The flora in the planktonic phase of the chemostat was compared for the three waters over a 6-month period; mean values are presented in Table 1. The lower dilution rate in the medium-hard river water resulted in highest num-

TABLE 1. Comparison of growth of flora within chemostat culture, using three different waters for growth media at 30°C

Sample	Organisms/ml	
	Nonlegionella	Legionellae
Softened river water	5×10^5	1×10^3
Medium-hard river water	2×10^6	7×10^2
Hard borehole water	4×10^5	2×10^3

bers of nonlegionellae; however the numbers of *L. pneumophila* were a lower proportion of the consortia in this water. The data suggest that the water chemistry modifies the growth of the microbial consortium and consequently modifies the proportion of *L. pneumophila* in the culture.

INFLUENCE OF TEMPERATURE ON BIOFILM DEVELOPMENT

Biofilm that develops within a plumbing system is greatly influenced by the materials present within the system. Copper has been shown to inhibit colonization and support less biofilm development than do plastics or elastomeric materials at 30°C in softened water (11). Of public health concern, several plastics were found to support high biofilm flora, and up to 10% of the biofilm consisted of legionellae (6a). Since polybutylene is a widely used plumbing material, a range of temperatures affecting colonization was investigated. The results of our temperature studies are shown in Fig. 1.

Growth at 20°C. When polybutylene was incorporated into the chemostat at 20°C, there was rapid biofilm development, with 5.30×10^5 CFU of total biofilm flora cm^{-2} after only 24 h. The total numbers in the biofilm gradually increased to a maximum of 9.50×10^5 CFU cm^{-2} at 14 days. The *L. pneumophila* organisms in the biofilm reached a maximum of 2,200 CFU cm^{-2} at 4 days, when they accounted for 0.3% of the total biofilm flora. The microbial flora of the biofilm at 20°C contained a diverse range of amoebae and protozoa, including predatory *Lacrymaria* spp. and *Hartmannella vermiformis,* an amoeba capable of supporting growth of *L. pneumophila* (9). The bacterial species present in the chemostat were also diverse and were predominated by *Pseudomonas paucimobilis* throughout biofilm development. Other pseudomonads, including *P. fluorescens* and *P. vesicularis,* were present in lower proportions. *Klebsiella, Aeromonas, Flavobacterium,* and *Actinomyces* spp. occurred in much lower proportions than the pseudomonads within the biofilms.

Growth at 40°C. At 40°C in hard borehole water, the plastics were rapidly colonized by the aquatic microflora after 24 h, with a total flora of 1.55×10^6 CFU^{-2}. The maximum total flora (3.25×10^6 CFU cm^{-2}) occurred after 14 days. There was 600 CFU of *L. pneumophila* cm^{-2} after only 24 h. As the total flora consolidated into biofilm, the numbers of *L. pneumophila* rapidly increased to 3.78×10^5 CFU cm^{-2}, accounting for 48% of the total biofilm flora. The polybutylene was initially colonized by pseudomonads, particularly *P. mendocina* and *P. testosteroni.* As the biofilm developed, the flora became increasingly diverse and other gram-nega-

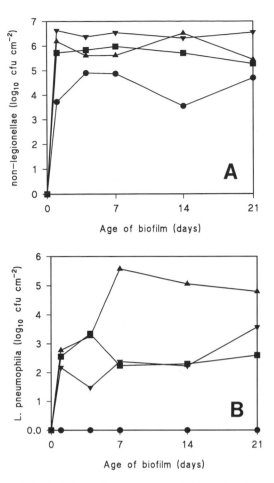

FIG. 1. Effects of temperature on biofilm development (A) and *L. pneumophila* colonization (B) on polybutylene at 20°C (■), 40°C (▲), 50°C (▼), and 60°C (●).

tive organisms, including *Acinetobacter* and *Klebsiella* spp., became more abundant. No amoebae or other protozoa were detected at 40°C, yet the numbers of legionellae remained high, suggesting that the biofilm consortium was amplifying the numbers of this pathogen.

Growth at 50°C. Biofouling was not reduced at 50°C, with a biofilm containing 4.64×10^6 CFU cm^{-2} developing after only 24 h; however, the diversity of flora within developing biofilm was greatly reduced. The biofilm was composed principally of a single species *P. hydrogenothermophila.* The numbers of *L. pneumophila* were reduced at 50°C to a maximum of 3,750 CFU cm^{-2} in the 21-day biofilm. *L. pneumophila* organisms do not appear to grow in the chemostat at this temperature; their increase in the biofilm was probably due to a gradual colonization over time from the inflowing culture of the first vessel. Viability appeared to be maintained within the biofilm over extended time periods suggesting that the biofilm in some way protected them from the high temperatures. These data indicate that water systems maintained at 50°C may contain a reservoir of viable *L. pneumophila* within biofilms.

Growth at 60°C. Biofilm was reduced at 60°C, with a maximum flora of 7.95×10^4 CFU cm^{-2} after 4 days. The biofilm was still able to form at this high temperature but contained the low diversity of organisms that was evident at 50°C. Legionellae were completely undetectable in biofilms developed at 60°C despite being constantly introduced from the first culture vessel. This result indicates that water systems that are maintained at 60°C remain free of *L. pneumophila* indefinitely (as recommended by the U.K. Department of Health Code of Practise).

REFERENCES

1. **Dennis, P. J., C. L. R. Bartlett, and A. E. Wright.** 1984. Comparison of isolation methods for *Legionellae* spp., p. 294–296. *In* C. Thornsberry, A. Balows, J. C. Feeley, and W. Jakubowski (ed.), *Legionella: Proceedings of the 2nd International Symposium.* American Society for Microbiology, Washington, D.C.
2. **Keevil, C. W., C. W. Mackerness, and J. S. Colbourne.** 1990. Biocide treatment of biofilms. *Intr. Biodeterior.* **26:**169–179.
3. **Keevil, C. W., A. J. West, J. T. Walker, P. J. Dennis, and J. S. Colbourne.** 1989. Biofilms: detection, implications and solutions, p. 367–374. *In* D. Wheeler, M. L. Richardson, and J. Bridges (ed.), *Watershed 89. The Fu-*ture *for Water Quality in Europe,* vol. 2. Pergamon Press, Oxford.
4. **Mauchline, W. S., and C. W. Keevil.** 1991. Development of the Biolog substrate utilization system for the identification of *Legionella* spp. *Appl. Environ. Microbiol.* **57:**3345–3349.
5. **Pasculle, A. W., J. C. Feeley, R. J. Gisbson, L. G. Cordes, P. L. Myerowitz, C. M. Patton, G. W. Gorman, C. L. Carmack, J. W. Ezzell, and J. N. Dowling.** 1980. Pittsburgh pneumonia agent: direct isolation from human lung tissue. *J. Infect. Dis.* **141:**727–732.
6. **Reasoner, D. J., and E. E. Geldrich.** 1985. A new medium for the enumeration and subculture of bacteria from potable water. *Appl. Environ. Microbiol.* **49:**1–7.
6a. **Rogers, J., A. B. Dowsett, J. V. Lee, and C. W. Keevil.** 1990. P. 458–460. *In* H. W. Rossmoore (ed.), *Biodeterioration and Biodegradation 8.* Elsevier, London.
7. **Rowbotham, T. J.** 1980. Preliminary report on the pathogenicity of *Legionella pneumophila* for freshwater and soil amoebae. *J. Clin. Pathog.* **33:**1179–1183.
8. **Tison, D. L., D. H. Pope, W. B. Cherry, and C. B. Fliermans.** 1980. Growth of *Legionella pneumophila* in association with blue-green algae (cyanobacteria). *Appl. Environ. Microbiol.* **39:**456–459.
9. **Wadowsky, R. B., L. J. Butler, M. K. Cook, S. M. Verma, M. A. Paul, B. S. Fields, G. Keleti, J. L. Sykora, and R. B. Yee.** 1988. Growth-supporting activity for *Legionella pneumophila* in tap water cultures and implication of hartmannellid amoebae as growth factors. *Appl. Environ. Microbiol.* **54:**2677–2682.
10. **Wadowsky, R. M., and R. B. Yee.** 1983. Satellite growth of *Legionella pneumophila* with an environmental isolate of *Flavobacterium breve. Appl. Environ. Microbiol.* **46:**1447–1449.
11. **West, A. A., R. Araujo, P. J. Dennis, J. V. Lee, and C. W. Keevil.** 1989. Chemostat models of *Legionella pneumophila*, p. 107–116. *In* B. Flannigan (ed.), *Airborne Deteriogens and Pathogens.* Biodeterioration Society, Kew, Surrey, England.

Microbiocides and the Control of *Legionella*

R. ELSMORE

Coalite Chemicals, P.O. Box 152, Buttermilk Lane, Bolsover, Chesterfield, Derbyshire S44 6AZ, United Kingdom

Microbiocides are chemical agents used to kill or inactivate microorganisms. They are used in a wide range of applications as preservatives, sanitizers, disinfectants, and sterilizers. In industrial applications, biocides are used to control microbial growth in such areas as petroleum products, constructional materials, textiles, and foodstuffs.

This report addresses one application, water treatment. In water treatment, biocides are used primarily to minimize biofouling. If not controlled, biofouling and microbial growth can lead to reduced efficiency and heat transfer, increased pumping costs, microbially induced corrosion, and the degradation of corrosion inhibitors and descalants. Severe microbial growth can even produce structural damage. In addition to these operational and economic considerations, the use of biocides to control potentially pathogenic microorganisms such as *Legionella* species has been highlighted in recent years.

Many of the industrial biocides used in recir-culating water systems have been tested for activity against *Legionella pneumophila* in laboratory studies. These biocides include chlorine (11, 17–19), isothiazolinones (2, 15, 17–19), quaternary ammonium compounds (2, 8, 18, 19), dibromonitrilopropionamide (2, 10, 18, 19), dichlorophen (2, 11), thiocarbamates (10, 18, 19), sodium pentachlorophenate (19), methylene-bis-thiocyanate (8), 2(thiocyanomethyl thio)benzthiazole (2), N-alkyl-1,3-propanediamine (8), 2-bromo-2-nitropropane-1,3-diol (1, 2, 17), bromochlorodimethylhydantoin (14), and several others.

No standard method has existed for the evaluation of biocides against legionellae. The report of the Expert Advisory Committee on Biocides (23) recommended that "[t]he preparation of a standard procedure should be expedited for the assessment of the efficacy of biocides against legionellae." The British Association for Chemical Specialities has been involved in the development of a standard method for assaying biocide activity in the laboratory.

DEVELOPMENT OF A STANDARD TEST METHOD

Any standard test protocol represents a compromise between a wide range of factors that will affect the performance of a chemical in a real-life situation. With respect to legionellae, this issue is further complicated by the wide variation in engineering design of the systems being treated.

Much research effort is currently being devoted to understanding the role of biofilms and the influence of other organisms on the ecology of legionellae in industrial systems. The role of free-living amoebae on the survival of legionellae and the effect of amoebae on the susceptibility of the bacteria to biocide treatment may also be important. It was felt that the current level of understanding of many of these questions is far from complete. In attempting to devise a biocide test protocol, the British Association for Chemical Specialities task force has adopted a simple time-kill bottle test, as this represents the current state of the art in terms of reproducible technology that is widely available to industrial and commercial laboratories.

The proposed test method is outlined in Table 1. Some of the parameters chosen deserve further discussion.

pH. A pH of 8.0 $\pm$ 0.2 was felt to be in accordance with the general trend of operating cooling towers at alkaline pH values.

Test medium. Water of standard hardness supplemented with iron and organic soiling represented the best approach to a typical cooling water that was possible. The range of nonbiocide water treatment chemicals that are used in cooling systems (corrosion and scale inhibitors, biodispersants, etc.) is so large and varied that it is impractical to include representatives in the test medium.

Contact time. In industrial water systems, the residence time or half-life of the water can vary tremendously from as little as a few hours to as long as several days. At the same time, it must be appreciated that water treatment biocides can be divided into two main groups (oxidizing and nonoxidizing) that have some major differences in the speed of kill. In trying to develop a test protocol, there is inevitably a compromise between a wide range of practical situations. Therefore, it was felt appropriate to introduce different contact times for

TABLE 1. Proposed test method

Component	Specification
Type of test	Bactericidal suspension test
Test medium	World Health Organization standard hard water containing $CaCl_2$ and $MgSO_4$ to a total hardness of 342 ppm. This medium was supplemented by the addition of 3 ppm of iron as ferric sulfate.
Test organism	*L. pneumophila* serogroup 1 type strain (NCTC 11192)
Test vol	10 ml in 1-oz (ca. 30-ml) glass universals
Contact temp	30 $\pm$ 1°C
pH	8.0 $\pm$ 0.2, achieved by the addition of a boric acid-borax buffer to the test medium
Organic soiling	5 ppm of yeast extract and 5 ppm of pulverized yeast cells
Contact time	Oxidizing biocides, 1 h; nonoxidizing biocides, 24 h, (additional contact times may be relevant to a particular system's operating conditions)
Inoculum level	The inoculum was adjusted to give an initial concentration of organisms in the contact bottle of 10^7 CFU/ml (range, 5×10^6–5×10^7 CFU/ml).
Inactivator	A broad-spectrum inactivating solution was developed based on the European suspension test inactivator.
Pass criteria	For a biocide concentration to have a satisfactory activity against *L. pneumophila* within the context of this test, a 4-log reduction in recoverable organisms is required after the appropriate contact time.
Expression of results	Results of biocide evaluations according to this test protocol were expressed either as "pass" or "fail." No intermediate grading is appropriate.

these fundamentally different classes of biocide.

Extrapolation from laboratory results. Extrapolation from laboratory studies to applications may not be realistic, given such factors as possible interaction with other water treatment chemicals and inactivation by slimes. This problem has been indicated by several workers who have shown that compounds deemed to be effective in the laboratory were less than effective in use (5, 16).

To date, few extensive field studies on the activity of biocides against *L. pneumophila* in recirculating water applications have been published (6, 7, 9, 12, 13, 22).

Factors affecting biocide activity. Several factors can affect biocidal activity; these include pH, temperature, concentration, and the presence of organic matter (e.g., slimes). The relationship between activity and stability can be an important factor in determining the suitability of a biocide for water treatment. For example, some biocides may be less stable under the alkaline conditions that most cooling systems use. However, legionellae may become more stressed as the pH rises above the optimum for growth (pH 6.9) and are more susceptible to certain biocides that are used (3).

Additional factors of importance are possible interactions between biocides and other water treatment chemicals, e.g., descalants and corrosion inhibitors. Obviously, any biocide should be tested for compatibility with a range of water treatment additives. Other parameters affecting the performance of biocides include the residence time in the system, which is affected by both bleed and drift.

Resistance development is another area that has received little attention. The Expert Advisory Committee on Biocides (23) advises investigation of the possibility that organisms can develop resistance to biocides. It is well known that under conditions of continuous use, microorganisms can become resistant to certain biocides. Consequently, it is common practice in many countries to alternate biocides on a regular basis to minimize the possibility of resistance development.

CONCLUSION

Many biocides have been shown to be active against legionellae in the laboratory. With the development of standard test methods, more unified results will be obtainable for the assessment of biocide activity. Care should be taken in extrapolating from laboratory to in-use applications, however, since there may be interactions with water treatment chemicals and biofilms. Further testing should therefore be carried out to determine whether these factors will affect the activity of the compounds in the field. In addition, experience with use of a biocide is important. For example, sodium dichlorophen (Panacide) has been used for

many years in water treatment and found effective in controlling both legionellae and biofouling.

It has also been shown that legionellae are more likely to be isolated from systems with high microbial counts (4), possibly because of the interaction of legionellae and other microorganisms. Therefore, it would be prudent to maintain microbial counts as low as possible by treatment with biocides that are active against a wide range of common water microorganisms (including algae and protozoa).

REFERENCES

1. **Coughlin, M., and G. Caplan.** 1987. Microbiocidal efficacy of BNPD against *Legionella pneumophila.* Technical Paper TP 87-18. Cooling Tower Institute Annual Meeting, New Orleans, La.
2. **Elsmore, R.** 1986. Biocidal control of legionellae. *Isr. J. Med. Sci.* **22:**647–654.
3. **Elsmore, R.** 1989. The activity of BNPD against *Legionella pneumophila* serogroup 1: the influence of pH, inoculum level and test media. *Int. Biodeterior.* **25:**107–113.
4. **Elsmore, R., R. J. Corbett, and E. J. Channon.** 1989. Relationship between the common water flora and isolation of *Legionella* species from water systems, p. 83–96. *In* B. Flannigan (ed.), *Airborne Deteriogens and Pathogens.* Biodeterioration Society, Kew, England.
5. **England, A. C., D. W. Fraser, G. F. Mallison, D. C. Mackel, P. Skaliy, and G. W. Gorman.** 1982. Failure of *Legionella pneumophila* sensitivities to predict culture results from disinfectant-treated air conditioning cooling towers. *Appl. Environ. Microbiol.* **43:**240–244.
6. **Fliermans, C. B., G. E. Bettinger, and A. W. Fynsk.** 1982. Treatment of cooling systems containing high levels of *Legionella pneumophila. Water Res.* **16:**903–909.
7. **Fliermans, C. B., and R. S. Harvey.** 1984. Effectiveness of 1-bromo-3-chloro-5, 5-dimethylhydantoin against *Legionella pneumophila* in a cooling tower. *Appl. Environ. Microbiol.* **47:**1307–1310.
8. **Grace, R. D., N. E. Dewar, W. G. Barnes, and G. R. Hodges.** 1981. Susceptibility of *Legionella pneumophila* to three cooling tower microbiocides. *Appl. Environ. Microbiol.* **41:**233–236.
9. **Grow, K. M., D. O. Wood, J. H. Cogging, and E. D. Leinbach.** 1984. Environmental factors influencing growth of *Legionella pneumophila* in operating biocide treated cooling towers, p. 316–318. *In* C. Thornsberry, A. Balows, J. C. Feeley, and W. Jakubowski (ed.), *Legionella: Proceedings of the 2nd International Symposium.* American Society for Microbiology, Washington, D.C.
10. **Hollis, C. G., and D. L. Smalley.** 1980. Resistance of *Legionella pneumophila* to microbiocides. *Dev. Ind. Microbiol.* **21:**265–271.
11. **Kobayashi, H., and M. Tsuzuki.** 1984. Susceptibility of *Legionella pneumophila* to cooling tower microbiocides and hospital disinfectants, p. 342–343. *In* C. Thornsberry, A. Balows, J. C. Feeley, and W. Jakubowski (ed.), *Legionella: Proceedings of the 2nd International Symposium.* American Society for Microbiology, Washington, D.C.
12. **Kurtz, J. B., C. Bartlett, H. Tillet, and U. Newton.** 1984. Field trial of biocides in control of *Legionella pneumophila* in cooling water systems, p. 340–342. *In* C. Thornsberry, A. Balows, J. C. Feeley, and W. Jakubowski (ed.), *Legionella: Proceedings of the 2nd International Symposium.* American Society for Microbiology, Washington, D.C.
13. **Kurtz, J. B., C. L. R. Bartlett, U. A. Newton, R. A. White, and N. Jones.** 1982. *Legionella pneumophila* in cooling water systems. *J. Hyg.* **88:**369–381.

14. **McCoy, W. F., and J. W. Wireman.** 1989. Efficacy of bromochlorodimethylhydantoin against *Legionella pneumophila* in industrial cooling water. *J. Ind. Microbiol.* **4:**403–408.

15. **McCoy, W. F., J. W. Wireman, and E. S. Laskens.** 1986. Efficacy of methyl chloro/methyl isothiazolone biocide against *Legionella pneumophila* in cooling tower water. *J. Ind. Microbiol.* **1:**49–56.

16. **Orrison, L. H., W. B. Cherry, and D. Milan.** 1981. Isolation of *Legionella pneumophila* from cooling tower water by filtration. *Appl. Environ. Microbiol.* **41:**1202–1205.

17. **Sawatari, K., K. Watanabe, H. Nakasato, H. Koga, N. Ito, K. Fujila, Y. Shigeno, Y. Suzuyama, K. Yumaguchi, A. Saito, and K. Hara.** 1984. Bactericidal effects of disinfectant against *Legionella pneumophila* and *Legionella bozemanii.* *Kansenshogaku Zasshi* **58:**130–136.

18. **Skaliy, P., T. A. Thompson, G. W. Gorman, G. K. Morris, H. V. McEachern, and D. C. Machel.** 1980. Laboratory studies of disinfectants against *Legionella pneumophila.* *Appl. Environ. Microbiol.* **40:**697–700.

19. **Soracco, R. J., H. K. Gill, C. B. Fliermans, and D. H. Pope.** 1983. Susceptibilities of algae and *Legionella pneumophila* to cooling tower biocides. *Appl. Environ. Microbiol.* **45:**1254–1260.

20. **Tobin, J. O., R. A. Swann, and C. L. R. Bartlett.** 1981. Isolation of *Legionella pneumophila* from water systems: methods and preliminary results. *Br. Med. J.* **282:**515–517.

21. **Watkins, I. D., J. O. Tobin, P. J. Dennis, W. Brown, R. Newnham, and J. B. Kurtz.** 1985. *Legionella pneumophila* serogrouping by monoclonal antibodies: an epidemiological tool. *J. Hyg.* **95:**211–216.

22. **Witherell, L. E., L. F. Novick, K. M. Stone, R. W. Duncan, L. A. Orciari, D. A. Jillson, R. B. Myers, and R. L. Vogt.** 1984. *Legionella pneumophila* in Vermont cooling towers, p. 315–316. *In* C. Thornsberry, A. Balows, J. C. Feeley, and W. Jakubowski (ed.), *Legionella: Proceedings of the 2nd International Symposium.* American Society for Microbiology, Washington, D.C.

23. **Wright, A. E.** 1989. *Report of the Expert Advisory Committee on Biocides.* H. M. Stationery Office, London.

Control of Nosocomial Legionellosis Based on Water System Disinfection by Heat and UV Light: a Four-Year Evaluation

MARC J. STRUELENS, FRANCIS ROST, NICOLE MAES, ANN MAAS, AND ELISABETH SERRUYS

Infection Control and Hospital Epidemiology Unit and Microbiology Laboratory Hôpital Erasme, University of Brussels, Brussels 1070, Belgium

Nosocomial legionellosis is most often acquired through exposure to contaminated domestic water, either by inhalation of aerosol or by aspiration following ingestion. Control measures, therefore, have attempted to reduce the level of *Legionella* contamination of hospital water systems or to prevent exposure of susceptible patients to water sources (1). Various chemical and physical methods have been investigated for *Legionella* decontamination of hospital water distribution systems. These include intermittent and continuous hyperchlorination, ozonization, metal ionization, heat treatment, and UV irradiation (1). In addition, good engineering practices should ensure that the system design and maintenance procedures prevent stagnation, corrosion, scale deposition, and the use of materials and water temperatures favoring the multiplication of legionellae (1). However, each hospital presents specific problems that require local evaluation of any of these measures or combination thereof. Each method has specific advantages and disadvantages in terms of efficacy, simplicity, cost of installation and maintenance, and untoward effects on the integrity of the plumbing and the safety of patients and hospital personnel. The long-term efficacy has been documented for some of these methods in a few hospitals, but the optimal modality is not yet established (1). An additional problem concerns the methods and interpretation of microbiological surveillance of

the water system to monitor the reduction of legionellae following the implementation of disinfection measures.

In Erasme Hospital, a 900-bed university hospital, surveillance of nosocomial legionellosis has been conducted since 1983. During the period from 1983 through 1991, 187,280 patients were admitted, 883 of whom received a solid organ (kidney, pancreas, liver, heart, or lung) transplant. At first outbreak of *Legionella pneumophila* serogroup 1 involved 12 kidney transplant recipients in 1983. This outbreak was controlled by administration of erythromycin prophylaxis to kidney recipients treated for graft rejection and to other immunosuppressed patients while reduction in *L. pneumophila* serogroup 1 in the water system was being attempted through use of departmentwide heat treatment (3). A second outbreak affected 32 patients in the period 1985 to 1987. The epidemiologic investigation indicated that the water system was the likely source of infection (2). Domestic water was heated at that time to 45°C by instantaneous heat exchange, and the reservoir for amplification of *Legionella* was found in corroded deadlegs in the central piping system and not in water tanks (2).

To control this outbreak, we introduced sequentially a series of technical modifications and physical disinfection procedures of the water system. This report evaluates the efficacy and safety of these measures after a follow-up of 4 years, based

TABLE 1. Incidence of nosocomial Legionnaires' disease in transplant recipients and other patients admitted to Erasme Hospital, 1983 through 1991

Period[a]	Comment	No. of cases of Legionnaires disease/no. of admissions (incidence/10,000)			Relative risk (95% CI), Transplant versus other patients
		Transplant recipients	Other patients	All admissions	
1983–85	Baseline	4/153 (261)	3/38,644 (0.8)	7/38,797 (1.8)	336 (76–1,500)
1985–87	Outbreak	17/202 (841)	15/44,133 (3.4)	32/44,335 (7.2)	248 (125–489)
1987–91	Water disinfection	5/528 (95)	4/103,620 (0.4)	9/104,148 (0.9)	245 (66–911)

[a]Time period is October through September.

on continuous water monitoring and disease surveillance using standard microbiological methods and case-definition during the 8-year study period.

In October 1987, modifications of the hot water system included removal of all faucet aerators, replacement of corroded pipes, and elimination of deadlegs. The flow rate was increased, and the temperature was raised to 50 to 55°C at the outlets. Pasteurization of the system was conducted by raising the water temperature to 65 to 85°C and by flushing all outlets for 30 min on 3 consecutive days. These procedures were repeated five times during the follow-up period, whenever the extent of *Legionella* colonization reached 30% of 62 surveillance sites. No scalding injury occurred. In January 1989, a 5-μm-pore-size filtration unit and a 500-W UV light treatment system were centrally installed to irradiate recirculating water at 45°C. In April 1990, corrosion control was implemented by continuous infusion of zinc orthophosphate (Permoset DP-4; Permo, Rueil-Malmaison, France). Overall, the incidence of major leaks decreased during the control period compared with previous years.

Active surveillance of nosocomial legionellosis was achieved through *Legionella* culture of respiratory specimens (mean, 52 specimens per month) and serologic testing (mean, 110 serum samples per month) in hospitalized patients with pneumonia. Nine cases were detected during the 4-year control period. Of these, seven (four infections with the epidemic subtype of *L. pneumophila* serogroup 1, two infections with *L. pneumophila* serogroup 6, and one infection with *L. longbeachae* serogroup 1) were documented by culture. The latter two organisms were not recovered from the hospital environment. Table 1 shows the incidence of nosocomial legionellosis according to the study period in transplant recipients and other patients. A similar risk reduction was noted for

both patient categories during the control versus epidemic period; 88% risk reduction (95% confidence interval [CI], 75 to 94%). There was a 94% risk reduction for documented infection with the epidemic strain (95% CI, 82 to 98%) (2).

Semiquantitative *Legionella* cultures of swabs performed on 62 pipework sites at monthly to bimonthly intervals allowed monitoring of the central hot water system and outlets in the intensive-care and transplant units. However, there was no systematic relationship either between the proportion of contaminated sites in the hospital and in individual units or between the density of growth and the occurrence of nosocomial legionellosis. For this reason, we are now adding quantitative monitoring of *Legionella* density in water samples from selected sites to determine the maximal level of contamination not associated with disease.

In summary, our experience illustrates the efficacy and safety of relatively low cost physical disinfection procedures for control of legionellosis, although the aim of nosocomial disease eradication will require the study of additional measures.

REFERENCES

1. **Muraca, P. W., V. L. Yu, and A. Goetz.** 1990. Disinfection of water distribution systems for legionella: a review of application procedures and methodologies. *Infect. Control Hosp. Epidemiol.* **11:**79–88.
2. **Struelens, M. J., N. Maes, F. Rost, A. Deplano, F. Jacobs, C. Liesnard, N. Bornstein, F. Grimont, S. Lauwers, M. P. MC. Intyre, and E. Serruys.** 1992. Genotypic vs phenotypic methods for the investigation of nosocomial *Legionella pneumophila* outbreak and efficacy of control measures. *J. Infect. Dis.* **166:**22–30.
3. **Vereerstraeten, P., J. C. Stolear, E. Schoutens-Serruys, N. Maes, J. P. Thys, C. Liesnard, F. Rost, P. Kinnaert, and C. Toussaint.** 1986. Erythromycin prophylaxis for Legionnaires' disease in immunosuppressed patients in contaminated hospital environment. *Transplantation* **41:**52–54.

Efficacy of UV Radiation for Eradicating
Legionella pneumophila from a Shower

T. MAKIN AND C. A. HART

Department of Medical Microbiology, University of Liverpool, P.O. Box 147, Liverpool L69 3BX, United Kingdom

This study was initiated after sporadic nosocomial cases of Legionnaires disease were diagnosed in patients on the renal transplant unit and leukemic unit in the Royal Liverpool University Hospital. In all cases for which epidemiological and environmental data were available, the potable water system was implicated as the likely source of infection.

A number of methods for controlling the growth of legionellae in potable water have been described. Continuous chlorination has been widely used but has not always proven effective (2, 16), and it has been contraindicated in some guidelines because of its corrosive action on metals and the potential for producing carcinogenic chlorinated organic compounds (6). Furthermore, chlorine added to mains cold water dissipates rapidly upon heating in a calorifier (3).

Raising the temperature of a hot water system to over 60°C at calorifiers and to over 50°C at outlets has been recommended for controlling legionellae and may be more effective when combined with regular flushing (11). However, the use of hot water introduces the risk of scalding and may fail to eradicate legionellae from some parts of a hot water system, notably deadlegs off the circulating hot water supply and the section of a shower between the mixer valve and the sprinkler. This area is shielded from contact with hot water by the action of the mixer valve and, in many showers, a thermal cutoff valve.

In previous studies, we have shown that a number of secondary control methods, including use of automatic drain valves, hyperchlorination of mixer valves and shower heads, use of trace heating elements, and regular flushing of showers, varied in the ability to control legionellae in shower water but at best only reduced the numbers normally present (9, 10).

We have reported a nosocomial case of Legionnaires disease in a kidney transplant recipient infected with *Legionella pneumophila* serogroup 12, even though this serogroup was isolated only rarely from the renal transplant unit and only in small numbers (12). Further control methods that may completely eradicate legionellae in potable water systems were therefore considered.

UV radiation at 254 nm is an effective bactericidal agent, and *L. pneumophila* is particularly susceptible with a 90% lethal dose of 2.04 mW-s/cm². Farr et al. (7) showed that UV irradiation was effective in controlling legionellae in the water system of a renal transplant unit, and Muraca et al. (13) reported that UV irradiation eradicated *L. pneumophila* from a model plumbing system.

In this study to assess the efficacy of UV radiation for eradicating microorganisms, including legionellae, from a shower, we used two adjacent showers on the same hot and cold water supply. The showers were known to be heavily colonized with *L. pneumophila*, amoebae, and non-*Legionella* bacteria, particularly in the mixer valve and in the deadlegs between the circulating hot water supply and the mixer valve.

Both showers were sampled weekly, and shower water was cultured for legionellae, amoebae, and non-*Legionella* bacteria. Legionellae were isolated on buffered charcoal-yeast extract agar with selective supplements and incubated for 10 days at 37°C. Amoebae were cultured on nonnutrient agar surface inoculated with approximately 10⁵ CFU of UV-killed *Escherichia coli* and *Klebsiella aerogenes* per ml. Plates were incubated for 5 days at 22, 30, and 37°C in a moist atmosphere and scanned for amoebic cysts and motile trophozoites by light microscopy using a low-power objective. Non-*Legionella* bacteria were isolated on 10% horse blood agar incubated at 30°C for 3 days. After each sampling, the showers were run for 5 min.

Six weeks into the study, both showers were dismantled after it had been established that they were both heavily colonized. The deadlegs and mixer valve components were sampled, and the pipework and most of the mixer valve components were autoclaved at 121°C and 15 psi for 15 min. Heat-sensitive parts of the mixer valve were disinfected by immersion in 50 mg of sodium hypochlorite per liter for 1 h.

The showers were reassembled with 10-μm-pore-size filters installed on the hot and cold water supply feeding both showers (Fig. 1) in order to remove large particulate material that could allow microorganisms to be shielded from the effects of UV irradiation. UV units were fitted to the hot and cold water supply feeding one shower only; the units contained a low-pressure mercury lamp that produced UV radiation at 254 nm and delivered a UV dose of 30 mW-s/cm² to water passing through the shower at maximum flow rate.

In the nonirradiated shower (Fig. 2) non-*Legionella* bacteria were detected in shower water 5 days after the showers were reassembled. *Pseudomonas stutzeri* appeared first, followed by a micrococcus at 4 weeks and a *Flavobacterium* sp. at 8 weeks. One week later, small numbers of *L.*

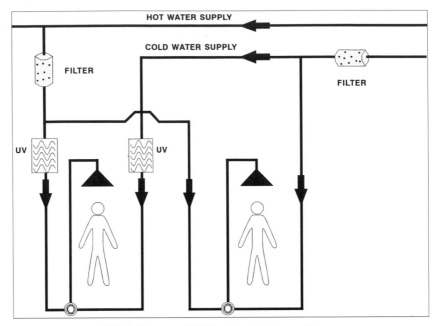

FIG. 1. Diagram of UV-irradiated and control showers.

pneumophila were detected simultaneously with free-living amoebae. Thereafter, *L. pneumophila* was present throughout the study and amoebae were isolated intermittently.

In the irradiated shower (Fig. 3), the same non-*Legionella* bacteria were detected in shower water within 3 weeks after the UV units were in-

stalled. It is not known whether these bacteria evaded or survived UV irradiation or whether they appeared as a result of incomplete disinfection during hyperchlorination.

No legionellae or amoebae were detected in shower water during the 8-month period for which the lamps were lit. Two weeks after the lamps

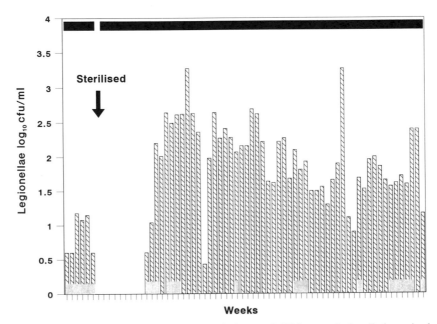

FIG. 2. Microorganisms isolated from a nonirradiated shower. Solid bar, nonlegionella bacteria; hatched bar, legionellae; shaded bar, amoebae.

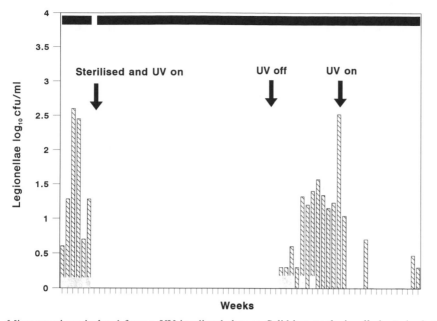

FIG. 3. Microorganisms isolated from a UV-irradiated shower. Solid bar, nonlegionella bacteria; hatched bar, legionellae; shaded bar, amoebae.

were turned off, *L. pneumophila* and amoebae were isolated simultaneously. Thereafter, amoebae were detected intermittently. *L. pneumophila* continued to be isolated until the UV lamp was relit, when the count declined significantly. If the mixer valve and deadlegs had become recolonized by *L. pneumophila* during the period when the lamp was off, the reduction in *L. pneumophila* detected in shower water after the lamp was relit may have been due to a residual disinfection activity of the water that had been UV irradiated.

UV radiation is normally considered a biocide lacking remnant activity; however, free radicals may be formed when water is UV irradiated, particularly at 185 nm, which is the other major wavelength produced by low-pressure mercury lamps (1). Although *L. pneumophila* possesses intracellular enzymes such as peroxidase and superoxide dismutase that may neutralize some free radicals, it has been reported that legionellae are susceptible to exogenous radicals, which are likely to be directed toward unprotected extracellular targets (8). However, some free radicals are relatively short lived, and it is not known whether, if formed, they would have survived for long enough to have an effect on the legionellae during this study.

Alternatively, long-term colonization of a site by legionellae may need periodic reseeding by fresh exogenous legionellae or by other microorganisms capable of promoting the growth of legionellae. UV irradiation in this study would have interfered with this process.

In conclusion, UV irradiation at 254 nm was effective in controlling *L. pneumophila* in shower water. UV prevented recolonization of the shower by *L. pneumophila* after it was initially eradicated by chlorination and autoclaving. Furthermore, UV irradiation was associated with a significant reduction in the number of *L. pneumophila* detected in shower water after *L. pneumophila* had been continuously isolated for a period of 12 weeks.

Amoebae were also not detected during the period when the UV lamp was first lit. Available data on the effects of UV on amoebae are limited, but cysts of *Acanthamoeba castellanii* have a 90% lethal dose with UV radiation of 40 mW-s/cm^2 (4), which exceeds the output of the lamp in our study. De Jonckheere (5) showed that UV-treated hydrotherapy pools contained high numbers of thermophilic *Naegleria,* although the specifications of his UV lamp were not disclosed. Failure to detect amoebae during the initial irradiation period in our study may therefore be largely attributable to the 10-μm-pore-size filter on the hot and cold water supplies. Free-living amoebae produce cysts from 4 to over 30 μm; however, the majority of amoebae produce cysts in excess of 10 μm in diameter (14). During the course of this study, the filters, particularly the filter on the hot water supply, became visibly discolored. Filtration of particulate material would reduce the effective pore size of the filters and further enhance retention of amoebic cysts. Trophozoites may pass through filters with pores of 2-μm diameter (18) but are likely to be more susceptible to UV irradiation, as trophozoites are consistently more sensitive than cysts to other forms of physical and chemical disinfection.

In both showers, *L. pneumophila* was initially detected concurrently with the isolation of amoebae. This observation supports the findings of Rowbotham (15) and others who have shown that amoebae may act as intermediary hosts to legionellae and can promote their multiplication. Furthermore, the ubiquity of legionellae in potable water systems appears to be matched by that of amoebae, which in a recent study were isolated from 84% of tank cold water supplies and 66% of the mains cold water supplies tested (17).

The appearance of *L. pneumophila* in the nonirradiated shower was preceded by a change in the non-*Legionella* bacteria present.

Others have demonstrated the growth-promoting activity of some non-*Legionella* bacteria on legionellae. In particular, Wadowsky and Yee reported satellite growth of *L. pneumophila* around colonies of *Flavobacterium breve* (19). The flavobacterium in this study was detected in the nonirradiated shower the week before *L. pneumophila* appeared. However, we were unable to demonstrate satellitism by *L. pneumophila* around colonies of the flavobacterium when the organism was grown on unsupplemented charcoal-yeast extract agar. The flavobacterium colonizing the showers in this study may therefore have acted primarily as a food source for amoebae.

One other noteworthy observation from the study was the failure of legionellae or amoebae to colonize the UV-irradiated shower by ingress through the shower head.

We conclude that UV irradiation can be an effective method of controlling *L. pneumophila* in showers, provided that the UV lamp and prefilters are appropriately sized and maintained and that the UV transmission value of the potable water remains high and stable. Furthermore, colonization of potable water systems by *L. pneumophila* in this study appeared to be facilitated by amoebae and non-*Legionella* bacteria.

REFERENCES

1. **Anghern, M.** 1984. Ultraviolet disinfection of water. *Aqua* **2**:109–115.
2. **Baird, I. M., W. Potts, J. Smiley, N. Click, S. Schleich, C. Connole, and K. Davison.** 1984. Control of endemic nosocomial legionellosis by hyperchlorination of potable water, p. 333. *In* C. Thornsberry, A. Balows, J. C. Feeley, and W. Jakubowski (ed.), *Legionella: Proceedings of the*

2nd International Symposium. American Society for Microbiology, Washington, D.C.
3. **Brundrett, G. W.** 1992. Guides on avoiding Legionnaires' disease, p. 346–373. *In* G. W. Brundrett (ed.), *Legionella and Building Services*. Butterworth-Heinemann Ltd., Oxford.
4. **Chang, J. C. H., S. F. Ossoff, D. C. Lobe, M. H. Dorfman, C. M. Dumais, R. G. Qualls, and J. D. Johnson.** 1985. UV inactivation of pathogenic and indicator microorganisms. *Appl. Environ. Microbiol.* **49**:1361–1365.
5. **De Jonckheere, J. F.** 1982. Hospital hydrotherapy pools treated with ultra violet light: bad bacteriological quality and presence of thermophilic *Naegleria. J. Hyg.* (Cambridge) **88**:205–214.
6. **Department of Health and Social Security.** 1988. The control of *Legionellae* in health care premises: a code of practice. Her Majesty's Stationery Office, London.
7. **Farr, B. M., J. C. Gratz, J. C. Tartaglino, S. I. Getchell-White, and D. H. M. Groschell.** 1988. Evaluation of ultra violet light for disinfection of hospital water contaminated with legionella. *Lancet* **ii**:669–672.
8. **Hoffman, P.** 1984. Bacterial physiology, p. 61–67. *In* C. Thornsberry, A. Balows, J. C. Feeley, and W. Jakubowski (ed.), *Legionella: Proceedings of the 2nd International Symposium.* American Society for Microbiology, Washington, D.C.
9. **Makin, T., and C. A. Hart.** 1990. The efficacy of control measures for eradicating legionellae in showers. *J. Hosp. Infect.* **16**:1–7.
10. **Makin, T., and C. A. Hart.** 1991. The effect of a self-regulating trace heating element on legionella within a shower. *J. Appl. Bacteriol.* **70**:258–264.
11. **Meenhorst, P. L., A. L. Reingold, D. G. Groothuis, G. W. Gorman, H. W. Wilkinson, R. M. McKinney, J. C. Feeley, D. J. Brenner, and R. V. Furth.** 1985. Water-related nosocomial pneumonia caused by *Legionella pneumophila* serogroup 1 and 10. *J. Infect. Dis.* **152**:356–363.
12. **Meigh, R. E., T. Makin, M. H. Scott, and C. A. Hart.** 1989. *Legionella pneumophila* serogroup 12 pneumonia in a renal transplant recipient: case report and environmental observations. *J. Hosp. Infect.* **13**:315–319.
13. **Muraca, P., J. E. Stout, and V. L. Yu.** 1987. Comparative assessment of chlorine, heat, ozone and UV light for killing *Legionella pneumophila* within a model plumbing system. *Appl. Environ. Microbiol.* **53**:447–453.
14. **Page, F. C.** 1976. *An illustrated Key to Freshwater and Soil Amoebae.* Scientific publication no. 34. Freshwater Biological Association, Ambleside, England.
15. **Rowbotham, T. J.** 1980. Preliminary report on the pathogenicity of *Legionella pneumophila* for freshwater and soil amoebae. *J. Clin. Pathol.* **33**:1179–1183.
16. **Shands, K. N., J. L. Ho, and R. D. Meyer.** 1985. Potable water as a source of legionnaires' disease. *JAMA* **253**:1412–1416.
17. **Stapleton, F., D. V. Seal, and J. Dart.** 1991. Possible environmental sources of *Acanthamoebae* species that cause keratitis in contact lens wearers. *Rev. Infect. Dis.* **13**(Suppl. 5):S392.
18. **Wadowsky, R. M., J. B. Lawrence, M. K. Cook, S. M. Verma, M. A. Paul, B. S. Fields, G. Keleti, J. L. Sykora, and R. B. Yee.** 1988. Growth-supporting activity for *Legionella pneumophila* in the tap water cultures and implication of hartmannellid amoebae as growth factors. *Appl. Environ. Microbiol.* **54**:2677–2682.
19. **Wadowsky, R. M., and R. B. Yee.** 1985. Effect of non-*Legionellaceae* bacteria on the multiplication of *Legionella pneumophila* in potable water. *Appl. Environ. Microbiol.* **49**:1206–1210.

The Physiological Status of *Legionella pneumophila* and Its Susceptibility to Chemical Inactivation

J. BARKER, M. R. W. BROWN, P. GILBERT, P. J. COLLIER, AND I. D. FARRELL

Regional Public Health Laboratory, East Birmingham Hospital, Birmingham B9 5ST, Department of Pharmaceutical Sciences, Pharmaceutical Sciences Institute, Aston University, Birmingham B4 7ET, and Department of Pharmacy, University of Manchester, Manchester M13 9PL, United Kingdom

Contributory to the recalcitrance of legionellae in water systems is its growth within an adherent biofilm composed of numerous other bacterial species, protozoa, and ciliates (10). Together, these organisms form a complex balanced ecosystem in which the legionellae may exist in several physiological states: as planktonic cells, as free-living components of the biofilm ecosystem, and also in association with amoebae that may become parasitized by this organism. While the majority of studies on the susceptibility of legionellae to disinfectants have used cells grown under ill-defined conditions, i.e., in complex, nutrient-rich media (5, 7, 14), there is recent evidence (9, 11) that intra-amoebal growth significantly enhances chlorine resistance of this organism. It is likely that engulfed *Legionella pneumophila* is subject to an amoeba-imposed iron restriction, which might affect the phenotype of the cells and affect the biocide susceptibility of the released organism (2).

Organism culture. Preparation of intra-amoebally grown *L. pneumophila* serogroup 1 subtype Knoxville for use in biocide susceptibility studies was performed in two stages. Axenically grown suspensions of *Acanthamoeba polyphaga* (13) (10^5 trophozoites per ml) were inoculated with broth cultures of *L. pneumophila* (10^2 bacteria per ml) grown in a defined synthetic medium, ABCD broth (12), and incubated for 10 days at 35°C. Viable counts were performed on buffered charcoal-yeast extract agar (4), and the mixed suspension was centrifuged ($200 \times g$, 6 min) to remove amoebal debris. Supernatants were harvested for legionellae by further centrifugation ($2,080 \times g$, 15 min). The resultant pellets were washed twice and resuspended in amoebal saline. Second-stage culture in the amoebae was as described above, with initial inoculum levels increased to 10^5 cells per ml for the legionellae. Cultures were monitored by phase-contrast microscopy, which indicated the presence of infective, highly motile intra- and extra-amoebal legionellae after 3 days of incubation. At this point, the bacterial cells were harvested as before and resuspended in one-quarter-strength Ringer's solution. For comparison, broth cultures were grown at 35°C (100 rpm) in ABCD broth (12). Iron restriction of growth was imposed upon the cells in ABCD broth by omitting the iron-containing components and passing the filtered medium through a Chelex 100 ion-exchange column as appropriate (3, 8). Such procedures were demonstrated to reduce the cell density of stationary-phase cultures and to induce siderophore production. Replacement of the iron restored the medium to its full growth potential.

Biocide susceptibility. Time-survival data were determined for variously grown *L. pneumophila* suspensions by exposure (24 h) of cells (10^5/ml) to various concentrations of polyhexamethylenebiguanides (PHMB), 5-chloro-*N*-methylisothiazolone (CMIT; the active ingredient of Kathon), Fentichlor, and tetradecyltrimethylammonium bromide (quat). Concentrations of the biocides were selected on the basis of their MBCs and recommended use levels. Volumes (0.1 ml) of suspension were taken at the commencement of the exposure and at 2, 4, 6, and 24 h. Serial dilutions, in neutralizers when appropriate, were made and spread onto the surfaces of predried buffered charcoal-yeast extract agar plates. Colony counts (9 days, 35°C) were expressed as log_{10} reduction relative to untreated controls.

The relative susceptibilities of ABCD broth-grown and amoeba-grown *L. pneumophila* to quat, Fentichlor CMIT, and PHMB are illustrated in Table 1. The activities of quat, CMIT, and PHMB were significantly lower against amoeba-grown cells than against broth-grown cells. Significantly, in broth-grown systems, PHMB was active at concentrations well below the recommended use concentrations for swimming pool applications (ca. 10 μg/ml). PHMB at 20 μg/ml gave 4-log cycles of killing within 6 h and no detectable survivors at 24 h, but these values were reduced to 0.6 log at 6 h and 2 log at 24 h for amoeba-grown organisms. Similarly, use concentrations of CMIT and quat, while effective at reducing the viability of broth-grown cells, were virtually ineffective against these intra-amoebally grown legionellae freed from the amoebal host. Fentichlor was notably active against intra-amoebally grown legionellae, achieving 5-log cycles of killing after 6 h of contact. A factor contributing to the general recalcitrance of the intra-amoebal legionellae might have been imposition of iron restriction. Table 1 also demonstrates the effects of iron deprivation upon the susceptibility of broth-grown cells. Surprisingly, expression of an iron-deprived phenotype increased susceptibility to all four biocides compared with iron-plentiful broth cultures. In the aquatic environment, *L. pneumophila* infects and multiplies within a wide

TABLE 1. Biocide susceptibility of *L. pneumophila* grown under various conditions

	Log_{10} reduction in viable count following exposure to biocides					
	Broth grown				Intra-amoebal	
	Fe-sufficient culture		Fe-depleted culture			
Treatment	2 h	6 h	2 h	6 h	2 h	6 h
Control	0.1	0.1	0.1	0.1	0	0.1
PHMB						
2 µg/ml	2.2	>4.5	3.2	>3.4	0.1	0.5
20 µg/ml	4.0	>4.5	3.5	>3.4	0.4	0.6
Quat						
10 µg/ml	0.2	0.1	0.2	1.4	0	0
50 µg/ml	2.6	3.3	4.1	>4.1	0.3	0.6
Fentichlor						
10 µg/ml	2.3	>4.1	4.3	>4.8	0	0.1
100 µg/ml	>4.1	>4.1	>4.8	>4.8	1.7	5.0
CMIT						
2 µg/ml	0.5	0.9	0.6	1.6	0.3	0.4
15 µg/ml	0.6	2.5	1.3	2.5	0.4	1.0

range of amoebal hosts (13). The environmental stresses imposed upon such cells and their physiologic response and phenotype are likely therefore to be unrepresented by typical broth cultures (1, 6). The recalcitrance of *L. pneumophila* when grown intra-amoebally might relate to increased levels of poly-β-hydroxybutyric acid inclusions (15) associated with this mode of growth. The lipophilic poly-β-hydroxybutyric acid will probably sequester the relatively hydrophobic biocides CMIT, quat, and Fentichlor and reduce their interaction with cytosolic components. Such inclusions are likely only to affect the activity of CMIT, which alone acts solely within the cytosol. In conclusion, these studies clearly indicate the profound effect that intra-amoebal growth has on the physiological status and antimicrobial susceptibility of *L. pneumophila* and suggest that such phenomena might account for the organism's recalcitrance in situ.

We acknowledge T. J. Rowbotham, Leeds Public Health Laboratory, for helpful advice and provision of the *Acanthamoeba* cultures.

REFERENCES

1. **Brown, M. R. W., P. J. Collier, and P. Gilbert.** 1990. Influence of growth rate on susceptibility to antimicrobial agents: modifications of the cell envelope and batch and continuous culture studies. *Antimicrob. Agents Chemother.* **34:**1623–1628.
2. **Brown, M. R. W., and P. Williams.** 1985. Influence of substrate limitation and growth phase on sensitivity to antimicrobial agents. *J. Antimicrob. Chemother.* **15**(Suppl. A):7–14.
3. **Domingue, P. A. G., B. Mottle, D. W. Morck, M. R. W. Brown, and J. W. Costerton.** 1990. A simplified and rapid method for the removal of iron and other cations from

complex media. *J. Microbiol. Methods* **12:**13–22.
4. **Edelstein, P. H.** 1981. Improved semiselective medium for isolation of *Legionella pneumophila* from contaminated clinical and environmental specimens. *J. Clin. Microbiol.* **14:**298–303.
5. **Elsmore, R.** 1986. Biocidal control of legionellae. *Isr. J. Med. Sci.* **22:**647–654.
6. **Gilbert, P., P. J. Collier, and M. R. W. Brown.** 1990. Influence of growth rate on susceptibility to antimicrobial agents: biofilms, cell cycle, dormancy, and stringent response. *Antimicrob. Agents Chemother.* **34:**1865–1868.
7. **Hollis, C. G., and D. L. Smalley.** 1980. Resistance of *Legionella pneumophila* to microbicides. *Dev. Ind. Microbiol.* **21:**265–271.
8. **Kadurugamuw, J. L., H. Anwar, M. R. W. Brown, G. H. Shand, and K. H. Ward.** 1987. Media for study of growth kinetics and envelope properties of iron-deprived bacteria. *J. Clin. Microbiol.* **25:**849–855.
9. **Kilvington, S., and J. Price.** 1990. Survival of *Legionella pneumophila* within cysts of *Acanthamoeba polyphaga* following chlorine exposure. *J. Appl. Bacteriol.* **68:**519–525.
10. **Lee, J. V., and A. A. West.** 1991. Survival and growth of *Legionella* species in the environment. *J. Appl. Bacteriol. Symp. Suppl.* **70:**121s–129s.
11. **Navratil, J. S., R. H. Palmer, S. States, J. M. Kuchta, R. M. Wadowsky, and R. B. Yee.** 1990. Increased chlorine resistance of *Legionella pneumophila* released after growth in amoeba *Hartmannella vermiformis*, Abstr. Q-82. *Abstr. Annu. Meet. Am. Soc. Microbiol.*
12. **Pine, L., P. S. Hoffman, G. B. Malcolm, R. F. Benson, and M. J. Franzus.** 1986. Role of keto acids and reduced oxygen-scavenging enzymes in the growth of *Legionella* species. *J. Clin. Microbiol.* **23:**33–42.
13. **Rowbotham, T. J.** 1983. Isolation of *Legionella pneumophila* from clinical specimens *via* amoebae and the interaction of those and other isolates with amoebae. *J. Clin. Pathol.* **36:**978–986.
14. **Skaliy, P., T. A. Thompson, J. G. W. Gorman, G. K. Morris, H. E. McEachern, and D. C. Mackel.** 1980. Laboratory studies of disinfectants against *Legionella pneumophila. Appl. Environ. Microbiol.* **40:**697–700.
15. **Vandenesh, F., M. Surgot, N. Bornstein, J. C. Paucod, D. Marmet, P. Isoard, and J. Fleurette.** 1990. Relationship between free amoeba and *Legionellae:* studies in-vitro and in-vivo. *Zentralbl. Bakteriol.* **272:**265–275.

Shock Absorbers as a Source of *Legionella pneumophila*

ZIAD A. MEMISH, CATHERINE OXLEY, JOCELYNE CONTANT, AND GARY E. GARBER

Ottawa General Hospital, 501 Smyth Road, Ottawa, Ontario K1H 8L6, Canada

Water distribution systems have been demonstrated to be a major source of nosocomial Legionnaires disease (1). Hot water supplies have been specifically implicated. Other studies have demonstrated that hospital potable water systems are also colonized with *Legionella pneumophila*, which has been isolated from shower heads, faucets, and whirlpool tanks. Water fittings were identified as a source of *L. pneumophila* in a hospital plumbing system causing an outbreak in London, England (2).

Our institution is a tertiary-care center that has 529 beds. It was built in 1980. Between March and December 1983, 10 cases of Legionnaires disease occurred. These cases were associated with positive cultures for *L. pneumophila* serogroup 1 from hot water tanks, shower heads, and faucets that correlated with the *L. pneumophila* strain isolated from the patients. Recommended infection control measures, including superheating of hot water tanks to 80°C, hyperchlorination to 2 ppm, decontamination of shower heads and faucets with quaternary ammonium, and flushing, were instituted, after which monthly surveillance was performed. There were no new cases until 1988, when three new cases were identified. Despite the previously mentioned control measures, the potable water continued to be positive for legionellae. This finding prompted a search for a possible reservoir in the plumbing system. Shock absorbers were identified, and their removal decreased the positivity of random water samples (4a).

Environmental surveillance was performed by sampling potable hot water from faucets in 20 patient rooms that were selected as surveillance sites for monthly cultures. Water samples were also collected on a random basis from the four existing hot water tanks in the institution. These water samples were inoculated on buffered charcoal-yeast extract (BCYE) medium, which is a standard *Legionella* medium. The samples were incubated at 35°C in an atmosphere with 2.5% CO_2 and examined at 3, 5, and 10 days. Suspicious colonies were transferred to BCYE agar and sheep blood agar. Colonies morphologically consistent with legionellae growing solely on BCYE agar were confirmed as *L. pneumophila* by direct immunofluorescence testing with polyvalent antisera (3).

To clear legionellae from the water system, flushing was carried out. This was done by raising the temperature of hot water tanks to 80°C and then flushing all faucets in patient and nonpatient areas for a period of 10 min. Shock chlorination was used for the same reason. This was done by introducing additional chlorine into the system to achieve a free chlorine residual level of between 10 and 20 ppm.

After the initial outbreak, control measures cleared the water system for 5 years, with no new cases identified. From December 1988 to March 1989, two new cases were detected at a time when 72% of the potable hot water samples were positive for legionellae. Shock chlorination and flushing cleared the system for 5 months. From October 1989 to January 1990, a third case was detected, with 15 to 30% of water samples being positive. This contamination was resistant to repeat flushing. Since cultures from the main tanks, faucets, and shower heads were negative, a source in the plumbing system was suspected. In consultation with the hospital engineers, two possible reservoirs (hot water risers and shock absorbers) were identified.

In February 1990, dead ends of hot water risers, which fed water from main pipelines to room faucets, were targeted. All existing risers were drained, and all of the 182 samples were negative for legionellae. In May 1990, shock absorbers located directly on the tap line were identified as another potential reservoir; of 125 shock absorbers that were removed, 13 (10%) yielded heavy growth of *L. pneumophila* (serogroup 1). After removal of the shock absorbers, the percent positivity of surveillance sites has dropped to 0 to 5, with no new cases identified.

Hospital plumbing systems are the primary source of *L. pneumophila* associated with most outbreaks reported (4, 5). The recommended control measures, including superheating to 80°C, hyperchlorination to 2 ppm, and disinfection of shower heads and faucets, worked for 5 years. The persistent contamination of water with legionellae led to the search for a possible reservoir and identification and removal of shock absorbers.

Shock absorbers are made of stainless steel and are present in the plumbing systems of many buildings, especially new facilities. They absorb noises from the hot and cold water system created primarily from valve opening and closing. There are many types; the one used in our facility has a dead end that allows collection of water and sediment and becomes a natural reservoir for *L. pneumophila*. When the shock absorbers were removed, sediment and dirt were found in direct contact with the water, and 13 of 125 shock absorbers were positive for legionellae (from direct swabbing).

The reason for persistent low-grade positivity may relate to the presence of other niches in the system or of some shock absorbers left in the system, as they were technically difficult to remove. However, over the past 6 months, all sentinal sites have been negative for legionellae.

Environmental control measures implemented to initially control outbreaks of legionellosis are known to be effective. However, maintaining the water supply free from legionellae can be problematic.

Our experience involving a secondary water supply contaminated with *L. pneumophila* suggests that hyperchlorination and superheating may not always be sufficient to eradicate the problem. If such measures prove to be inadequate in other facilities, an assessment of the role of shock absorbers as a potential source of contamination should be considered.

REFERENCES

1. **Best, M., J. Stout, R. R. Muder, V. L. Yu, A. Goetz, and F. Taylor.** 1983. Legionellaceae in the hospital water-supply. Epidemiological link with disease and evaluation of a method for control of nosocomial Legionnaires' disease and Pittsburgh pneumonia. *Lancet* **ii:**307–310.
2. **Colbourne, J. S., D. J. Pratt, M. G. Smith, S. P. Fischer-Hoch, and D. Harper.** 1987. Water fitting as source of *Legionella pneumophila* in a hospital plumbing system. *Lancet* **i:**210–213.
3. **Edelstein, P. H.** 1985. *Legionella*, p. 373–381. *In* E. H. Lennette, A. Balow, W. J. Hausler, Jr., and H. J. Shadomy (ed.), *Manual of Clinical Microbiology*, 4th ed. American Society for Microbiology, Washington, D.C.
4. **Meenhorst, P. L., A. L. Reingold, D. G. Groothuis, et al.** 1985. Water-related nosocomial pneumonia caused by *Legionella pneumophila* serogroup 1 and 20. *J. Infect. Dis.* **152:**356–364.
4a. **Memish, Z., C. Oxley, J. Contant, and G. Garber.** *Am. J. Infection Control,* in press.
5. **Stout, J., V. L. Yu, R. M. Vickers, J. Zuravleff, M. Best, et al.** 1982. Ubiquitousness of *L. pneumophila* in the water supply of a hospital with endemic Legionnaire's disease. *N. Engl. J. Med.* **306:**466–468.

Environmental Regulation of the Virulence and Physiology of *Legionella pneumophila*

W. S. MAUCHLINE, R. ARAUJO, R. B. FITZGEORGE, P. J. DENNIS, AND C. W. KEEVIL

Division of Pathology, Public Health Laboratory Service Centre for Applied Microbiology and Research, Porton Down, Salisbury, Wiltshire SP4 0JG, United Kingdom; Departamento de Microbiologia, Universidad de Barcelona, Barcelona 08071, Spain; and Thames Water Utilities, Spencer House Laboratory, Reading, RG2 0JN, United Kingdom.

Although legionellae are commonly found in man-made water systems (1), in natural surface water (9), and even in potable water (5), the incidence of Legionnaires disease is relatively low (accounting for only around 2% of community-acquired pneumonias in the United Kingdom). Host factors, size of challenge dose, intrastrain differences in the virulence, and presentation in a respirable aerosol are all factors in whether infection occurs or not. It is, however, conceivable that some aspect of the growth environment either selects for subpopulations of virulent legionellae or stimulates the expression of a pathogenic phenotype; when such an event occurs, the potential for an outbreak exists.

Most pathogenic bacteria spend at least some of their time external to their host, or at least in some other host species, and so have to adapt to different environments. Expressions of virulence factors in external environments is unnecessary and may put the bacterium at a selective disadvantage. Therefore, it is advantageous for bacteria to exercise the same level of control over the expression of virulence genes as over the expression of genes encoding metabolic pathways. Genetic control of virulence can be divided into two categories: random and nonrandom. Random forms of control

include phase or antigenic variation, in which a fraction of the population have a different phenotype that imparts some advantage in colonizing the host environment and are thus selected for during infection; nonrandom regulation requires the pathogenic bacterium to sense signals in the environment and to regulate virulence gene expression accordingly. Coordinate regulation of virulence genes has been reported for a number of pathogens, including *Shigella* and *Yersinia* spp., *Vibrio cholerae*, *Bordetella pertussis,* and *Staphylococcus aureus*. These bacteria respond to specific environmental stimuli such as temperature, pH, concentration of specific ions, osmolarity, or some combination of these factors (12, 13). In general, temperature is a strong candidate for a potential environmental stimulus, since the constant internal temperature of mammals is for the most part higher than that of the external environment. Growth temperature has been shown to affect the virulence of a number of bacterial pathogens (12).

Legionellae are thermotolerant organisms; *Legionella pneumophila* has been isolated from water between 5.7 and 63°C (9) and has been shown to grow between 25 and 45°C (18). It is therefore evident that legionellae are exposed to a wide variety of growth temperatures. With these considerations in mind, we investigated the effect of growth temperature on the virulence of *L. pneumophila*. To isolate the effects of growth temperature from those of growth rate, we used continuous culture. In continuous culture, the specific growth rate is fixed by the rate of addition of the growth-limiting nutrient and is independent of other culture conditions (15). Continuous culture also provides a defined and reproducible environment, which can be maintained as long as is desired.

In independent chemostat experiments, two different strains of *L. pneumophila* serogroup 1 monocolonal subgroup Pontiac (an environmental strain [74/81] and a clinical isolate [Corby]) were grown in *N*-(2-acetamido)-2-aminoethanesulfonic acid (ACES)-buffered chemically defined (ABCD) broth (14). This medium contains 20 amino acids; serine, at approximately 20 times the concentration of the other amino acids (except cysteine), acts as the main carbon and energy source. The chemostat was a modified Series 500 fermentor (LH Fermentation) as described by Keevil et al. (10), with the substitution of a titanium top plate for the one previously made of nylon. Provisional experiments showed that the best yield was obtained at a dissolved oxygen concentration of 0.3 mg liter^{-1}, and this concentration was used in all subsequent experiments. The strains used to inoculate the chemostat were stored in individual aliquots at $-80°C$ and were grown on buffered charcoal-yeast extract (BCYE) agar for 72 h prior to inoculation of the chemostat. The oxygen concentration in the chemostat medium was reduced to approximately 0.1 mg of oxygen liter^{-1} with nitrogen before inoculation. The culture was allowed to grow in batch until an optical density at 540 nm (OD_{540}) of 0.4 had been reached before medium addition was started, to give an initial dilution rate of 0.03 h^{-1}, and then increased to 0.08 h^{-1} when the OD_{540} was greater than 1. The culture conditions were tightly controlled by using Anglicon fermentation controllers (Brighton Systems Limited, Newhaven, United Kingdom); the pH was maintained at 6.9, the dissolved oxygen concentration was kept at 0.3 mg of O_2 liter^{-1}, and the dilution rate was set at 0.08 h^{-1}, giving a mean generation time of 8.7 h. The cultures were grown at various temperatures until steady state had been achieved, as determined by constant OD_{540} and dry weight measurements (after 8 to 10 generations). Samples were then taken for analysis.

To assess the virulence of *L. pneumophila* grown at different temperatures, steady-state samples were used to provide aerosol challenges for guinea pigs as described by Baskerville et al. (2) and Fitzgeorge et al. (8). Quantification of inhaled dose of bacteria was performed by viable counts carried out on lung macerate from animals killed

immediately after challenge; guinea pigs received either this dose or 10-fold serial dilutions of it.

ABCD broth proved to be a good medium for continuous culture of *L. pneumophila*, giving yields of between 0.6 and 1.3 g (dry weight) liter^{-1}, depending on culture conditions and strain. Also, since ABCD is a defined medium, its use has allowed investigation of the physiology of *L. pneumophila* under different growth conditions. Protease activity, consistent with that of tissue-destructive protease, and phospholipase C activity were detected in culture supernatants. Fifty percent lethal dose (LD_{50}) values obtained for strain 74/81 grown in continuous culture using ABCD broth as the medium were similar to those obtained when this strain was grown on BCYE agar; however, when strain Corby was grown in a chemostat, there was between a 1- and 2-log increase in the value of the LD_{50} obtained (Table 1 and unpublished data). Nevertheless, the LD_{50} values obtained for both 74/81 and Corby grown in a chemostat were reproducible for independent experiments (with fresh inocula) and after restoration of culture conditions following a temperature change. It was therefore concluded that both continuous culture of *L. pneumophila* and the maintenance of virulence were possible in our system over extended periods of time. Both 74/81 and Corby were significantly less virulent when the culture temperature was decreased from 37 to 24°C in the chemostat. Steady-state samples from the cultures at 24°C caused no mortality in the test animals, which was in contrast to the results obtained for the same cultures grown at 37°C (Table 1). When cultures were returned to 37°C, LD_{50} values similar to those in Table 1 were restored. Edelstein et al. (6) also reported a change in LD_{50} according to growth temperature; however, they found that *L. pneumophila* was more virulent when grown at 25°C than when grown at 37 or 41°C. The contrasting findings of these two studies might be due to either the difference in method of culture used (in that study, the growth rate would not have been fixed nor would culture conditions have been constant and defined during the growth of the bacteria) or the difference in the route of infection in the animal models used.

TABLE 1. Comparison of LD_{50} values obtained by aerosol challenge of guinea pigs with *L. pneumophila* grown on BCYE agar at 37°C or in continuous culture at 37°C

Strain	LD_{50} (no. of bacteria)	
	BCYE agar[a]	ABCD broth in chemostat
74/81	$10^{4.5}$	$10^{3.7b}$
Corby	$10^{2.5}$	$10^{4.0}$

[a]From Baskerville et al. (3).
[b]From West et al. (21).

A number of researchers have reported the presence of electron-translucent inclusions in *Legionella* spp. and have suggested that they resemble polyhydroxybutyrate (PHB) granules (4, 16). Since our chemostat-grown cells contained similar granules, we investigated whether the *L. pneumophila* cells contained PHB and, if so, how much. Extraction and purification of PHB was carried out by a modification of the method of Findlay and White (7). The product was characterized by gas chromatography mass spectrometry and ^{13}C nuclear magnetic resonance spectroscopy (19, 20). PHB content of cells was measured by a modification of the method of Slepecky and Law (17). *L. pneumophila* was found to accumulate PHB, and the proportion of the cell dry weight that it accounted for varied according to growth temperature. Since legionellae are able to metabolize β-hydroxybutyrate (the monomer of PHB) and PHB is accumulated by *L. pneumophila*, it is clear that this polymer may play a significant role as a carbon and energy storage compound for survival in low-nutrient environments (11).

The availability of the trace nutrient iron is restricted both in vivo (due to host lactoferrin and transferrin) and in vitro (due to insoluble oxide and hydroxide formation above neutral pH). Since the chemostat, medium bottle, and all associated tubing and connectors, being either glass, titanium, plastic, or silicone rubber, we are currently growing *L. pneumophila* under iron-limited conditions in modified ABCD broth and investigating the effects of iron restriction on the virulence and physiology of this pathogen.

REFERENCES

1. **Bartlett, C. L. R., J. B. Kurtz, J. G. P. Hutchinson, G. C. Turner, and A. E. Wright.** 1983. *Legionella* in hospital and hotel water supplies *Lancett* ii:1315.
2. **Baskerville, A., R. B. Fitzgeorge, M. Broster, P. Hambleton, and P. J. Dennis.** 1981. Experimental transmission of Legionnaires' disease by exposure to aerosols of *Legionella pneumophila. Lancet* ii:1389–1390.
3. **Baskerville, A., R. B. Fitzgeorge, D. H. Gibson, J. W. Conlan, L. A. E. Ashworth, and A. B. Dowsett.** 1984. Pathological and bacteriological findings after aerosol *Legionella pneumophila* infection of susceptible, convalescent, and antibiotic-treated animals, p. 131–132. *In* C. Thornsberry, A. Balows, J. C. Feeley, and W. Jakubowski (ed.), *Legionella: Proceedings of the 2nd International Symposium.* American Society for Microbiology, Washington, D.C.
4. **Chandler, F. W., J. A. Blackmon, M. D. Hicklin, R. M. Cole, and C. S. Callaway.** 1979. Ultrastructure of the agent of Legionnaires' disease in the human lung. *Am. J. Clin. Pathol.* 71:43–50.
5. **Colbourne, J. S., and P. J. Dennis.** 1989. The ecology and survival of *Legionella pneumophila. J. Inst. Water Environ. Manage.* 3:345–350.
6. **Edelstein, P. H., K. B. Beer, and E. D. DeBoynton.** 1987. Influence of growth temperature on virulence of *Legionella pneumophila. Infect. Immun.* 55:2701–2705.
7. **Findlay, R. H., and D. C. White.** 1983. Polymeric beta-hydroxyalkanoates from environmental samples and *Bacillus megaterium. Appl. Environ. Microbiol.* 45:71–78.
8. **Fitzgeorge, R. B., A. Baskerville, M. Broster, P. Hambleton, and P. J. Dennis.** 1983. Aerosol infection of animals with strains of *Legionella pneumophila* of different virulence: comparison with intraperitoneal and intranasal routes of infection. *J. Hyg.* 90:81–89.
9. **Fliermans, C. B., W. B. Cherry, L. H. Orrison, S. J. Smith, D. L. Tison, and D. H. Pope.** 1981. Ecological distribution of *Legionella pneumophila. Appl. Environ. Microbiol.* 41:9–16.
10. **Keevil, C. W., D. B. Davies, B. J. Spillane, and E. Mahenthiralingam.** 1989. Influence of iron-limited and replete continuous culture on the physiology and virulence of *Neisseria gonorrhoeae. J. Gen. Microbiol.* 135:851–863.
11. **Mauchline, W. S., and C. W. Keevil.** 1991. Development of the BIOLOG substrate utilization system for identification of *Legionella* spp. *Appl. Environ. Microbiol.* 57:3345–3349.
12. **Maurelli, A. T.** 1989. Temperature regulation of virulence genes in pathogenic bacteria: a general strategy for human pathogens? *Microb. Pathog.* 7:1–10.
13. **Miller, J. F., J. J. Mekalanos, and S. Falkow.** 1989. Coordinate regulation and sensory transduction in the control of bacterial virulence. *Science* 243:916–922.
14. **Pine, L., P. S. Hoffman, G. S. Malcom, R. F. Benson, and M. J. Franzus.** 1986. Role of keto acids and reduced oxygen-scavenging enzymes in the growth of *Legionella* species. *J. Clin. Microbiol.* 23:33–42.
15. **Pirt, S. J.** 1972. Prospects and problems in continuous flow culture of microorganisms. *J. Appl. Chem. Biotechnol.* 22:55–64.
16. **Rodgers, F. G., and M. R. Davey.** 1979. Ultrastructure of the cell envelope layers and surface details of *Legionella pneumophila. J. Gen. Microbiol.* 128:1547–1557.
17. **Slepecky, R. A., and J. H. Law.** 1960. A rapid spectrophotometric assay of alpha, beta-unsaturated acids and beta-hydroxy acids. *Anal. Chem.* 32:1697–1699.
18. **Wadowsky, R. M., R. Wolford, A. M. McNamara, and R. B. Yee.** 1986. Effect of temperature, pH, and oxygen level on the multiplication of naturally occurring *Legionella pneumophila* in potable water. *Appl. Environ. Microbiol.* 49:1197–1205.
19. **Wait, R., W. S. Mauchline, R. Araujo, and C. W. Keevil.** 1990. *Abstr. 15th Annu. Sci. Conf. Public Health Lab. Serv. United Kingdom,* p. 118, abstr. G119.
20. **Wait, R.** Personal communication.
21. **West, A. A., R. Araujo, P. L. J. Dennis, and C. W. Keevil.** 1989. Chemostat models of *Legionella pneumophila,* p. 107–116. *In* B. Flannigan (ed.), *Airborne Deteriogens and Pathogens.* Biodeterioration Society, Kew, United Kingdom.

In Vitro Antagonistic Activity of *Pseudomonas aeruginosa,* *Klebsiella pneumoniae,* and *Aeromonas* spp. against *Legionella* spp.

R. GOMEZ-LUS, E. LOMBA, P. GOMEZ-LUS, M. S. ABARCA, S. GOMEZ-LUS, A. MARTINEZ, E. DURAN, AND M. C. RUBIO

Department of Microbiology, School of Medicine, University of Zaragoza, C/ Domingo Miral s/n, 50009 Zaragoza, Spain

In previous studies (2, 3), we found that clinical and environmental isolates of *Pseudomonas* spp., *Aeromonas hydrophila,* and seven genera of the family *Enterobacteriaceae* (*Escherichia, Klebsiella, Enterobacter, Citrobacter, Serratia, Proteus,* and *Salmonella*) were active against the majority of 104 clinical and environmental *Legionella pneumophila* serogroup 1 strains (Lp1). In 1980, Rowbotham (5) reported that growth of *L. pneumophila* on solid media is inhibited by certain members of the oral flora, a *Bacillus* species, and *Pseudomonas aeruginosa.* In the same year, Flesher et al. (1) reported that several bacteria (*Streptococcus* spp. and *Staphylococcus saprophyticus*) isolated from human pharyngeal cultures specifically inhibited the growth of five strains of Lp1 and one strain each of Lp2, Lp3, and Lp4.

This study examines the interaction of *Legionella* spp. with bacteriocins produced by environmental *P. aeruginosa* and clinical *Klebsiella pneumoniae* isolates, and with bacteriocin-like substances (BLS) synthesized by clinical and environmental *Aeromonas* spp. Aeromonads may be specially interesting because they are widely distributed in stagnant and flowing fresh waters and in water supplies (even chlorinated ones). A total of 89 clinical and environmental isolates of *Aeromonas* spp. (50 *A. caviae,* 10 *A. hydrophila,* and 29 *A. sobria* isolates), 12 *K. pneumoniae* isolates, and 22 *P. aeruginosa* isolates were used to test which produced bacteriocins or BLS with activity against the following *Legionella* species (the number of isolates is given in parentheses): Lp1 (73), Lp2 (1), Lp3 (3), Lp4 (1), Lp5 (1), Lp6 (12), Lp7 (1), Lp8 (1), *L. dumoffii* (1), *L. gormanii* (1), *L. longbeachae* (1), *L. oakridgensis* (1), and *L. wadsworthii* (1). Eighty environmental and clinical isolates of Lp1 (73), Lp3 (5), and Lp6 (12) were collected at the Zaragoza University Hospital and other local buildings. Ten *Legionella* strains were obtained from the National Center for Microbiology, CNMVIS, Mahadahonda, Madrid, Spain.

To detect the bacteriocin activity against *Legionella* spp., the producer strain is inoculated on the surface of buffered charcoal-yeast extract (BCYE) α-ketoglutarate agar (spot inoculation or strip) and incubated at 36°C for 14 to 18 h. The

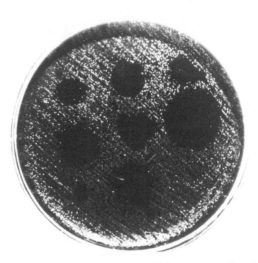

FIG. 1. Spotting method. Inhibition zones produced by eight bacteriocinogenic strains (four *P. aeruginosa,* three *K. pneumoniae,* and one *Citrobacter freundii*) against an *L. pneumophila* strain isolated from a patient.

plate is then inverted, and the petri dish is tapped sharply on the bench so that the agar disk falls into the lid and the *Legionella* strain(s) can be inoculated. After 2 to 4 days of incubation, zones of inhibition are clearly visible. Inhibition zones due to high-molecular-weight (R-type) bacteriocins ranged from 5 to 7 mm in diameter, while low-molecular-weight (S-type) bacteriocins produced zones of 9 to 12 mm or more in diameter. Examples of plates prepared by the spotting and cross-streaking methods are shown in Fig. 1 and 2.

In addition, we used the diffusion assay method for bacteriocins, improved by means of a prediffusion for 18 h at 4°C. BCYE agar plates are swabbed with the *Legionella* strain. Plugs of blood agar containing bacteriocins are placed with a forceps on the BCYE agar plates. The plates are kept at 4°C for 18 h and then incubated at 36°C for 2 to 4 days.

Eighteen *P. aeruginosa* strains producing S-type pyocins and four isolates producing R-type pyocins were active against Lp1 (73), Lp2 (1), Lp3 (3), Lp4 (1), Lp5 (1), Lp6 (12), Lp7 (1), Lp8 (1), *L. dumoffii* (1), *L. gormanii* (1), *L. long-*

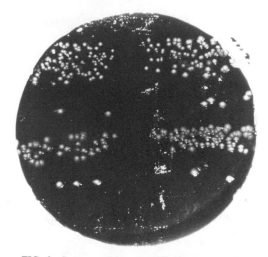

FIG. 2. Cross-streaking method. Bacteriocin activity of one *P. aeruginosa* strain against one environmental and one clinical *L. pneumophila* strain.

TABLE 1. Numerical breakdown of gram-negative bacilli producing bacteriocins for clinical and environmental *Legionella* strains

Microorganism	Total no. tested	No. (%) inhibiting
P. aeruginosa	22	22 (100)
K. pneumoniae	12	12 (100)
A. caviae	50	27 (54)
A. hydrophila	10	6 (60)
A. sobria	29	22 (75.8)

beachae (1), *L. oakridgensis* (1), and *L. wadsworthii* (1) (the number of isolates is given in parentheses). All clinical isolates of *K. pneumoniae* produced klebocins with activity against Lp1 (14), Lp3 (5), Lp6 (12), *L. oakridgensis* (1), and *L. wadsworthii* (1). High percentages of the *A. sobria* (74%), *A. hydrophila* (59%), and *A. caviae* (55%) appear to produce low- and high-molecular-weight BLS for Lp1 (4), Lp3 (1), Lp4 (1), Lp5 (1), *L. oakridgensis* (1), and *L. wadsworthii* (1). The temperature of *Aeromonas* incubation (22 or 35°C) does not influence BLS production. BLS or bacteriocin (aeromonacin) synthesis correlated with aerolysin and lysine decarboxylase production. The results are shown in Tables 1 and 2.

Because of the comparatively low density of microorganisms in drinking water, it is unlikely that bacteriocins would play a significant role in the suppression of *Legionella* spp. by gram-negative bacilli. It is difficult to demonstrate experimentally that bacteria produce bacteriocins under natural conditions, and in situ synthesis has not yet been quantified. Studies supporting the single-hit hypothesis of bacteriocin function improve the possibility that low levels of bacteriocin production might cause bacterial injury or death in situ. On the other hand, bacterial colonization of pipe surfaces in water distribution systems has been demonstrated (4). Such colonization might create a situation in which bacteriocin inhibition is more plausible. These microcolonies could be important sites of production of *Legionella*-specific bacteriocins by gram-negative bacilli.

Conclusions. (i) Members of three different families (*Enterobacteriaceae, Pseudomonada-*

TABLE 2. Sensitivity of six *Legionella* strains to 89 strains of *Aeromonas* spp. producing bacteriocin

Organism	Inhibition zone (mm)	No. of isolates sensitive to bacteriocin from:			
		A. caviae	*A. hydrophila*	*A. sobria*	% Sensitive
L. pneumophila					
Serogroup 1 L46	0	8	3	1	13.5
	≤7	19	4	15	42.7
	≥9	23	3	13	43.8
Serogroup 3	0	30	3	9	47.2
	≤7	17	5	14	40.4
	≥9	3	2	6	12.3
Serogroup 4	0	35	5	10	56.1
	≤7	12	4	10	29.2
	≥9	3	1	9	14.6
Serogroup 5	0	30	4	11	50.5
	≤7	12	4	12	31.4
	≥9	8	2	6	17.9
L. oakridgensis	0	20	4	4	31.4
	≤7	30	5	22	64.0
	≥9	0	1	3	4.4
L. wadsworthii	0	10	4	5	21.3
	≤7	25	4	11	44.9
	≥9	15	2	13	32.7

ceae, and *Vibrionaceae*) have the ability to inhibit legionellae. (ii) We have demonstrated that six *Legionella* species and eight serogroups of *L. pneumophila* are susceptible to a variety of bacteriocins. In addition, what has been termed bacterial antagonism may be related to low- and high-molecular-weight pyocins, klebocins, and BLS. (iii) It is clear from this research that *P. aeruginosa, K. pneumoniae,* and *Aeromonas* spp. bacteriocins have the potential to suppress detection of legionellae in clinical and environmental cultures. (iv) High percentages of the *A. sobria* (75.8%), *A. hydrophila* (60%), and *A. caviae* (54%) appear to produce low- and high-molecular-weight bacteriocins with activity against *Legionella* spp. (v) The differences in susceptibility of legionellae to the low- and high-molecular-weight bacteriocins produced by *Aeromonas* spp. suggest the possible existence of two classes of receptors in *Legionella* spp. (vi) Differences in sensitivity of legionellae to bacteriocins and BLS produced by gram-negative bacilli could support use of these substances in the classification of Lp1

as an alternative method for subtyping.

This research was sponsored by the Diputación General de Aragon (project PCM-5/88).

REFERENCES

1. **Flesher, A. R., D. L. Kasper, P. A. Modern, and E. Mason, Jr.** 1980. *Legionella pneumophila:* growth inhibition by human pharyngeal flora. *J. Infect. Dis.* **142:**313–317.
2. **Gomez-Lus, R., M. L. Gomez-Lus, M. S. Abarca, E. Duran, C. Garcia, A. Rezusta, and M. C. Rubio.** 1987. *Program Abstr. 3rd Eur. Congr. Clin. Microbiol.,* abstr. 227.
3. **Gomez-Lus R., M. L. Gomez-Lus, M. Sanchez-Gimeno, M. S. Abarca, and M. C. Rubio.** 1989. *Program Abstr. 29th Int. Congr. Antimicrob. Agents Chemother.,* abstr. 260.
4. **Means, E. G., and B. H. Olson.** 1981. Coliform inhibition by bacteriocin-like substances in drinking water distribution systems. *Appl. Environ. Microbiol.* **42:**506–512.
5. **Rowbotham, T. J.** 1980. Preliminary report on the pathogenicity of *Legionella pneumophila* for freshwater and soil amoebae. *J. Clin. Pathol.* **33:**1179–1183.
6. **Stout, J. E., V. L. Yu, and M. B. Best.** 1985. Ecology of *Legionella pneumophila* within water distribution systems. *Appl. Environ. Microbiol.* **49:**221–228.

The Influence of the Sessile Population in the *Legionella* Colonization of Cooling Towers

R. H. BENTHAM, C. R. BROADBENT, AND L. N. MARWOOD

Repatriation General Hospital, Daw Park, Adelaide, South Australia 5041, Federal Department of Administrative Services, Canberra, Phillip Act 2606, and Australian Construction Services, Adelaide, South Australia, Australia

Frequently, legionellae have been isolated in high numbers from sediments and slimes in cooling water systems (3) and have been shown to grow in biofilms adherent to a variety of surfaces, including aluminum, copper, stainless steel, galvanized steel, glass, wood, rubber, and polyvinyl chloride (9). Biofilm populations have been shown to be much more stable than planktonic populations (4) and to have greater resistance to the effects of biocides (6).

Three conclusions from a 4-year field study of *Legionella* colonization in cooling towers (2) prompted investigation of the role of the sessile population on the planktonic concentrations. These conclusions were as follows: (i) system water temperature was a major predictor of planktonic *Legionella* concentrations, (ii) the frequency of operation showed significant correlation with *Legionella* concentrations, and (iii) cleaning was ineffective in controlling the *Legionella* population in the cooling water, and hyperchlorination with cleaning had only a short-term effect. These observations indicated the possible importance of the pipework and other inaccessible warm areas of the system in *Legionella* colonization.

Samples of water were taken from a tower basin at half-hourly intervals over a 6.5-h period while water was bled from the system and replaced from the mains supply. Basin water temperature was recorded at each sample collection. This procedure was repeated with altered bleed rates and no bleed in operation.

Sediment samples and biofilm samples were taken from 25 cooling towers and cultured for *Legionella* species. Sediment and biofilm samples were collected from artificial dead legs attached to the pipework of the cooling towers. Additional biofilm samples were collected from the water line of the tower basin.

Legionellae were enumerated by culture on Oxoid buffered charcoal-yeast extract agar (5) and Oxoid modified Wadowsky-Yee agar (10). Water samples were heat pretreated by the method of Dennis (5). Sediment and biofilm samples were acid pretreated by the method of Bopp et al. (1), and the modified Wadowsky-Yee medium was supplemented with 8 mg of aztreonam per liter. All plates were incubated at 37°C in 5% CO_2 for 7 days.

Hourly bleed rates of 0, 25, 33, and 95% of the

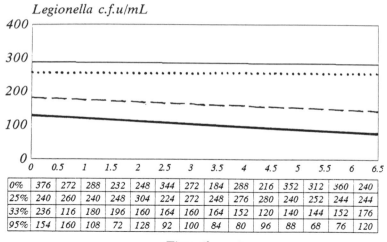

	0	0.5	1	1.5	2	2.5	3	3.5	4	4.5	5	5.5	6	6.5
0%	376	272	288	232	248	344	272	184	288	216	352	312	360	240
25%	240	260	240	248	304	224	272	248	276	280	240	252	244	244
33%	236	116	180	196	160	164	160	164	152	120	140	144	152	176
95%	154	160	108	72	128	92	100	84	80	96	88	68	76	120

Time (hours)

FIG. 1. *Legionella* counts in cooling towers with various hourly bleed rates. The tabulated data indicate *Legionella* CFU per milliliter at each sampling. Plots present lines of best fit for the data sets. Bleed rates: thin line, 0%; dotted line, 25%; dashed line, 33%; thick line, 95%.

system volume all resulted in no significant decrease in *Legionella* concentrations (Fig. 1). In all cases, *Legionella* concentrations remained within 1 log of the initial concentration over the 7-h duration of sampling. The highest hourly bleed rate (95%) reduced the planktonic *Legionella* concentrations by less than 40% in 7 h, though the system water was replaced more than six times from the mains supply, where *Legionella* were undetected in 1-liter samples (11). *Legionella* counts significantly higher (by 2 logs) than those in the bulk water were recorded in some sediment and biofilm samples (Table 1).

The results indicate that in cooling towers in which the circulating water is colonized by legionellae, there is commonly an extensive sessile population of legionellae in sediments and bio-

films. In some cases, this sessile population may be present when planktonic populations are undetectable.

The bleed rate investigations indicate that the sessile *Legionella* population in cooling water systems is the major site of *Legionella* multiplication within the system. In systems in which this sessile population is well established, it is unlikely that water treatments focusing only on the planktonic population will have a major effect on the overall *Legionella* population of the system and may be ineffective in controlling the planktonic population (4). Chemical treatments which are penetrant and have surface-active properties would seem best suited for this purpose, combined with mechanical cleaning when indicated.

At the temperatures recorded, the dilution rate of the legionellae exceeds documented mean generation times for the bacteria in complex media at 37°C (7, 8, 12). It can be assumed that the planktonic concentrations are maintained by seeding from the sessile population. For *Legionella* concentrations to remain constant at variable bleed rates, an equilibrium between sessile and planktonic population must exist.

The results from this study suggest that the contribution of biofilm bacteria is of greater significance than that of the planktonic population in colonization of the system. This conclusion indicates that the planktonic population in cooling water systems may not necessarily be derived from intracellular multiplication within amoebae. A reduction in the internal surface area of cooling water systems (e.g., reduced pipe lengths to and from the heat exchanger) may reduce the maximum potential concentration of free-floating le-

TABLE 1. Summary of positive results from sediment and biofilm sampling of cooling towers for legionellae

	No. of bacteria in[a]:			
Tower	Basin water	Basin biofilm	Dead leg sediment	Dead leg biofilm
A	36	12	NS	NS
B	24	NS	0	0
C	0	NS	1,400	2,000
D	0	NS	2,400	OG
E	4	NS	2,400	2,200
F	136	280	160	NS
G	136	24,000	NS	10,000
H	0	NS	28	0
I	252	NS	24	220

[a]NS, not sampled; OG, overgrowth by other organisms.

gionellae in the water by reducing sites for biofilm formation.

REFERENCES

1. **Bopp, C. A., J. W. Sumner, G. K. Morris, and J. G. Wells.** 1981. Isolation of *Legionella* spp. from environmental water samples by low-pH treatment and use of a selective medium. *J. Clin. Microbiol.* **13:**714–719.
2. **Broadbent, C. R., L. N. Marwood, and R. H. Bentham.** 1991. *Legionella* in cooling towers: report of a field study in South Australia, p. 55–61. *In* R. A. Parsons (ed.), *ASHRAE Far East Conference on Environmental Quality.* American Society of Heating, Refrigerating and Air-Conditioning Engineers, Atlanta.
3. **Colbourne, J. S., and P. J. Dennis.** 1988. *Legionella:* a biofilm organism in engineered water systems? *Biodeterioration* **7:**36–42.
4. **Costerton, J. W., K.-J. Cheng, G. G. Geesey, T. I. Ladd, J. C. Nickel, M. Dasgupta, and T. J. Marrie.** 1987. Bacterial biofilms in nature and disease. *Annu. Rev. Microbiol.* **41:**435–464.
5. **Dennis, P. J.** 1988. Isolation of legionellae from environ- mental specimens, p. 31–171. *In* T. G. Harrison and A. G. Taylor (ed.), *A Laboratory Manual for Legionella,* vol. 4. John Wiley & Sons, New York.
6. **Dennis, P. J.** 1990. Biofilms: detection, implications and solutions. *Health Est. J.* **October:**1–13.
7. **Pope, D. H., R. J. Soracco, H. K. Gill, and C. B. Fliermans.** 1982. Growth of *Legionella pneumophila* in two-membered cultures with green algae and cyanobacteria. *Curr. Microbiol.* **7:**319–322.
8. **Rodgers, F. G., A. O. Tzianabos, and T. S. J. Elliott.** 1990. The effect of antibiotics that inhibit cell-wall, protein, and DNA synthesis on the growth and morphology of *Legionella pneumophila. J. Med. Microbiol.* **31:**37–44.
9. **Schofield, G. M., and R. Locci.** 1985. Colonization of components of a model hot water system by *Legionella pneumophila. J. Appl. Bacteriol.* **58:**151–162.
10. **Wadowsky, R. M., and R. B. Yee.** 1981. Glycine-containing selective medium for isolation of *Legionellaceae* from environmental specimens. *Appl. Environ. Microbiol.* **42:**768–772.
11. **Walters, O.** Personal communication.
12. **Warren, W. J., and R. D. Miller.** 1979. Growth of Legionnaires' disease bacterium (*Legionella pneumophila*) in chemically defined medium. *J. Clin. Microbiol.* **10:**50–55.

Bactericidal Effect of Inhibitory Non-*Legionella* Bacteria on *Legionella pneumophila*

SIMON TOZE, LINDSAY SLY, CHRIS HAYWARD, AND JOHN FUERST

CSIRO Division of Water Resources, Private Bag, P.O. Wembley, Perth, W. A. 6014, Australia, and Department of Microbiology, University of Queensland, Brisbane 4072, Australia.

Several researchers have demonstrated that non-*Legionella* bacteria are capable of inhibiting the growth of legionellae on solid media (4, 6, 9). Flesher et al. (4), Makin (6), and Toze et al. (9) have all proposed that the presence of inhibitory bacteria in water containing legionellae could prevent the growth of *Legionella* colonies on isolation media. Nothing is known, however, about the influence of inhibitory bacteria on the growth and survival of *Legionella* cells in the aquatic environment. The aim of this study was to examine the ability of an *Aeromonas* strain, known to be inhibitory to *Legionella pneumophila* growth on solid agar, to actively reduce the number of viable cells of an *L. pneumophila* strain in conditions resembling natural aquatic systems.

The *Legionella* strain used, *L. pneumophila* UQM 3336, was a cooling tower isolate that had been passaged a maximum of four times on artificial media and was maintained as a tap water culture in filter-sterilized tap water at 20°C. The maintenance in filter-sterilized tap water was used to keep the *L. pneumophila* cells in a nutritional and physical condition similar to that of cells in the environment.

The inhibitory non-*Legionella* strain, M94, was an *Aeromonas* strain that had been isolated from chlorinated drinking water. M94 had been ob- served to produce a diffusible, bactericidal compound that was active against *L. pneumophila*. It was maintained aerobically on R2A medium.

All inhibitory coculture experiments were carried out in coculture vessels. The design of a coculture vessel is shown in Fig. 1.

Known concentrations of *L. pneumophila* and M94 cells were placed on apposing separate sides of a coculture vessel. A 0.2-μm-pore-size cellulose acetate filter was used to separate the *L. pneumophila* and M94 cells to prevent physical contact between them. Control cocultures were constructed in exactly the same manner as the experimental cocultures except that no M94 cells were added.

The inhibitory strain, M94, was tested for its ability to reduce the number of viable *L. pneumophila* cells in cocultures containing (i) an unsupplemented buffered charcoal-yeast extract agar (UNBCYEA) slope overlaid with tap water, (ii) tap water containing 0.025% yeast extract, (iii) tap water containing 0.0025% yeast extract, and (iv) tap water plus tap water sediment. The total organic carbon content of tap water plus 0.025% yeast extract was determined to be 82.8 μg liter^{-1}.

The coculture vessels were incubated at 28°C and sampled daily. The ability of the M94 cells to

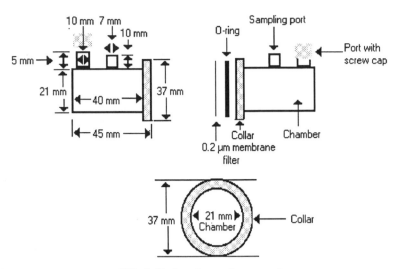

FIG. 1. Design of a coculture vessel.

reduce the number of viable *L. pneumophila* cells was determined by the decrease in the number of *L. pneumophila* colonies recovered from the coculture compared with the control.

The M94 strain was observed to actively decrease the number of viable *L. pneumophila* cells in the model cultures that contained the UN-BCYEA slope and 0.025 and 0.0025% yeast extract solutions as nutrient sources (Fig. 2A to C). No bactericidal action was observed to occur in the coculture containing tap water plus tap water sediment (Fig. 2D).

M94 cells were observed to multiply in all nutrient sources except the 0.0025% yeast extract–tap water suspension (Fig. 2A to C). In this solution, a steady decrease in the number of viable M94 cells was noted after day 4 (Fig. 2C).

The detection of *Legionella* cells in a variety of aquatic niches (5, 6, 8) and the ability of the cells to multiply in some of these niches (3, 10) have led to the study of how *Legionella* cells grow and survive in their natural habitat. These studies have included the interactions of legionellae with other microorganisms (1, 3, 10). It has been considered possible that non-*Legionella* bacteria present with legionellae in such niches may have a positive or negative effect on the survival of the *Legionella* cells (3, 6).

Previous studies of the inhibition of legionellae by non-*Legionella* bacteria have observed inhibition of *Legionella* growth only on solid media (4, 6, 9). The results of the experiments presented here suggest that, given suitable conditions, some inhibitory bacteria may be capable of decreasing the survival of *Legionella* cells in suitable aquatic niches. *Aeromonas* is a bacterial genus whose members are also commonly found in water and are known to produce a number of exotoxins (3).

Use of the membrane filter demonstrated that the bactericidal effect on the *L. pneumophila* cells was due to a compound, produced by the M94 cells, that was able to diffuse across the membrane. It was noted that when sufficient nutrients were available and the M94 cells were able to multiply, the inhibiting compound began to have an effect several days after the M94 cells had reached stationary phase (Fig. 2A and B). This finding could suggest that the inhibiting compound produced by the inhibitory strain was a secondary metabolite.

No reduction of the number of viable *L. pneumophila* cells was noticed in the tap water plus tap water sediment despite the slow growth of the M94 cells (Fig. 2D). This inability of the M94 cells to kill the *L. pneumophila* cells in the presence of tap water sediment could be due to the ability of the sediment to protect the *L. pneumophila* cells from the bactericidal action of the compound(s) released by the M94 cells.

The rapid decrease of the *L. pneumophila* cells in the coculture containing the 0.0025% yeast extract-tap water solution was noted despite the lack of growth of the M94 cells. This finding may be explained by the fact that in the low-nutrient conditions of the coculture, the M94 cells would have remained in the stationary phase that they had reached when growing on the R2A plate. If the inhibiting compound produced was a secondary metabolite produced under nutrient limitation during stationary phase, it was likely that the M94 cells were producing it when added to the coculture and continued to produce the inhibiting com-

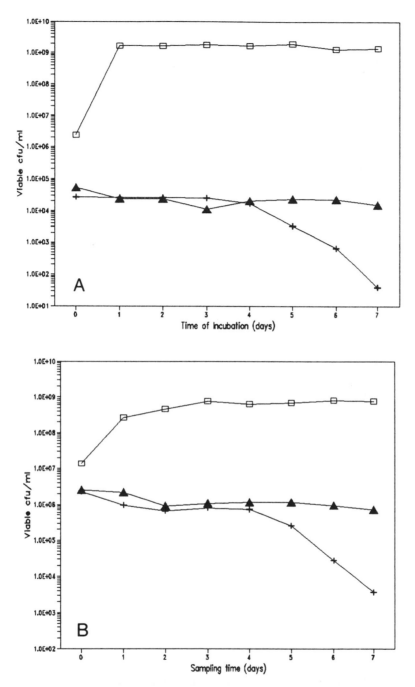

FIG. 2. Ability of *Aeromonas* strain M94 to reduce the number of viable *L. pneumophila* cells in coculture in tap water plus (a) UNBCYEA slope, (b) 0.025% yeast extract, (c) 0.0025% yeast extract, and (d) tap water sediment. Symbols: □, number of M94 cells per milliliter; +, number of viable *L. pneumophila* cells present in the *L. pneumophila*-M94 coculture; ▲, number of viable *L. pneumophila* cells in the control coculture.

pound over the incubation time in the coculture vessel.

Keevil (5a) has also noticed that the introduction of *Aeromonas* cells to a biofilm known to contain viable *L. pneumophila* cells results in the inability to recover *L. pneumophila* cells from the biofilm or reintroduce *L. pneumophila* cells into the biofilm.

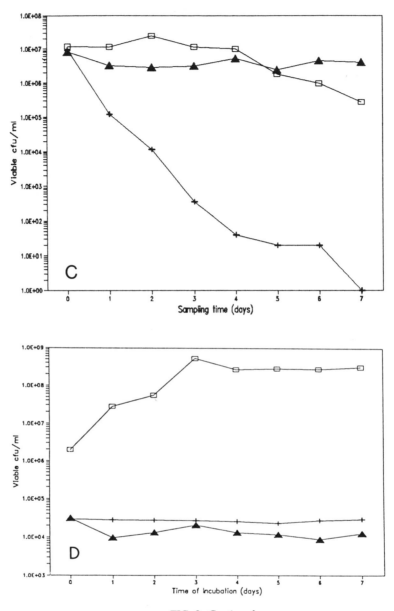

FIG. 2. *Continued.*

In conclusion, the results presented here demonstrate that non-*Legionella* bacteria originally isolated from environmental water samples are capable of decreasing the survival of *L. pneumophila* cells in conditions approaching those found in aquatic environments. Further work is needed to determine (i) what factors would influence the production of these inhibitory effects produced by inhibitory bacteria in the natural, nonsterile aquatic environment and (ii) the identities and modes of action of the inhibiting compounds produced by inhibitory non-*Legionella* bacteria.

REFERENCES

1. **Bohach, G. A., and I. S. Snyder.** 1983. Cyanobacterial stimulation of growth and oxygen uptake by *Legionella pneumophila. Appl. Environ. Microbiol.* **46:**528–531.
2. **Cahill, M. M.** 1990. Virulence factors in motile *Aeromonas* species. *J. Appl. Bacteriol.* **69:**1–16.
3. **Fields, B. S., G. N. Sanden, J. M. Barbaree, W. E.**

Morrill, R. M. Wadowsky, E. H. White, and J. C. Feeley. 1989. Intracellular multiplication of *Legionella pneumophila* in amoebae isolated from hospital hot water tanks. *Curr. Microbiol.* **18**:131–137.

4. Flesher, A. R., D. L. Kasper, P. A. Modern, and E. O. Mason. 1980. *Legionella pneumophila*: growth inhibition by human pharyngeal flora. *J. Infect. Dis.* **142**:313–317.

5. Fliermans, C. B., W. B. Cherry, L. H. Orrison, and L. Thacker. 1978. Isolation of *Legionella pneumophila* from non-epidemic environments. *Appl Environ. Microbiol.* **41**:9–16.

5a. Keevil, W. Personal communication.

6. Makin, T. 1986. Inhibition of *Legionella* by other organisms. *Med. Lab. Sci.* **43**:S54.

7. Ortiz-Roque, C. M., and T. C. Hazen. 1987. Abundance and distribution of *Legionellaceae* in Puerto Rican waters. *Appl. Environ. Microbiol.* **53**:2231–2236.

8. Stout, J. E., and M. G. Best. 1985. Ecology of *Legionella pneumophila* within water distribution systems. *Appl. Environ. Microbiol.* **49**:221–228.

9. Toze, S., L. I. Sly, I. C. MacRae, and J. A. Fuerst. 1990. Inhibition of growth of *Legionella* species by heterotrophic plate count bacteria isolated from chlorinated drinking water. *Curr. Microbiol.* **21**:139–143.

10. Wadowsky, R. M., and R. B. Yee. 1985. Effect of non-*Legionella* bacteria on the multiplication of *Legionella pneumophila* in potable water. *Appl. Environ. Microbiol.* **49**:1206–1210.

Rapid Thermal Disinfection of *Legionella*-Contaminated Water with a Drip Coffee Maker

WILLIAM E. MAHER, BARBARA HACKMAN, AND JOSEPH F. PLOUFFE

Department of Internal Medicine, Division of Infectious Diseases, The Ohio State University College of Medicine, 410 West 10th Avenue, Columbus, Ohio 43210-1228

Nosocomial Legionnaires disease has been linked to *Legionella pneumophila* contamination of hospital potable water systems, although the exact route of transmission has not been firmly established. There is evidence to support airborne transmission, but these associations may have been confounded, and cases have occurred without exposure to any of these factors. Both oropharyngeal colonization with subsequent aspiration and dissemination from the gastrointestinal tract have been suggested by epidemiologic, pathologic, and animal model data. Ingestion of potable water contaminated with *L. pneumophila* has not been excluded as a major route of transmission of nosocomial Legionnaires disease (7).

Extrapulmonary legionellosis has been reported as an unusual complication of concurrent or recent pulmonary infection with *L. pneumophila* (2, 3, 5). Extrapulmonary infection has been reported without coexistent or prior pulmonary infection (1, 6, 11), and in two cases (1, 6), the probable route of infection was soiling of wounds with potable water contaminated with legionellae.

Provision of *Legionella*-free water for patient consumption and routine nursing care may be underutilized in efforts to control the incidence of nosocomial legionellosis. Our previous experience with in-line filtration as a method of tap water sterilization (12) and concern for the cost and quality of bottled water led us to explore alternative methods for providing *Legionella*-free water for these purposes. We conducted a pilot study, rapid decontamination of 1- to 2-liter volumes of *Legionella*-seeded water in a drip coffee maker.

A Koffee King coffee maker (Bloomfield Industries, Chicago, Ill.) was used in all experiments. This type of coffee maker has an internal reservoir (approximately 2,700 ml) in which water is held at an elevated temperature. Once the reservoir is filled with tap water and the green "ready to brew" light on the front panel is lit, rapid dumping of a pot of cold tap water (approximately 1.6 liters) into the machine delivers an equal volume of hot water (approximately 82°C) over a 2- to 3-min interval. All coffee pots were sterilized prior to use.

Environmental *L. pneumophila* serogroup 1 strain UH-1 (8) was isolated and subcultured on buffered charcoal-yeast extract (BCYE) plates (Remel, Lenexa, Kans.). This isolate was passaged at most four times prior to these experiments.

Legionellae were grown on a BCYE plate for 72 h in air at 35°C and suspended in sterile H_2O. From this suspension, three separate 5-liter inocula were prepared by dilution with double-distilled water (approximately 10^5, 10^6, and 10^7 CFU/ml, respectively). In all cases, legionellae were enumerated by serial dilution in sterile water and spread plating on BCYE plates.

Legionella inocula were poured a pot at a time into the coffee maker, the effluent was collected, and the temperature was noted. Five milliliters of effluent was placed in a capped polypropylene tube. This sample was allowed to cool to room temperature, and a 0.1-ml aliquot was cultured on a BCYE plate. The remainder of the effluent, approximately 1.6 liters, was allowed to cool to 61 to 65°C and was filtered through a 0.45-μm-pore-

TABLE 1. Isolation of *L. pneumophila* from a coffee maker[a]

Log$_{10}$ *L. pneumophila* inoculum	Temp (°C) of effluent	CFU/0.1 ml of effluent	CFU/1.6 liters of effluent filtrate	CFU/0.1 ml of effluent 24 h at 22°C	Log$_{10}$ CFU of *L. pneumophila*/ml after 24 h at 22°C
5.2	79	0	3 *Bacillus* sp.	0	5.1
	82	0	1 *Bacillus* sp.	0	5.1
	82	1 GNR	0	0	5.1
6.2	82	0	1 GNR	0	6.1
	82	0	1 *Bacillus* sp., 1 GNR	0	6.1
	83	0	1 GNR	1 *Bacillus* sp.	6.1
7.2	83	0	1 *Bacillus* sp.	0	7.2
	81	0	0	1 *Bacillus* sp., 2 GPC	7.2
	82	1 GPC, 1 GNR	2 *Bacillus* sp.	0	7.2

[a]GNR, gram-negative rod, not *Legionella* sp.; GPC, gram-positive coccus. No legionellae were isolated from effluent, effluent filtrate, or effluent after 24 h of incubation at 22°C.

size filter (Metricel; Gelman, Ann Arbor, Mich.). This filter was then placed on a BCYE plate and incubated at 35°C for 7 days (as were all BCYE plates). The remainder of the 5-ml sample was incubated at room temperature (22°C) for 24 h, when another 0.1 ml was cultured on a BCYE plate. Colonies were counted and identified by standard techniques to the extent necessary.

Results are displayed in Table 1. Effluent temperatures were in the range of 79 to 83°C. Despite inocula in excess of 10^{10} organisms, no legionellae were isolated from any cultures. The only bacterial isolates were *Bacillus* sp. and nonfermentative oxidase-negative gram-negative rods and gram-positive cocci (0 to 3 CFU). Incubation of effluents for 24 h at room temperature did not result in regrowth of bacteria. Parallel incubation of unprocessed inocula showed minimal if any decline in titer of the *L. pneumophila* over the same time period. Pretreatment of 0.45-μm-pore-size filters with 10 ml of hot (78°C) sterile water had no impact on the quantitative recovery of organisms from a standardized *L. pneumophila* suspension via this filtration technique (data not shown).

The data presented above indicate that a Koffee King coffee maker can rapidly decontaminate water that has been seeded with rather large numbers of *L. pneumophila*. Absence of organisms in the immediate culture of 0.1 ml indicates as much as a 6-log$_{10}$ kill of legionellae by passage through the coffee maker. This finding is consistent with published thermal labilities of legionellae (10). Absence of organisms in the whole-pot filtrates supports killing of all legionellae (up to 10^{10} organisms) by this process. That preheating the filters had no impact on recovery of legionellae from a standard suspension suggests that this observation is not a methodologic artifact. It is important to stress these quantitative aspects, as potable water may be heavily contaminated with legionellae at times (> 10^4 CFU/ml [9]), and sternotomy infections may have been caused by contamination

levels as low as 20 to 50 CFU/50 ml of tap water (6). Lack of regrowth of organisms, i.e., a negative culture of a 0.1-ml aliquot after 24 h of incubation at 22°C, is reassuring as well, but filtration of a larger volume of water may have been a more appropriate assay. Our data cannot totally exclude the possibility that low levels of organisms (10 CFU/ml or less) recovered from the heat stress at 24 h, but given the temperatures and times used, this seems unlikely (10).

Coffee maker processed hot water could be mixed with smaller amounts of sterile water to make appropriate temperature bath water or could be stored and used when it has reached the appropriate temperature for bathing or drinking. Depending on the volumes needed, tap water processed through such a coffee maker could be used to fill whirlpool baths or to replace sterile water in nebulizers used in the home. It is doubtful that the low numbers of nonpathogenic organisms isolated from effluent cultures would be of any clinical significance in these contexts. Because water temperatures in excess of 80°C are used, care to avoid scalding must be taken, and this factor must enter into any consideration of routine use of this form of disinfection (4).

Other, more conventional human pathogens have thermal labilities similar to those of legionellae (10). It is foreseeable, then, that coffee maker disinfection of potable water could be used to control transmission of other waterborne diseases (e.g., enteric diseases).

We used the Koffee King coffee maker because of the rapid delivery of hot water afforded by the reservoir design. A survey of other, less expensive coffee makers such as a Mr. Coffee showed that effluent temperatures were similar to that provided by the Koffee King, although the lack of a reservoir resulted in longer delivery times. Coffee maker disinfection of contaminated water may be an inexpensive and readily available means of microbiologic water purification for a variety of applications.

REFERENCES

1. **Brabender, W., D. R. Hinthorn, M. Asher, N. J. Lindsey, and C. Liu.** 1983. *Legionella pneumophila* wound infection. *JAMA* **250**:3091–3092.
2. **Dorman, S. A., N. J. Hardin, and W. C. Winn, Jr.** 1981. Pyelonephritis associated with *Legionella pneumophila* serogroup 4. *Ann. Intern. Med.* **93**:835–837.
3. **Kalweit, W. H., W. C. Winn, Jr., T. A. Rocco, Jr., and J. C. Girod.** 1982. Hemodialysis fistula infections caused by *Legionella pneumophila. Ann. Intern. Med.* **96**:173–175.
4. **Katcher, M. L.** 1981. Scald burns from hot tap water. *JAMA* **246**:1219–1222.
5. **Landes, B. W., G. W. Pogson, G. D. Beauchamp, R. K. Skillman, and J. H. Brewer.** 1982. Pericarditis in a patient with Legionnaires' disease. *Arch. Intern. Med.* **142**:1234–1235.
6. **Lowry, P. W., R. J. Blankenship, W. Gridley, N. J. Troup, and L. S. Tompkins.** 1991. A cluster of legionella sternal-wound infections due to postoperative topical exposure to contaminated tap water. *N. Engl. J. Med.* **324**:109–113.
7. **Muder, R. R., V. L. Yu, and A. H. Woo.** 1986. Mode of transmission of *Legionella pneumophila,* a critical review. *Arch. Intern. Med.* **146**:1607–1612.
8. **Plouffe, J. F., M. F. Para, W. E. Maher, B. Hackman, and L. Webster.** 1983. Subtypes of *Legionella pneumophila* serogroup 1 associated with different attack rates. *Lancet* **ii**:649–650.
9. **Snyder, M. B., M. Siwicki, J. Wireman, D. Pohlod, M. Grimes, S. Bowman-Riney, and L. D. Saravolatz.** 1990. Reduction in *Legionella pneumophila* through heat flushing followed by continuous supplemental chlorination of hospital hot water. *J. Infect. Dis.* **162**:127–132.
10. **Stout, J. E., M. G. Best, and V. L. Yu.** 1986. Susceptibility of members of the family *Legionellaceae* to thermal stress: implications for heat eradication methods in water distribution systems. *Appl. Environ. Microbiol.* **52**:396–399.
11. **Tompkins, L. S., B. J. Roessler, S. C. Redd, L. E. Markowitz, and M. L. Cohen.** 1988. Legionella prosthetic-valve endocarditis. *N. Engl. J. Med.* **318**:530–535.
12. **Webster, L. R., M. F. Para, B. A. Hackman, and P. A. Kulich.** 1985. Effectiveness of in-line and terminal filtration for sterilization of potable water for compromised patients. *Abstr. 12th Annu. Assoc. Pract. Infect. Control Educ. Conf.*

Phenotypic and Genotypic Variability of *Legionella pneumophila* Populating Potable Waters and Patients of a Tertiary-Care Hospital over a Five-Year Period

G. S. BEZANSON, J. JOLY, S. M. BURBRIDGE, R. D. KUEHN, D. J. M. HALDANE, AND T. J. MARRIE

Departments of Microbiology and Medicine, Dalhousie University and Victoria General Hospital, Halifax, Nova Scotia, B3H 1V8, and Department of Microbiology, Université Laval, Quebec G1K 7P4, Canada

During the period 1983 to 1989, 43 cases of Legionnaires disease occurred among patients in the Victoria General Hospital. In a case control study, we established that aspiration of potable water was the most likely source of infection in a significant number of these patients (8). Serologic and molecular analysis of sets of patient and environmental isolates of *Legionella pneumophila* matched for isolation date and room number supported this conclusion. We now have completed the characterization of a much larger number of isolates from both sources. As described below, the data define the composition of the two populations, establish their relatedness, and provide a measure of their long-term stabilities.

For environmental sampling, approximately 200 ml of mixed hot and cold water was drawn from each of 20 sampling sites in the two main patient care buildings (10 sites in each building) at intervals of 3 to 5 weeks. The specimens from patients included bronchial washings, sputa, and lung tissue. Standard methods were used to isolate *L. pneumophila*. Direct fluorescent antibody staining and failure to grow on blood agar were used as confirmatory tests. Isolates were maintained on buffered charcoal-yeast extract agar or frozen at -70°C. Monoclonal antibody (MAb) subtyping by indirect immunofluorescence microscopy was conducted as described by Joly et al. (6) Plasmids were extracted from buffered charcoal-yeast extract-grown cells by using a modified alkaline detergent procedure (3). Chromosomal DNA for use as a substrate for restriction endonuclease digestion was prepared according to the guanidium isothiocyanate procedure of Pitcher et al. (10). Endonucleases were used as recommended by the manufacturers. Electrophoretic separations were completed in vertical 0.75% agarose slab gels.

A total of 406 *Legionella* isolates were obtained during the 1983 to 1989 sampling period. The vast majority (>99%) of these were *L. pneumophila* serogroup 1 (Lp1). Only one isolate each of *L. micdadei* and *L. bozemanii* was recovered. Representative numbers of Lp1 from each yearly period were characterized as to MAb subtype, plasmid type (PT), and chromosomal endonuclease fragmentation pattern (FP). The first parameter was considered to delineate phenotype; the others considered to delineate genotype. In combination, they defined a particular strain-type. Because systematic sampling did not commence until 1986, the few (i.e., 16) isolates recovered between 1983 and 1985 were treated as a single group.

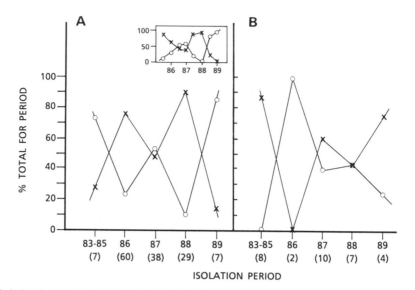

FIG. 1. Variation in the incidence of isolates displaying MAb subtypes OLDA (×) and Oxford (○) among *L. pneumophila* isolates recovered from hospital potable water (A) and patients (B) during 1983 to 1989. The small number of isolates available from 1983 to 1985 necessitated their being grouped for purposes of analysis. The insert in panel A represents the same data plotted in 6-month steps in order to verify the 12-month pattern. Numbers in parentheses indicate the total sample size for each period.

Thirty-four patient and 141 water isolates were subjected to MAb subtyping. Four subtypes were detected, the two most prevalent of which were OLDA and Oxford (65 and 33% of the total). Subtypes Camperdown and Philadelphia each occurred once, in water and a patient, respectively. Lp1 isolates displaying the OLDA and Oxford subtypes were detected concurrently in both sources. The prevalence of these two subtypes varied considerably over the study period, regardless of their origin (Fig. 1). Within each source group, an increase in the incidence of one subtype was accompanied by a decrease in the other. Changes in the environmental types (Fig. 1A) were not reflected in the patient population (Fig. 1B).

Eight distinct patterns were observed among the 314 water and 34 patient isolates screened for their plasmid contents. The plasmids ranged in mass from 20 to 103 MDa, with a maximum of two plasmids per isolate. No plasmidless isolates were detected. Specimens that yielded more than 10 colonies per plate were homogeneous with regard to the PT of the Lp1 recovered. Each environmental site tended to be colonized continuously by Lp1 of a particular PT (7). The three most prominent PTs, II (20-MDa plasmid), III (72- and 96-MDa plasmids), and VI (100-MDa plasmid), accounted for 59, 24, and 14%, respectively, of the types seen. All three PTs were isolated concurrently from patients and potable waters. The prevalence of each type varied with time (Fig. 2). In contrast to the MAb subtypes, the change in the

prevalence of each PT was more gradual and less cyclic and was mirrored in each source group. Isolates belonging to PT VI were detected in potable water 18 months prior to their appearance in patients.

The 81 water and 34 patient isolates examined displayed four distinct endonuclease FPs upon digestion of their chromosomes with *Eco*RI or *Bgl*II. The two most prominent FPs, b and d, were detected in 67 and 29%, respectively, of the Lp1 isolates. Strains with these FPs occurred concurrently in both water and patients. Because the b and d patterns were very closely related, double digestion with endonucleases *Hpa*I and *Hpa*II was used to resolve discrepancies (13). As observed with the first genotypic parameter, the change in the prevalence of the two FPs was gradual and of long periodicity (Fig. 3). Change in the two patterns within the environmental isolates was reflected in the patient isolates only after a delay of approximately 24 months (compare Fig. 3A and B). The relative incidence of the two types appeared to be inversely related.

By combining the single phenotype with the two genotypes, we were able to assign strain types to 39 water and 27 patient isolates. Of the resultant 18 types, 6 were recovered from both water and patients, but only 4 of them (IIb/OLDA, IIb/Oxford, IId/OLDA, and IId/Oxford) were detected in both sources concurrently. Strain-types IIb/OLDA and IIb/Oxford were the most prevalent, accounting for 33 and 22% of the isolates grouped this way.

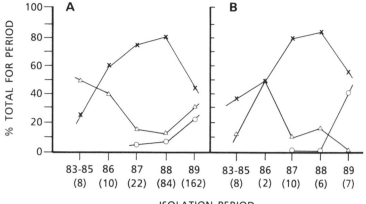

FIG. 2. Variation in the incidence of isolates displaying PTs II (×), III (△), and VI (○) among the *L. pneumophila* isolates recovered from hospital potable water (A) and patients (B) during 1983 to 1989. Numbers in parentheses indicate the total sample size for each period.

Together, these data indicate that the *Legionella* population of our hospital is heterogeneous in composition. However, just two MAb subtypes, three PTs, and two FPs consistently formed greater than 90% of the whole (patient plus water) population. We have completed a similar analysis of the Lp1 populations of four other health care institutions in our area (1). With one exception, they too display such limited heterogeneity.

Although the number of types constituting our Lp1 population remained constant, their proportions relative to each other varied over time. MAb reactivity, the only phenotypic property monitored, changed its predominant type most frequently. The more gradual, but persistent, shifts observed in PTs and FPs also attest to this dynamic nature. However, this variability (lack of stability?) was tempered by the apparent limitation

on the number of alternatives available for use. Such controlled variability might produce an effective homogeneity within the whole population.

The data also provide support for potable water being the most likely source of patient infections in our hospital. Lp1 possessing the same genotypic and phenotypic properties occurred simultaneously in patients and hospital waters. The particular trait displayed varied with time, but a type corresponding to that recovered from the patient was always present in the environment. Further, in the case of the genotypic traits, the variations themselves were significant. Changes in the relative proportion of certain isolate types within the water system were mirrored in the patient population. This was particularly evident with PTs. It is noteworthy in this regard that PT VI did not appear among patient isolates until it

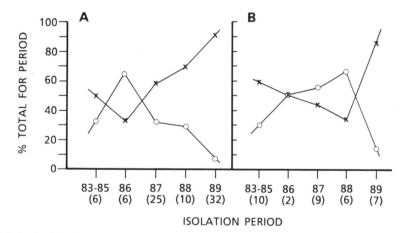

FIG. 3. Variation in the incidence of isolates displaying restriction endonuclease FPs b (×) and d (○) among the *L. pneumophila* isolates recovered from hospital potable water (A) and patients (B) during 1983 to 1989. Numbers in parentheses indicate the total sample size for each period.

had become well established in the environment (20% incidence). The clonal nature of this spread was established by extensive endonuclease analysis of the 100-MDa plasmid after its extraction from selected patient and water isolates (not shown).

The high prevalence of MAb subtypes OLDA and Oxford appears to be unique to our area. Subtypes Pontiac, Allentown, and Philadelphia predominated among the *Legionella* isolates obtained from patients and the environment in Los Angeles, Pittsburgh, and Iowa, respectively, during the period 1980 to 1986 (5, 9, 12). In the United Kingdom and Europe, Watkins et al. (14) found subtype Pontiac to be predominant in patients and in buildings in which infections had occurred, while subtype OLDA prevailed in buildings without human infections. The Iowa study detected subtype Oxford in only 4 of 35 environmental isolates and OLDA in one community-acquired pneumonia.

L. pneumophila isolates belonging to MAb subtypes Pontiac, Allentown, and Philadelphia react with MAb 2 of the international panel (6). The high association between these particular subtypes and human infection has prompted the suggestion that reactivity with MAb 2 be used as a virulence marker for Lp1 (4, 12). Neither subtype OLDA nor subtype Oxford reacts with MAb 2, yet they were the only subtypes isolated from patients in our hospital. Studies to be reported elsewhere demonstrate that these subtypes are as virulent in guinea pigs as those reacting with MAb 2 (1a). Clearly other markers for Lp1 virulence are needed.

A number of authors have presented data that suggest that plasmid carriage may be negatively correlated with *Legionella* virulence (2, 11, 12). They have observed that patient isolates (that is, "virulent" strains) were more likely to be plasmid-free than those from the environment. Since there were no plasmidless Lp1 organisms detected among the 352 isolates examined in our study, including the 34 recovered from patients, this finding does not appear to apply in our area.

In summary, our data reveal that the Lp1 population of the Victoria General Hospital is heterogeneous in nature but of restricted membership. The results suggest that the imposition of such limits on constituent types determines the long-term stability of the population. Finally, our data confirm the potable water supply of the hospital as the most likely source of patient infections.

This work was supported by grant MT-10577 from the Medical Research Council of Canada. The enthusiastic assistance of the VGH Infection Control nurses, the staff of the Respiratory Microbiology Laboratory, and D. Ramsay, Laval University, is gratefully acknowledged.

REFERENCES

1. **Bezanson, G. S., S. Burbridge, D. Haldane, C. Yoell, and T. Marrie.** 1992. Diverse populations of *Legionella pneumophila* present in geographically clustered institutions served by the same water reservoir. *J. Clin. Microbiol.* **30:**570–576.

1a. **Bezanson, G. S., et al.** Unpublished data.

2. **Brown, A., R. M. Vickers, E. M. Elder, M. Lema, and G. M. Carrity.** 1982 Plasmid and surface antigen markers of endemic and epidemic *Legionella pneumophila* strains. *J. Clin. Microbiol.* **16:**230–235.

3. **Dillon, J. R., G. S. Bezanson, and K. H. Yeung.** 1985. Basic techniques, p. 1–126. *In* J. R. Dillon, A. Nasim, and E. Nestman (ed.), *Recombinant DNA Methodology.* J. Wiley & Sons, Inc., Toronto.

4. **Dournon, E., W. F. Bibb, P. Rajogophan, N. Desplaces, and R. M. McKinney.** 1988. Monoclonal antibody reactivity as a virulence marker for *Legionella pneumophila* serogroup 1 strains. *J. Infect. Dis.* **157:**496–501.

5. **Edelstein, P. H., C. Nakahama, J. Tobin, K. Calarco, K. B. Berr, J. R. Joly, and R. K. Selander.** 1986. Paleo-epidemiologic investigation of Legionnaires' disease at Wadsworth Veterans Administration Hospital by using three typing methods for comparison of legionellae from clinical and environmental sources. *J. Clin. Microbiol.* **23:**1121–1126.

6. **Joly, J. R., R. M. McKinney, J. O. Tobin, W. F. Bibb, I. D. Watkins, and D. Ramsay.** 1986. Development of a standardized subgrouping scheme for *Legionella pneumophila* serogroup 1 using monoclonal antibodies. *J. Clin. Microbiol.* **23:**768–711.

7. **Marrie, T. J., D. Haldane, G. Bezanson, and R. Peppard.** Each outlet is a unique ecological niche for *Legionella pneumophila. Epidemiol. Infect.* **108:**261–270.

8. **Marrie, T. J., D. Haldane, S. MacDonald, K. Clarke, C. Fanning, S. LeFort-Jost, G. Bezanson, and J. Joly.** 1991. Control of endemic nosocomial Legionnaires' disease by using sterile potable water for high risk patients. *Epidemiol. Infect.* **107:**591–605.

9. **Pfaller, M., R. Hollis, W. Johnson, R. M. Massaneri, C. Helms, R. Wenzel, N. Hall, N. Moyer, and J. Joly.** 1989. The application of molecular and immunologic techniques to study the epidemiology of *Legionella pneumophila* serogroup 1. *Diagn. Microbiol. Infect. Dis.* **12:**295–302.

10. **Pitcher, D. G., N. A. Saunders, and R. J. Owen.** 1989. Rapid extraction of bacterial genomic DNA with guanidium thiocyanate. *Lett. Appl. Microbiol.* **8:**151–156.

11. **Plouffe, J. F., M. F. Para, W. E. Maher, B. Hackman, and L. Webster.** 1983. Subtypes of *Legionella pneumophila* serogroup 1 associated with different attack rates. *Lancet* **55:**649–650.

12. **Stout, J. E., J. Joly, M. Para, J. Plouffe, C. Ciesilski, M. J. Blaser, and V. L. Yu.** 1988. Comparison of molecular methods for subtyping patients and epidemiologically linked environmental isolates of *Legionella pneumophila. J. Infect. Dis.* **157:**486–495.

13. **van Ketel, J. R.** 1988. Similar DNA restriction endonuclease profiles in strains of *Legionella pneumophila* from different serogroups. *J. Clin. Microbiol.* **26:**1838–1841.

14. **Watkins, I. D., J. O. Tobin, P. J. Dennis, W. Brown, R. Newnham, and J. B. Kurtz.** 1985. *Legionella pneumophila* serogroup 1 subgrouping by monoclonal antibodies—an epidemiological tool. *J. Hyg.* **95:**211–216.

Reducing Risks Associated with *Legionella* Bacteria in Building Water Systems

B. G. SHELTON, G. K. MORRIS, AND G. W. GORMAN

Pathcon Laboratories, Norcross, Georgia 30092

Building water systems may serve as amplifiers of *Legionella* bacteria and as a source of outbreaks. We analyzed data on 900 samples from buildings where outbreaks of Legionnaires disease had occurred, buildings thought to be associated with sporadic cases of Legionnaires disease, and buildings with no disease. The numbers of legionellae in water samples were determined, and results were categorized by source. Hazard categories were developed for each source, with category 5 being the highest and corresponding to the upper 5th percentile. We analyzed samples from three outbreaks, and all three contained numbers of legionellae in hazard level 5. Therefore, we suggest that the risk of Legionnaires disease outbreaks is associated with amplified numbers of legionellae in building water systems and that the incidence may be reduced by taking steps to reduce the numbers of legionellae when the hazard level is high.

Public health officials usually do not recommend environmental sampling for *Legionella* bacteria in the absence of an outbreak, partially because no data are available to predict the efficacy or cost-benefit of such efforts for sporadic cases (5). Water samples from cooling towers and evaporative condensers were collected from across the country. Most potable waters in this study were pre- and postflush samples collected from the hot water systems through outlets capable of emitting an aerosol (shower or spray nozzles, faucets, etc.). These methods included direct inoculation of the sample on buffered charcoal-yeast extract agar containing selective antibiotics and glycine (1). Depending on the preliminary microbiological analysis, samples were sometimes concentrated by filtration or acid treated to suppress competing microflora (3) and then analyzed further.

Positive samples were summarized according to the building water source (Table 1). Although 45% of cooling towers and evaporative condensers and 20% of potable water samples were positive, it is rare to find legionellae in humidifiers, air washers, and condensate waters. Some of the samples yielded legionellae from a hospital cooling tower that was determined to be associated with an outbreak of three cases. The cooling water was shown to have *Legionella pneumophila* serogroup 1 monoclonal antibody subtypes 1, 6 and 1, 2, 5, 6 at levels over 3,000 CFU/ml. No legionellae were recovered from any samples from inside the hospital, even after a thorough investigation of the potable water system. The patient isolates of all three cases were *L. pneumophila* serogroup 1 monoclonal antibody subtype 1, 2, 5, 6.

Some samples were received from potable water sources in a community care home where a confirmed outbreak of multiple cases of Legionnaires disease occurred. *L. pneumophila* serogroup 1 of the same monoclonal antibody subtype as the outbreak strain was isolated from water samples from multiple sites in the community care home. The numbers ranged from less than 1 to 1,500 CFU/ml (average, 162 CFU/ml).

A reservoir water sample was received from a mister/fogger device that was epidemiologically associated with an outbreak of Legionnaires disease among adult shoppers who came in close contact with the mist. *L. pneumophila* serogroup 1 of the same monoclonal antibody subtype as the outbreak strain was isolated from the reservoir water. The number of legionellae in the sample was 10 CFU/ml.

Many people with the responsibility for maintaining the air quality in buildings and industrial settings require programs designed to detect po-

TABLE 1. Quantitative analysis of *Legionella* bacteria in environmental samples

Water source	% of samples in each category					Total % positive
	<1 CFU/ml	1–9 CFU/ml	10–99 CFU/ml	100–999 CFU/ml	≥1,000 CFU/ml	
Cooling tower (*n* = 244)	4	7	22	8	4	45
Potable hot water (*n* = 342)	7	2	6	4	1	20
Mister/foggers[a] (*n* = 28)	0	0	22	4	4	29
Condensates (*n* = 44)	0	0	0	0	0	0
Humidifiers/air wash (*n* = 87)	0	0	0	0	0	0
Other nonpotable (*n* = 82)	5	4	2	2	0	13

[a]Most were reservoir type.

TABLE 2. Suggested remedial action criteria for legionellae

Legionellae/ml	Remedial action[a] if detected in:		
	Cooling towers and evaporative condensers	Potable water	Humidifier/fogger
Detectable, but < 1	1	2	3
1–9	2	3	4
10–99	3	4	5
100–999	4	5	5
≥ 1,000	5	5	5

[a]See Table 3.

tential problems with legionellae. We have developed quantitative criteria for legionellae and propose remedial actions (Tables 2 and 3). These quantitative data are based on numbers of viable legionellae because the health risk from nonviable legionellae has not been documented. These criteria are based on the presumption that the likelihood of human infections is dose related; i.e., the higher the number of organisms to which people are exposed, the more likely that they will become infected. Best and coworkers (2) noted an association of Legionnaires disease with the prevalence of legionellae in the environment. They found that the incidence of Legionnaires disease decreased when environmental *Legionella* levels were lowered. These criteria take into consideration the number of *Legionella* bacteria in the building water system and the type of building water system involved.

Outbreaks were associated with building equipment representing each of the three building equipment system categories in Table 2. For each of the three outbreaks, the environmental samples contained legionellae in hazard level 5, indicating that hazard level 5 (amplified *Legionella* levels representing approximately the upper 5th percentile) may be associated with outbreaks. It is highly significant that none of the three outbreaks were in hazard levels 1 through 4. It is noteworthy that for all three outbreaks, once the implicated source was removed or treated to reduce the levels, no further cases had occurred as of at least April 1990.

The presence of legionellae in building water

TABLE 3. Remedial actions

Hazard level	Actions
1	Review routine maintenance program recommended by the manufacturer of the equipment to ensure that the recommended program is being followed. The presence of barely detectable numbers of legionellae represents a low level of concern.
2	Implement action 1. Conduct follow-up analysis after a few weeks for evidence of further *Legionella* amplification. This level of legionellae represents little concern, but the number of organisms detected indicates that the system is a potential amplifier for legionellae.
3	Implement action 2. Conduct review of premises for direct and indirect bioaerosol contact with occupants and health risk status of people who may come in contact with the bioaerosols. Depending on the results of the review of the premises, action related to cleaning and/or biocide treatment of the equipment may be indicated. This level of legionellae represents a low but increased level of concern.
4	Implement Action 3. Cleaning and/or biocide treatment of the equipment is indicated. This level of legionellae represents a moderately high level of concern, since it is approaching levels that may cause outbreaks. It is uncommon for samples to contain numbers of legionellae that fall in this category.
5	Immediate cleaning and/or biocide treatment of the equipment is definitely indicated. Conduct posttreatment analysis to ensure effectiveness of the corrective action. The level of legionellae represents a high level of concern, since it poses the potential for causing an outbreak. It is very uncommon for samples to contain numbers of legionellae that fall in this category.

systems at hazard level 5 is not necessarily a danger to building occupants. Some of the samples that we found to be in hazard level 5 were not associated with human disease. In these situations, the water source may not be aerosolized and disseminated in such a way that viable bacteria will reach the lungs of the target person, or the contaminated source may be sufficiently distant from the target person that exposure to an infectious dose does not occur. Of utmost importance, however, is the fact that most cases of Legionnaires disease occur as sporadic cases, not as outbreak clusters. It is possible that long-term exposure to low levels of legionellae causes some of the sporadic cases. It is also possible that some sporadic cases are associated with an outbreak, with the outbreak and its source being unrecognized. It has been recommended that immunocompromised individuals not be exposed to any legionellae (4). Results of this study suggest a strong association of exposure to amplified legionellae with Legionnaires disease outbreaks. Therefore, we think it is prudent for building and hospital managers to err on the side of safety, taking preventative maintenance steps when amplified levels of legionellae are detected.

REFERENCES

1. **Barbaree, J. M., G. W. Gorman, W. T. Martin, B. S. Fields, and W. E. Morrill.** 1987. Protocol for sampling environmental sites for legionellae. *Appl. Environ. Microbiol.* **53**:1454–1458.
2. **Best, M., V. L. Yu, J. Stout, A. Goetz, R. R. Muder, and F. Taylor.** 1983. Legionellaceae in the hospital water supply. Epidemiologic link with disease and evaluation of a method for control of nosocomial Legionnaires' disease and Pittsburgh pneumonia. *Lancet* **ii**:307–310.
3. **Bopp, C. A., J. W. Summer, G. K. Morris, and J. G. Wells.** 1981. Isolation of *Legionella* spp. from environmental water samples by low-pH treatment and use of a selective medium. *J. Clin. Microbiol.* **13**:714–719.
4. **Helms, C. M., R. M. Massanari, R. Zeitler, S. Streed, M. J. R. Gilchrist, N. Hall, W. J. Hausler, Jr., J. Sywassink, W. Johnson, L. Wintermeyer, and W. J. Hierholzer, Jr.** 1983. Legionnaires' disease associated with a hospital water system: a cluster of 24 nosocomial cases. *Ann. Intern. Med.* **99**:172–178.
5. **Redd, S. C., and M. L. Cohen.** 1987. Legionella in water: what should be done? *JAMA* **257**:1221–1222.

Investigation and Control of Nosocomial Legionnaires Disease in Zaragoza, Spain

R. GOMEZ-LUS, P. GOMEZ-LUS, C. GARCIA, L. GOMEZ-LOPEZ, AND M. C. RUBIO

Department of Microbiology, School of Medicine, University of Zaragoza, C/ Domingo Miral s/n, 50009 Zaragoza, Spain

The incidence of nosocomial legionellosis has varied greatly, but we know that *Legionella* infection is widespread throughout the world and is particularly prevalent in the Mediterranean countries. Legionellosis acquired by foreign tourists during visits to Spain has been frequently documented (1–3, 5, 7, 8). To our knowledge, data on Legionnaires disease (LD) acquired by tourists in the Comunidad Autonóma de Aragon have not been included in any of the publications cited above. This paper reports the first two outbreaks of nosocomial LD (NLD) diagnosed at our hospital between October 1984 and July 1985. We also report an investigation of the plumbing system in a military residence (MR) after 30 cases of LD occurred.

Hospital discharge records, laboratory records, and infection surveillance data were reviewed to identify cases of legionellosis. In our study, one case of NLD was defined as acute pneumonia associated with a fourfold rise in *Legionella* antibody titer to 125, a single convalescent titer of ≥256, or a positive culture of respiratory secretions for *Legionella pneumophila* and onset of symptoms of pneumonia 2 to 10 days after exposure to the hospital environment. Two outbreaks of NLD occurred in a 900-bed university hospital during October and November 1984 (seven cases) and during May and July 1985 (seven cases). The ages of the patients ranged from 29 to 87 years (mean, 51 years); the male/female ratio was 1. Eleven (78.5%) of the patients were receiving immunosuppressive therapy. Fatality rates were 42.8% for the first outbreak and 57.1% for the second outbreak.

Hot water taps from patient areas in the hospital were cultured for the presence of *L. pneumophila*. For each culture, taps were turned on and the initial 500 ml of water was collected. The inside of the tap was swabbed, and the swab was inoculated onto a buffered charcoal-yeast extract–0.1% α-ketoglutarate (BCYE) agar plate. In addition, 250 ml of each sample was filtered through a 0.45-μm-pore-size Millipore membrane, and then the membrane was placed on the BCYE agar plate. Serogroup 1 strains of *L. pneumophila* were isolated from the 13 shower heads and the 52 faucets in the patient rooms and in other bathrooms at the hospital (Table 1). The hot water circuit was positive more often and usually contained larger

TABLE 1. Cultures of *L. pneumophila* in hot water samples from taps and showers related to the two small outbreaks of NLD[a]

Date	No. of samples	No. (%) negative	No. (%) positive		No. of cases
			≤ 10² CFU/liter	> 10³ CFU/liter	
November 1984	39	29 (74.35)	4	6 (15.4)	
					7
December 1984	26	18 (69.3)	1	7 (26.9)	
January 1985	30	30 (100)	0	0	
February 1985	40	27 (67.5)	11	3 (50)	
					0
March 1985	28	19 (67.8)	6	3 (10.5)	
April 1985	23	16 (69.5)	3	4 (17.3)	
May 1985	30	20 (66.6)	3	5 (16.6)	
					7
June 1985	28	19 (67.8)	5	4 (14.2)	

[a]Treatment consisting of hyperchlorination (6 mg/liter), continuous chlorination (1 to 2 mg/liter), and heating (60 to 70°C) was introduced between December 1984 and 1985 and between June and July 1985.

numbers of organisms than did the cold water system. All strains were screened for plasmids by the method of Kado and Liu (6). Molecular masses of plasmids were estimated from their electrophoretic mobilities relative to those of Sa (23 MDa), RP4 (36 MDa), R1 (62 MDa), and R40a (96 MDa) (Fig. 1). All serogroup 1 strains contained one plasmid with a molecular mass of 15 MDa and had identical *Bam*HI and *Pst*I fragment patterns (4) (Fig. 2).

Hyperchlorination (6 mg/liter), continuous chlorination (1 to 2 mg/liter), and heat treatment of the hospital's water systems, introduced at the peak of the outbreak in 1984, reduced the level of

L. pneumophila-positive water samples by 100% (December 1984). However, sampling of the hospital environment in January 1985 revealed that the hot water system was contaminated with *L. pneumophila* serogroup 1. No additional cases of NLD were found to occur from January to April 1985 despite intensive surveillance, but from May to July, the second outbreak occurred.

Since we began hyperchlorination and continuous chlorination in 1986 by using an automated chlorinator/analyzer, there had been only 35 sporadic cases of NLD through July 1991 (Fig. 3), with persistence of *L. pneumophila* serogroup 1 in the potable water supply (≥ 10² CFU/liter). One

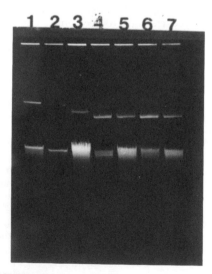

FIG. 1. Agarose gel (0.7%) electrophoresis of plasmid DNA from clinical and environmental isolates during a university hospital NLD outbreak. Lanes: 1 to 3, plasmids RP4, N3, and Sa: 4, *L. pneumophila* E7; 5 to 7, *L. pneumophila* C4, C5, and C17.

FIG. 2. Agarose gel (0.7%) electrophoresis of a restriction endonuclease digest of *L. pneumophila* serogroup 1 purified plasmid DNA. Lanes: 1 and 8, *Hin*dIII fragments of lambda DNA; 2 to 7, strains E3, C4, E7, E9, C5, and C17.

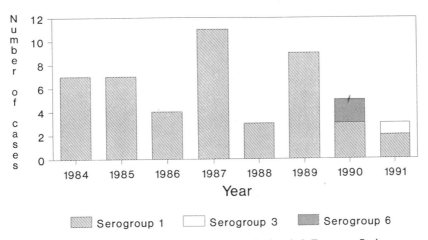

FIG. 3. Annual incidence of LD in the university hospital, Zaragoza, Spain.

interesting finding was the postchlorination occurrence of environmental and clinical isolates of *L. pneumophila* serogroups 3 and 6. In addition, strains of *L. pneumophila* serogroups 3 and 6 were found in samples obtained from the municipal main.

On the other hand, an extensive study of the plumbing system in an MR was made over the 8 years following the 1983 outbreak of LD (23 cases). Hot tap water specimens from 14 (27.4%) of the 51 rooms contained *L. pneumophila* serogroup 1 at concentrations of 10^3 CFU/liter or greater. All of these environmental isolates harbored a single 34-MDa plasmid and had identical restriction fragment patterns. Unfortunately, no patient isolate was available for comparison with the environmental strains. The MR was closed, the components in the fittings were replaced, and the hyperchlorination and continuous chlorination treatment was introduced, with intermittent heating of the water (60 to 70°C). We were unable to isolate *L. pneumophila* serogroup 1 from the water system, and the absence of further cases of LD after the opening of the MR might be interpreted as evidence of the success of eradication measures. It is noteworthy that the domestic water of the university hospital and MR is supplied by the same municipal main.

In summary, our results showed that most nosocomial cases of LD at Zaragoza University Hospital were caused by a single type of *L. pneumophila* serogroup 1; after 6 years of hyperchlorination and continuous chlorination, there have been only sporadic cases of LD. During 1990 through 1991, we found clinical and environmental isolates of *L. pneumophila* serogroups 3 and 6. These serogroups were also isolated from the municipal drinking water system, which serves as the pathway for the dissemination of legionellae. Finally, after 4 years of surveillance in the MR, we were unable to isolate *L. pneumophila* from water supplies.

This research was sponsored by the Diputación General de Aragon (project PCM-5/88).

REFERENCES

1. **Bartlett, C. L. R., R. A. Swann, J. Casal, L. Canada Royo, and A. G. Taylor.** 1984. Recurrent Legionnaires disease from a hotel water system, p. 237–239. *In* C. Thornsberry, A. Balows, J. C. Feeley, and W. Jakubowski (ed.), *Legionella: Proceedings of the 2nd International Symposium.* American Society for Microbiology, Washington, D.C.
2. **Bouza, E., and M. Rodriguez-Creixems.** 1984. Legionnaires disease in Spain, p. 15–17. *In* C. Thornsberry, A. Balows, J. C. Feeley, and W. Jakubowski (ed.), *Legionella: Proceedings of the 2nd International Symposium.* American Society for Microbiology, Washington, D.C.
3. **Boyd, J. F., W. M. Buchanan, T. I. F. McLeod, R. I. Shaw-Donn, and W. P. Weir.** 1978. Pathology of five Scottish deaths from pneumocin illnesses acquired in Spain due to Legionnaires' disease agent. *J. Clin Pathol.* **31**:809–816.
4. **Gomez-Lus, R., C. Martin, M. C. Rubio, A. Rezusta, and M. L. Gomez-Lus.** 1986. *Program Abstr. IXth Int. Congr. Infect. Dis. Parasitic Dis.*
5. **Jenkins, P., A. C. Miller, J. Osman, S. B. Pearson, and J. M. Rowley.** 1978. Legionnaires' disease: a clinical description of thirteen cases. *Br. J. Dis. Chest* **73**:31–38.
6. **Kado, C. I., and S. T. Liu.** 1981. Rapid procedure for detection and isolation of large and small plasmids. *J. Bacteriol.* **145**:1365–1373.
7. **Lawson, J. H., N. R. Grist, D. Reid, and T. S. Wilson.** 1977. Legionnaires' disease. *Lancet* **i**:1083.
8. **Reid, D., N. R. Grist, and R. Najera.** 1978. Illness associated with "package tours", a combined Spanish-Scottish study. *Bull. W.H.O.* **56**:117–122.

Association of *Legionella pneumophila* with Natural Ecosystems

CARL B. FLIERMANS AND RICHARD L. TYNDALL

Savannah River Laboratory, Aiken, South Carolina 29801, and Oak Ridge National Laboratory, Oak Ridge, Tennessee 37831

The Savannah River Site is a 768-km² restricted access area in South Carolina set aside by the U.S. government in the 1950s for the production of national defense materials. The facility is currently operated by Westinghouse Savannah River Co. for the Department of Energy. The site offers myriad habitats in which the ecological relationships can be investigated in detail over an extended period of time. Early work on the ecology of *Legionella* species centered at this facility and helped to determine and to expand the physiological and ecological characteristics of these bacteria (2, 4), habitats most suitable for the organism, temperature relationships, and relationships with other, more complex aquatic organisms (8). Of all the species of *Legionella*, *Legionella pneumophila* serogroup 1 is the most widely understood in terms of its ecology, physiology, and epidemiology. Ecological investigations over the last decade have dealt with defining not only the niche of *L. pneumophila* but also its association with blue-green algae, submerged aquatic plants, and protozoa from natural and man-made aquatic habitats. *L. pneumophila* has been observed and isolated from naturally occurring algal colonies, protozoan enrichments, and moribund aquatic plants.

In 1985, the U.S. Department of Energy established a research program, called "Microbiology of the Deep Subsurface," that focused on detecting microorganisms at greater depths, establishing fundamental scientific information, which included microbial ecology, and exploring the use of microbial systems in the cleanup of contaminated deep terrestrial sediments and groundwater environments associated with energy and defense activities (3).

Groundwaters in sections of the Savannah River Site have been affected by effluents from the site's manufacturing and processing facilities. Unconsolidated sediments extend to depths of 400 m and are underlaid by crystalline metamorphic rock of consolidated mudstone (7). In conjunction with this program, aseptic microbiological sediment samples were collected in sterilized Plexiglas insert tubes sealed with Teflon inside a sampling barrel in order to keep the cored sediments away from the drilling fluid (5). Retrieved material was immediately removed from the sampling barrel, transported to a mobile laboratory adjacent to the drill site, and extruded into a nitrogen-flushed glove bag. The outer two-thirds of each 7.5-cm-diameter core was aseptically pared away, and only the core's center portion was used for micro-biological investigations. Sediments were sonicated, vortexed, and centrifuged as previously described (5), which yielded a clear supernatant. A 10-μl aliquot of the supernatant was spotted into each well of an alcohol-washed toxoplasmosis slide preheated to 65°C. Each spotted sample was overlaid with a nonspecific fluorescent antibody (FA) blocking fluid (2% hydrolyzed gelatin or 5% dry milk in phosphate-buffered saline at pH 9.0), stained with customized serospecific monovalent antibodies, washed, mounted, and evaluated by epifluorescence microscopy.

To effectively use the direct FA technique for environmental samples, several modifications of the technique are of paramount importance. These include sample preparation, blocking of any nonspecific FA adsorption, use of serospecific monovalent antibodies, the proper use of false-negative and false-positive results and controls, as well as specific adsorption of any cross-reacting antigens derived from total viable count screening.

Samples that contained more than 10^4 fluorescing *L. pneumophila* serogroup 1 per g (dry weight) were cultured onto *Legionella* selective agar (BBL), which contained vancomycin, colistin, and anisomycin, after the sample was treated for 15 min at 55°C to reduce the competing bacteria while allowing the more thermally tolerant *Legionella* organisms to remain viable. Isolations were not generally successful at lower concentrations; however, the use of sterile *Fisherella* extract (6) usually enhanced the growth and subsequent isolation of legionellae.

Our study indicates that legionellae are present in terrestrial subsurface environments, although in low numbers. The density of the organisms in the subsurface with respect to the total bacterial population is much lower than one observes in the aquatic community. On occasion, one can observe legionellae comprising as much as 5% of the total bacterial population, as measured by direct FA and acridine orange direct count epifluorescence techniques. The terrestrial subsurface samples often exceed 10^7/g (dry weight), while legionellae are often near the level of detectability or, on occasion, present in concentrations greater than 10^4/g (dry weight). While the aquatic ecosystems are far more homogeneous than the terrestrial habitats, it is clear that a definite patchiness occurs with legionellae in terrestrial sediments, even in sediments collected aseptically from wells that are as close as a few hundred feet from each other.

Terrestrial habitats have remained a potential

source of legionellae (1), but their isolation from terrestrial subsurface environments has not been confirmed until now. Initial ecological investigations conducted on *L. pneumophila* indicated that the organism was somewhat unusual in its temperature relationships in that it could span a tremendous range of natural temperature habitats and remain viable. Thus, it should not be too surprising that *L. pneumophila* is able to inhabit a wide variety of habitats, including terrestrial subsurface environments.

The investigations reported here demonstrate that *L. pneumophila* serogroup 1 is indeed present in terrestrial subsurface environments but at low numbers compared with the total bacterial population. Isolates of *L. pneumophila* serogroup 1 have been recovered from depths of up to 190 ft (ca. 57 m) in terrestrial subsurface sediments. While we believe that the major ecological niche of legionellae continues to be aquatic habitats, the fact that the organism is part of the subsurface terrestrial community must now be recognized.

Finally, one wonders whether the writer of Ecclesiastes was not right in that there is indeed "nothing new under the sun" and that *Legionella* species have been associated with natural habitats for a very long period of time. The finding of the bacteria in terrestrial subsurface environments lends credence to such a suggestion in that one of the more tenable hypotheses for the presence of organisms at great depths in the terrestrial subsurface is that they were trapped in the sediments at the time the sediments were laid down (4). Only

recently, when humans have provided extensive man-made habitats suitable for the amplification, growth, and dissemination of the bacteria, have the niches of humans and legionellae had extensive overlap. Therein lies part of the story of Legionnaires disease and the autecology of *Legionella* species.

REFERENCES

1. **Cherry, W. B., B. Pittman, P. P. Harris, G. A. Herbert, B. M. Thomason, L. Thacker, and R. E. Weaver.** 1978. Detection of Legionnaires' disease bacterium by direct immunofluorescent staining. *J. Clin. Microbiol.* **8:**329–338.
2. **Fliermans, C. B.** 1985. Ecological niche of *Legionella pneumophila*, p. 75–116. *In* R. S. Katz (ed.), *Legionellosis*, vol. II. CRC Press, Inc., Boca Raton, Fla.
3. **Fliermans, C. B., and D. L. Balkwill.** 1989. Life in the terrestrial deep subsurface. *BioScience* **39:**370–377.
4. **Fliermans, C. B., W. B. Cherry, L. H. Orrison, S. J. Smith, D. L. Tison, and D. H. Pope.** 1981. Ecological distribution of *Legionella pneumophila*. *Appl. Environ. Microbiol.* **41:**9–16.
5. **Phelps. T. J., C. B. Fliermans, T. Garland, S. M. Pfiffner, and D. C. White.** 1989. Recovery of deep subsurface material for microbiological studies. *J. Microbiol. Methods* **9:**267–279.
6. **Pope, D. H., R. J. Soracco, H. K. Gill, and C. B. Fliermans.** 1982. Growth of *Legionella pneumophila* in two membered cultures with green algae and cyanobacteria. *Curr. Microbiol.* **7:**319–322.
7. **Sargent, K. A., and C. B. Fliermans.** 1989. Microbiology and geological comparisons of the terrestrial deep subsurface. *Geomicrobiol. J.* **7:**1–11.
8. **Tyndall, R. L., K. Ironside, P. Metler, E. Tan, T. C. Hazen, and C. B. Fliermans.** 1989. Effect of thermal additions on the distribution of thermophilic amoebae and pathogenic *Naegleria fowleri* in a newly created cooling lake. *Appl. Environ. Microbiol.* **55:**722–738.

Strategies for Prevention and Control of Legionellosis in Australia

CLIVE R. BROADBENT

Federal Department of Administrative Services, Phillip ACT 2606, Australia

The implementation of control measures to minimize or prevent the health hazards associated with air and water systems in buildings has legislative backing throughout Australia, although the means of enactment may differ from state to state. The primary reference document used to facilitate this legislative process is the Australian Standard, AS 3666—1989, "Air-Handling and Water Systems of Buildings, Microbial Control." This standard is a product of the Standards Association of Australia, the peak standards-setting body in this country. The standards that are set generally result from known needs, deliberation by representatives of government and industry groups affected by the proposed standard, and then a commitment to production of practical documents. Standards are

made available in draft form for public review before being finalized by the working committee. A standard that is concerned with the safety of life or property usually finds compulsory application through reference in statutory regulations, i.e., the acts, ordinances, and regulations administered by municipal, state, and federal authorities.

AS 3666—1989 was produced by a committee comprising experts in engineering, medicine, microbiology, and public health as well as building owners. This standard addresses not only the problems created by *Legionella* species but also those presented by other microorganisms that are not life threatening but may cause allergic illnesses such as humidifier fever.

AS 3666—1989 has now been written into the

statutory law applying in most Australian states. Even if this were not so, it would still have authority within the framework of common law as applied in Australia. This is so because a plaintiff must always particularize the complaint of negligence against the defendant. AS 3666—1989 provides an important reference document, and even a ready-made catalog, for the things that should have been carried out by the defendant to prevent injury to the plaintiff.

Legislation currently being enacted in the state of New South Wales is considerably more extensive than that applying in other states largely because Australia's worst outbreak of legionellosis occurred, in the city of Wollongong in 1987, in that state. The legislation is enacted under the public health act and seeks to regulate the installation, operation, and maintenance of those systems that may encourage growth of microorganisms able to cause legionellosis and other diseases. The regulations, which are to be read in conjunction with AS 3666—1989, require that all water cooling systems be registered and that only licensed people execute work on these systems.

Such systems are not to operate unless an approved "process of disinfection" is installed. Acceptable bacteriological tests have been formulated and included in the Health Department guidelines that accompany the legislation. The tests are associated with approval of products or processes of disinfection. An approval can be withdrawn should the relevant test standards not be met. These test standards actually specify the maximum permissible *Legionella* concentrations and total bacterial counts. The inclusion of these limits in such legislation has not been without controversy. However, the purpose of specifying acceptable concentrations is to ensure that the process of disinfection that is in place is effective. Once effective procedures have been established for each system, regular monitoring is no longer needed. The guidelines recommend against routine testing for *Legionella* populations.

While the New South Wales approach has been described in some quarters as draconian, it must be appreciated that this and all other preventive strategies in Australia arise from a heightened awareness of the hazard to health presented by legionellae, a community expectation that the occurrence of epidemics is unacceptable, and a knowledge that the means are at hand to greatly reduce the risk of such outbreaks.

The words in the legislation applying in each state differ, but the overall intent is the same. In Queensland, it is the Workplace Health and Safety Act 1989 that is the legislative means of implementing control measures. This act refers to AS 3666—1989, thereby giving it regulatory status. Air conditioning units that incorporate cooling tower devices are required to be registered. The

duties of the various parties that may have health and safety responsibility are listed. These parties are owners of plant, manufacturers of plant (including installation of plant), designers (the placement of a cooling tower next to a fresh air intake would be regarded as a breech of the regulations), persons in control of workplaces, employees, and, employers. Inspectors are empowered to issue warning or prohibition notices for failure to comply.

In the state of Victoria, the Health Department has taken an administratively simple approach. First, the department spent considerable effort in developing a high-quality guideline booklet, "Guidelines for the Control of Legionnaires' Disease." The document preparation committee included wide professional representation from industry as well as the government sector. The guidelines complement AS 3666—1989 and describe not only what is required but also the reasons for and means of implementing the practical control measures recommended. Second, the legislative requirements are contained in the Health (Infectious Diseases) Regulations 1990, which simply state that the owner of a cooling water (or warm water) system must maintain it in a manner as set out in the guidelines. Penalties apply if an audit by a health official subsequently finds that such equipment is not being properly attended to.

An interesting approach has been taken by the Wollongong City Council in the aftermath of the major outbreak that occurred there, an outbreak that caused considerable suffering and also loss of business and retail confidence. The council did not wait for state legislation to be introduced but rather instituted direct actions of its own by keeping a detailed inventory of all cooling towers in its jurisdiction and by requiring monthly reports on their bacteriological status. Generally, total bacterial counts only are required, but a large number of cooling tower owners have instituted programs of routine testing for legionellae to allay possible public anxiety. The reports required by the council are effective as a means of overcoming complacency and neglect, which can all too easily reappear.

Authority for the direct action by the Wollongong City Council derives from a clause in the local government act applying in New South Wales which states that "the council may control and regulate the sanitation of premises and the use and occupation of premises so as to avoid any insanitary condition thereon or any interference therefrom with the healthiness of the vicinity."

The council supported establishment of a *Legionella* testing laboratory at the University of Wollongong's Department of Applied Biology. The laboratory's functions, in addition to research, include analysis of water samples by postgraduate students under direction. This approach has minimized costs while maintaining high standards and levels of confidence by the Wollongong community.

While the drafting of appropriate legislation is of importance, it can never be regarded as the panacea or even the main means of control. Some of the other initiatives under way in Australia are industry-to-government liaison committees that meet regularly; up-to-date control guidelines; educational material for use at seminars; training workshops for industry representatives, community groups, and others (including politicians); development of accredited course material for use in universities and other educational institutions; production of additional standards by the Standards Association to cover the methodology for laboratory culturing and enumeration of legionellae in environmental samples, field measurement of drift loss from cooling towers, and requirements for water treatment at cooling towers; and standards for health care facilities, e.g., the "Code of Practice for Thermostatic Mixing Valves" produced by the Department of Health in New South Wales. Within industries such as air conditioning and whirlpool spa manufacture, every effort has been made to improve equipment design for ease of maintenance.

All of these strategies illustrate the deep concern in Australia about the hazards presented by *Legionella* colonization. These hazards have been firmly addressed by all interested parties to help ensure that the community at large has the best available protection against the likelihood of further outbreaks of legionellosis in Australia.

VI. SUMMARIES OF STRATEGY SESSIONS

Prevention and Control of Legionellosis

JEAN R. JOLY

Groupe de Recherche en Épidémiologie de l'Université Laval, Hôpital du Saint-Sacrement, 1050 Chemin Sainte-Foy, Quebec, Quebec G1S 4L8, and Département de Microbiologie Faculté de Médecine, Université Laval, Quebec G1K 7P4, Canada

The purpose of this session was to discuss primary and secondary prevention of legionellosis. At the end of the session, topics of future research in specific areas related to prevention and control were identified.

PRIMARY PREVENTION

Primary prevention refers to the prevention of legionellosis in an environment where no known cases have occurred, as opposed to secondary prevention, which relates to actions taken after cases of Legionnaires disease have been identified and epidemiologically related to a given environment. During the meeting, it was generally agreed that the large majority of cases of legionellosis are sporadic. It was suggested that between 7,000 and 8,000 such cases occur each year in the United States, an estimate that was challenged by some participants. (These numbers were extrapolated from a study of patients hospitalized for pneumonia.) In the United Kingdom, more than three-fourths of all patients with pneumonia are never hospitalized. If the proportions of legionellosis are similar in hospitalized and ambulatory subjects with pneumonia, then the true incidence of Legionnaires disease is grossly underestimated by these figures. A similar proportion of hospitalized versus ambulatory pneumonia patients is likely in the United States. In addition, there were questions as to the exact spectrum of the infection, an issue that will be dealt with below (see Future Research). Since by definition these sporadic cases cannot be related to a common source of exposure, an important issue before primary prevention can be considered as a viable alternative is the identification of the risk attributable to exposure to different environmental sources of legionellae. Unfortunately, this information is largely unknown.

A few ongoing studies were presented, and preliminary data were discussed. The importance of domestic exposure and occurrence of legionellosis is currently being examined in a study in Columbus, Ohio. In this investigation, it was found that only 8 of 62 sporadic cases of legionellosis could be related to domestic exposure. In only 3 of the 91 selected controls could legionellae be found in the domestic environment, suggesting that domestic exposure is an important risk factor for Legionnaires disease. In the remaining 54 cases,

however, no known source of *Legionella* infection could be identified. In this study, the investigators were unable to identify any cluster of cases among the 62 investigated. Thus, at least in Columbus, the large majority of infections (>85%) could not be related to any given environmental source. Could these cases be related to exposure in the workplace, to contaminated drifts from cooling towers, or some other unknown source(s)? Although the relative importance of these known and possibly unknown sources is currently ignored, a recent report showed that in Glasgow, Scotland, houses associated with sporadic cases of legionellosis were closer to cooling towers than were houses of control subjects. This finding suggests that drifts from these towers could be a source of sporadic Legionnaires disease.

It was suggested during the meeting that primary prevention should be restricted to high-risk subjects. Numerous participants challenged that proposition, arguing that in many studies a substantial proportion of cases of legionellosis occur in subjects with no known risk factors. Restricting our attention to subjects with known risk factors would lead to poor primary prevention strategies.

The issue of primary prevention is closely related to that of an approved code of practices for the design and maintenance of cooling towers, plumbing systems, and other known amplifiers or disseminators of legionellae in both the public and private sectors. Emphasis was placed on hospitals and institutions caring for chronically ill subjects as well as nursing homes. Experiences of different countries with these regulations were examined.

The British experience was reviewed first. The largely publicized outbreaks that occurred at the British Broadcasting Corporation (79 cases and 2 deaths) and in Staffordshire (100 cases and 28 deaths) were the main impetus for the preparation of the approved code of practice. The code came into effect only 2 weeks prior to this meeting (January 15, 1992); one of its key features was that it was noncompulsory but strongly incentive in nature. The preface to the document states that "although failure to comply with any provision of this Code is not in itself an offense, that failure may be taken by a court in criminal proceedings as proof that a person has contravened the legal requirement to which the provision relates. In such a case, it will be open to that person to satisfy a court that he has complied with the requirement in some other way" (1). This statement was interpreted to mean that the burden of proof will be on the victims if employers or institutions comply with the code of practice. Otherwise, the burden of proof will be on the employers or the institutions. These are fairly good reasons to comply with the code.

The code itself, although extensive, is fairly simple. It is divided into sections on (i) the identification and assessment of risk, (ii) the prevention or minimization of risk from exposure to legionellae, (iii) the management, selection, training, and competence of personnel, (iv) record keeping, and (v) responsibilities of designers, manufacturers, importers, suppliers, and installers. A cost-benefit analysis of this approved code of practice estimated that the cost/benefit ratio varied between 8:1 and 17:1, the critical factor in the variation being the actual number of cases of legionellosis occurring yearly in the United Kingdom.

In Australia, where outbreaks of Legionnaires disease have occurred in the last few years, regulations have also been adopted. The Australian Standard Association code of practice is generally considered the best. Each Australian state is, however, responsible for the formulation and implementation of its own regulations. This approach has resulted in different codes of practice, some of which are very stringent. Enumeration of legionellae has been adopted by one or more of the states, and this has resulted in "intolerable situations." Indeed, the small number of legionellae present in one building resulted in closure of the building until eradication procedures had proven successful. It was emphasized that we do not know the exact numbers of legionellae that might be harmful and that until studies on this and related issues are available, no standard of acceptable potable or environmental water quality should be accepted for legionellae. Finally, because of the nature of the Australian outbreaks, a major emphasis was placed on drift control in that country. This effort has resulted in improved drift eliminators in cooling towers.

In the United States, the regulations were last revised by the Environmental Protection Agency in 1988. It was felt that a major revision of these guidelines was warranted in light of our greatly expanded knowledge about legionellae.

SECONDARY PREVENTION

Three questions were raised by one of the moderators: (i) What should be done about a single case in your neighborhood? (ii) What should be done if there are two cases in 2 weeks in the workplace? (iii) What should be done if the city councilors are worried because legionellae have been found in the cooling tower of the city hall?

To the first of these questions, answers of the participants were ambiguous. A recent report showed that an environmental source could be found in 40% of sporadic cases of legionellosis. Participants were uncertain about the meaning of these results as applied to the issue of secondary prevention, especially when few individuals were likely to be exposed to the same source. Should immediate action be taken? How far should we go in identifying these sources in routine practice? Would these efforts be cost-effective? To none of these issues were adequate answers provided.

The second of these questions raised a heated debate. The British approach was presented. If only one case can be related to exposure in the workplace, then no special measures are taken except to speak to the engineer responsible for maintenance of the building. If the approved code of practice is followed or if similar procedures are already in place, then no further action is taken. Otherwise, the engineer is instructed on the importance of these good housekeeping procedures and the employer's or institution's liabilities. If other cases have occurred previously or simultaneously, then a full inquiry is initiated and appropriate measures are taken.

In the United States, a similar course of action is followed. Quite frequently, however, there is intense pressure from union representatives to initiate a full inquiry even if only one case is identified. Because of these pressures, an inquiry was recently initiated under such circumstances. Of the 10 subjects complaining of lower respiratory tract infections in the preceding few months, 60% had a *Legionella* antibody titer of $\geq 1:256$, whereas only 6% of employees without lower respiratory tract infections and 10% of normal blood donors had similar titers. These results, if confirmed, suggest that numerous *Legionella* infections cause no or relatively minor symptoms and thus are either misdiagnosed or overlooked. Should this be the case, the incidence of legionellosis and Legionnaires disease might be far greater than previously estimated. Finally, if this is the case, then the whole strategy that has governed our secondary intervention measures would have to be rethought. It was pointed out that Occupation Safety and Health Administration regulations are nonspecific and that "general industry knowledge" is the accepted standard; i.e., if an employer has knowledge of the hazard, the employer is likely to be held responsible.

The last question raised by the moderator was left largely unanswered since no one really knows what to do about a contaminated cooling tower that has not yet been associated with legionellosis. Since the likelihood that a sporadic case will be related to a contaminated cooling tower is low, it will be difficult to convince the owners of their duties. Additional epidemiological studies similar to the one done in Glasgow will have to be relied upon. If the results obtained in Glasgow are confirmed, preventive measures, such as aerosol reduction through improved drift eliminators or decontamination and adequate maintenance of the towers, will have to be implemented. Whether or not monitoring of cooling towers and other environmental sources of legionellae for the presence of these bacteria should be implemented is highly debatable.

The final issue raised related to an increase in water temperature to 60°C and the possibility of scalding. Mixed opinions were expressed. Participants working in institutions where the water temperature was raised after cases were identified mentioned that scalding was not an issue, whereas an emergency room physician mentioned that for children 1 to 5 years of age, scalding is the second cause of death in the United States. He urged that participants exercise prudence when suggesting an increase in water temperature to 60°C in different environments, including the home.

Everyone agreed that Legionnaires disease should be kept in perspective. Legionellosis is only one of numerous infectious diseases that are transmitted from the environment in hospitals and elsewhere. Hospital and state epidemiologists are reluctant to add to the already long list of infections they must deal with. Most are already overburdened with addressing human immunodeficiency virus, infections caused by multiply resistant *Staphylococcus aureus,* hepatitis B, and all other preventable infections. Adding *Legionella* infections to this list might lead to allocation of resources to an issue that is not a major problem. Additional information on the incidence of legionellosis is urgently needed.

FUTURE RESEARCH

The following issues were thought to be of primary importance with respect to prevention and control. First, the epidemiology of sporadic Legionnaires disease, as well as the source of exposure for these cases, should be better defined. From these studies, more focused intervention strategies can be defined and more aggressive prevention programs can be directed to the most important sources of infection.

Attributable risk due to exposure in the domestic and nondomestic environments should be determined. Within each of these environments, and especially when the attributable risk is high, identification of the most likely reservoirs, amplifiers, and disseminators should be attempted. The exact role of primary prevention in institutions that are known to be areas at high risk for the acquisition of legionellosis (e.g., hospitals) should be defined. For travel-associated cases, the logistics of surveillance from local through international levels should be enhanced. For this effort, the case definition proposed by the World Health Organization, although restrictive, should be followed.

The exact spectrum of the infection should be better defined. As one participant pointed out, it is unlikely that all or most of the nonpulmonary cases of legionellosis are occurring in a single institution. It is also probable that, as is the case with so many infectious diseases, identified and reported cases of legionellosis represent only the tip of the iceberg. We need to identify and assess the frequency and importance of less severe infections. Virulence and ecological factors that contribute to virulence should be identified. Finally, our interventions and especially the design of new strategies should always place emphasis on multidisciplinarity. Public health officers, physicians, microbiologists, and engineers are all part of the solution. Strategies designed by only one of these groups of professionals are unlikely to succeed.

REFERENCE

1. **Health and Safety Commission.** 1991. *The Prevention or Control of Legionellosis (Including Legionnaires' Disease). Approved Code of Practice.* HMSO Publications, London.

Evolution of Chemotherapy and Diagnostic Tests

JOSEPH F. PLOUFFE

Division of Infectious Diseases, Ohio State University Hospitals, 410 West 10th Avenue, Columbus, Ohio 43210-1228

The main goal of our session was to define research needs related to the diagnosis and treatment of Legionnaires disease. The mainstay of the tests for legionellosis is the culture of respiratory secretions. If a *Legionella*-positive culture is obtained, then a firm diagnosis can be made.

With respect to what needs to be done differently in the area of culture media, one of the points raised was the development of multiresistant gram-negative and gram-positive organisms that grow in semiselective or selective plates. Further research needs to be done to continually refine these selective media with newer antibiotics that have a broader spectrum of activity and thus prevent overgrowth.

Another topic deserving of research is the competency of laboratories to culture legionellae. It was fairly obvious from the data presented by Paul Edelstein that many laboratories are attempting to address this problem. To this end, resources are needed to support the development of programs to provide better training for laboratory personnel, establish regional laboratories, or use reference laboratories that are now in existence.

The treatment of specimens with acid prior to culture was brought up. Approximately 60% of the participants stated that they use an acid wash treatment and feel that it gives a significant improvement in culture of *Legionella* organisms compared with non-acid-treated specimens.

The final point on culture was the problem of recognizing non-*Legionella pneumophila* species. Perhaps additions to media such as are used in Australia to identify *Legionella longbeachae* can be adopted for clinical specimens.

Measurement of urine antigen by radioimmunoassay was felt to be a very rapid and helpful procedure. Again, regional laboratories must be relied on since this test is not performed frequently in hospitals. The point was made that many bacteriology laboratories do not want to use radioisotopic procedures, although chemistry laboratories usually perform such tests. But again, considering the numbers involved, it might be wiser to use regional and reference laboratories for such tests. More research is required to simplify assays to the level of the enzyme-linked immunosorbent assay. A less complicated assay would facilitate use by hospitals and could be used to identify organisms other than just *Legionella pneumophila* serogroup 1.

With respect to serology, it would be useful to have a serum bank of samples from culture-positive cases. One investigator said that sera from patients with infections caused by strains other than *L. pneumophila* serogroup 1 need to be examined thoroughly to improve our serologic diagnostic abilities.

The participants thought that it should be clear whether we were talking about the academic or the clinical definition of Legionnaires disease. Speaking from the academic viewpoint, most participants felt that a single serologic test, no matter what the titer rate, in the nonoutbreak situation was of questionable use in making a definitive diagnosis. But it was pointed out that those titers can be occasionally helpful to the clinician in the early stage of the disease.

A test that is in the process of being developed is the polymerase chain reaction using respiratory secretions. Although cultures will still need to be done, resources should be allocated to this effort so as to develop another, more rapid technique.

Another goal for this session was to develop a standardized case definition of Legionnaires disease to be used in the evaluation of chemotherapy. The case definition of Legionnaires disease, adopted by the World Health Organization, specifies a person with acute respiratory disease as evidenced by an abnormal chest X-ray examination and a *Legionella*-positive culture and/or a fourfold rise in antibody to *L. pneumophila* serogroup 1. Presumptive cases include those with positive results with urine antigens and direct fluorescent antibody stains. There is no mention of single titers in that definition.

The final topic was antibiotic therapy for Legionnaires disease. Virtually everyone agreed that the current drug of choice is erythromycin, followed by rifampin if the patient does not respond. Tom File reviewed the studies in the literature on erythromycin efficacy. It appears that in community-acquired cases, mortality is relatively low and erythromycin works reasonably effectively. The mortality rate for nosocomial cases is fairly high, as would be expected for infections of people who are already very ill. But are there other agents that would be more efficacious? Animal studies have shown that at least on a concentration basis, quinolones have much more activity than does erythromycin.

There was much discussion of how to design a clinical study, since such a study has not been carried out since 1976. The suggestions included creating retrospective chart reviews such as was done by Dr. Germaine in Paris. Back-matching cases has obvious difficulties because of the problems in interpreting results but still provides some information. The preferred alternative, an erythromycin-controlled study, would take several years and a considerable amount of money, but could be done by screening all cases of community-acquired pneumonia as well as those of nosocomial pneumonia.

One tool suggested for evaluating therapy in an outbreak situation was a preprogrammed package that could be ready for use at the time of the outbreak and had approval of a national institutional review board. In this situation, the group in charge of the program, potentially the Centers for Disease Control, would identify large groups of patients in a relatively short period of time.

There was some sense of frustration in that many of the questions addressed were the same ones that we have been discussing for many years. We hope that some of the concepts set forth will encourage cooperation so that we can make even more advances before the 5th International Symposium.

Prospects for Vaccine Development

MARCUS A. HORWITZ, BARBARA J. MARSTON, CLAIRE V. BROOME, AND ROBERT F. BREIMAN

UCLA School of Medicine, Los Angeles, California 90024, and Centers for Disease Control and Prevention, Atlanta, Georgia 30333

Participants in the session on Prospects for Vaccine Development discussed a broad range of topics relevant to vaccination against Legionnaires disease, including clinical, epidemiologic, immunologic, feasibility, safety, and cost-benefit considerations.

With respect to clinical considerations, the participants fully appreciated that Legionnaires disease is a relatively common, serious, and frequently fatal disease that often requires very expensive hospitalization. The participants also understood that Legionnaires disease is an important cause of nosocomial pneumonia and death. Thus, the participants felt that prevention of Legionnaires disease by immunization merits serious consideration.

Central to the topic of vaccination is an assessment of the risk of acquiring vaccine-preventable disease. Unfortunately, accurate information on the incidence of Legionnaires disease is extremely limited. Estimates of the incidence of Legionnaires disease have ranged from 10,000 to 100,000 cases annually in the United States. However, the scientific basis for these estimates is not clear. Cases reported to the Centers for Disease Control via the usual reporting mechanisms are unquestionably a minute fraction of the total that occur. Consequently, accurate estimates of incidence are likely to derive instead from carefully conducted epidemiologic studies. In this regard, the study presented at this conference by Barbara Marston and her colleagues on the incidence of community-acquired pneumonia in Ohio has provided data on hospitalized cases of Legionnaires disease. If extrapolated to the United States as a whole, which may or may not be a valid exercise, the Ohio incidence data yield an estimate of 11,000 hospitalized cases of Legionnaires disease annually in the United States. This estimate does not include cases of serious pneumonia not leading to hospitalization.

A vaccine against Legionnaires disease might be targeted against high-risk groups, i.e., smokers; persons with chronic cardiopulmonary disease, chronic renal disease, and diabetes mellitus; the elderly; transplant recipients; alcoholics; immunocompromised patients; and persons on corticosteroid medications; etc. In addition to data on overall incidence of Legionnaires disease, more information is needed on the incidence of Legionnaires disease in high-risk groups.

With respect to immunologic considerations and feasibility, four prototypic vaccines have been reported that induce protective immunity in the guinea pig model of Legionnaires disease: an avirulent mutant *Legionella pneumophila strain; L. pneumophila* membranes; the major secretory protein of *L. pneumophila*; and the major cytoplasmic membrane protein of *L. pneumophila*, a genuscommon antigen and member of the Hsp60 family of heat shock proteins. In the guinea pig model, animals infected with aerosolized *L. pneumophila* develop a pneumonic illness that mimics Legionnaires disease in humans both clinically and pathologically, and thus this animal model is a superb one for studies of vaccine efficacy. All of the reported prototypic vaccines induce cell-mediated immunity, which is generally believed to play a central role in host defense against Legionnaires disease in humans. Since immunocompromised patients are among those at high risk for Legionnaires disease and many of these persons may have diminished cell-mediated immune responses, some participants in this session felt that an evaluation of the efficacy of prototypic vaccines in an immunocompromised animal model would be useful. Once promising vaccine candidates are identified, investigators must address production of the material in a form acceptable for clinical studies.

Studies on the efficacy of vaccines in the human population would probably need to focus on high-risk groups. Accurate estimates of disease incidence will be crucial to determine the sample size needed for a vaccine efficacy study. A multicenter trial would likely be required to enroll a sufficiently large study population.

With respect to safety, a successful vaccine would obviously need to be safe as well as effective. A vaccine consisting of one or a few molecules would seem less likely to cause toxic or other adverse reactions than one consisting of a whole organism or large multimolecular components of an organism.

With respect to cost-benefit considerations, the lack of good epidemiologic data on the incidence of Legionnaires disease in high-risk groups renders accurate cost-benefit analysis very difficult. Nevertheless, it seems likely from available information that a safe, effective, and moderately priced vaccine targeted against high-risk groups, e.g., renal transplant recipients or patients with chronic renal disease, would be extremely cost-beneficial.

A vaccine against Legionnaires disease might be combined with other vaccines targeted against diseases such as influenza, for use with high-risk groups that overlap with those at risk for Legionnaires disease. This should favorably affect the cost-benefit ratio.

In summary, the participants of this session felt that Legionnaires disease is a serious and highly fatal disease with a relatively high incidence, and that development of a vaccine to prevent Legionnaires disease is desirable. Given the success of prototypic vaccines in an animal model, a safe and effective vaccine against Legionnaires disease in humans seems feasible. Development and use of a safe and effective vaccine against Legionnaires disease would likely result in substantial reductions in mortality, morbidity, and medical expenditures; however, additional epidemiologic studies will need to be conducted to optimally target risk populations and define cost-benefit ratios.

VII. OVERVIEW

OVERVIEW

Ten Years of Progress in *Legionella* Research: Summary of the Fourth International Symposium on *Legionella*

ROBERT F. BREIMAN AND JAMES M. BARBAREE

Respiratory Diseases Branch, Division of Bacterial and Mycotic Diseases, National Center for Infectious Diseases, Centers for Disease Control, Atlanta, Georgia 30333, and Botany and Microbiology, Auburn University, Auburn University, Alabama 36849-5407

Ten years of research since the Centers for Disease Control-sponsored *Legionella* symposium in 1983 have produced many notable advances in knowledge of *Legionella* species and legionellosis. This progress leads to speculation about what new advances we can expect in the next ten years. However, the actual course of future research is often not foreseeable, and the significance of new findings is often either overstated or unrecognized. For instance, although data on a relationship between amoebae and legionellae were presented in 1983, amoebae were deemed by some investigators to be unlikely to have an important role in amplifying legionellae in the environment. In the 1992 International Symposium on *Legionella*, more than 10 papers and one state of the art lecture on the role of amoebae were presented. Understanding the dependence of legionellae on amoebae now appears crucial for the development of approaches to control *Legionella* infections. In contrast, in 1983, a DNA probe that could detect small numbers of legionellae in clinical specimens generated a great deal of excitement. Sidney Finegold suggested that this procedure should "revolutionize not only the diagnosis of Legionnaires disease but that of infectious diseases in general." While this procedure is helpful in confirming culture results, it has not yet achieved the potential anticipated nine years ago.

While the true significance of scientific developments often is not immediately appreciated, not all forecasting is inconsistent with subsequent events. At the 1983 symposium, James Feeley recognized newly introduced molecular marker systems for their potentially immense epidemiologic value. Since then, monoclonal antibody subtyping and enzyme electrophoresis, as well as newer molecular epidemiologic techniques such as restriction fragment length polymorphism and ribosomal DNA analysis, have contributed information to investigations of outbreaks of legionellosis. Likewise, detection of antigens of *Legionella pneumophila* serogroup 1 in urine was recognized as a potentially valuable test; ten years later, a radioimmunoassay method for urinary antigen detection is a rapid, highly specific test that is a very useful part of our diagnostic capacities. At this meeting, Tang and colleagues presented data on a promising, simpler method (enzyme-linked immunosorbent assay) for detecting a broader spectrum of *Legionella* antigens in urine.

A course can be charted for future research (confidently, if not accurately) based on several exciting advances presented at the 1992 symposium. New work was presented from the laboratories of Engleberg, Cianciotto, and Horwitz on factors related to virulence, such as the *Legionella mip* gene and iron-binding proteins, and newly applied methods for assessing virulence factors, such as use of transposons and macrophage models to study expression of *Legionella* proteins. Sahney and colleagues demonstrated that oxidative burst and chemotaxis of phagocytes were depressed by the *Legionella* major secretory protein, a protease shown by Horwitz to provide protective immunity when injected in guinea pigs. These studies should increase our understanding of the pathogenesis of infection due to intracellular pathogens, including *Legionella* species.

A number of reports focused on the use of DNA amplification techniques for diagnosis of legionellosis and for detection of the bacteria in the environment. Polymerase chain reaction has not yet achieved its promise for diagnosis of infectious diseases, in part because of problems with contamination in the laboratory. However, this technique will become very useful because of the significance of finding legionellae, which are noncommensal organisms, in human secretions, tissues, and fluids. A great deal of information will be needed before the method can be applied to environmental studies, since the significance of finding low numbers of this ubiquitous organism in water specimens is not known.

An ongoing population-based study in Ohio of community-acquired pneumonia, presented by Marston, has provided a clear description of incidence rates for pneumonia due to *Legionella* infection and has shown that the disease is markedly underdiagnosed and occurs mostly sporadically. Systematic studies on incidence are important for identifying the true magnitude of disease, so that resources for studies related to prevention and control can be appropriately allocated. Additional studies in other sites should be done to confirm the findings from Ohio and provide data useful for extrapolating incidence for entire regions. A description of an ongoing study evaluating risk factors for sporadically occurring legionellosis among patients identified during the Ohio study was presented by Straus during the strategy session on prevention and control. Identifying risk factors and sources for sporadically occurring disease will be the key to developing coherent and effective prevention and control strategies.

Papers on control of *Legionella* colonization of potable water systems also were presented. Studies evaluated the use of heat, hyperchlorination, and UV light for disinfection. The role of routine monitoring for the bacteria was discussed but not, unfortunately, clarified. Use of "levels" or concentrations of legionellae in water specimens would be an attractive approach to identify sources at highest probability for causing disease, because identified sources could be targeted for aggressive primary control efforts; however, conclusions could not be drawn from data presented from the study by Shelton and colleagues because too few outbreak-related water sources were studied. Nonetheless, a systematic approach is needed to evaluate the concentration of legionellae in specimens from multiple water sources implicated by outbreak investigations and the concentration in water collected from non-outbreak-related

sources. Since legionellae can multiply within amoebae in water in specimen containers, these studies will need to be done prospectively, using consistent sample collection methodology.

It is likely that studies in the near future will clarify the role of monitoring and the optimal methods for disease prevention and control. Once these data are available, it should be possible to develop a coherent, comprehensive, and cost-effective strategy to dramatically reduce the incidence of legionellosis. In addition, as discussed during the strategy sessions, vaccines for prevention of disease appear promising. Cost-effectiveness analyses, using updated estimates of disease incidence and risk factor information, may be useful for pharmaceutical companies as they decide whether to pursue development of what has previously been a most improbable vaccine.

The preponderance of papers presented at this meeting were from the fields of molecular and cellular biology and prevention and control, reflecting continuing intensive research in these areas. Because legionellae are intracellular bacteria (and models for studying a vast array of other intracellular pathogens) transmitted via environmental sources, research on these organisms brings together a curious combination of molecular biologists and environmental scientists. Participation at this meeting reflected the particularly dynamic and diverse nature of *Legionella* research. We hope that the work in progress from the many capable scientists participating in this symposium will continue, even in the face of dwindling research resources, and lead to improved understanding of this fascinating genus of microorganisms.

AUTHOR INDEX

SUBJECT INDEX